Behavioral Emergencies for Healthcare Providers

Leslie S. Zun • Kimberly Nordstrom
Michael P. Wilson
Editors

Behavioral Emergencies for Healthcare Providers

Second Edition

Springer

Editors
Leslie S. Zun
Department of Emergency Medicine
Rosalind Franklin University of Medicine and Science/ The Chicago Medical School
North Chicago, IL
USA

Kimberly Nordstrom
Department of Psychiatry
University of Colorado Anschutz
Aurora, CO
USA

Michael P. Wilson
Department of Emergency Medicine
University of Arkansas for Medical Sciences
Little Rock, AR
USA

ISBN 978-3-030-52519-4 ISBN 978-3-030-52520-0 (eBook)
https://doi.org/10.1007/978-3-030-52520-0

This Springer imprint is published by the registered company Springer Nature Switzerland AG
The registered company address is: Gewerbestrasse 11, 6330 Cham, Switzerland

Les Zun: "I would like to dedicate the book to my children, Amy and Rachel."

Michael Wilson: "I would like to thank Kristi Wilson, who even in my most challenging moments always said, 'Why don't you give it a shot?' It is because of her that I have hit more targets than I thought possible."

Kimberly Nordstrom: "This work is dedicated to my two Bs, with love."

Acknowledgments

We would like to thank all of the authors who gave their time and shared their expertise in creating this book. A very special thank you to: Carly Eastin, Jagoda Pasic, Lynn Roppolo, Scott Simpson, Ambrose Wong, Lara Chepenik, and Jon Cole for their extraordinary work as Section Editors. Thank you for your dedication in seeing this project through. Lastly, we would like to acknowledge Jade Beshears for her copyediting help throughout the book.

Contents

Contributors

Editors

Kimberly Nordstrom, MD, JD Department of Psychiatry, University of Colorado Anschutz, Aurora, CO, USA

Michael P. Wilson, MD, PhD Department of Emergency Medicine, University of Arkansas for Medical Sciences, Little Rock, AR, USA

Leslie S. Zun, MD Department of Emergency Medicine, Rosalind Franklin University of Medicine and Science/ The Chicago Medical School, North Chicago, IL, USA

Section Editors

Lara Chepenik, MD, PhD Department of Psychiatry, Yale University School of Medicine, New Haven, CT, USA

Jon Cole, MD Department of Emergency Medicine, Hennepin County Medical Center, Minneapolis, MN, USA

Carly Eastin, MD Department of Emergency Medicine, University of Arkansas for Medical Sciences, Little Rock, AR, USA

Jagoda Pasic, MD, PhD Department of Psychiatry and Behavioral Sciences, University of Washington School of Medicine, Seattle, WA, USA

Lynn P. Roppolo, MD Department of Emergency Medicine, Parkland Health and Hospital System, Dallas, TX, USA

Scott A. Simpson, MD, MPH Department of Behavioral Health Services, Denver Health & Hospital Authority, Denver, CO, USA

Ambrose Wong, MD, MSEd Department of Emergency Medicine, Yale University School of Medicine, New Haven, CT, USA

Authors

Zakaria Abdulnabi, MD Department of Emergency Medicine, Carle Foundation Hospital, Urbana, IL, USA

James Ahn, MD, MPHE Department of Emergency Medicine, University of Chicago, Chicago, IL, USA

Eric L. Anderson, MD, FAPA Luminis Health, J. Kent McNew Family Medical Center, Annapolis, MD, USA

Kristen Baker, MD Department of Emergency Medicine, University of Arkansas for Medical Sciences, Little Rock, AR, USA

Jon S. Berlin, MD Department of Psychiatry and Behavioral Medicine, Department of Emergency Medicine, Medical College of Wisconsin, Wauwatosa, WI, USA

Vint Blackburn, MD Department of Psychiatry, University of Pittsburgh Medical Center, Pittsburgh, PA, USA

Garrett K. Blumberg, MD Department of Emergency Medicine, University of Texas Southwestern Medical Center, Dallas, TX, USA

Benjamin L. Bregman, MD Department of Psychiatry and Behavioral Health, George Washington University of Medicine, Washington, DC, USA

Suzanne Bruch, MD Psychiatry, Northern California, CA, USA

Lynn Barkley Burnett, MD, EdD, JD(c) Department of Clinical Specialties, Community Regional Medical Center, Fresno, CA, USA

Margaret A. Cashman, MD, FAASM Department of Psychiatry and Behavioral Sciences, University of Washington School of Medicine, Seattle, WA, USA

Jamie C. Christensen, BA Public Health Department of Acute Psychiatry, Vituity, Reno, NV, USA

Bryan Corbett, MD Department of Emergency Medicine, Division of Medical Toxicology, University of California Health Sciences, San Diego, CA, USA

Ashley Curry, MD Psychiatric Emergency Services, Denver Health Medical Center, Denver, CO, USA

Abigail Dahan, MD, FAPA Department of Psychiatry, Bellevue Hospital, New York, NY, USA

Paul H. Desan, MD, PhD Director, Psychiatric Consultation Service, Yale New Haven Hospital, New Haven, CT, USA

Associate Professor, Department of Psychiatry, Yale School of Medicine, New Haven, CT, USA

Suzanne Dooley-Hash, MD Department of Emergency Medicine, University of Michigan, Ann Arbor, MI, USA

Thom Dunn, PhD Behavioral Health Service, Denver Health, Denver, CO, USA

School of Psychological Sciences, University of Northern Colorado, Greeley, CO, USA

Carly Eastin, MD Department of Emergency Medicine, University of Arkansas for Medical Sciences, Little Rock, AR, USA

Steven W. Flynn, MD, BA Department of Emergency Medicine, Methodist Hospitals, Gary, IN, USA

Rachel L. Glick, MD Psychiatry, University of Michigan, Ann Arbor, MI, USA

Ross Heller, MD Department of Emergency Medicine, Saint Louis University School of Medicine, St. Louis, MO, USA

Jeffrey D. Ho, MD Department of Emergency Medicine, Hennepin County Medical Center, Minneapolis, MN, USA

David Hoyer, MD First Choice ER, First Texas Hospital, Houston, TX, USA

Andy Jagoda, MD Department of Emergency Medicine, Mount Sinai Health System, New York, NY, USA

Abhishek Jain, MD Board Certified Forensic Psychiatrist, New York, NY, USA

Lauren R. Klein, MD Department of Emergency Medicine, Hennepin County Medical Center, Minneapolis, MN, USA

Gregory Luke Larkin, MD, MSPH, FACEP, FACEM Department of Emergency Medicine and Psychiatry, Northeast Ohio Medical University, Akron, OH, USA

Rachel Littlefield, MD Department of Emergency Medicine, University of Arkansas for Medical Sciences, Little Rock, AR, USA

Marc L. Martel, MD Department of Emergency Medicine, Hennepin County Medical Center, Minneapolis, MN, USA

Anna K. McDowell, MD Department of Mental Health, Rocky Mountain Regional VA Medical Center, Aurora, CO, USA

Samuel Mullinax, BA Department of Emergency Medicine, University of Arkansas for Medical Sciences, Little Rock, AR, USA

Mark Newman, MD Department of Psychiatry, University of Washington Medical Center, Seattle, WA, USA

Barbara Nightingale, MD, FAAFP Department of Family Medicine and Psychiatry, University of Pittsburgh Medical Center, Pittsburgh, PA, USA

Kimberly Nordstrom, MD, JD Department of Psychiatry, University of Colorado Anschutz, Aurora, CO, USA

Jagoda Pasic, MD, PhD Department of Psychiatry and Behavioral Sciences, University of Washington School of Medicine, Seattle, WA, USA

Jennifer M. Peltzer-Jones, PsyD, RN Department of Emergency Medicine, Henry Ford Health System, Detroit, MI, USA

Seth Powsner, MD Department of Psychiatry, Yale University School of Medicine, New Haven, CT, USA

Arjun Prabhu, MD, MBE Department of Emergency Medicine, Mount Sinai Health System, New York, NY, USA

Divy Ravindranath, MD, MS, FACLP Department of Psychiatry, Palo Alto Veterans Affairs Health Care System, Palo Alto, CA, USA

Janet S. Richmond, MSW Department of Psychiatry, VA Boston Healthcare System, Boston, MA, USA

McLean Hospital, Belmont, MA, USA

Tufts University School of Medicine, Boston, MA, USA

Megan Riddle, MD, PhD, MS Eating Recover Center, Bellevue, WA, USA

Silvana Riggio, MD Department of Psychiatry and Neurology, Icahn School of Medicine at Mount Sinai, New York, NY, USA

Alicia Romeo, MD Department of Psychiatry, Atrium Health Behavioral Health Charlotte, Charlotte, NC, USA

Linda Ronquillo, PsyD Alliant International University, San Diego, CA, USA

Lynn P. Roppolo, MD Department of Emergency Medicine, Parkland Health and Hospital System, Dallas, TX, USA

John S. Rozel, MD, MSL Department of Psychiatry, UPMC Western Psychiatric Hospital, Pittsburgh, PA, USA

Department of Psychiatry, University of Pittsburgh School of Medicine, Pittsburgh, PA, USA

Naomi A. Schmelzer, MD, MPH Department of Psychiatry, Brigham and Women's Faulkner Hospital, Harvard Medical School, Boston, MA, USA

Carmen R. Serpa, MD Macomb County Community Mental Health Services, Clinton Twp, MI, USA

Common Ground, Pontiac, MI, USA

Scott A. Simpson, MD, MPH Department of Behavioral Health Services, Denver Health & Hospital Authority, Denver, CO, USA

Layla Soliman, MD Department of Psychiatry, Atrium Health Behavioral Health, Charlotte, NC, USA

Susan Stefan, M.Phil., JD Rutland, MA, USA

Victor G. Stiebel, MD Department of Emergency Medicine, University of West Virginia, Morgantown, WV, USA

Brian Strickland, MD Department of Emergency Medicine, Massachusetts General Hospital, Boston, MA, USA

Scott Sulik, MD Department of Emergency Medicine, Ochsner Medical Center, Jefferson, LA, USA

Alifiya Tahir, MPH, BDS Tisch MS Research Center, New York, NY, USA

Julie Taub, MD Department of Medicine, Denver Health & Hospital Authority, Denver, CO, USA

Vaishal Tolia, MD, MPH Department of Emergency Medicine, Internal Medicine-Division of Hospital Medicine, University of California Health Sciences, San Diego, CA, USA

Samidha Tripathi, MD Department of Psychiatry, University of Arkansas for Medical Sciences, Little Rock, AR, USA

Gary M. Vilke, MD Department of Emergency Medicine, University of California Health Sciences, San Diego, CA, USA

Michael Ward, MD Department of Emergency Medicine, University of Wisconsin School of Medicine and Public Health, Madison, WI, USA

Michael P. Wilson, MD, PhD Department of Emergency Medicine, University of Arkansas for Medical Sciences, Little Rock, AR, USA

Mark Z. Zacharia, Esq. Corporate Legal Department, University of Pittsburgh Medical Center, Pittsburgh, PA, USA

Scott L. Zeller, MD Department of Psychiatry, University of California-Riverside, Emeryville, CA, USA

Department of Acute Psychiatry, Vituity, Reno, NV, USA

Leslie S. Zun, MD Department of Emergency Medicine, Rosalind Franklin University of Medicine and Science/ The Chicago Medical School, North Chicago, IL, USA

Author Biography

Leslie S. Zun, MD, MBA Dr. Zun is a Professor in the Clinical Sciences Department, Emergency Medicine discipline, with a secondary appointment in Psychiatry at Rosalind Franklin University of Medicine and Science/Chicago Medical School in North Chicago, Illinois. He is Medical Director of the Lake County Health Department/Community Health Center. Dr. Zun's background includes a medical degree (MD) from Rush Medical College and a business degree (MBA) from Northwestern University's School of Management. He has presented his research and lectured on behavioral emergencies topics both nationally and internationally. Dr. Zun is Past President of the American Association for Emergency Psychiatry and prior board member of American Academy of Emergency Medicine. He is Chief Editor of the textbook *Behavioral Emergencies for Emergency Physicians* and Course Director of the National Update on Behavioral Emergencies Conference.

Michael P. Wilson, MD, PhD, FAAEM, FACEP Dr. Wilson is an Assistant Professor in the Division of Research and Evidence-Based Medicine at the University of Arkansas for Medical Sciences, Department of Emergency Medicine, with a secondary appointment in the Department of Psychiatry. He currently serves on board of directors of the American Association for Emergency Psychiatry, as the Director of the UAMS Department of Emergency Medicine Behavioral Emergencies Research (DEMBER) lab, as the Director of the UAMS Emergency Medicine Research Associates program, and as Associate Conference Director of the annual National Update on Behavioral Emergencies Conference. He is a reviewer for several academic journals and is published broadly in the field of behavioral emergencies and agitation.

Kimberly Nordstrom, MD, JD, DFAPA Dr. Nordstrom has degrees in medicine and law, stemming from her interest in health policy and legislation. She is an Associate Professor of Psychiatry at the University of Colorado, School of Medicine. Dr. Nordstrom works clinically at the University of Colorado as an Emergency Psychiatrist and administratively with Colorado Access as Medical Director for Health Strategy & Behavioral Health. She serves as Associate Conference Director of the National Update on Behavioral Emergencies Conference. Dr. Nordstrom is Past President of the American Association for Emergency Psychiatry and immediate Past Chairperson of the Coalition on Psychiatric Emergencies. She has published widely in psychiatric and emergency medicine journals and texts and has lectured nationally and internationally on various topics regarding behavioral emergencies.

Part I

General Considerations

The Magnitude of the Problem of Psychiatric Illness Presenting in the Emergency Department

1

Gregory Luke Larkin and Alifiya Tahir

Introduction

Mental illness is ubiquitous and increasingly recognized as a growing problem throughout the world [1]. The purpose of this chapter is to describe the magnitude of the problem of mental illness, both globally and in terms of specific mental-health-related visits encountered in emergency department (ED) settings.

While emergency departments may not be the optimal location to manage the growing burden of mental illness, they generally constitute the only 24/7 access for the preponderance of patients in crisis.

Global Burden

The global burden of mental illness supersedes that of all other diseases. Recent estimates place mental illness first in the proportion of both global years of life lost due to disability (YLDs; 32.4%) and in terms of disability-adjusted life years lost (DALYs; 13%) [2]. More conservative and somewhat incomplete metrics from WHO in 2013 suggested mental illness constituted only 21.2% and 7.1% of all global YLDs and DALYs, respectively [3]. The following two graphics from Vigo et al. [2] highlight two different ways mental health burden may be estimated, giving significantly different results (Figs. 1.1 and 1.2).

Regardless of the yardstick, the burden of mental illness is increasing. Escalation of mental illness is attributed to an increase in psychosocial and environmental stressors in many parts of the world, combined with the epiphenomenon of mental illnesses becoming less stigmatized in many advancing societies and patriarchal cultures. Indeed, a substantial increase in measured prevalence comes less from new biological challenges and much more from an increase in diagnoses; the latter diagnostic contagion has been generated in part by improved training and recognition, the proliferation of clinical psychologists, the widespread availability of structured diagnostic tools, and a penchant to pathologize symptoms formerly regarded as nonpsychiatric.

Prevalence

Diagnostic trends notwithstanding, the worldwide prevalence of mental illness remains profound. The growing extent of the problem has been well described in the psychiatric epidemiologic studies of the World Health Organization's (WHO) World Mental Health Surveys conducted

G. L. Larkin (✉)
Department of Emergency Medicine and Psychiatry, Northeast Ohio Medical University, Akron, OH, USA

A. Tahir
Tisch MS Research Center, New York, NY, USA

L. S. Zun et al. (eds.), *Behavioral Emergencies for Healthcare Providers*,
https://doi.org/10.1007/978-3-030-52520-0_1

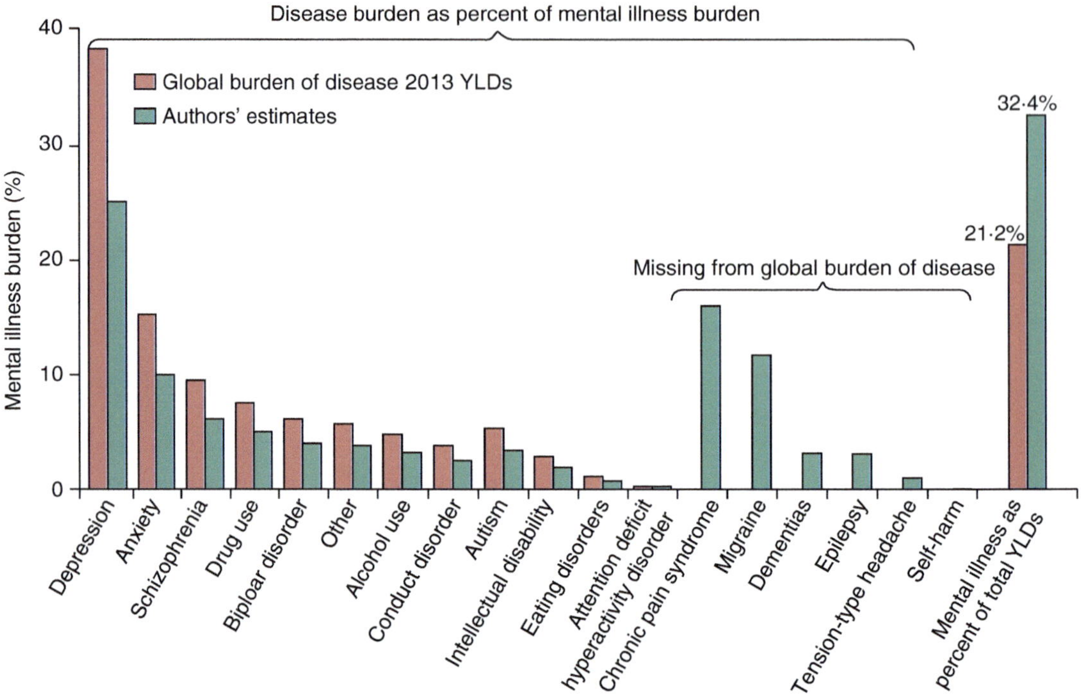

Fig. 1.1 Comparison of global burden of disease 2013: years lived with disability (YLDs) with the authors' estimates. Analysis based on data from Global Burden of Disease Study 2013 Collaborators [3]

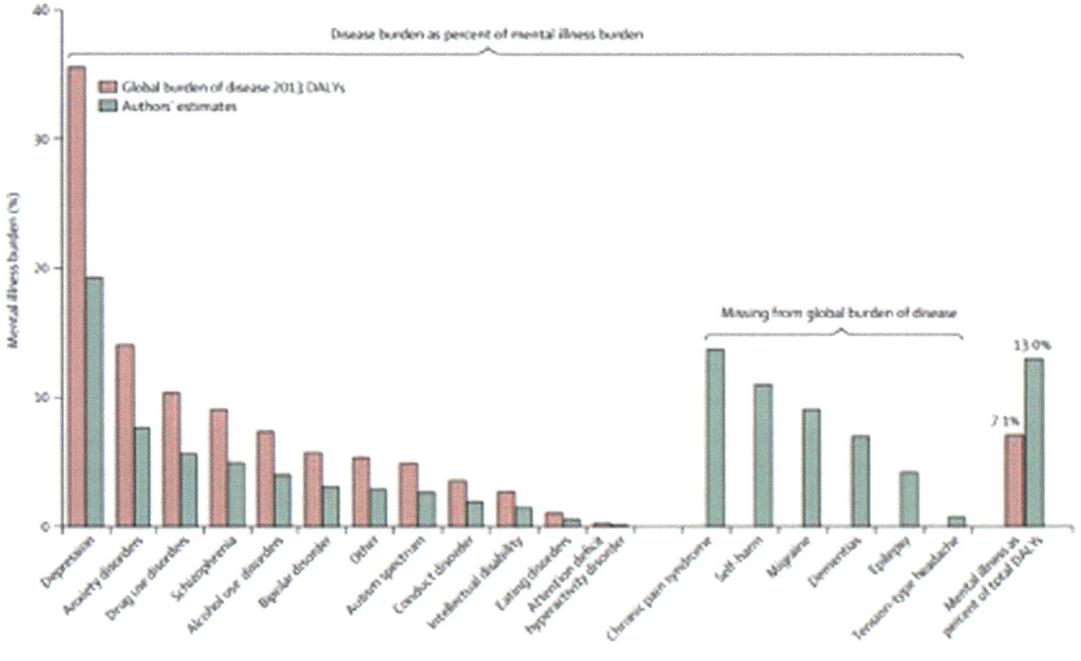

Fig. 1.2 Comparison of global burden of disease 2013: disability-adjusted life years (DALYs) with the authors' estimates of years lived with disability (YLDs); analysis based on data from GBD 2013 DALYs and HALE Collaborators [3, 4]

in 28 countries [1]. The WHO's cross-national comparisons show a globally high prevalence of major mental disorders (defined by Diagnostic and Statistical Manual of Mental Disorders, Fourth Edition (DSM-IV): anxiety disorders, mood disorders, impulse-control disorders, and substance-use disorders). Combined, one or more of these disorders impacts one in four persons; the 25th–75th interquartile prevalence range (IQR) is 18.1–36.1% of the total population. These WHO-sponsored data also reveal cross-nationally consistent findings of early ages at onset, high comorbidity, significant chronicity, widespread unmet treatment needs, significant delays between illness onset and treatment, and inadequate frequency and quality of mental health care [1].

In the United States, the National Survey on Drug Use and Health (NSDUH) estimates 43.4 million adults, or 18% of the US adult population, has had a mental illness in the past year [5] (Fig. 1.3). The World Mental Health Survey (WMHS) found that lifetime prevalence of major DSM-IV mental disorders was highest in the United States, with almost half (47.4%) the population having a lifetime risk of at least one mental illness [6]. The 12-month WMHS-based prevalence estimate for any disorder varied widely and was also highest in the United States at 24.6% (6% higher than US estimates from NSDUH), but lowest in Shanghai, China (4.3%) [7].

All four major classes of DSM-IV disorders are important components of overall prevalence. Anxiety disorders (IQR, 9.9–16.7%) and mood disorders (IQR, 9.8–15.8%) are the most prevalent lifetime illnesses. Impulse-control disorders (IQR, 3.1–5.7%) and substance-use disorders (IQR, 4.8–9.6%) are generally less prevalent in global samples, despite their relatively high frequency among emergency department patients in the English-speaking world [6].

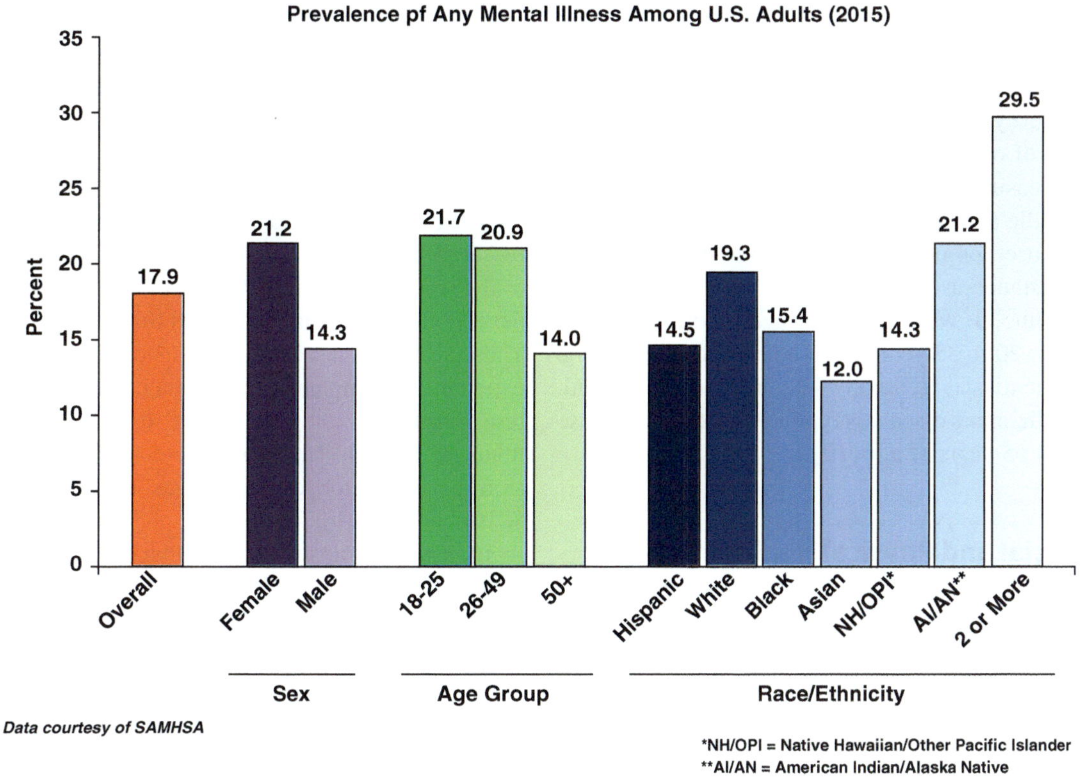

Fig. 1.3 Prevalence of any mental illness among U.S. adults (2015)

Extent of Mental Illness Across the Life Cycle

Most mental disorders begin early in life and often have a chronic, fulminating course. They have much earlier ages of onset than most chronic non-psychiatric disorders. In the US sample of the World Mental Health Survey, approximately 50% of psychiatric disorders existed by age 14 and 75% by age 24 [8]. Very early age of onset occurs for some anxiety disorders, notably phobias and separation anxiety disorder (SAD), with a median age of onset in the range of 7–14 years [6]. Early onsets are also typical for the externalizing disorders, with 80% of all lifetime attention-deficit/hyperactivity disorder beginning in the age range of 4–11, and the clear majority of oppositional-defiant disorder and conduct disorder beginning between ages 5 and 15 [6]. Serious mental illnesses such as schizophrenia typically first manifest in the late teenage years or early adulthood, typically in the range of 15–35 years of age [9].

Adult onsets are seen for the other common anxiety disorders (panic disorder, generalized anxiety disorder, and post-traumatic stress disorder), with median onset in the age range of 25–50 years old. Mood disorders have a similar age of onset to the later-onset anxiety disorders, increasing linearly from the early teens until late middle age, and then declining. The median age of onset for mood disorders ranges from 25 to 45. Substance-use disorders also begin in young adulthood, with a median age of onset ranging from 20 to 35 years [6]. The age of onset for the dementias is generally late in older adulthood. Alzheimer's disease is typically first seen in those over 65 years of age [10].

Social and Physical Health Impacts

WHO data from both the World Mental Health Survey and the Global Burden of Disease Study show that mental disorders impose enormous personal and economic costs. These enduring costs arise in part from the combination of early onset, high prevalence, high disability, and chronicity of mental health disorders [11]. Early-onset mental disorders are associated with a wide array of adverse outcomes over the life course, including lowered educational attainment, early marriage, marital instability, and low occupational and financial status [11]. In addition, and particularly relevant to emergency medicine, early-onset mental disorders increase the risk of onset and persistence of a wide range of physical disorders, including heart disease, asthma, diabetes mellitus, arthritis, chronic back pain, and chronic headache [12, 13]. Adult-onset mood, substance, and anxiety disorders are also associated with significant role impairment and are often comorbid with physical illnesses.

Economic Burden: United States

In any given year, an estimated one in four (26.2%) of the United States population has a diagnosable mental or substance-use disorder [14]. Of those with a disorder, 22% are classified as serious, 37% as moderate, and 40% as mild. To address this burden, the total US national health expenditures for mental health services has increased exponentially during the last three decades, from $33 million in 1986 to $147.4 billion in 2009 [5, 15]. Projections based on the SAMHSA findings estimate an increase in expenditures to $238 billion by 2020 (Fig. 1.4) [5, 16].

Most of the World Mental Health Survey research undertaken to calculate the magnitude of the short-term societal burden of mental disorders has been done in the United States [17, 18]. These studies count costs in terms of health care expenditures, impaired functioning, and premature mortality, and reveal an overwhelming financial burden. The economic cost of depression in 2010, for example, was estimated at $210.5 billion [19].

Industrial analyses suggest that one-third of all health-related days lost from work or home responsibilities in the United States (totaling in the billions) are due to mental disorders [20]. Major depressive disorder alone impacts 6.4% of US workers annually and results in an average of >5 weeks of absenteeism and lost work productivity, costing employers around $51 billion. The burden of depression-associated presenteeism—when workers are present at the workplace in

Fig. 1.4 Total U.S. expenditure for mental health services from 1986 to 2020 (in billion U.S. dollars)

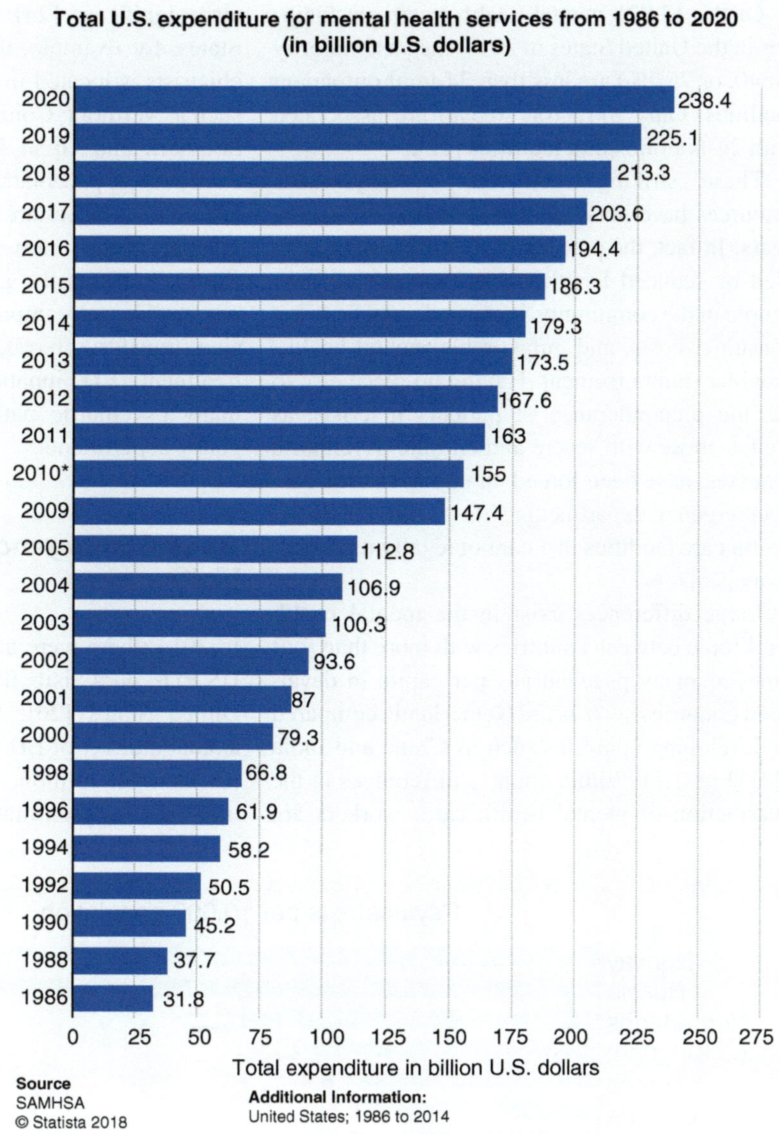

body but not in mind—is even more costly, estimated at more than $84 billion annually in the United States [21].

Changes in Mental Health Care Infrastructure

Globally, the burden of escalating numbers of mental health patients has been exacerbated by negative changes in mental health infrastructure that have resulted in reduced resources and restricted access for patients. In the United States, psychiatric inpatient facilities have been closed, numbers of psychiatrists have declined, and numbers of psychiatric beds have decreased, both in state hospitals and in general. For example, from 1986 to 2004, the number of mental health organizations in the United States has contracted, from 3512 to 891; the total number of psychiatric beds has fallen by 20%, from 267,613 to 212,231; the number of psychiatric beds in state and county mental hospitals has halved, from 119,033 to 57,034; and the number of beds per 100,000 civilian population decreased from 111.7 in 1986 to 71.2 in 2004 [21].

Of the 12,826 mental health treatment facilities in the United States in 2015, the vast majority (9640, or 75.2%) are less than 24-hour outpatient facilities. Only 2115 (or 16.5%) are associated with 24-hour hospital facilities [22].

These striking reductions in psychiatric resources have not been reversed in more recent years. In fact, the problems are worse, accompanied by reduced lengths of stay, moves to treat people in the community, increased out-of-pocket consumer costs, and unfavorable mental-health-provider reimbursement. Having no place else to go, the preponderance of patients in crisis, as well as those with severe and chronic psychiatric illnesses, have been forced en masse to seek care at emergency departments (EDs)—the only 24/7 health care facilities that cannot legally turn them away [26].

Large differences exist in the mental health workforce between countries with more than four times as many psychiatrists per capita in developed countries such as the Netherlands compared to developing countries such as China and India [23] (Fig. 1.5). Within country differences in the distribution of mental health care, workers are also significant [24] (Fig. 1.6). In the United States, for example, the highest density of psychiatrists is located in small New England states such as Vermont, Connecticut, and Rhode Island. Southern and Great Plains states have significantly fewer psychiatrists per capita. Similar distribution variances are observed for other types of mental health care providers as well [25] (Fig. 1.7). Naturally, access to local mental health resources greatly impacts the disposition (admission, transfer, referral, and discharge home) and treatment (ED, inpatient, and/or outpatient) of many psychiatric patients presenting to emergency departments.

Overall Emergency Department Visits

In 2014, there were almost 141 million visits to US EDs, 44.4 visits for every 100 persons in the United States [26]. From 1994 to 2014, the annual number of ED visits increased 52%, from 93 to 141 million, representing an average increase of approximately 2.4 million (2.6%) vis-

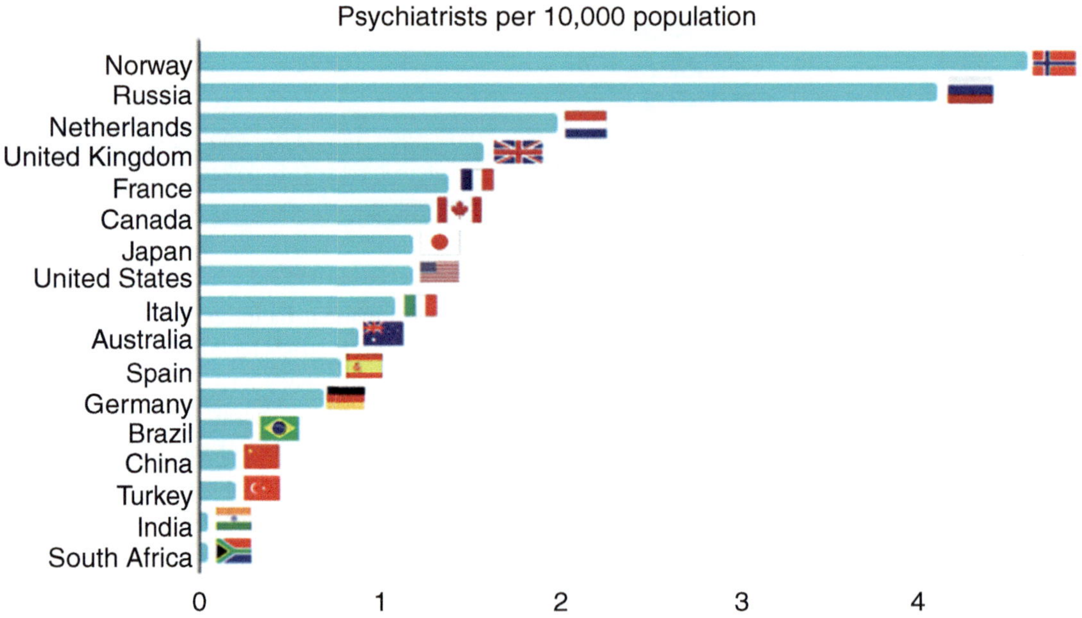

Fig. 1.5 Psychiatrists per 10,000 population (Data source: Mental Health Atlas 2014 [23]). (*Number of psychiatrists in India and South Africa are <0.05 per 10,000 population)

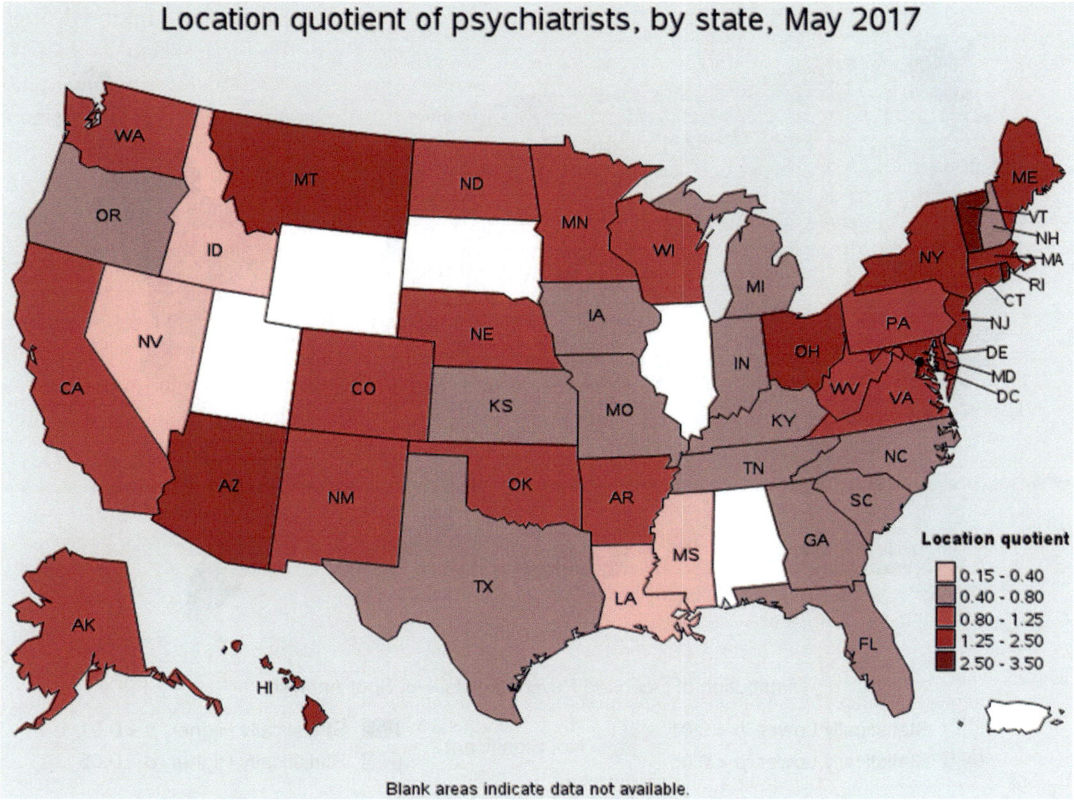

Fig. 1.6 (Source: US Bureau of Labor Statistics [24]). (*The location quotient is the ratio of the area concentration of occupational employment to the national average concentration. A location quotient greater than one indicates the occupation has a higher share of employment than average, and a location quotient less than one indicates the occupation is less prevalent in the area than average)

its every year [26, 27]. However, as the number of visits has increased, the number of hospital-based EDs has decreased, from 4960 in 1994 to 4408 in 2014, and this trend shows no sign of reversal [28] (Fig. 1.8). The net effect of increasing visit rates and a reciprocal decline in the number of EDs is a 20% increase in ED volume and concomitant overcrowding. Mental health patients have played an increasing role in ED oversubscription, and we describe this below.

Increased Mental Health Visits to Emergency Departments

An increasing fraction of annual ED visits are for mental health presentations [29]. Indeed, while overall use of US ED services increased by 52% from 1994 to 2014, the number of documented mental-health-related visits increased at an even faster rate—100% over the same 20 years [27, 29]. For the past two decades, mental disorders have been the fastest growing component of emergency medical practice, while psychiatric services have diminished.

Nearly one in three adults in the noninstitutionalized community has a diagnosable mental or addictive disorder; in the ED, this figure climbs to at least 40%. In 2006, the National Center for Health Statistics (NCHS) reported that 4.7 million patients presented to American Eds with a primary psychiatric diagnosis. However, this number does not include codes for psychiatric reasons for the visit, comorbid mental health issues, substance-related visits, and the many patients in whom psychiatric reasons for the visit

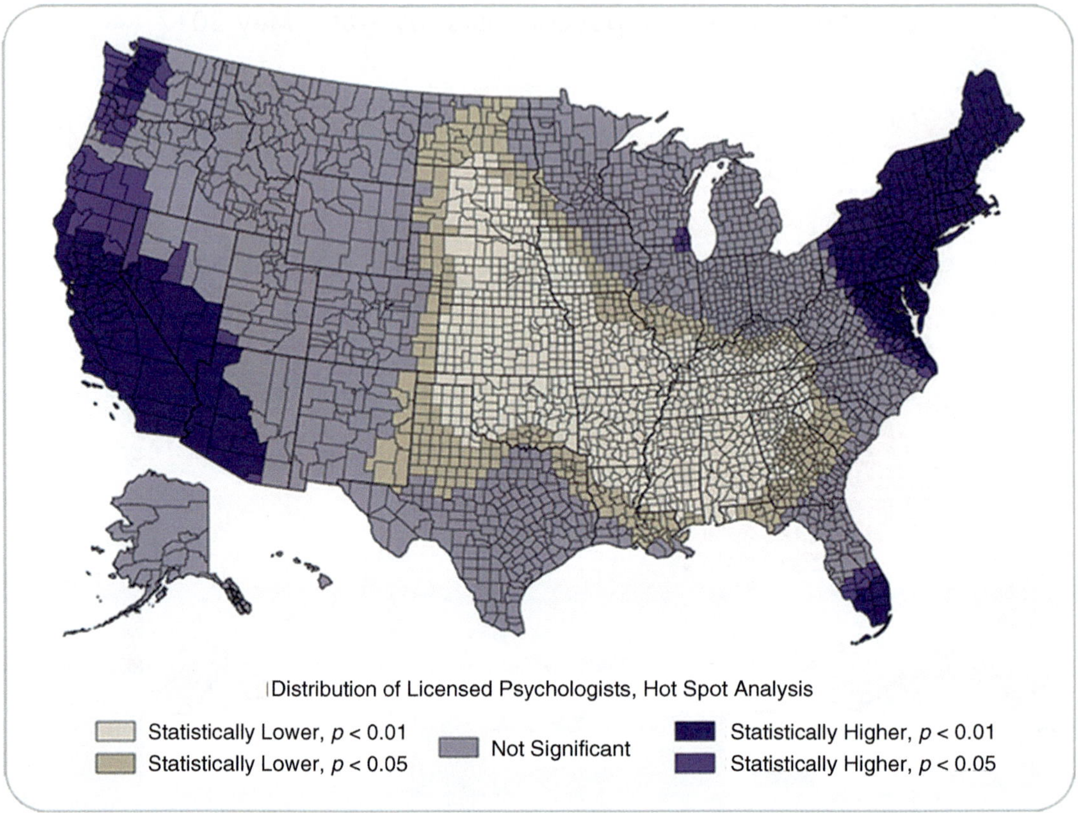

Fig. 1.7 Hot-spot analysis on the number of licensed psychologists, 2012–2015. (Source: American Psychological Association [25]). (Note: This map was based on the Getis-Ord statistic generated from the hot-spot analysis. The number of licensed psychologists was statistically compared to the national mean. Counties in Hawaii, Oklahoma, and Utah were included in the analysis based on state means of licensed psychologists per county)

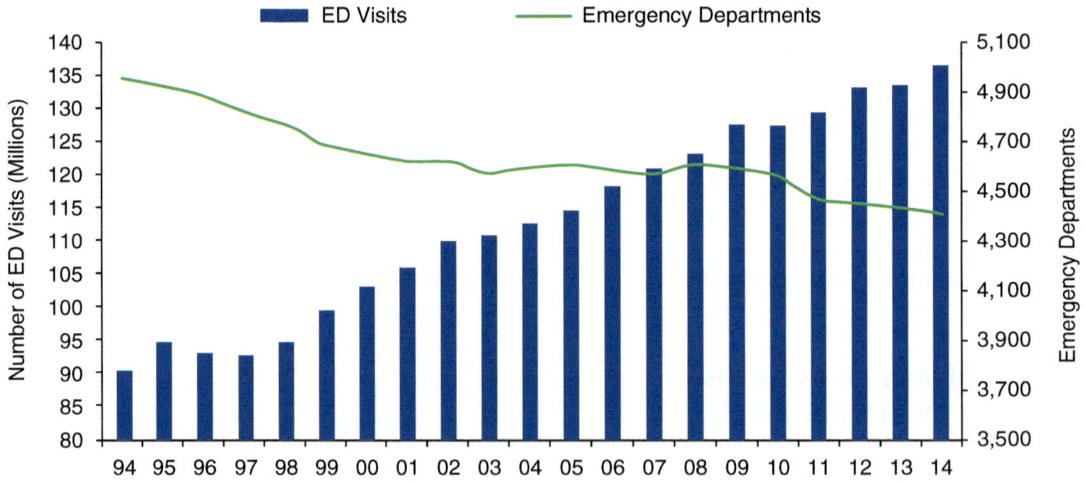

Fig. 1.8 US emergency department visits and hospital-based emergency departments, 1994–2014. (Source: American Hospital Association TrendWatch ChartBook [28]). (*Defined as hospitals reporting ED visits in the AHA Annual Survey)

are secondary; hence, NCHS numbers are a gross underestimate.

The Emergency Medical Treatment and Active Labor Act (EMTALA) legislation and mental health insurance exclusions, as well as changes in the mental health infrastructure, mean that Eds have become the default option for urgent and acute contact for many psychiatric patients, including high severity patients and those who are suicidal. For some, the ED is their sole source of health care [26]. While many of those who present to Eds with mental health problems are uninsured, underinsured, homeless, and of racial and ethnic minorities who have no easy access to health care, the largest increase in mental health visits in the past decade comes from those who are insured [30]. As states reduce mental health care expenditure and the US health care system becomes inaccessible to an increasing fraction of the American population, the 100% increase in ED psychiatric visits observed between 1994 and 2014 is likely to continue.

As a result of these trends, emergency medicine is being forced to assume a growing responsibility for providing both primary and acute mental health care. Paradoxically, however, while ED visits increase every year, both the number of general and psychiatric EDs are declining. Only approximately 146 EDs with specialized psychiatric emergency units remain (American Association for Emergency Psychiatry, 2009, "personal communication").

The Epidemiology of Mental Health Visits to Emergency Departments

Emergency department use for psychiatric reasons has expanded over the past two decades and now accounts for 3.5% of all US emergency department visits by adults [27, 29]. Despite these recent trends, which have resulted in record-breaking numbers of patients seeking emergency services nationwide, there have been few methodologically and epidemiologically sound studies of mental-health-related emergency visits in the United States.

The most comprehensive study used National Hospital Ambulatory Medical Care Survey (NHAMCS) data relevant diagnostic fields, including psychiatric reason-for-visit codes, DSM-based ICD diagnoses, Supplementary Classification of Factors Influencing Health Status and Contact with Health Services (V codes), and external cause-of-injury codes (E codes) for all appropriate mental-health-related disorders [30]. This study found that from 1992 to 2001, a total of 53 million visits to US EDs were made primarily for mental-health-related reasons. Of these, an estimated 17 million visits were for a mental-health-related primary complaint (i.e., as conveyed to the clinician by the patient), but many more involved a psychiatric diagnosis (i.e., the assessment of the patient's condition by the clinician). Among the estimated 53 million mental-health-related visits overall, the most common diagnoses were substance-related disorders (30%), mood disorders (23%), and anxiety disorders (21%). Psychoses constituted 10%, and suicide attempts 7%, of all documented mental-health-related visits. These five major subgroups accounted for 79% of all mental-health-related visits [30].

The remaining visits included all other Diagnostic and Statistical Manual of Mental Disorders (DSM) diagnostic codes and reason-for-visit codes referable to other psychological and mental disorders. Rates of these miscellaneous mental-health-related visits increased significantly over the decade. Rates of presentation to EDs for the most serious mental health problem (suicidal behavior) increased by almost 50% from 1992 to 2001. As well as suicidal behavior, increased rates of visits were significant for all of the most prevalent disorders (mood, substance use, and anxiety disorders). According to the Nationwide Emergency Department sample, mental health ED visits increased from 2006 to 2014 by 44.1% [32]. However, rates of psychoses-related visits remained stable over this period from 0.6% in 2009 to 0.7% in 2014 in the adult male population [27, 33].

Specific Mental Disorders

The goal of the following section is to describe the magnitude of the problem of ED presentations for specific mental disorders. The most prevalent conditions are highlighted. While the prevalence and illness burden of each condition are worthy of discussion, prevalence data are not available for all mental illnesses, particularly those that are less common. While some disorders are increasingly recognized (ADHD, e.g., 2.8% prevalence), their relative lack of ED treatment-seeking often keeps them out of the discussion of emergency mental health [34].

Anxiety Disorders

Anxiety disorders are the most common psychiatric disorders in the general population. Studies suggest that as many as one in four ED patients screen positive for anxiety disorders [35]. Many patients with anxiety disorders visit emergency departments, either to seek help for the anxiety symptoms explicitly or because they have physical symptoms related to anxiety. While anxiety symptoms rarely constitute a life-threatening emergency, severe anxiety is a common presenting problem in emergency department patients, consuming many resources. Specific anxiety disorders include (based on DSM-5):

- Anxiety disorders
  - Separation anxiety disorder
  - Selective mutism
  - Specific phobia
  - Social anxiety disorder
  - Panic disorder
  - Panic attack specifier
  - Agoraphobia
  - Generalized anxiety disorder
  - Anxiety disorder due to another medical condition
  - Other specified anxiety disorder
  - Unspecified anxiety disorder
- Obsessive-compulsive disorders
  - Obsessive-compulsive disorder
  - Body dysmorphic disorder
  - Hoarding disorder
  - Trichotillomania
  - Excoriation disorder
  - Substance/medication-induced obsessive-compulsive and related disorder
  - Obsessive-compulsive and related disorder due to another medical condition
  - Other specified obsessive-compulsive and related disorder
  - Unspecified obsessive-compulsive and related disorder
- Trauma and stressor-related disorders
  - Reactive attachment disorder
  - Disinhibited social engagement disorder
  - PTSD
  - Acute stress disorder
  - Adjustment disorders
  - Other specified trauma-and-stressor-related disorder
  - Unspecified trauma-and-stressor-related disorder

In any given year, anxiety disorders affect 25% of the US adult population, making them the most prevalent type of mental disorders [36]. Of these cases, 22.8% (4.2% of the total adult population) are classified as "severe" [8]. The mean age of onset of anxiety disorders is 11 years, and these disorders are more common in females than males and less common in non-Hispanic Blacks and in Hispanics than in non-Hispanic Whites.

Despite the high prevalence rates of anxiety disorders, they are often underrecognized and undertreated clinical problems in the general population and in primary care. Of all cases each year, only one-third (36.9%) receive treatment, and for only one-third of those (12.7% of those with the disorder) is the treatment effective or adequate [37]. Anxiety disorders have a strong comorbidity with depression and substance-use disorders; the risk of suicidal behavior in anxiety-disordered patients is often underestimated [38].

Anxiety-related presentations accounted for 16% of emergency department mental health visits from 1992 to 2001, increasing from 4.9% to 6.3% of all emergency department visits across the decade [38]. While not always used for anxiety, the anxiolytics/sedatives/hypnotics prescriptions escalated from 9.6M in 2006 to 13.5M in 2014 [27, 33]. This growth may reflect a rise in anxiety-related emergency department care-seeking, an increase in anxiety awareness among patients and practitioners, or both. Of all mental health visits to the ED, anxiety disorders are the least likely to result in admission, with an overall hospitalization rate of 20% [38].

The European Study of the Epidemiology of Mental Disorders (ESEMeD) based on more than 21,000 adults across Belgium, France, Germany, Italy, Netherlands, and Spain estimated that only one-fifth of anxiety patients seek help. Of those that reach out for health services, 23% receive no treatment, 31% receive only drugs, 20% receive only psychotherapy, and 27% are treated with both pharmacotherapy and psychotherapy [39].

Panic Disorder

The estimated lifetime prevalence of panic disorder in the US adult population is 4.7% [40, 41]. Twelve-month prevalence is estimated at 2.7%. The lifetime prevalence of panic disorder is twice as high among females (6.2%) than males (3.1%). Twelve-month prevalence is 3.8% for females and 1.6% for males. The age of onset for panic disorder is typically is early to mid-20s, and panic disorder is seen most commonly in people aged 15–24 years [42]. However, these population estimates may not reflect the characteristics of panic disorder patients seen in emergency department settings. For example, it has been found that panic patients in an ED were older and more likely to be male than patients seen in psychiatric clinics. One study found ED panic patients were also significantly more likely to be on Medicare and less likely to be uninsured [43].

Patients with panic disorder have high rates of use of both ED services and 911 emergency services, as well as high rates of ED recidivism. Panic patients seek emergency care not only because of the sudden, severe, and frightening onset of symptoms but also because anxiety disorders often occur in association with somatic complaints. The direction of association is unclear but is likely to be bidirectional.

A series of ED studies have focused on patients who present with chest pain [43]. Chest pain is the most common reason for ED presentation for those over 65 and the second most common reason for those aged 15–64 years, accounting in 2008 for 4.7 million ED visits [15]. Studies of ED chest pain patients consistently report that panic disorder can be diagnosed in two-thirds of all patients presenting to an ED with medically unexplained chest pain. In several studies, the vast majority (98%) of ED patients with panic disorder were undiagnosed. These patients often receive costly cardiac workups to exclude coronary artery disease, yet they are seldom, if ever, screened for panic disorder [44].

Underdiagnosis of panic disorder is unfortunate, not only because identification of these patients might reduce their economic burden in the ED by avoiding unnecessary and expensive investigative tests, and minimizing rates of medical care usage, use of 911 services, and overall ED use, but also because effective pharmacological and psychotherapeutic treatments are available. Untreated, panic patients tend to develop depression, agoraphobia, alcohol and substance abuse problems, and impaired social and occupational functioning. Panic disorder is also associated with an elevated risk of suicidal behavior. Although only 60% of people with panic disorder seek care, 32% of these patients present to EDs, rendering EDs an appropriate site for detection and possibly early treatment and referral of panic disorder patients [44].

Posttraumatic Stress Disorder (PTSD)

While the nosology of posttraumatic stress disorder is still being debated, the estimated lifetime prevalence of PTSD among adult Americans is 6.8% [14]. The 12-month PTSD prevalence estimate is 3.5%. PTSD is significantly more common in women than men; the lifetime prevalence of PTSD among men is 3.6%, and among women, 9.7%. The 12-month prevalence is 1.8% among men and 5.2% among women.

PTSD is often unrecognized in the general population, as well as in emergency departments, which are routine reception zones for trauma and disaster victims. Emergency departments receive many patients who have experienced mass-casualty events, natural disasters, serious accidents, assault or abuse, sudden and major deaths, as well as deep emotional losses that put them at risk of PTSD. The ED as an ideal setting for PTSD prevention is being increasingly recognized.

Generalized Anxiety Disorder

The lifetime prevalence of generalized anxiety disorder (GAD) is estimated at 5.7% in the United States, which is higher than the estimated 3.7% lifetime prevalence globally [14, 40, 45]. The 12-month US prevalence is 2.7%. The lifetime prevalence of generalized anxiety disorder is estimated to be 7.1% in females and 4.2% among males. Past-year prevalence is 3.4% among females and 1.9% in males. Generalized anxiety disorder rarely occurs in isolation from other psychiatric disorders, with an estimated 90% of people with GAD meeting criteria for another psychiatric disorder over the course of their lifetime. The most common comorbid illnesses are depression, alcohol abuse, and other anxiety disorders [46]. In the emergency department, GAD is likely to be a secondary diagnosis both to these comorbid mental disorders as well as to physical illnesses.

Phobic Disorders

The global estimates for phobia report a 3.6% lifetime prevalence [47]. The estimates for the adult US population are much higher, at 12.5% [14]. In any year, one in every ten adults reports having a specific phobia. The lifetime prevalence is estimated at 15.8% in females and 8.9% in males. While phobias are the most prevalent anxiety disorders, they are much less likely than panic disorder, PTSD, and GAD to be the primary reason for ED presentation.

Mood Disorders

After anxiety disorders, mood disorders are the second most common psychiatric disorder in the general population, occurring in 10% of the US adult population each year [14, 48]. Of these cases, 45% (4.3% of the total population) are classified as severe. The mean age of onset is 30 years, and women are 50% more likely than men to suffer a mood disorder during their lifetime. Non-Hispanic Blacks and Hispanics are less likely than non-Hispanic Whites to experience a mood disorder during their lifetime.

Mood disorders are the most expensive mental illness in the general population because they are frequently undiagnosed, underdiagnosed, or misdiagnosed, and, even if detected, often inadequately treated. Each year, half of those in the general population with a mood disorder receive treatment, and for 40% (20% of those with any mood disorder), this treatment is minimally adequate [42].

The economic burden of depression in the general population is derived not only from the health care costs of inadequate diagnosis and treatment but also from workplace absenteeism and loss of productivity, lost earnings due to premature death, and the costs incurred by social agencies (including law enforcement, the justice system, and shelters), as well as personal costs in terms of reduced quality of life.

After substance-use disorders, mood disorders (including major depressive disorder, bipolar disorder, and dysthymia) are the most common mental illnesses seen in the emergency department, accounting for 17% of US ED visits for mental-health-related reasons from 1992 to 2001 [31]. More recent data reveal a 34% increase in the rate of mood disorder presentations to the ED as a first-listed diagnosis, from 1.1M in 2006 to 1.5M in 2014 [32].

Major Depression

Major depression was estimated to affect 322 million, or 4.4% of the world's population, in the year 2015 [49]. Currently, 16.1 million adults in the United States are considered to suffer from MDD [5]. Each year, 6.7% of US adults suffer a major depressive episode (MDE) [14, 50] (Fig. 1.9). The prevalence of MDE among young adults aged 18–25 in the United States has increased significantly in recent years, and overall, this prevalence is higher than all other age groups [5] (Fig. 1.10). Of all major depressive episodes, one-third (2% of all the US adult population) are classified as severe. The mean age of onset is 32 years. Women are 70% more likely than males to have a major depressive episode during their lifetime, and MDD is 40% less common in non-Hispanic Blacks than non-Hispanic Whites. Of all those with MDD each year, only half receive treatment, and of those receiving treatment, 38% (20% of those with the disorder) are receiving minimally adequate treatment.

The use of antidepressants for treating depression has risen sharply in the years 2001–2011, showing an increase of 98% [51]. This increase is much higher than the 6% increase over the previous decade, which ended in 2001 [30]. The rise in antidepressant prescriptions accompanies a general awareness of treatment for depression, with a 220% increase since the 1980s [52]. Although more individuals are seeking treatment, a gradual decline in the use of psychotherapy can be appreciated in the 2000s compared to the 1980s (54–43%) [52].

Untreated depression imposes a severe economic burden, resulting largely from inadequate diagnosis and treatment. In the majority (50–60%) of those with depression, the disorder is not accurately diagnosed [53]. Wells and colleagues found that depressed medically ill patients have significantly more pain and functional impairment than matched patients having chronic medical conditions alone [54]. Only advanced coronary artery disease accounts for more bed disability days (defined as days during which a person stayed in bed for more than half a day because of illness or injury) than depression, and only arthritis causes more pain. In terms of

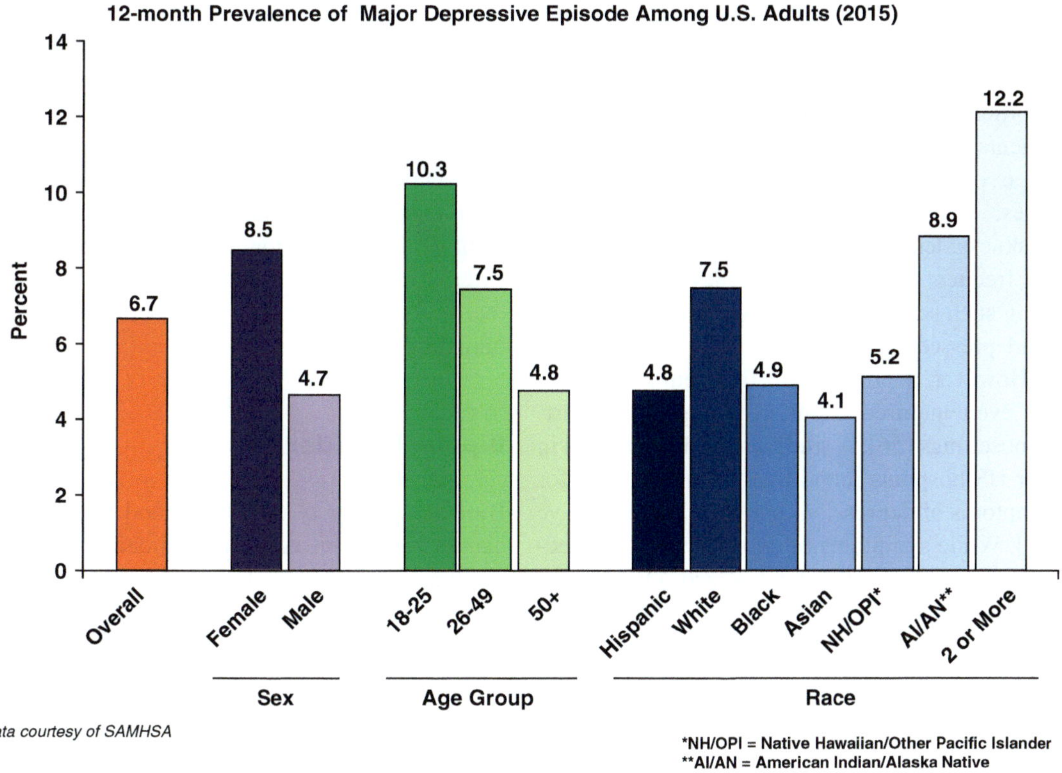

Fig. 1.9 Twelve-month prevalence of major depressive episodes among US adults (2015). (Source: SAMHSA [50])

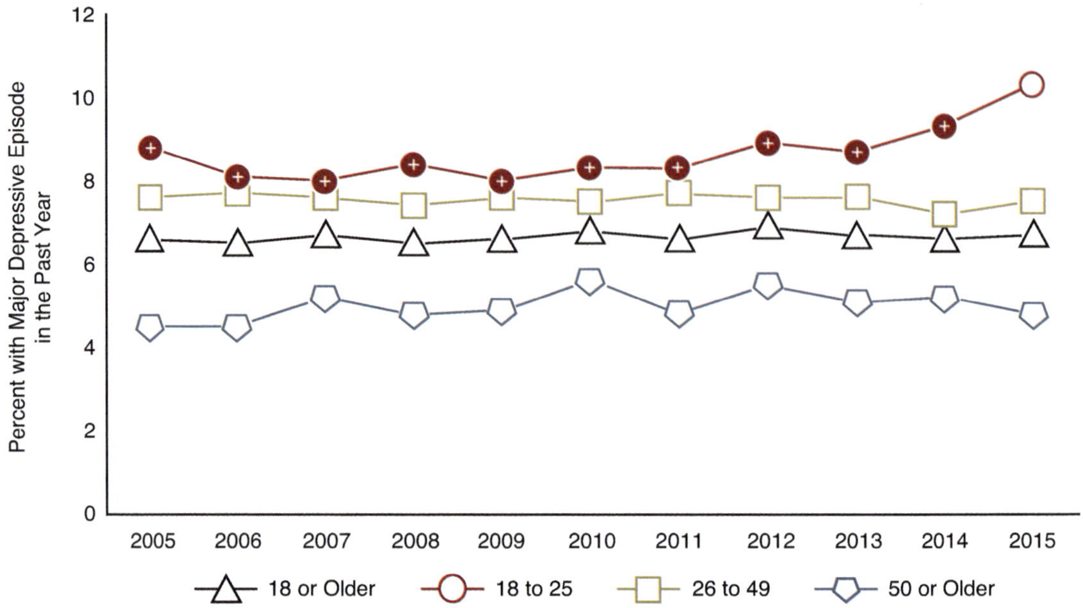

Fig. 1.10 Major depressive episode in the past year among adults aged 18 or older, by age group: percentages, 2005–2015. (Source: Center for Behavioral Health Statistics and Quality [5])

impaired physical functioning and ability to work, to function socially, and to care for home and family, depression is more disabling than hypertension, diabetes, arthritis, gastrointestinal disorders, or back pain problems. Depressed patients have high rates of medical usage for a range of somatic complaints, including headaches, backaches, gastrointestinal disorders, weakness, lethargy, fatigue, and insomnia. They are frequent users of emergency departments, using such services three to five times more than nondepressed patients [55].

However, depression is often neither detected nor even inquired about in emergency department settings [56]. A study of 476 ED patients in four US hospitals found that, when screened for symptoms of depression, one-third were positive [57]. While symptoms of depression do not necessarily equate with standardized DSM-based diagnoses of depression, these results suggest that depression in ED patients may be approximately six times higher than in general population samples.

Depression is often comorbid with anxiety disorders, substance dependence, and other mental disorders, as well as a range of somatic complaints. It may be obscured in ED presentations by these other concerns unless explicit screening for depression is undertaken. However, if ED screening for depression is implemented, then there is a need to develop a range of ED-based interventions to either provide ED-delivered interventions or to link all those who screen positive for depression to appropriate services external to the ED and, furthermore, to ensure that no one falls through gaps between ED and outpatient services.

Bipolar Disorder

Bipolar disorder is a chronic mood disorder that causes significant economic burden to patients, families, and society [14, 58]. The 12-month prevalence of bipolar disorder in the US adult population is 2.6%. Prevalence estimates may vary from 2.4% to 15.1%, depending upon how inclusive the diagnostic categories employed. For example, the highest prevalence of 15.1% would comprise manic episode, hypomanic episode, and soft hypomanic episode [59–65]. The majority of these cases (83%) are classified as severe. Half of those with the disorder receive treatment each year, and of those, 40% receive minimally adequate treatment.

Bipolar disorder is characterized by recurrent manic (or hypomanic) and depressive episodes that cause functional impairment and reduce the quality of life [66]. At least 25–50% of patients with bipolar disorder also attempt suicide [67]. People with bipolar disorders are 20–30 times more likely to commit suicide than the general population [69, 70]. Bipolar patients may present to the ED in either depressed or manic states; some will have attempted suicide. There are few studies of the epidemiology of bipolar disorder visits to the ED, but one small study found that almost 7% of ED patients screened positive for bipolar disorder, considerably higher than population estimates of 1.3% [68]. As with anxiety disorders, bipolar disorders carry significant comorbidity with substance-use disorders [69].

Dysthymic Disorder

The DSM-5 characterizes dysthymia as a "Persistent Depressive Disorder." This category is a consolidation of the DSM-IV defined chronic major depression and dysthymia. Persistent Depressive Disorder is characterized by a depressed mood for most of the day for at least 2 years. If individuals meet the MDD criteria for 2 years, they are classified as having both MDD and Persistent Depressive Disorder. People with dysthymia may also experience one or more episodes of major depression during their lifetime [14]. The lifetime prevalence of dysthymic disorder is estimated to be 2.5% [14]. The 12-month prevalence is 1.5%. Lifetime estimates are 3.1% among females and 1.8% in males. Twelve-month estimates are 1.9% among females and 1.0% in males. Dysthymia may underlie many ED visits, but it is frequently undetected, and many outpatients with dysthymia may be receiving inadequate treatment.

Suicidal Behavior

Suicidal behavior is a proposed DSM-5 disorder assigned to those who have attempted suicide in the past 2 years. Suicidal behavior is closely associated with most mental disorders and is one of the most common and arguably the most serious psychiatric emergency presentation to the ED. Suicide ideation and suicide attempts are strongly linked to death by suicide and predict further suicidal behavior [71]. The lifetime prevalence of suicide ideation is 9%, and the lifetime prevalence of suicide attempts is 3%. Twelve-month prevalence rates of suicide ideation, plans, and attempts are, respectively, 2%, 0.6%, and 0.3% for developed countries [72].

Recently, suicide has surpassed transport-related crashes as the most common cause of injury-related deaths in the United States. In 2004, suicide was responsible for approximately 32,000 deaths, and motor vehicles for 47,000 deaths. By 2014, the numbers reversed: Suicide became responsible for 43,000 deaths compared to 38,000 deaths due to motor vehicle crashes [73].

Suicide attempts accounted for approximately 2.5 million (5.9%) injury-related US ED visits in 2012 [30]. The rate of presentation for suicide-related visits to US EDs increased by 73%, from 0.3M in 1994 to 0.5M in 2014 [27, 29]. Yet these figures underestimate the prevalence of suicide-related visits to the ED. A study by Claassen and Larkin (2005), for example, found that a significant fraction of those who present to EDs for non-mental-health reasons often have occult or silent suicide ideation (estimated at 8–12%) [74].

Three clusters of ED patients can be identified as being at risk of suicide ideation and behavior: (i) those who present to ED with suicide ideation or threats, or following suicide attempts; (ii) those who present with the mental health problems with which suicide is associated; and (iii) those who present with specific physical problems but who have occult or silent suicide risk [75–77].

Almost all mental disorders have an increased risk of suicide apart from mental retardation and dementia [77]. Outside of China, psychological autopsies reveal that approximately 90% of individuals who attempt or commit suicide meet diagnostic criteria for a mental disorder, most commonly mood disorders, substance-use disorders, psychoses, and personality disorders. However, both the mental disorders with which suicide is associated and the subtle levels of suicide ideation are frequently underrecognized and undertreated in ED settings.

Those who make suicide attempts also present to ED services for a range of medical problems and have increased risks of homicide, accidents, disease, and premature death in general [79]. Patients who present to the ED with suicide ideation (without attempt) also have risks of returning to the ED with further ideation or with suicide attempts; in fact, those with SI have as much risk as those who present with attempts [74].

EDs have an unmatched burden of responsibility for suicidal patients. EDs are thoroughfares for a range of endophenotypes at high risk of suicidal behavior, including not only those with frank or occult suicidal behavior but also young people; males; prisoners; gun owners; the homeless; the psychiatrically ill; binge drinkers, illicit drug users, and substance abusers; older adults; victims of abuse, trauma, and assault; perpetrators of crime, assault, and violence; substance-abusing youth; violent youth; youth with conduct disorder and those in foster and welfare care; patients with severe, chronic mental disorders, including those with depression, psychosis, and personality disorders; older adults with physical health problems, persistent pain, disability, and/or depression; and adults and young adults with degenerative illnesses. Given that emergency departments are in frequent contact with suicidal patients, EDs represent underutilized sites for suicide prevention [74]. Potentially, EDs are sites that could identify and engage at-risk patients into accessible outpatient care management and suicide prevention programs.

Substance-Use Disorders

One person in three in the US population has a lifetime substance-use disorder, and the lifetime risk is higher among males (41.8%) than females (29.6%) [14]. The 12-month prevalence is 13.4%—again, higher in males (15.4%) than females (11.6%).

Substance abuse is the most common mental health reason for ED presentations. The primary diagnosis of substance abuse was responsible for 30% of psychiatric-related ED visits in the United States from 1992 to 2001 [30]. In 2015, substance abuse constituted 7% of all ED visits (NHAMCS-ED 2015). Substance abuse is often comorbid with other mental disorders, including mood and anxiety disorders in particular. Patients with comorbid major psychiatric diagnoses and substance-abuse diagnoses are overrepresented in those who are frequent recidivists to EDs.

Substance abuse is also commonly involved in injury-related ED presentations, including violence, falls, drownings, motor vehicle crashes, and suicide attempts. Substance misuse is also associated with hazardous and costly social consequences, including driving under the influence of alcohol or drugs, arrest, and violent behavior.

Alcohol Abuse or Dependence

In 2000, 16.2% of deaths and 13.2% of disability-adjusted life years (DALYs) from injuries globally were estimated to be attributed to alcohol. The lifetime prevalence of alcohol abuse or dependence in the US population is estimated to be 13.2% [14]. The 12-month estimate is 3.1%. Lifetime prevalence is estimated at 19.6% among males and 7.5% among females. The 12-month estimates are 4.5% among males and 1.8% among females. The apparent prevalence of alcohol-use disorder in the United States has decreased significantly in recent years, especially among those aged 18–25 [5] (Fig. 1.11).

Alcohol-related disorders presenting to EDs as first-listed diagnoses increased by 76%, from 0.8M to 1.5M in the years 2006 to 2014 [32]. This inflation, however, represents only the tip of an iceberg. An important caveat to these numbers

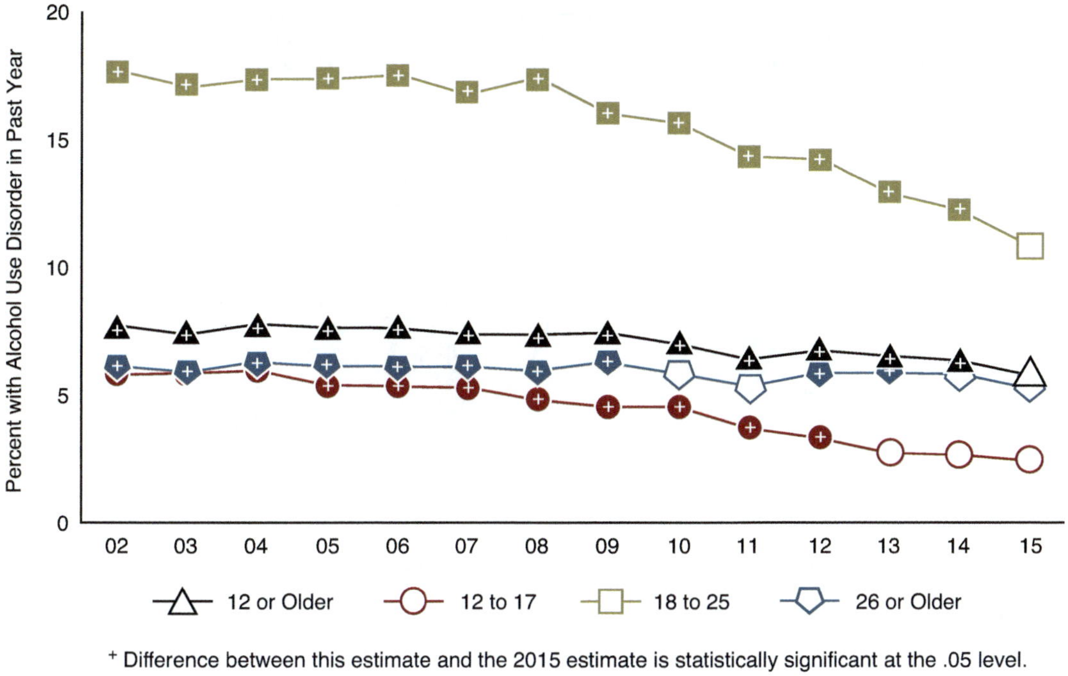

Fig. 1.11 Alcohol-use disorder in the past year among people aged 12 or older, by age group: Percentages, United States (2002–2015). (Source: Center for Behavioral Health Statistics and Quality [5])

is a systematic underestimation due in part to patient and provider denial. Trauma patients who are intoxicated are often underdiagnosed with substance abuse in order to maximize the likelihood that a claim will not be denied. Frequent alcohol recidivists rarely have their alcohol levels checked, in order to expedite their disposition. Numerous patient, provider, and systemic issues conspire, leading to an underdiagnosis of alcohol abuse and dependence.

Alcohol-related visits impose a significant burden on emergency departments. As mentioned, patients often withhold information about their drinking habits and drinking history; hence, the role of alcohol in many ED visits is likely underestimated. Nevertheless, alcohol abuse is often implicated in ED visits for violence and injury. Half of all drug abuse/misuse visits made to EDs by individuals under 20 years old involve alcohol [80]. Indeed, there is a significant overlap among persons with illicit drug-use disorders and alcohol-use disorders [5] (Fig. 1.12).

Drug Abuse or Dependence

An estimated 8% of the US adult population has a lifetime drug abuse or dependence disorder [14]. The 12-month estimate is 1.4%. Lifetime estimates are 11.6% among males and 4.8% among females. The 12-month estimates are 2.2% for males and 0.7% for females. Drug-related ED visits include those made for drug abuse and misuse, suicide attempts, adverse reactions, and accidental ingestions. Adverse effects from drug abuse represent almost half of all drug-related ED visits [81] (Fig. 1.13). Drug abuse also spawned increased violence during the crack-cocaine epidemic of the 1990s, followed in the United States by prescription opiate abuse (e.g., oxycodone) and ultimately in the last decade by a resurgence in heroin and related substance abuse.

The number of drug abuse-related ED visits have skyrocketed by 161% in 7 years, from 1,545,136 in 2004 to 4,032,571 in 2011 [80]. A resurgence of methamphetamine abuse has led to an increase in methamphetamine-related ED vis-

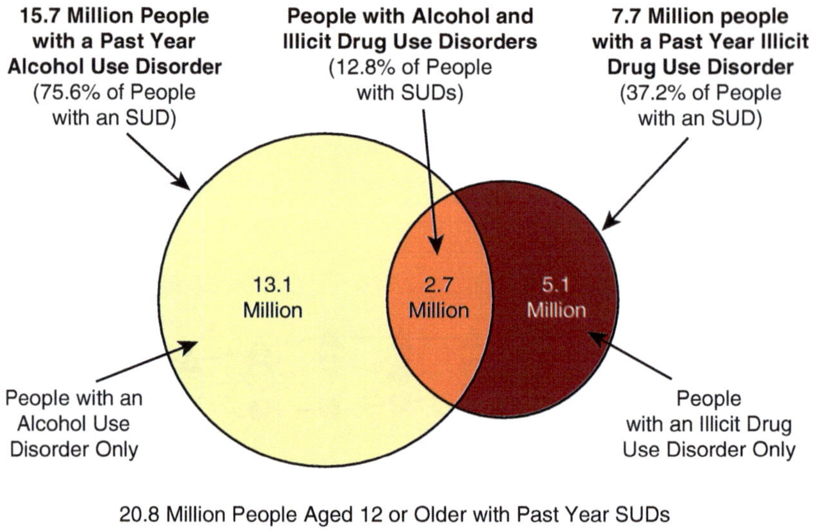

Fig. 1.12 Alcohol-use disorder and illicit-drug-use disorder in the past year among people aged 12 or older, with a past-year substance-use disorder (SUD): United States (2015). (Source: Center for Behavioral Health Statistics and Quality [5])

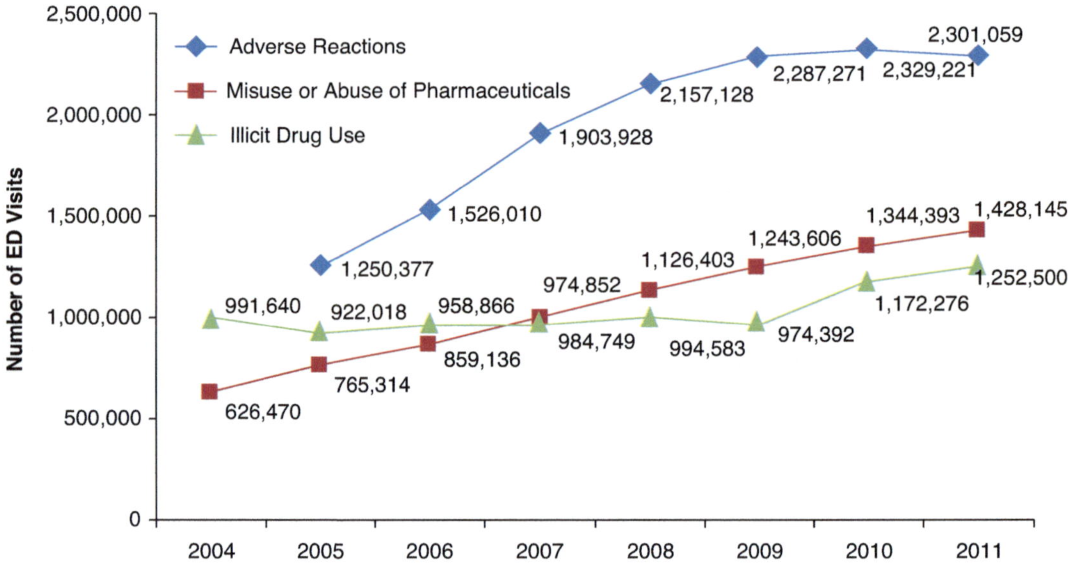

Fig. 1.13 Trends in drug-related emergency department visits by type: United States (2004–2011). (Source: Substance Abuse and Mental Health Services Administration [81])

its by 61%, from 64,117 in 2009 to 102,961 in 2011. Substance abuse and dependence remains a central reason for visiting the ED for many patients in the United States. However, opiate abuse has tremendous regional variation both within and between countries. Opiate abuse, for example, is much less of an ED issue in more socialized systems like New Zealand.

Schizophrenia and Other Psychotic Disorders

Schizophrenia-spectrum diagnoses account for approximately two-thirds of all psychotic disorders. The estimated lifetime prevalence of schizophrenia in the US adult population is 1.1% [14]. Twelve-month healthcare use is estimated at 60%.

Schizophrenia is a serious mental illness with high economic and social costs for families and for society. The overall US 2013 cost of schizophrenia was estimated to be $155.7 billion, of which the largest components were excess costs associated with unemployment (38%), productivity loss due to caregiving (34%), and direct health care costs (24%) [82].

A population-based study of ED mental health visits, using NHAMCS data, found that psychosis-related ED visits accounted for approximately 10% of all mental health ED visits during the decade from 1992 to 2001 [83]. Notably, while overall mental-health-related ED visits increased by more than a third over this time, and rates of ED visits for other major mental health problems (including suicidal behavior, substance-use disorders, mood disorders, and anxiety disorders) all increased, the rate of psychosis-related ED visits per capita did not change. Psychoses-related ED visits formed 0.4% of all ED visits in 2004 and remained at 0.3% in 2014 [84]. This stability may reflect the results of recent substantial investment in early intervention and intensive case management for the seriously mentally ill.

Some patients with schizophrenia may present to EDs in a psychotic crisis that requires immediate management and may not have been diagnosed with psychiatric illness previously. They often present diagnostic dilemmas involving organic versus psychiatric etiology and primary psychotic versus affective disorder diagnosis. Treatment may be complicated further by the presence of alcohol or drug intoxication. Previously diagnosed patients with serious mental illness may also present to the ED with a complication of treatment (e.g., adverse effects of medication) or a psychotic crisis that may arise from gaps in treatment or socioeconomic challenges engendered by serious mental illness (e.g., poverty, homelessness, social isolation, failure of support systems).

Eating Disorders

Both obesity and the fear of obesity are on the rise. The lifetime prevalence of anorexia nervosa is 0.6% of the US adult population; only one-third of anorexia nervosa patients receive treatment [14]. Similarly, the lifetime prevalence of bulimia nervosa is 0.6%; 43.2% receive treatment. The 12-month prevalence is bulimia is 0.3%, and only 15.6% receive treatment over that year.

Binge eating is much more common, with a lifetime prevalence of 28%, of whom 43.6% receive treatment. The 12-month prevalence of binge eating is 1.2% of US adults, of whom 28% receive treatment [85]. As many as 5% of young women exhibit symptoms of anorexia but do not meet full diagnostic criteria, and some studies show disordered eating behavior in 13% of adolescent girls in the United States.

Patients with anorexia nervosa may present to the ED with extreme weight loss, food refusal, dehydration, electrolyte abnormalities, weakness, acute abdominal pain, or shock. They are frequent users of the emergency department; they may often present at the urging of family members or friends and may often deny their disorder and their malnutrition. Major depression and dysthymic disorder have been reported in up to 50% of patients with anorexia nervosa, and these patients have an elevated risk of suicide.

Impulse Control Disorders

An estimated one in four of the US adult population has one of the impulse control disorders (oppositional defiant disorder, conduct disorder, attention-deficit/hyperactivity disorder, or intermittent explosive disorder) [14]. The 12-month estimate is 10.5%. Lifetime estimates are higher for males (28.6%) than females (21.6%). Twelve-month estimates are 11.7% for males and 9.3% for females. These disorders are likely associated with ED presentations for violence and injury, and with high rates of medical usage, but are rarely assessed in the ED setting.

Personality (Axis II) Disorders

Almost one in ten of the adult US population is estimated to have an Axis II personality disorder in any year [14]. People with personality disorders have high rates of comorbid mental disorders, including anxiety disorders, mood disorders, impulse control disorders, and substance abuse or dependence, and may present to the ED with these mental illnesses. Although DSM-IV defines ten categories of personality disorder, population prevalence, and ED visit data are lacking for most classifications, they are available for the most common disorders: borderline personality disorder and antisocial personality disorder.

Borderline personality disorder (BPD) is a personality disorder seen frequently in EDs, and BPD patients are high users of ED services and psychiatric services. The 12-month prevalence of borderline personality disorder is estimated to be 1.6%, of whom 42.4% receive treatment. From 10% to 20% of all psychiatric patients are diagnosed with this disorder, which is approximately three times more common in women than men.

The major feature of BPD patients is that they are emotionally unstable and chaotic. They are often also impulsive and frequently self-harming. They tend to present to the ED in emotional crisis and/or having made a suicide attempt or gesture by overdose or cutting their wrists in response to some emotional stressor. The majority (approximately 75%) of BPD patients attempt suicide or display self-mutilating behaviors like cutting or burning. The risk of suicide is approximately 10%.

Antisocial personality disorder (ASPD) is a condition in which an individual chronically manipulates others and violates their rights, disregarding their feelings without remorse. ASPD is more common in males than females, and ASPD is often comorbid with substance-abuse disorders, depression, anxiety disorders, attention-deficit/hyperactivity disorder, and legal problems. Patients with ASPD may be high users of ED services and may present to the ED with comorbid psychiatric conditions, but also with substance-abuse-, injury-, or violence-related problems. While the 12-month prevalence of ASPD in the general population is only 1%, it is likely to be much higher in the ED population.

Miscellaneous/Occult Mental Health Disorders

The prevalence and ED burden of many less common mental disorders remain unknown. Studies conducted by our laboratory and by others on the prevalence of occult, unmeasured, and often unrecognized mental disorders suggest that large segments of the ED patient population have relatively severe comorbid mental health problems, in addition to other somatic maladies. These relatively undercounted mental health conditions include delirium; dementia and amnestic and other cognitive disorders; somatoform disorders; dissociative disorders; conversion disorders; and factitious disorders. While many of these disorders, such as the somatoform and factitious disorders, are counted among the so-called ER frequent flyers, they are also seen in patients with asthma, diabetes, malignancies, and other nonpsychiatric health conditions. A significant proportion of ED patients with abdominal pain, chest pain, back pain, and headache are not ultimately diagnosed with somatic diseases that account for their typical symptoms. However, taking a better accounting of patients with somatoform and factitious disorders would be a first step toward targeting those who frequently use and sometimes misuse or abuse ED services.

Most mental health patients do not abuse ED services, however, and many ED patients suffer silently from occult and comorbid mental illnesses, resulting in significant diagnostic and treatment delays at the local level, as well as a systematic epidemiologic undercounting of mental-health-related ED visits on the global level. Efforts to screen more aggressively for mental illness would certainly improve psycho-epidemiologic estimates of the prevalence and true magnitude of the mental health problem. Uncovering more comorbid psychopathology may also benefit patients. However, many emergency departments and psychiatric services are currently too oversubscribed and underresourced to adequately manage those currently suffering in silence.

Conclusion

This chapter outlined the psychoepidemiology of mental illness, both in global terms and in terms of the reigning acute care system in most developed countries: emergency departments. Decreased stigmatization, enhanced legitimization, and increased public and clinical recognition of mental illness have led to significant, record-breaking, global increases in the point prevalence, and incidence of mental illness in the general population. These population increases in mental illnesses have, in turn, increased the census of mentally unwell emergency department patients in need of care at the local level.

Paradoxically, psychiatric patient population expansion has developed during a time of ED overcrowding and sharp reductions in both the total number of EDs and psychiatric beds in many communities. In addition, the willingness of mental health providers to make new DSM diagnoses appears to be out of step with either a systemic unwillingness or a provider inability to provide acute psychiatric and crisis care. Gaps in crisis care and the overall lack of affordable, 24/7 access to cost-effective mental health care services have fostered continued and increasing reliance on ED services. Unchecked, the growing tidal wave of mental health patients in need of care can be expected to rise significantly, flooding EDs throughout the world for the foreseeable future.

References

1. Kessler RC, Aguilar-Gaxiola S, Alonso J, et al. The global burden of mental disorders: an update from the WHO World Mental Health (WMH) surveys. Epidemiol Psichiatr Soc. 2009;18:23–33.
2. Vigo D, Thornicroft G, Atun R. Estimating the true global burden of mental illness. Lancet Psychiatry. 2016;3(2):171–8. https://doi.org/10.1016/S2215-0366(15)00505-2.
3. Global Burden of Disease Study Collaborators. Global, regional, and national incidence, prevalence, and years lived with disability for 301 acute and chronic diseases and injuries in 188 countries, 1990–2013: a systematic analysis for the Global Burden of Disease Study 2013. Lancet. 2015;386(9995):743–800. https://doi.org/10.1016/S0140-6736(15)60692-4.
4. GBD 2013 DALYs and HALE Collaborators. Global, regional, and national disability-adjusted life years (DALYs) for 306 diseases and injuries and healthy life expectancy (HALE) for 188 countries, 1990–2013: quantifying the epidemiological transition. Lancet. 2015. Published online Aug. 27. https://doi.org/10.1016/S0140-6736(15)61340-X.
5. Center for Behavioral Health Statistics and Quality. Key substance use and mental health indicators in the United States: results from the 2015 National Survey on Drug Use and Health (HHS Publication No. SMA 16-4984, NSDUH Series H-51). 2016. Accessed on http://www.samhsa.gov/data/.
6. Kessler RC, Angermeyer M, Anthony JC, et al. Lifetime prevalence and age-of-onset distributions of mental disorders in the World Health Organization's World Mental Health Survey Initiative. World Psychiatry. 2007;6:168–76.
7. Demyttenaere K, Bruffaerts R, Posada-Villa J, et al. Prevalence, severity, and unmet need for treatment of mental disorders in the World Health Organization World Mental Health Surveys. JAMA. 2004;291:2581–90.
8. Kessler RC, Berglund P, Demler O, Jin R, Walters EE. Lifetime prevalence and age-of-onset distributions of DSM-IV disorders in the National Comorbidity Survey Replication. Arch Gen Psychiatry. 2005;62:593–602.
9. Morgan C, Lappin J, Heslin M, Donoghue K, Lomas B, Reininghaus U, Onyejiaka A, et al. Reappraising the long-term course and outcome of psychotic disorders: the AESOP-10 study—CORRIGENDUM. Psychol Med. 2014;44(13):2727. https://doi.org/10.1017/s0033291714000890.
10. Qiu C, Kivipelto M, von Strauss E. Epidemiology of Alzheimer's disease: occurrence, determinants, and strategies toward intervention. Dialogues Clin Neurosci. 2009;11(2):111–28.
11. Kessler RC, Ustun TB, editors. The WHO world mental health surveys: global perspectives on the epide-

miology of mental disorders. New York: Cambridge University Press; 2008.
12. Scott KM, Von Korff M, Angermeyer MC, et al. Association of childhood adversities and early-onset mental disorders with adult-onset chronic physical conditions. Arch Gen Psychiatry. 2011;68: 838–44.
13. Ormel J, Von Korff M, Burger H, et al. Mental disorders among persons with heart disease—results from World Mental Health surveys. Gen Hosp Psychiatry. 2007;29:325–34.
14. Kessler RC, Chiu WT, Demler O, Merikangas KR, Walters EE. Prevalence, severity, and comorbidity of 12-month DSM-IV disorders in the National Comorbidity Survey Replication. Arch Gen Psychiatry. 2005;62:617–27.
15. National Center for Health Statistics. Health, United States, 2010: with special feature on death and dying. Hyattsville, MD: National Center for Health Statistics; 2011.
16. Statista. 2017. Total US expenditure for mental health services from 1986 to 2020 (in billion US dollars). Available at https://www.statista.com/statistics/252393/total-us-expenditure-for-mental-health-services/.
17. Greenberg PE, Birnbaum HG. The economic burden of depression in the US: societal and patient perspectives. Expert Opin Pharmacother. 2005;6:369–76.
18. Greenberg PE, Sisitsky T, Kessler RC, et al. The economic burden of anxiety disorders in the 1990s. J Clin Psychiatry. 1999;60:427–35.
19. Greenberg PE, Fournier AA, Sisitsky T, Pike CT, Kessler RC. The economic burden of adults with major depressive disorder in the United States (2005 and 2010). J Clin Psychiatry. 2015;76(2):155–62. https://doi.org/10.4088/JCP.14m09298.
20. Alonso J, Petukhova M, Vilagut G, et al. Days out of role due to common physical and mental conditions: results from the WHO World Mental Health surveys. Mol Psychiatry. 2011;16:1234–46.
21. Evans-Lacko S, Knapp M. Global patterns of workplace productivity for people with depression: absenteeism and presenteeism costs across eight diverse countries. Soc Psychiatry Psychiatr Epidemiol. 2016;51(11):1525–37. https://doi.org/10.1007/s00127-016-1278-4.
22. Ting SA, Sullivan AF, Boudreaux ED, Miller I, Camargo CA. Trends in US emergency department visits for attempted suicide and self-inflicted injury, 1993–2008. Gen Hosp Psychiatry. 2012;34(5):557–65. https://doi.org/10.1016/j.genhosppsych.2012.03.020.
23. Mental Health Atlas 2014. Geneva: World Health Organization; 2014.
24. US Bureau of Labor Statistics. 2017. Occupational employment and wages, May 2016: psychiatrists. Available at https://www.bls.gov/oes/current/oes291066.htm.
25. American Psychological Association, 2012–2015 State Licensing Board Lists; US Census Bureau, 2014 County Cartographic Boundary Shape files.
26. Fields WW, Asplin BR, Larkin GL, et al. The emergency medical treatment and labor act as a federal health care safety net program. Acad Emerg Med. 2001;8:1064–9.
27. Rui P, Kang K. National Hospital Ambulatory Medical Care Survey: 2014 Emergency Department Summary Tables. Available at http://www.cdc.gov/nchs/data/ahcd/nhamcs_emergency/2014_ed_web_tables.pdf
28. American Hospital Association TrendWatch ChartBook 2016.
29. Stussman BJ. National Hospital Ambulatory Medical Care Survey: 1994 emergency department summary. Adv Data. 1996(275):1–20.
30. Larkin GL, Claassen CA, Emond JA, Pelletier AJ, Camargo CA. Trends in U.S. emergency department visits for mental health conditions, 1992 to 2001. Psychiatr Serv. 2005;56:671–7.
31. Regier DA, Narrow WE, Rae DS, et al. The de facto US mental and addictive disorders service system: epidemiologic catchment area prospective 1-year prevalence rates of disorders and services. Arch Gen Psychiatry. 1993;50:85–94.
32. Moore BJ (IBM Watson Health), Stocks C (AHRQ), Owens PL (AHRQ). Trends in emergency department visits, 2006–2014. HCUP Statistical Brief #227. September 2017. Agency for Healthcare Research and Quality, Rockville, MD. Available at http://www.hcup-us.ahrq.gov/reports/statbriefs/sb227-Emergency-Department-Visit-Trends.pdf
33. Pitts SR, Niska RW, Xu J, Burt CW. National Hospital Ambulatory Medical Care Survey: 2006 emergency department summary. National health statistics reports; no 7. Hyattsville, MD: National Center for Health Statistics; 2008.
34. Fayyad J, Sampson NA, Hwang I, Adamowski T, Aguilar-Gaxiola S, Kessler RC. The descriptive epidemiology of DSM-IV adult ADHD in the World Health Organization World Mental Health Surveys. ADHD Atten Defic Hyperact Disord. 2016;9(1):47–65. https://doi.org/10.1007/s12402-016-0208-3.
35. Schriger DL, Gibbons PS, Langone CA, Lee S, Altshuler LL. Enabling the diagnosis of occult psychiatric illness in the emergency department: a randomized, controlled trial of the computerized, self-administered PRIME-MD diagnostic system. Ann Emerg Med. 2001;37:132–40.
36. Kessler RC, Petukhova M, Sampson NA, Zaslavsky AM, Wittchen HU. Twelve-month and lifetime prevalence and lifetime morbid risk of anxiety and mood disorders in the United States. Int J Methods Psychiatr Res. 2012;21(3):169–84. https://doi.org/10.1002/mpr.1359.
37. Wang PS, Lane M, Olfson M, et al. Twelve-month use of mental health services in the United States: results from the National Comorbidity Survey Replication. Arch Gen Psychiatry. 2005;62:629–40.
38. Smith RP, Larkin GL, Southwick SM. Trends in U.S. emergency department visits for anxiety-related mental health conditions, 1992–2001. J Clin Psychiatry. 2008;69:286–94.

39. Alonso J, Lepine JP, ESEMeD/MHEDEA Scientific Committee. Overview of key data from the European study of the epidemiology of mental disorders (Esemed). J Clin Psychiatry. 2007;68(Suppl. 2):3–9.
40. Kessler RC, Wang PS. The descriptive epidemiology of commonly occurring mental disorders in the United States. Annu Rev Public Health. 2008;29:115–29.
41. Kessler RC, Ruscio AM, Shear K, Wittchen HU. Epidemiology of anxiety disorders. Curr Top Behav Neurosci. 2010;2:21–35.
42. Kessler RC, Amminger GP, Aguilar-Gaxiola S, et al. Age of onset of mental disorders: a review of recent literature. Curr Opin Psychiatry. 2007;20:359–64.
43. Katerndahl DA. Chest pain and its importance in patients with panic disorder: an updated literature review. Prim Care Companion J Clin Psychiatry. 2008;10:376–83.
44. Coley KC, Saul MI, Seybert AL. Economic burden of not recognizing panic disorder in the emergency department. J Emerg Med. 2009;36:3–7.
45. Ayelet R, Lauren H, Carmen L, Sergio A-G, Ali A-H, Jordi A, Laura A, et al. Cross-sectional comparison of the epidemiology of DSM-5 generalized anxiety disorder across the globe. JAMA Psychiat. 2017;74(5):465. https://doi.org/10.1001/jamapsychiatry.2017.0056.
46. Back SE, Brady KT. Anxiety disorders with comorbid substance use disorders: diagnostic and treatment considerations. Psychiatr Ann. 2008;38(11):724–9. https://doi.org/10.3928/00485713-20081101-01.
47. Stein DJ, Lim CCW, Roest AM, de Jonge P, Aguilar-Gaxiola S, Al-Hamzawi A, Alonso J, et al. The cross-national epidemiology of social anxiety disorder: data from the world mental health survey initiative. BMC Med. 2017;15(1):143.
48. Kessler RC, Berglund P, Demler O, et al. The epidemiology of major depressive disorder: results from the National Comorbidity Survey Replication (NCS-R). JAMA. 2003;289:3095–105.
49. Depression and other common mental disorders: global health estimates. Geneva: World Health Organization; 2017. Licence: CC BY-NC-SA 3.0 IGO.
50. SAMHSA. Major depression among adults. 2015. Available at https://www.nimh.nih.gov/health/statistics/prevalence/major-depression-among-adults.shtml
51. Lindsley CW. 2012 trends and statistics for prescription medications in the United States: CNS therapeutics continue to hold leading positions. ACS Chem Nerosci. 2013;4(8):1133–5. https://doi.org/10.1021/cn400127u.
52. Olfson M, Marcus SC. National patterns in antidepressant medication treatment. Arch Gen Psychiatry. 2009;66(8):848. https://doi.org/10.1001/archgenpsychiatry.2009.81.
53. Greenberg PE, Stiglin LE, Finkelstein SN, Berndt ER. The economic burden of depression in 1990. J Clin Psychiatry. 1993;54:405–18.
54. Wells KB, Stewart A, Hays RD, et al. The functioning and well-being of depressed patients. Results from the medical outcomes study. JAMA. 1989;262:914–9.
55. Katon W, Sullivan MD. Depression and chronic medical illness. J Clin Psychiatry. 1990;51(Suppl):3–11; discussion 2–4.
56. Harman JS, Scholle SH, Edlund MJ. Emergency department visits for depression in the United States. Psychiatr Serv. 2004;55:937–9.
57. Boudreaux ED, Clark S, Camargo CA Jr. Mood disorder screening among adult emergency department patients: a multicenter study of prevalence, associations and interest in treatment. Gen Hosp Psychiatry. 2008;30:4–13.
58. Kessler RC, Rubinow DR, Holmes C, Abelson JM, Zhao S. The epidemiology of DSM-III-R bipolar I disorder in a general population survey. Psychol Med. 1997;27:1079–89.
59. Jansen K, Ores L, Cardoso T, Lima R, Souza LD, Magalhaes PV, Pinheiro RT, da Silva RA. Prevalence of episodes of mania and hypomania and associated comorbidities among young adults. J Affect Disord. 2011;130(1–2):328–33.
60. Moreno DH, Andrade LH. The lifetime prevalence, health services utilization and risk of suicide of bipolar spectrum subjects, including subthreshold categories in the Sao Paulo ECA study. J Affect Disord. 2005;87(2–3):231–41. https://doi.org/10.1016/j.jad.2005.04.010.
61. Merikangas KR, Akiskal HS, Angst J, Greenberg PE, Hirschfeld RM, Petukhova M, Kessler RC. Lifetime and 12-month prevalence of bipolar spectrum disorder in the National Comorbidity Survey replication. Arch Gen Psychiatry. 2007;64(5):543–52. https://doi.org/10.1001/archpsyc.64.5.543.
62. Merikangas KR, Jin R, He JP, Kessler RC, Lee S, Sampson NA, Zarkov Z, et al. Prevalence and correlates of bipolar spectrum disorder in the world mental health survey initiative. Arch Gen Psychiatry. 2011;68(3):241–51. https://doi.org/10.1001/archgenpsychiatry.2011.12.
63. Lee S, Ng KL, Tsang A. A community survey of the twelve-month prevalence and correlates of bipolar spectrum disorder in Hong Kong. J Affect Disord. 2009;117(1–2):79–86. https://doi.org/10.1016/j.jad.2008.12.003.
64. Zutshi A, Eckert KA, Hawthorne G, Taylor AW, Goldney RD. Changes in the prevalence of bipolar disorders between 1998 and 2008 in an Australian population. Bipolar Disord. 2011;13(2):182–8. https://doi.org/10.1111/j.1399-5618.2011.00907.x.
65. Dell'Aglio JC Jr, Basso LA, de Lima Argimon II, Arteche A. Systematic review of the prevalence of bipolar disorder and bipolar spectrum disorders in population-based studies. Trends Psychiatry Psychother. 2013;35(2):99–105. https://doi.org/10.1590/S2237-60892013000200002.
66. Kessler RC, Akiskal HS, Ames M, et al. Considering the costs of bipolar depression. Behav Healthc. 2007;27:45–7.
67. Jamison KR. Suicide and bipolar disorder. J Clin Psychiatry. 2000;61(Suppl. 9):47–51.

68. Boudreaux ED, Cagande C, Kilgannon JH, Clark S, Camargo CA. Bipolar disorder screening among adult patients in an urban emergency department setting. Prim Care Companion J Clin Psychiatry. 2006;8:348–51.
69. Lewinsohn PM, Klein DN, Seeley JR. Bipolar disorders in a community sample of older adolescents: prevalence, phenomenology, comorbidity, and course. J Am Acad Child Adolesc Psychiatry. 1995;34(4):454–63. https://doi.org/10.1097/00004583-199504000-00012.
70. Pompili M, Gonda X, Serafini G, Innamorati M, Sher L, Amore M, Rihmer Z, Girardi P. Epidemiology of suicide in bipolar disorders: a systematic review of the literature. Bipolar Disord. 2013;15(5):457–90. https://doi.org/10.1111/bdi.12087.
71. Institute of Medicine. Reducing suicide: a national imperative. In: Goldsmith SK, Pellmar TC, Kleinman AM, Bunny WE, editors. Washington, DC: National Academies Press; 2002.
72. Borges G, Nock MK, Haro Abad JM, et al. Twelve-month prevalence of and risk factors for suicide attempts in the World Health Organization World Mental Health Surveys. J Clin Psychiatry. 2010;71:1617–28.
73. Kochanek KD, Murphy SL, Xu JQ, Tejada-Vera B. Deaths: final data for 2014. National vital statistics reports, vol. 65, no 4. Hyattsville, MD: National Center for Health Statistics; 2016.
74. Claassen CA, Larkin GL. Occult suicidality in an emergency department population. Br J Psychiatry. 2005;186:352–3.
75. Larkin GL, Smith RP, Beautrais AL. Trends in US emergency department visits for suicide attempts, 1992–2001. Crisis. 2008;29:73–80.
76. Larkin GL, Beautrais AL. Emergency departments are underutilized sites for suicide prevention. Crisis. 2010;31:1–6.
77. Harris EC, Barraclough B. Suicide as an outcome for mental disorders. Br J Psychiatry. 1997;170:205–28.
78. Larkin GL, Beautrais AL, Gibb SJ, Laing S. The epidemiology of presentations for suicide ideation to the Emergency Department. Acad Emerg Med. 2008;15:S208–9.
79. Beautrais AL. Further suicidal behavior among medically serious suicide attempters. Suicide Life Threat Behav. 2004;34:1–11.
80. Center for Behavioral Health Statistics and Quality. Drug abuse warning network methodology report. 2010 update. Rockville, MD: Substance Abuse and Mental Health Services Administration; 2012.
81. Substance Abuse and Mental Health Services Administration. Drug Abuse Warning Network, 2004–2011.
82. Cloutier M, Aigbogun M, Guerin A, Nitulescu R, Ramanakumar A, Kamat A, DeLucia M, et al. The economic burden of schizophrenia in the United States in 2013. J Clin Psychiatry. 2016;77(6):764–71. https://doi.org/10.4088/jcp.15m10278.
83. Pandya A, Larkin G, Randles R, Beautrais A, Smith RP. Epidemiological trends in psychosis-related Emergency Department visits in the United States, 1992–2001. Schizophr Res. 2009;110:28–32.
84. McCaig LF, Nawar EN. National Hospital Ambulatory Medical Care Survey: 2004 Emergency Department summary: advance data from vital and health statistics, no. 372. Hyattsville, MD: National Center for Health Statistics; 2006.
85. Hudson JI, Hiripi E, Pope HG Jr, Kessler RC. The prevalence and correlates of eating disorders in the National Comorbidity Survey Replication. Biol Psychiatry. 2007;61:348–58.

Part II

Evaluation of the Psychiatric Patient

2 The Medical Screening Process for Psychiatric Patients Presenting Acutely to Emergency Departments

Vaishal Tolia and Michael P. Wilson

Introduction

Mental-health-related visits to emergency departments are common and steadily increasing [1–3]. More than ever, emergency departments (EDs) have become burdened with longer wait times, overcrowding, and complex patient safety issues. Patients with primary psychiatric complaints, numbering approximately 53 million from 1992 to 2001 in the United States, now constitute 12.5% of all adult ED visits [1, 4]. This rise in mental health visits corresponds to a 38% increase [5]. At the same time, there has been an increasing shortage of inpatient psychiatric beds nationally, with a decline in a number of inpatient beds per capita of 62% from 1970 to 2003 [6]. Frequently, there is an inherent challenge or even fear in dealing with these patients and their behavioral symptoms due to discomfort in diagnosing and managing psychiatric conditions, such that the medical aspects of psychiatric care are overshadowed in order to arrange a rapid disposition. Sigmund Freud once famously noted, "When I treat a psychoneurotic, for instance, hysterical patient … I am compelled to find explanations for the first symptoms of the malady, which have long since disappeared, as well as for those existing symptoms which have brought the patient to me; and I find a former problem easier to solve than the more exigent one of today" [7].

Although Freud's words are by now a century old, the search for the medical causes of existing psychiatric problems is still common. This screening, usually performed by emergency physicians, has become known as "medical clearance." The clearance process is enigmatic and, at best, an imperfect science. The discrimination and depth of this screening, such as which patients require extensive workup and which laboratory tests are most useful, is controversial without much high-quality evidence to support various practices [8–10]. Even the goals of screening, such as whether to identify all possible medical causes of psychiatric illness or simply to identify medical conditions that either contribute to or supersede the psychiatric emergency, are often disagreed upon by specialists in psychiatry and emergency medicine.

Furthermore, the term "medical clearance" itself is controversial and often misinterpreted [11]. In general, emergency department screening is not designed to evaluate all possible coexisting illnesses. Thus, some authors have argued

V. Tolia (✉)
Department of Emergency Medicine, Internal Medicine-Division of Hospital Medicine, University of California Health Sciences, San Diego, CA, USA
e-mail: vtolia@ucsd.edu

M. P. Wilson
Department of Emergency Medicine, University of Arkansas for Medical Sciences, Little Rock, AR, USA
e-mail: mpwilso1@outlook.com

L. S. Zun et al. (eds.), *Behavioral Emergencies for Healthcare Providers*,
https://doi.org/10.1007/978-3-030-52520-0_2

that there is no such entity as being completely "medically clear" from the emergency department, preferring instead to use the terms "focused medical assessment" or "medically stable," or simply listing the screening procedures performed in a discharge summary [11–13].

Areas of Consensus

Despite the controversy surrounding this process, both research and expert consensus agree upon important principles of the medical screening process. First, regardless of the details of the screening, the millions of emergency department patients who make a mental-health-related visit deserve at a minimum an adequate history, an adequate physical exam, and a measurement of vital signs. Second, emergency physicians are obligated to discover medical etiologies that may be the cause for new psychiatric symptoms or exacerbate psychiatric conditions. These signs and symptoms—often referred to as "medical mimics" but more appropriately characterized as a delirium state—may be missed by initial evaluators, particularly in the elderly [14]. Third, emergency physicians should seek to identify and treat life-threatening medical conditions that supersede the psychiatric emergency. Even medical urgencies are best identified prior to psychiatric admission, as most psychiatric facilities are neither equipped with the resources nor do they have appropriately trained staff to treat these conditions [15]. Failure to identify these conditions can lead to dangerously bad outcomes for the patient [13]. Fourth, guidelines and protocols may help streamline the medical screening process in the emergency department [16–18].

This chapter serves to introduce and describe the process of medical evaluation, also termed "medical screening," of the psychiatric patient in a typical United States emergency department. The term "screening" is deliberate, as "medically clear" is often too ambiguous. In addition, "medical clearance" implies a detailed history, a thorough physical exam, laboratory testing, and observation beyond the timeframe of a typical ED visit. The diagnosis of medical mimics is discussed first, along with the utility of both the patient history and physical exam and laboratory evaluations. The second half of the chapter discusses the use of standardized screening algorithms, which have been shown in several studies to decrease testing costs for emergency department patients undergoing medical screening. Though there are no uniform guidelines for this process, attention to detail while minimizing resource overutilization, all while providing the best care for the individual patient, will likely yield the best outcome for both the patient and the institution.

Medical Mimics

Ralph Waldo Emerson once said, "Every man is a borrower and a mimic, life is theatrical, and literature a quotation" [19]. Although Emerson was not referring to the medical mimicry of psychiatric conditions, he might as well have been. The evaluation that an emergency physician conducts is an extremely important and albeit limited chance for the patient to be treated for a medical condition that may be causing their symptoms.

The Role of the History and Physical in Recognizing Medical Mimics

Although the often-taught truism is that a thorough history and physical exam (H&P) is the key to making a diagnosis, the ability of the H&P to discover all disease during medical screening is controversial. In part, this is because the important elements of the H&P have not yet been fully quantified [20]. In a 1994 study, for instance, Henneman and colleagues analyzed the standard medical evaluation of 100 consecutive adult emergency department patients with new psychiatric symptoms [21]. Although 63 of these 100 patients were eventually noted to have a medical etiology for their symptoms, the H&P was only significant in 33/63 patients. The authors, therefore, recommended performing additional laboratory evaluations along with the H&P. Unfortunately, neither the quality of the

H&P performed nor the most revealing portions of the H&P for these patients were analyzed.

Other authors have noted that mental status changes (i.e., disorientation) are often associated with medical causes of psychiatric illness. Counterintuitively, mental status changes are sometimes surprisingly difficult to discover on physical exam, and cases of delirium are missed by emergency providers 12.5–75% of the time [14, 22]. As a result, many authors have also advised formal mental status screenings as part of the standard H&P [9]. Although a prospective randomized trial of the additional benefit of mental status screenings over and above a standard H&P has never been performed, the performance of mental status screenings may nonetheless be reasonable in the assessment of psychiatric patients, particularly for patients at higher risk of delirium, such as the elderly. One study by Kaufman and Zun found that a six-item questionnaire had a 72% sensitivity and a 95% specificity in identifying impaired mental status [23]. This test was noted to take only a few minutes and rated useful by the clinicians using it. Expert guidelines, such as those by the American College of Emergency Physicians, also recommend an assessment of mentation as part of medical screening in emergency departments [24]. By definition, symptoms of delirium wax and wane, necessitating frequent patient reevaluation and observation by experienced providers for maximum diagnostic sensitivity.

The Role of Laboratory Testing in Recognizing Medical Mimics

There has been considerable disagreement between emergency physicians and psychiatrists on the necessity for laboratory screening, with conflicting evidence about its utility [25]. In a study by Hall and colleagues, for instance, the authors performed blood work, an ECG, an EEG, and detailed medical and neurologic exams on 100 consecutive patients admitted to an inpatient psychiatric unit [26]. The authors found that 46% of these patients had an unrecognized medical illness that caused or exacerbated their symptoms, with an additional 34% of patients having an unrelated physical illness. After medical treatment, 28 of the 46 patients had rapid clearing of their psychiatric symptoms. The authors concluded that patients should have laboratory evaluations and detailed physical exams. A 1994 study by Henneman and colleagues reached similar conclusions [21]. Finally, Schillerstrom and colleagues noted that patients who were emergently medicated for agitation were more likely to have abnormal laboratory values and suggested that these patients were medically different from unagitated patients [27].

Other authors, however, have found that routine laboratory evaluations are of low yield. In a 1997 study, for instance, Olshaker and colleagues retrospectively investigated 345 patients with psychiatric symptoms [28]. The sensitivity of the history, physical exam, vital signs, and laboratory testing for indicating disease were calculated as 94%, 51%, 17%, and 20%, respectively. The authors concluded that the vast majority of medical problems of psychiatric patients in the emergency department could be identified by routine H&P and vital-sign measurement. In a 2000 study, Korn, Currier, and Henderson retrospectively investigated 212 patients with psychiatric complaints in the emergency department [29]. In this study, patients presenting with psychiatric complaints underwent routine testing, including electrolytes, blood urea nitrogen/creatinine, complete blood count (CBC), urine and blood toxicology screens, chest x-ray, and a pregnancy test. Patients with a psychiatric history, normal physical findings, stable vital signs, and no current medical problems did not have abnormal laboratory findings. The authors concluded that routine laboratory testing was of low yield. Janiak and Atteberry also retrospectively reviewed 502 charts of psychiatric patients who received routine laboratory testing by the psychiatric service and found, with only one exception, no labs ordered routinely would have changed emergency department management [30]. A similar conclusion was reached in a prospective study of 375 patients by Amin and Wang [31].

Nonetheless, routine testing is often required for patients in the emergency department with mental-health complaints. In a 2002 survey of emergency physicians by Broderick and colleagues, for instance, 35% of respondents indicated that they were required by consultants to obtain routine tests [32]. Many respondents believed that at least some of these tests were unnecessary, with urine toxicology screening and serum alcohol testing felt to be more necessary than blood work or an EKG.

Unfortunately, it is difficult to draw firm conclusions from existing studies such as these, since none of the above studies documented the comprehensiveness of their history, physical, or mental status examinations. In addition, none of these studies investigated whether the testing of high-risk groups increases the number of positive laboratory investigations or whether inpatient treatment by the psychiatry service (as opposed to emergency department management and disposition) would have changed as a result of obtaining labs. However, based on evidence of this type, the American College of Emergency Physicians recently stated in a clinical guideline on the evaluation of adult psychiatric patients that routine laboratory testing for asymptomatic, alert, cooperative patients was unnecessary [24]. However, it remains unknown whether the identification of chronic comorbidities, such as diabetes, HIV, or chronic kidney disease, impacts the patient after ED discharge [9].

The Role of Urine Drug Screens in Recognizing Medical Mimics

As with laboratory values, the utility of routine urine drug screens has also been questioned, since many psychoactive substances are not tested for in the "drugs of abuse" urine assays. Some studies, such as those by Schuckman and colleagues, have indicated self-reporting of illicit drug use is unreliable in the emergency department [33]. However, several emergency department studies have indicated that urine drug screens, even when positive, do not often change emergency department management or disposition of psychiatric patients [34–37]. Schiller and colleagues, for instance, prospectively investigated 392 patients presenting to a psychiatric emergency service [34]. The researchers found 20.8% of patients who denied substance use actually had positive screens, but dispositions did not change between patients in whom a routine urine drug screen was ordered and patients in whom it was not. Similar results have been found by both Fortu and colleagues in a retrospective review of 652 charts [35] and Eisen and colleagues in a prospective study of 133 patients [36].

Concerns have also been raised about the accuracy of urine drug screens. In a 2009 study, Bagoien and colleagues compared a commercially available urine drug screen against liquid chromatography/mass spectrometry analysis of the same urine samples [38]. The standard urine drug screen was correct for all five drugs of abuse included on the panel only in 75.2% of cases, with sensitivities of 43–90% depending on the drug of interest.

Based primarily on evidence of this type, the American College of Emergency Physicians stated in a recent clinical policy that routine urine drug testing is unnecessary in the emergency department [24]. However, these types of studies have not investigated whether or not the requirement for urine drug screen testing is influenced by the type of patient, the facility to which the patient is being transferred, or by demand for payment from insurers [37].

Tips to Improve the Accuracy of Medical Screening Exams

Examine Thoroughly, Test Selectively

Despite the conflicting evidence about routine laboratory testing, most experts agree that emergency physicians can improve their diagnostic accuracy both by selective testing of certain patient groups and by increasing their knowledge of medical mimics of psychiatric disease. Obtaining an adequate history is often the first and most important step. Although most astute clinicians rely primarily on the history as the most useful information when formulating a diagnosis and care plan, missing pieces of vital information regarding the history, as well as inadequate physical examinations, are far too common in the evaluation of the psychiatric patient. In a study in 2000, for instance, Reeves et al. found inadequate history, physical exam, and the almost universal failure of obtaining a mental status exam in those patients in whom a medical diagnosis was missed [22]. Inadequate H&P were also cited by Koranyi and Potoczny as the leading contributor to missed diagnoses [39].

Search for Collateral Information

Incomplete history and physicals are not always the fault of the clinician; it is not uncommon for psychiatric patients to be unable to provide a clear detailed history [13]. Both delirium and underlying psychosis can make it difficult for the provider to obtain accurate information, and there may be an additional degree of fear or shame that prevents some patients from being fully forthcoming regarding their symptoms [40]. Obtaining a collateral history from family, friends, other providers, and prehospital personnel is important. In addition, previous or outside medical records should be carefully reviewed. Review of the patient's medication list is also important, as this can be a significant contributor to the patient's symptoms [41, 42].

Stratify Risk with H&P, Including Mental Status Exam

In order to best identify patients with a medical cause for their psychiatric symptoms, it is important to recognize patients at the highest risk of illness. In general, existing studies have noted that patients with a new onset of psychiatric symptoms have a high rate of medical illness [12, 16, 17, 21]. However, it is reasonable to suspect a high rate of medical illness in other groups, as well, such as patients with preexisting comorbid medical conditions, especially immunosuppressive disease and active substance abuse, and those without regular access to health care (i.e., those from lower socioeconomic situations) or the elderly [15]. Given the difficulty of obtaining a history from agitated patients and the numerous causes of agitation, these patients may form an additional high-risk group [43].

Along with obtaining a thorough medical history, a focused yet appropriately detailed physical examination can be informative. The physical exam should always begin with an assessment of vital signs, as these are more likely to be abnormal with an underlying medical cause, but should also include an assessment of general appearance, affect, a mental status examination, and a thorough neurologic examination. The physical examination should also note evidence of encephalitis, thyroid disease, signs of liver disease, seizures, trauma, toxidromes, or withdrawal syndromes, as each can present with psychiatric symptoms [44–47].

Specifically Exclude Delirium and Treat Its Causes

The goal of the mental status exam is to exclude delirium, which is defined as an acute medical condition resulting in a state of confusion or disturbance of consciousness [47, 48]. Delirium, which often presents with a short period of symptom onset and fluctuating mental status, is not a diagnosis in itself. Rather, it is a common symptom of impaired brain functioning. As such, it is often accompanied by disorientation or memory deficit. This is in contrast to patients with dementia, who often have a gradual onset of symptoms without changes in consciousness. A good delirium assessment is important, particularly in senior patients [49].

Delirium has numerous causes, which are listed in Table 2.1 [50, 51]. Several of these conditions require prompt recognition and treatment, and so delirium is regarded as a potential medical emergency. Despite this, emergency physicians often overlook the recognition of delirium. In a 2010 study, Reeves et al. found that elderly patients with delirium are more likely to be admitted to psychiatric units and less likely to complete a medical assessment than patients admitted to the inpatient service [51].

Table 2.1 Medical conditions: delirium

Causes of delirium due to underlying medical conditions
Intoxication with drugs—Many drugs implicated especially anticholinergic agents, anticonvulsants, anti-parkinsonism agents, steroids, cimetidine, opiates, sedative hypnotics. Don't forget alcohol and illicit drugs
Withdrawal syndromes—Alcohol, sedative hypnotics, barbiturates
Metabolic causes
Hypoxia, hypoglycemia, hepatic, renal or pulmonary insufficiency
Endocrinopathies (such as hypothyroidism, hyperthyroidism, hypopituitarism, hypoparathyroidism, or hyperparathyroidism)
Disorders of fluid and electrolyte balance
Rare causes (such as porphyria, carcinoid syndrome)
Infections
Head trauma
Epilepsy—Ictal, interictal, or postictal
Neoplastic disease
Vascular disorders
Cerebrovascular (such as transient ischemic attacks, thrombosis, embolism, migraine)
Cardiovascular (such as myocardial infarction, cardiac failure)

Reproduced from Brown and Boyle [47]. Used with permission from BMJ Publishing Group Ltd

Table 2.2 The brief mental status exam

Questions	Score number of errors × weight
What year is it now?	(0 or 1) × 4
What month is it?	(0 or 1) × 3
Repeat this phrase after me and remember it: "John Brown, 42 Market Street, New York"	
About what time is it? (Correct if within 1 hour)	(0 or 1) × 3
Count backwards from 20 to 1	(0, 1, or 2) × 2
Say the months in reverse	(0, 1, or 2) × 2
Repeat the memory phrase (each underlined portion is 1 point)	(0, 1, 2, 3, 4, or 5) × 2

Final score is the sum of total errors in each box. 0–8 normal; 9–19 mildly impaired; 20–28 severely impaired

Table 2.3 The quick confusion scale

Quick confusion scale	Scoring
What year is it now?	2 points
What month is it?	2 points
Repeat this phrase: "John Brown, 42 Market Street, New York"	
About what time is it?	2 points
Count backwards from 20 to 1	2 points
Say the months in reverse	2 points
Repeat the memory phrase	5 points

Final score is the sum of the total in each box. Impaired is <11

Assume a Medical Cause in the Absence of Previous Psychiatric History

Given the number of potentially life-threatening causes of infection and studies such as those by Henneman and colleagues in which a high percentage of patients with new psychiatric symptoms were found to have medical illness [21], a thorough workup is generally advisable for any patient with first-time onset of psychiatric symptoms [9]. In addition, medical screening should include an assessment for delirium. Both the brief mental status exam and the quick confusion scale (see Tables 2.2 and 2.3) have been shown to be useful in the emergency department setting [23, 52]. Although each asks similar questions, scoring is different for each test. The Brief Mental Status Exam has been shown to have a sensitivity of 72% when compared against emergency physician judgment. The Quick Confusion Scale has been shown to have a sensitivity of 64% for detecting cognitive impairment when compared against the Mini-Mental Status Exam [23]. The 3D CAM is another brief screening tool with a sensitivity in one study of 95% [53].

In summary, there are a number of ways that clinicians can improve their diagnostic accuracy when medically screening patients with psychiatric complaints. All physicians should be aware of the numerous medical causes of psychiatric illness and should seek to exclude these illnesses in their history and physical examination. Laboratory testing should be based on the results of an adequate history and physical exam [54]. *Clinicians should have a low threshold for a broader workup in patients in whom an adequate history and physical cannot be obtained; in patients with no prior psychiatric history; or in patients at higher risk of medical illness*. As part of the physical exam, emergency physicians should obtain both an assessment of mental status and a neurologic examination; validated assessment tools can be useful. Universal routine laboratory testing is not supported, especially in patients with a known psychiatric history, a presentation consistent with that psychiatric history, normal vitals, and a normal history and physical examination [20, 24, 54].

The Utility of Guidelines and Protocols

Given the frequent disagreement between emergency medicine and psychiatry over the scope of the medical workup, many authors have argued for the use of standard protocols that have been agreed upon in advance by all specialties involved. One algorithm was created by Zun and colleagues in their work with the Illinois Mental Health Task Force [16]. This protocol is implemented by asking five binary questions:

1. Does the patient have any new psychiatric condition?
2. Does the patient have any history of active illness needing evaluation?
3. Does the patient have any abnormal vital signs?
4. Does the patient have an abnormal physical exam (unclothed)?
5. Does the patient have any abnormal mental status?

If the answer to all five questions was no, the patient could be safely transferred without further evaluation. Zun and Downey then performed a retrospective chart review of all emergency department patients with psychiatric complaints who were transferred to a psychiatric facility both before and after the adoption of this protocol. The total cost was $269 per patient after the adoption of the protocol but $352 before [16]. The return rate of patients to the emergency department for further evaluation after the protocol, however, was similar.

Another screening algorithm was recently proposed by Shah and colleagues [18]. In this study, the authors retrospectively reviewed the charts of 485 patients who had been screened in the emergency department with a five-item questionnaire (stable vital signs, no prior psychiatric history, alert/oriented × 4, no evidence of acute medical problem, no visual hallucinations). Only six patients (1.2%) with a "yes" to all five questions were transferred back to the emergency department for further medical workup, and none of these patients required medical or surgical admission.

A quick glance at these two screening tools finds them remarkably similar, yet the reported effectiveness differed. Local processes, such as coordination of care, trust between providers, wait times for subsequent psychiatric admission, facility overcrowding, and subgroup demographics, may play a strong role in acceptance and accuracy of the emergency medicine evaluation process. Perhaps for these reasons, a simple medical screening algorithm has not yet been widely accepted. This is unfortunate, as medical protocols have the potential to resolve many conflicts between psychiatric receiving facilities and emergency departments. Agreed-upon protocols also maintain a high standard of care for patients, reduce the cost of testing, and provide a structured format for quality improvement activities and clinical research.

Conclusions

Emergency physicians are commonly expected to evaluate patients presenting with psychiatric symptoms. Medical screening of these patients, to stabilize medical conditions, to facilitate psychiatric evaluation, and to safely transfer them to an appropriate treatment facility, is indicated. Evidence-based limitations of these assessments should be recognized.

1. Emergency physicians should not use the phrase "medical clearance," as this implies that the patient is medically free from all disease. Instead, this phrase should be replaced

by "medical stability" or by a concise discharge note listing the screening procedures performed.

2. Emergency physicians should be aware of the medical mimics of psychiatric disease. All patients with psychiatric complaints should receive an adequate history and physical exam, including both a neurologic exam and an assessment of mental status.
3. Emergency physicians should have a low threshold to obtain laboratory testing on high-risk patients. Commonly encountered high-risk patients in the emergency department include those with a new onset of psychiatric symptoms; those with preexisting comorbid medical conditions (especially immunosuppressive disease); the elderly; patients with active substance abuse; and patients without access to health care (i.e., those from lower socioeconomic situations). Agitated patients may also be an additional underrecognized high-risk group.
4. Psychiatry services should recognize the indications and limits of routine testing. In particular, laboratory testing does not reveal significant disease in young patients with known psychiatric disease who have normal vitals, a normal H&P, and a presentation consistent with their psychiatric illness.
5. Prospectively developed protocols that are collaboratively derived by emergency medicine and psychiatry specialists can decrease the amount of testing while preserving a high level of care.

As the number of visits to emergency departments increases, the number of screenings of psychiatric patients by emergency physicians will also continue to increase. A systematic approach, focused medical assessment, and appropriate laboratory testing guided by the history and physical examination and followed by clear communication between providers will achieve a high quality of care, control costs, and guide improvement activities. Further research may help refine the medical screening process even further, by identifying the most sensitive and specific parts of the history and physical exam, by determining the groups at highest risk for medical disease, and by validating the most efficient medical screening protocols.

References

1. Larkin GL, Claassen CA, Emond JA, Pelletier AJ, Camargo CA. Trends in U.S. emergency department visits for mental health conditions, 1992 to 2001. Psychiatr Serv. 2005;56(6):671–7.
2. Wilson MP, Zeller SL. Introduction: reconsidering psychiatry in the emergency department. J Emerg Med. 2012;43(5):771–2.
3. Vilke GM, Wilson MP. Agitation: what every emergency physician should know. Emerg Med Rep. 2009;30(19):233–44.
4. Owens PL, Mutter R, Stocks C. Mental health and substance abuse-related emergency department visits among adults, 2007: statistical brief #92. Healthcare Cost and Utilization Project (HCUP) Statistical Briefs. Rockville; 2006.
5. Pitts SR, Niska RW, Xu J, Burt CW. National hospital ambulatory medical care survey: 2006 emergency department summary. 2006.
6. President's New Freedom Commission on Mental Health Report of the Subcommittee on Acute Care. Meeting Minutes, March 5, 2003. Available at: http://govinfo.library.unt.edu/mentalhealthcommission/minutes/march03.htm. Accessed 13 Nov 2017.
7. Freud S. The Brill dictionary of religion. Brill Academic Publishers. 2007; ISBN: 978-90-04-15100-0.
8. Anderson EL, Nordstrom K, Wilson MP, Peltzer-Jones JM, Zun L, Ng A, et al. American Association for Emergency Psychiatry Task Force on medical clearance of adults part I: introduction, review and evidence-based guidelines. West J Emerg Med. 2017;18(2):235–42.
9. Wilson MP, Nordstrom K, Anderson EL, Ng AT, Zun LS, Peltzer-Jones JM, et al. American Association for Emergency Psychiatry Task Force on medical clearance of adult psychiatric patients. Part II: controversies over medical assessment, and consensus recommendations. West J Emerg Med. 2017;18(4):640–6.
10. Chennapan K, Mullinax S, Anderson E, Landau MJ, Nordstrom K, Seupaul RA, et al. Medical screening of mental health patients in the emergency department: a systematic review. J Emerg Med. 2018;55(6):799–812.
11. Tintinalli JE, Peacock FW, Wright MA. Emergency medical evaluation of psychiatric patients. Ann Emerg Med. 1994;23(4):859–62.
12. Zun LS. Evidence-based evaluation of psychiatric patients. J Emerg Med. 2005;28(1):35–9.
13. Sood TR, McStay CM. Evaluation of the psychiatric patient. Emerg Med Clin North Am. 2009;27(4):669–83, ix
14. Han JH, Zimmerman EE, Cutler N, Schnelle J, Morandi A, Dittus RS, et al. Delirium in older emer-

gency department patients: recognition, risk factors, and psychomotor subtypes. Acad Emerg Med. 2009;16(3):193–200.
15. Gregory RJ, Nihalani ND, Rodriguez E. Medical screening in the emergency department for psychiatric admissions: a procedural analysis. Gen Hosp Psychiatry. 2004;26(5):405–10.
16. Zun LS, Downey L. Application of a medical clearance protocol. Prim Psychiatry. 2007;14(1):47–51.
17. Downey L, Zun LS, Gonzales SJ. Utilization of emergency department by psychiatric patients. Prim Psychiatry. 2009;16(4):60–4.
18. Shah SJ, Fiorito M, McNamara RM. A screening tool to medically clear psychiatric patients in the emergency department. J Emerg Med. 2012;43(5):871–5.
19. Emerson RW. Society and solitude. Boston: Houghton, Osgood, and Company; 1870.
20. Chennapan K, Mullinax S, Brennan JJ, Vilke GM, Oliveto A, Wilson MP. Screening tools validated in the outpatient setting poorly predict opioid misuse in the emergency department. Submitted. J Emerg Med. 2019;56(6):601–10.
21. Henneman PL, Mendoza R, Lewis RJ. Prospective evaluation of emergency department medical clearance. Ann Emerg Med. 1994;24(4):672–7.
22. Reeves RR, Pendarvis EJ, Kimble R. Unrecognized medical emergencies admitted to psychiatric units. Am J Emerg Med. 2000;18(4):390–3.
23. Kaufman DM, Zun L. A quantifiable, brief mental status examination for emergency patients. J Emerg Med. 1995;13(4):449–56.
24. Lukens TW, Wolf SJ, Edlow JA, Shahabuddin S, Allen MH, Currier GW, et al. Clinical policy: critical issues in the diagnosis and management of the adult psychiatric patient in the emergency department. Ann Emerg Med. 2006;47(1):79–99.
25. Zun LS, Hernandez R, Thompson R, Downey L. Comparison of EPs' and psychiatrists' laboratory assessment of psychiatric patients. Am J Emerg Med. 2004;22(3):175–80.
26. Hall RC, Gardner ER, Popkin MK, Lecann AF, Stickney SK. Unrecognized physical illness prompting psychiatric admission: a prospective study. Am J Psychiatry. 1981;138(5):629–35.
27. Schillerstrom TL, Schillerstrom JE, Taylor SE. Laboratory findings in emergently medicated psychiatry patients. Gen Hosp Psychiatry. 2004;26(5):411–4.
28. Olshaker JS, Browne B, Jerrard DA, Prendergast H, Stair TO. Medical clearance and screening of psychiatric patients in the emergency department. Acad Emerg Med. 1997;4(2):124–8.
29. Korn CS, Currier GW, Henderson SO. "Medical clearance" of psychiatric patients without medical complaints in the Emergency Department. J Emerg Med. 2000;18(2):173–6.
30. Janiak BD, Atteberry S. Medical clearance of the psychiatric patient in the emergency department. J Emerg Med. 2012;43(5):866–70.
31. Amin M, Wang J. Routine laboratory testing to evaluate for medical illness in psychiatric patients in the emergency department is largely unrevealing. West J Emerg Med. 2009;2:97–9.
32. Broderick KB. Emergency physician practices and requirements regarding the medical screening examination of psychiatric patients. Acad Emerg Med. 2002;9(1):88–92.
33. Schuckman H, Hazelett S, Powell C, Steer S. A validation of self-reported substance use with biochemical testing among patients presenting to the emergency department seeking treatment for backache, headache, and toothache. Subst Use Misuse. 2008;43(5):589–95.
34. Schiller MJ, Shumway M, Batki SL. Utility of routine drug screening in a psychiatric emergency setting. Psychiatr Serv. 2000;51(4):474–8.
35. Fortu JM, Kim IK, Cooper A, Condra C, Lorenz DJ, Pierce MC. Psychiatric patients in the pediatric emergency department undergoing routine urine toxicology screens for medical clearance: results and use. Pediatr Emerg Care. 2009;25(6):387–92.
36. Eisen JS, Sivilotti MLA, Boyd KU, Barton DG, Fortier CJ, Collier CP. Screening urine for drugs of abuse in the emergency department: do test results affect physician's patient care decisions? Can J Emerg Med. 2004;6(2):104–11.
37. Wilson MP, Frenkel S, Brennan JJ, Simanjuntak J, Deen J, Vilke GM. Patients with suicidal ideation and evidence of alcohol use are discharged at higher rates from the emergency department. Int J Psychol Psychoanal. 2017;3(2):1–5.
38. Bagoien G, Morken G, Zahlsen K, Aamo T, Spigset O. Evaluation of a urine on-site drugs of abuse screening test in patients admitted to a psychiatric emergency unit. J Clin Psychopharmacol. 2009;29(3):248–54.
39. Koranyi EK, Potoczny WM. Physical illnesses underlying psychiatric symptoms. Psychother Psychosom. 1992;58(3–4):155–60.
40. Kalogerakis MG. Emergency evaluation of adolescents. Hosp Community Psychiatry. 1992;43(6):617–21.
41. Gardner ER, Hall RC. Psychiatric symptoms produced by over-the-counter drugs. Psychosomatics. 1982;23(2):186–90.
42. Blanda MP. Pharmacologic issues in geriatric emergency medicine. Emerg Med Clin North Am. 2006;24(2):449–65, viii
43. Nordstrom K, Zun LS, Wilson MP, Md VS, Ng AT, Bregman B, et al. Medical evaluation and triage of the agitated patient: consensus statement of the American Association for emergency psychiatry project Beta medical evaluation workgroup. West J Emerg Med. 2012;13(1):3–10.
44. Hall RC, Popkin MK, DeVaul R, Hall AK, Gardner ER, Beresford TP. Psychiatric manifestations of Hashimoto's thyroiditis. Psychosomatics. 1982;23(4):337–42.
45. Talbot-Stern JK, Green T, Royle TJ. Psychiatric manifestations of systemic illness. Emerg Med Clin North Am. 2000;18(2):199–209, vii–viii

46. Pitzele HZ, Tolia VM. Twenty per hour: altered mental state due to ethanol abuse and withdrawal. Emerg Med Clin North Am. 2010;28(3):683–705.
47. Brown TM, Boyle MF. ABC of psychological medicine: delirium. BMJ. 2002;325(7365):644–7.
48. Fong TG, Tulebaev SR, Inouye SK. Delirium in elderly adults: diagnosis, prevention and treatment. Nat Rev Neurol. 2009;5(4):210–20.
49. Orimo H. Reviewing the definition of elderly. Nihon Ronen Igakkai Zasshi. 2006;43(1):27–34.
50. Cole MG, Ciampi A, Belzile E, Zhong L. Persistent delirium in older hospital patients: a systematic review of frequency and prognosis. Age Ageing. 2009;38(1):19–26.
51. Reeves RR, Parker JD, Burke RS, Hart RH. Inappropriate psychiatric admission of elderly patients with unrecognized delirium. South Med J. 2010;103(2):111–5.
52. Stair TO, Morrissey J, Jaradeh I, Zhou TX, Goldstein JN. Validation of the quick confusion scale for mental status screening in the emergency department. Intern Emerg Med. 2007;2(2):130–2.
53. Marcantonio ER, Ngo LH, O'Connor M, Jones RN, Crane PK, Metzger ED, et al. 3D-CAM: derivation and validation of a 3-minute diagnostic interview for CAM-defined delirium: a cross-sectional diagnostic test study. Ann Intern Med. 2014;161(8):554–61.
54. American College of Emergency Physicians Clinical Policies Subcommittee on the Adult Psychiatric P, Nazarian DJ, Broder JS, Thiessen MEW, Wilson MP, Zun LS, et al. Clinical policy: critical issues in the diagnosis and management of the adult psychiatric patient in the emergency department. Ann Emerg Med. 2017;69(4):480–98.

3 The Modern Emergency Psychiatry Interview

Jon S. Berlin

Introduction

Varied and complex, the clinical interview is the most important technical procedure in emergency psychiatry. It is also one that benefits only modestly from didactic instruction.

The prospective interviewer is well advised to consider ahead of time what his or her goals for the interview are and what the approach will be. Cognitive rehearsing and anticipatory mastery can be helpful. But interviews take place in real time, with an unpredictable partner, and if they are to be any good, they are semi-structured and semi-improvised, responsive to the unknown other, containing an element of suspense [1], and not perfunctory or formulaic.

Reading on this subject is as useful as it is with other fast-paced, kinetic activities requiring skill, such as downhill skiing or playing a form of music that requires improvisation, which is to say it is helpful up to a point: in getting started, avoiding major mistakes, and gradually achieving proficiency. With these other nonclinical endeavors, however, one has the ability to select the conditions or material depending on the particular skills one wishes to practice, and the level of difficulty, whereas with emergency psychiatry we control neither, and the stakes in terms of professional responsibility are very different. The best teacher is clinical experience combined with direct clinical supervision [2].

Review of Literature

There is a vast literature on the initial psychiatric interview in general practice, including some classics [2–5]. There are also excellent descriptions of the necessary modifications of the standard interview to fit the modern emergency setting, such as brevity and focus [6], stabilization [7], and sensitivity to anxiety in the patient and oneself [8]. There are useful writings on topics particularly relevant to the emergency interview. To name a few: suicidality [9], resistant and difficult patients [10], therapeutics [11, 12], and engaging the underlying real self [9, 13, 14]. As a rule, these authors articulate the need for the practitioner to have goals but emphasize or assume that the first goal is finding out what the patient is like and what he thinks and wants, which usually requires leading off with active listening and an unstructured approach. Yet one must also speak up early on if dangerousness or patient nonengagement demands.

One can also learn from the work of interviewers in other fields, such as Terry Gross, whose naturalness and instinct for candor and authenticity are exemplary [15].

J. S. Berlin (✉)
Department of Psychiatry and Behavioral Medicine,
Department of Emergency Medicine,
Medical College of Wisconsin, Wauwatosa, WI, USA

L. S. Zun et al. (eds.), *Behavioral Emergencies for Healthcare Providers*,
https://doi.org/10.1007/978-3-030-52520-0_3

Ten Interview Goals

Table 3.1 lists goals for the emergency psychiatry interviewer to consider. It is a personal distillation of useful concepts accumulated over time. Experienced practitioners often remember the first case that taught each of them. Repetition of similar cases makes the inclusion of these goals in one's performance second nature, yet one also learns from novel experiences and inevitable mistakes. Experienced readers will have their own ways of thinking about this material and not hesitate to refashion this list to suit their style and purpose.

The discussion in this chapter will touch briefly on each of the ten goals. Other sections of this textbook address one or more of them in greater detail. The reader is referred to the pertinent chapters.

Table 3.1 Ten goals of the emergency interview

1. From the beginning, set the overarching goal of the interview or interviews as eventually turning an acute patient into an outpatient [16].
2. Ensure one's own personal safety.
3. Ensure the person's comfort and safety, both medical and psychiatric. [a]Stabilize before probing; emergency practice is very much an iterative process. Be "trauma-informed."
4. Ascertain what the consumer wants and needs, and find something to agree with.
5. Attempt to engage the individual in a working doctor-patient (practitioner-consumer) relationship. (In disaster work, start with Psychological First Aid and avoid pathologizing extreme but normal, transitory reactions.)
6. Prevent iatrogenic deterioration and make even brief encounters a good experience. Psychiatric conditions are very dynamic and sensitive to here-and-now interactions, power dynamics, and latent cultural influences. Recover from mistakes.
7. Be aware of, tolerate, and put into perspective one's own intense feelings that a patient can engender [17].
8. Gather enough information to determine why the individual is here now and to form one's own opinion about what the real problem is, including the amount of risk for harming self or others. Making a diagnosis is only one part of the assessment.
9. Search for a patient narrative that is coherent and authentic, while appreciating the ever-present tension between resistance and the human need to be understood. This may require having to intuit people's underlying concerns and drawing them out.
10. Triage as service conditions demand but always attempt to begin treatment and to collaborate on disposition. (Remember goal #1: In a well-run psychiatric emergency service with active treatment orientation, as many as 70% of patients can go home in 24 hours or less [18].)

[a]Psychiatric conditions are medical. We use the term "medical" here to refer to "nonpsychiatric medical".

Medical Status

The interview can be a critical first step in determining medical status.

Case Example 1

A 45-year-old man came to a busy psychiatric emergency service (PES) with a friend for moral support. The gentleman reported decreased mood secondary to trouble thinking clearly and remembering things. He was worried and discouraged about early-onset dementia. Vital signs were stable, and history and exam were otherwise unremarkable except for a below-average performance on short-term memory testing. Following a formal mental status exam, the psychiatrist re-reviewed the patient's history and learned of a blow to the head 1 month earlier. He referred the patient to the emergency department (ED), where a head CT scan revealed a large subdural hematoma.

Case Example 2

A 56-year-old African American gentleman with schizophrenia was brought into PES by his case manager for recent onset of decreased interest in things and daytime sleepiness. His vital signs were stable, and he had no known medical problems. UDS was negative. He was affable and cooperative with the interview. Auditory hallucinations were constant but stable. The only out-of-the-ordinary mental status finding was his tendency to look sleepy on and off as they spoke. He reported sleeping well at night and believably denied overdosing or taking his medication, some of which could be sedating, any other way except as prescribed. The psychiatrist referred him to a busy ED for medical evaluation.

An hour later, the ED physician called to send him back, saying the patient had been alert and oriented the whole time, and the medical evaluation was negative. The psychiatrist reiterated the abnormal finding of excessive sleepiness. The EM physician admitted his evaluation had consisted only of a history and physical, and offered to check a few blood tests. He called back a few minutes later. The serum hemoglobin was 4, and stool guaiac was positive. The patient was admitted for a GI bleed.

In both of these cases, the interview was crucial, and the interviewers did not allow the low psychiatric acuity to lull them into a false sense of security. In the second case, the psychiatrist had to trust his own mental status findings and assert his belief that the presenting symptom was likely to be nonpsychiatric in origin. (He had not noticed an ashen-gray tinge to the dark skin, suggesting anemia.)

Challenge of Engagement

The remainder of this chapter takes up two of the greatest clinical challenges facing the interviewer, neither of which is unusual in the emergency setting: (1) a demand for a level of care opposite the one recommended and (2) the individual who refuses to talk. These interviews are fraught from the start, and many practitioners terminate them prematurely.

Our final case example involves both of these contentious elements. The dialogue is nearly a verbatim recreation, with some identifiers altered, and minimal poetic license taken. It highlights how a spontaneous yet purposeful approach can help an interviewer avoid becoming discouraged or derailed and salvage a seemingly hopeless interaction with a very difficult person.

Case Example 3

Mr. E. was a 45-year-old, one-legged man on crutches who called 911 on himself one night and was taken to the ED for an acetaminophen overdose. He admitted to an ingestion of somewhere between 12 and 15 grams. Serial acetaminophen levels decreased and were just below the toxic level on the nomogram. His only other medical problem was chronic pancreatitis that was subacute. He denied suicidality but was intoxicated and irritable, and his old chart was positive for multiple suicide attempts by acetaminophen overdoses in the past, as well as chronic, episodic alcohol abuse.

Mr. E. was medically cleared and slated for acute psychiatric hospitalization, but there were no open beds in the community. He would have gone along with a prompt transfer, but he refused to wait for one and tried to walk out of the ED against medical advice. When the staff blocked his exit, he swung his crutches at them, and they ended up restraining him. Police were called and filed a mental health hold. Mr. E. spent the night strapped to a hospital gurney. He was treated for mild alcohol withdrawal that resolved by midafternoon.

That evening, he was still waiting for a bed when the emergency psychiatrist from the night before was back on duty and showed up to see him. He found Mr. E. leaning back in a wheelchair, a glum look on his face, with a one-to-one sitter.

The following is their 10-minute conversation:

MD	Hello. How are you?
Mr. E.	F___ off.
MD	Remember me? We met last night. How are you?
Mr. E.	[Looks away and closes his eyes.]
MD	Need anything?
Mr. E.	[Silence.]
MD	Anything?
Mr. E.	[Turns and glares.] Man, I said f___ the f___ off!
MD	I'm serious. You okay? How was your night? Didn't have to sleep in that wheelchair, I hope.
Mr. E.	I got nothin' to say to you.

MD Mm-hmm. I heard that from day shift too. You wouldn't talk to them either.

Mr. E. F____n' idiots. Real gems you got working here.

MD What can we do for you?

Mr. E. You can't do sh__.

MD What do you want?

Mr. E. [Silence.]

MD What do you need?

Mr. E. F___ outta my face, m____f____. [Makes a half fist with one hand, but doesn't attempt to get up.]

MD [Backing up slightly] That's what I'm trying to do. I'm trying to get me out of your face, and everyone like me. I take it you still want to go. Fine. Let's start getting you out of here.

Mr. E. Start? Quit dicking around. Please, I ain't got the time.

MD Unfortunately, you have plenty of time—too much, in fact. Sorry about the wait. Plus, you looked bored. I'm trying to make things a little more interesting.

Mr. E. [Looks away.]

MD Look, I'm treating you with respect and trying to be useful. What's wrong with that? I'm trying.

Mr. E. Yeah, very trying.

MD If you're thinking about last night, I'm sorry about that, too, but we can't just let you go and kill yourself.

Mr. E. [Closes his eyes and pretends to sleep.]

MD Please, if I say or do anything you think is wrong or disrespectful, let me know.

Mr. E. [Silence.]

MD [Pause.] Well, we're making progress. You're ticked off and you're expressing yourself without getting physical. The threatening glares could ease up a little, but the nonviolence is good. I can work with that.

Mr. E. [Opens his eyes.] You're pissin' in my ear. Where do you even come up with this sh__? You sound like a f______ textbook.

MD Clear up just one thing for me.

Mr. E. Gimme my crutches back.

MD I'd like to.

Mr. E. [Silence.]

MD One thing I really don't understand.

Mr. E. [Silence.]

MD One thing I really don't understand.

Mr. E. Oh, really? Just one? F____ genius.

MD You said last night you're not suicidal. "Never have been," I think I heard you say. Yet you keep coming in with Tylenol overdoses. I don't get it.

Mr. E. [Silence.]

MD I don't get it.

Mr. E. Not my problem.

MD Might be able to help you better if I did.

Mr. E. Sure.

MD I'm serious.

Mr. E. Nobody believes me.

MD Try me.

Mr. E. You wouldn't understand.

MD Try me.

Mr. E. [Silence.]

MD Come on. Try me. I'm not as dumb as you think [19].

Mr. E. You couldn't be [19].

MD [Laughs.] Look. You don't particularly look suicidal to me, either. I'd like to let you go.

Mr. E. So what's stopping you? Oh, wait. No, that would mean you'd have to make a decision, take a chance. But, nooo, you chickenshit c___ s____r, I'm on a hold. You're looking for a bed. Go. F____' find your f____' bed. Take the easy way out. Man, you're a lazy m____f____. Thought I was lazy. You're lazier than I am. Leave me the f___ alone.

MD Man, you got a temper. Look, I'll make this real simple: I take it you're saying you're not suicidal. Great. You don't look suicidal. You don't act suicidal, at least not right now. You're having a great time putting me down, enjoying life, at least this part of it, and you have skills. Beautiful. You have some self-control, at least when you're sober. All that on one side. But then there's the other side: the Tylenol overdoses. Not just one but several. It doesn't make sense. I'm trying to reconcile these two totally different things. It would be lazy for me not to. We can banter all day if you want to. It's kind of fun. You're good at it. But it won't get you outta here. If that is what you want. Unless maybe you really do like it here and you don't want to leave—is that it? I don't know. So, you tell me, what's the deal? What have you got to lose?

Mr. E. I've told people before, and they didn't believe me.

MD And you're sick of it. Pisses you off. Why take a chance with me, right?

Mr. E. Right.

MD Okay, I get it. [Thinking.] Though, you know, you just told me not to be afraid to take chance. Why don't you take a chance?

Mr. E. F___ you. [Long pause.] Okay, professor. You want it? Here it is. I'll make this real simple: I love to drink. Love. I live to drink, and I drink to live. But I have this f____ chronic pancreatitis that makes my pancreas hurt like crap whenever I drink. So I take Tylenol ahead of time. High doses. Doctors tell me it shouldn't work, but it does. I take high doses, and then I drink, and then I come into hellholes like this to get that Mucus sh__ to save my f____n' liver. That's my sorry-ass life."

MD So that's it?

Mr. E. That's it.

MD Never tried to kill yourself.

Mr. E. Never.

MD You just drink to make life tolerable.

Mr. E. Einstein.

MD Interesting. [Pause.] You care about your liver? Ever consider that alcohol—

Mr. E. Save it. Heard that speech before. Nothing's perfect.

MD Okay. I think I believe you. You can probably go, but I do have to corroborate your story with someone that knows you. Who can I call?

Mr. E. My mother.

MD She'll confirm it?

Mr. E. She'll confirm.

MD All right. Pending that, you can go. Want any counseling or alcohol treatment?

Mr. E. Seriously?

MD Have to ask.

Mr. E. [Shakes his head.]

MD Need anything?

Mr. E. Yeah. I need a tall, cold one. After sitting in this sh__hole all night."

MD Naturally.

Mr. E. Couple four-packs.

MD Forty-ouncers, huh? That's a case. Malt liquor, too, I suppose.

Mr. E. Not as dumb as I thought. And some shots. Half pint. Maybe more.

MD F___, you'll be right back here with another Tylenol overdose! Some gratitude.

Mr. E. So?

MD Come on.

Mr. E. I'll go to another ER.

MD If you're in a mood to return the favor, how about drinking a little less?

Mr. E. No way.

MD You're really pushing your luck. There has to be another way. Plan B.

Mr. E. You could give me some Xanax or some oxy's.

MD Seriously?

Mr. E. Okay, then, Plan A.

MD What's the Xanax for?

Mr. E. Anxiety, of course. Then I wouldn't have to drink as much.

MD Maybe there's a Plan C.

Mr. E. What would that be?

MD I don't know. We should talk about it sometime. Next time you come—

Mr. E. There won't be a next—

MD Yes, there will.

Mr. E. Heh. Just forget it. I'm good.

MD All right. At least let me give you the number for AA.

Mr. E. AA?! Then I really would have to kill myself. Take a f____g header into the Grand Canyon.

MD Okay, then, good luck.

Mr. E. Whatever.

Discussion

The lessons of this interview may be self-evident, but consider how interview goals informed the approach (Table 3.1):

1. *Turn an Acute Patient into an Outpatient*

This goal was partially achieved. It was possible to release Mr. E. back home, and he showed a hint of interest in therapy when he asked what Plan C would be. High utilizers are sometimes just slow to engage in the idea of treatment, and this is what the first inklings of engagement look like. (See #5 below.)

Readers who deal regularly with the frustrations of boarding in the ED will appreciate that, regardless of whether community linkage was achieved, a good 10-minute interview resulted in a reasonable discharge. This is a major accomplishment for any ED. Mr. E.'s desire to get out of the wheelchair is a good sign too.

2. *Ensure Personal Safety*

The doctor took a risk trying so hard to start a conversation, but he did keep his distance, and he did take a step back when Mr. E. started to clench his fist. Mr. E. was not very mobile, and the doctor knew he could push him back down in his chair if he had to. He also knew the sitter could quickly summon help if the situation escalated. He liked the idea of giving back the crutches, but not until he was more certain he would not get hit.

3. *Ensure the Patient's Comfort and Safety; Stabilize Before Probing; Be Trauma-Informed*

The doctor's first question addressed any needs that Mr. E. might have, including physical comfort. The sitter was there to address immediate physical safety from suicide. Emergency practice is an iterative process, and the first round of evaluation and treatment the night before had stabilized Mr. E. to permit the possibility of a more definitive examination the next day. The gently probing interview should not be attempted when an individual is unstable or disinhibited. If a person needs to be on an antipsychotic medication, give that first. Remember the prevalence of trauma. Mr. E. has lost a leg. He probably feels vulnerable.

4. *Find out What the Patient Wants and Needs*

Mr. E. emphatically said he wanted to be left alone. The doctor interpreted this in a broader sense, that Mr. E. wanted freedom from people meddling in his life, and he wanted all authority figures to get away. This became the basis of a goal they could both work toward. "Let me go" is the usual request of involuntary patients, and it is a perfect place to start—with the proviso "as long as it's safe to go." (Note that the focus on what Mr. E. wants invokes an approach at the foundation of both Solution-Focused Brief Therapy and Motivational Interviewing.)

5. *Attempt to Establish a Working Alliance*

A frequent obstacle to real engagement is a disagreement about the level of care. There are patients who want to go but need to stay, and patients who want to stay but need to go. An interview of the type described here can sometimes resolve such impasses. The case at hand is a little atypical in that the doctor initially believed that, with regard to the most appropriate level of care, the doctors were right, but discovered that actually, the patient was probably right.

In trying to establish a rapport, the doctor did not rule out that, along with the desire to be left alone, Mr. E. also had an underlying desire for professional help. The doctor remained determined to engage, especially now that Mr. E. was sober. This was a potential opening. Patients with trust issues only consider trusting a physician or therapist when the person seems trustworthy and can be helpful in some way. It may take more than one conversation. But it can happen.

Here, as the doctor persisted despite the attacks, Mr. E.'s remarks became less caustic and more playful. An unacknowledged early connection occurred when he called out the doctor on sounding stilted like a textbook. The turning point, though, may have been his great zinger,

"You couldn't be." This momentarily gave him the upper hand, and he must have appreciated that the doctor could laugh at himself. The doctor took it as a sign of a good mind at work and a protective factor against imminent suicide. It broke the tension and was a bonding moment. Toward the end, their comments start to mirror each other's, an indication that they are starting to speak the same language.

In future episodes, this doctor can indeed be very useful to Mr. E. by reassuring ED personnel that, despite how it may look, he is probably not suicidal. Long-term, this will earn him points. In fact, following this interview, Mr. E. did tell people, "If you don't believe me, call up Dr. So-and-so and ask him."

6. *Prevent Iatrogenic Deterioration; Recover from Mistakes*

The situation had quickly deteriorated the night before, with Mr. E. ending up in restraints. Sometimes, such events are iatrogenic—for example, when a person on the brink of full-scale agitation is left sitting in the waiting room for a long time without treatment or updates, or when staff self-restraint succumbs to a smart remark. Patients can be very provocative, but still, these are mistakes that we need to learn from.

However, decompensation is also very difficult to avoid when a person is intoxicated and furious at an adverse disposition decision. Depending on how that was presented to him, and depending on the skill of verbal de-escalation, this episode of out-of-control behavior may or may not have been preventable. Nonetheless, later, when people do not have any acute or chronic brain impairment, approaching them respectfully, with appropriate caution but also determination, does tend to mitigate their unraveling.

7. *Be Aware of, Tolerate, and Put into Perspective One's Own Intense Feelings*

Going back for a moment to the very start of this interview, it would have been totally normal for the doctor to feel anger at being verbally assaulted. Considering that Mr. E. was on a mental health hold, it would have been easy to respond coolly and cut it short. Mr. E. is not a nice person, and perhaps he deserves just to sit and wait.

Here, though, the doctor was able to recognize and process his own anger, reminding himself that Mr. E. had been in crisis the night before, possibly to the point of wanting to end his life. Mr. E. also had some valid reasons to be mad. Regardless, there was still more to the story, and responding in kind to Mr. E. would not help to discover it. Perhaps Mr. E. was using anger to avoid dealing with more hopeless and helpless sorts of feelings. Perhaps he had an undisclosed history of present illness, or life history, worth taking into account—not that it excused his nastiness, but it did put it into a different perspective.

The end of the interview again challenged the doctor's equanimity, when Mr. E. announced his intention to go out and drink and, presumably, overdose again. The doctor had the option of changing his mind and waiting for the psychiatric hospital bed after all. He did allow himself an expression of honest exasperation, but ultimately calculated that he should reward Mr. E.'s pivotal self-disclosure with freedom and that pressing forward with involuntary hospitalization at this point would accomplish little except to undo their good work. Giving Mr. E. a break this time also strengthened the doctor's argument should he choose not to give Mr. E. a break the next time. The doctor is building a therapeutic relationship.

8. *Determine Why the Patient Is Here Now and What the Real Problem Is*

The doctor never found out why Mr. E.'s drinking was worse yesterday than another day. It could have been a psychosocial stressor, a worsening of a biological mental illness, a payday that put spending money in his pocket, or just thirst. But he did gain a much better understanding of the acetaminophen ingestion, and the new information revised the risk assessment, aligning it more closely with Mr. E.'s own self-assessment, and changing the disposition.

9. *Search for a Patient Narrative That Is Coherent and Authentic, While Appreciating the Ever-Present Tension Between Resistance and the Need to be Understood*

Mr. E.'s first narrative was neither coherent nor authentic-sounding. This motivated the interviewer to point out how incomplete the story was and use his leverage with the mental health hold to keep at it. He sensed that Mr. E. both needed to be understood and needed to defend himself against it. Asking Mr. E. what he had to lose is known as analyzing the resistance. Mr. E. did not like being poked and prodded. He was also defending against being judged, ridiculed, lectured, disbelieved, and made to take a painful look in the mirror. The doctor's sensitivity eased these fears, and Mr. E. revealed something new about himself that sounded like the truth. His denial of suicidal risk became believable, and the mental status exam became a more reliable part of the risk assessment. The doctor's own realness seems to increase in the course of the interview too.

10. *Triage as Needed, but Always Attempt to Begin Treatment*

Historically, patients like Mr. E. were always triaged and transferred to an inpatient setting. The modern approach is to treat and try for discharge. In Mr. E.'s case, he did not appear to need much more stabilization the day after admission, but he did need a more definitive evaluation to be released, which required a good interview. The doctor also attempted to make the interview therapeutic, in order to lay the foundation for future engagement. Admittedly, 10 minutes feels like an eternity to fast-paced, nonpsychiatric practitioners, but the dialogue presented here demonstrates that these situations can be interesting puzzles to solve and, in their own way, quite satisfying.

Conclusion

The goal of this chapter is to give the reader a new idea or two on what the emergency interview should consist of and generate interest in practicing or teaching emergency psychiatry interview technique. We do see cases where the interview seems wholly unproductive, but one should assume that on some level, it is always appreciated, and it remains a sine qua non of our work. Emergency medicine practitioners are beginning to realize that it belongs in their armamentarium too. It is the key to working more efficiently overall and to helping even the most difficult individuals make the transition to a nonacute level of care.

References

1. Dewey J. Art as experience. New York, NY: Penguin Group; 1934. p. 44–5.
2. MacKinnon RA, Michels R. The psychiatric interview in clinical practice. Philadelphia, PA: W.B. Saunders Co.; 1971. p. ix–x.
3. Gabbard GO. Psychodynamic psychiatry in clinical practice. 4th ed. Washington, DC: American Psychiatric Publishing, Inc.; 2005. p. 69–81.
4. Waldinger RJ. The clinical interview: fundamentals of technique. In: Psychiatry for medical students. 2nd ed. Washington, DC: American Psychiatric Press, Inc.; 1990.
5. Waldinger R, Jacobson AM. The initial psychiatric interview. Available at https://www.brown.edu/Courses/BI_278/Other/Clerkship/Didactics/Readings/THE%20INITIAL%20PSYCHIATRIC%20INTERVIEW.pdf. Accessed on 27 Sept 2017.
6. Riba MB, Ravindranath D. Clinical manual of emergency psychiatry. Washington, DC: American Psychiatric Press, Inc.; 2010, p. 12–5.
7. Petit JR. Handbook of emergency psychiatry. Philadelphia, PA: Lippincott Williams & Wilkins; 2004. p. 1.
8. MacKinnon RA, Michels R, Buckley PJ. The emergency patient. In: The psychiatric interview in clinical practice. 2nd ed. Washington, DC: American Psychiatric Press, Inc.; 2006.
9. Shea SC. The practical art of suicide assessment. Hoboken, NJ: John Wiley & Sons; 2002, 1999.
10. Giovacchini PL, Boyer LB, editors. The technical factors. In: The treatment of the severely disturbed patient. New York, NY: Jason Aronson; 1982.
11. Castelnuovo-Tedesco P. The twenty-minute hour. Washington, DC: American Psychiatric Press, Inc.; 1965.
12. Dewan MJ, Steenbarger BN, Greenberg RP. The art and science of brief psychotherapies: an illustrated guide. 2nd ed. Arlington, VA: American Psychiatric Press, Inc.; 2012.
13. Berlin JS, Gudeman J. Interviewing for acuity and the acute precipitant. In: Glick RL, Berlin JS, Fishkind AB, Zeller SL, editors. Emergency psychiatry: principles & practice. Philadelphia, PA: Lippincott Williams & Wilkins; 2008.

14. Berlin JS. Advanced interviewing techniques for psychiatric patients in the emergency department. In: Zun LS, Chepenik LG, Mallory MNS, editors. Behavioral emergencies for the emergency physician. 1st ed. New York, NY: Cambridge University Press; 2013.
15. Burton S. Terry gross and the art of opening up. NY Times. 21 Oct 2015.
16. Sederer LI. This goal is adapted from Sederer's overarching goal for inpatient psychiatry. In: Inpatient psychiatry: diagnosis and treatment. 3rd Sub ed. Lippincott Williams & Wilkins; 1991.
17. Semrad EV. This goal is adapted from Semrad's triad of goals for the person in psychotherapy. In: Buskirk DV, editor. Teaching psychotherapy of psychotic patients. New York, NY: Grune & Stratton; 1969.
18. Zeller S, Calma N, Stone A. Effects of a dedicated regional psychiatric emergency service on boarding of psychiatric patients in area emergency departments. West J Emerg Med. 2014;15(1):1–6.
19. These two lines of dialogue courtesy of Bob and Ronna Berlin, personal conversation. 2012.

General Management of the Poisoned Patient

4

Bryan Corbett

Introduction

Accidental death was the fourth leading cause of mortality in the United States in 2014. Within causes of accidental deaths, unintentional poisoning has been at the top since 2011 [1]. This does not include deaths from intentional self-poisoning and thus underestimates the total number of deaths related to poisoning. This information underscores the importance of developing adequate treatment strategies for the poisoned patient.

A systematic approach to the management of various medical situations is now commonplace. One such example is that of Advanced Trauma Life Support (ATLS). Studies of ATLS have shown an improvement in knowledge, clinical skills, and decision-making among participants compared to non-ATLS trained individuals [2]. While reviews on the benefit of ATLS on mortality are mixed, we believe that an organized approach to the management of various medical conditions is, nonetheless, of great benefit [2]. Such a systematic approach can readily be applied to the poisoned patient. Like other systematic approaches, management of the poisoned patient can be guided by the ABCs: airway, breathing, and circulation. Toxicologists frequently include D and E in this mnemonic, which stands for decontamination and elimination, respectively. This chapter will cover the initial management of the suspected poisoned patient, followed by workup and diagnosis, and finally, definitive treatment and antidote administration where appropriate.

B. Corbett (✉)
Department of Emergency Medicine, Division of Medical Toxicology, University of California Health Sciences, San Diego, CA, USA

Initial Management of the Poisoned Patient: The ABCs

As mentioned above, a conventional mantra in the initial management of acutely ill patients is the ABCs. This means assessing and intervening where necessary to stabilize the airway, breathing, and circulation. Not only is the assessment of the ABCs critical in the initial stabilization of patients, but it can also provide clues as to the specific poison involved. Intravenous access (IV), supplemental oxygen, cardiac monitoring, and blood sugar assessment are often piggybacked onto the ABCs, making the full mantra ABCs, IV, O2, monitor, and "fingerstick" to measure the blood glucose. These interventions will be mentioned peripherally in the discussion of the ABCs below, but their importance in assessment and stabilization of the patient cannot be overstated.

L. S. Zun et al. (eds.), *Behavioral Emergencies for Healthcare Providers*,
https://doi.org/10.1007/978-3-030-52520-0_4

Initially, the airway should be assessed for patency. Local trauma and thermal or caustic injury may lead to edema and loss of the airway. Cholinergic toxicity, as occurs with organophosphate poisoning, causes significant oropharyngeal secretions which may compromise the airway. Patients with severe central nervous system (CNS) depression may be unable to maintain their airway, and a decreased or absent gag reflex increases the risk for aspiration. Jaw thrust, suction, and nasopharyngeal and oropharyngeal airways can be used to improve airway patency temporarily. These interventions may not be possible in the setting of trauma, do not address lower airway edema from thermal or caustic injury, and do not protect against aspiration. In these settings, the establishment of a secure airway (i.e., intubation) should be considered and performed as the clinical context dictates.

Once a stable airway has been identified or secured, attention should be moved to the patient's breathing. First, is the patient breathing at all? If not, this necessitates immediate intervention, at least initially, with bag valve mask (BVM) ventilation if not already addressed during the assessment of the airway. If the patient is breathing, is he or she hypoxic and in need of supplemental oxygen? Does the hypoxia improve with supplemental oxygen? A persistently low oxygen saturation despite intervention might be a clue that the patient is suffering from methemoglobinemia. In addition to the above, assessment of the quality of breathing is essential as well. Is the patient's breathing fast or slow, deep or shallow? Slow and shallow respirations may be a clue that the patient has ingested an opioid or other sedative-hypnotic drug. Rapid breathing may be compensatory in the setting of metabolic acidosis or the result of direct respiratory stimulation in the brainstem, as occurs with salicylates. Real-time end-tidal carbon dioxide monitoring is particularly helpful in determining the adequacy of rate and depth of breathing and thus, ventilation.

Finally, circulation should be assessed. Of note, some now advocate for the assessment of circulation before airway or breathing (a CAB approach). Regardless of the order, the following holds true. Assessment of a pulse is the priority, as its absence necessitates chest compressions and initiation of cardiopulmonary resuscitation. If a pulse is present, a blood pressure reading should be obtained and hypotension addressed (usually initially with IV fluids). The patient should also be placed on a cardiac monitor, as this will aid in the assessment of rate and rhythm. Significant rate disturbances (bradycardia and tachycardia) can be a cause of hypotension and should be addressed. Also, these rate disturbances can give clues as to the etiology of the poisoning, such as with opioids and other sedative-hypnotics causing bradycardia, and sympathomimetics and anti-muscarinic drugs causing tachycardia. Rhythm is also essential, as it can give clues to the etiology of rate disturbances (examples being heart block in bradycardia or atrial fibrillation with a rapid ventricular response in tachycardia). Any significant rate or rhythm disturbances should be addressed as per advanced cardiovascular life support (ACLS) guidelines.

Diagnosis and Workup

After the initial stabilization of the patient, the focus should be turned to workup and diagnosis. As with much of medicine, a thorough history and physical exam are essential for accurate diagnosis. Unfortunately, the specific substance ingested is often unknown, or the patient may be unwilling or unable to give history. In these cases, assessment for the presence of a toxidrome may help at least identify an etiologic class of drug or toxin. A toxidrome is a specific grouping of signs and symptoms that indicate a type of or a particular poison [3–7]. Please see Table 4.1 for a list of particular toxidromes and their findings. Not all signs or symptoms delineated in the table are necessarily present at any one time. This is particularly true when the patient has ingested multiple drugs or toxins, which may make it difficult to identify a particular toxidrome.

Laboratory testing, imaging, and other ancillary testing are also helpful in the management and diagnosis of the poisoned patient. A complete metabolic panel (CMP) is useful in assessing electrolytes, the presence of an acidosis (gap or otherwise), kidney function, and transaminase levels. Many toxins cause acidosis, and arterial

Table 4.1 Toxidromes

Toxidrome (associated drug class)	Signs and Symptoms
Anti-muscarinic (antihistamines, tricyclic antidepressants, atropine)	Tachycardia, dry mucous membranes, decreased sweating, delirium, mydriasis, hyperthermia, urinary retention, decreased bowel sounds
Cholinergic (organophosphate insecticides, nerve agents)	Miosis, bronchorrhea, bronchospasm, urination, defecation, diaphoresis, emesis, lacrimation, bradycardia (theoretically, in practice often tachycardic)
Opioid	Miosis, sedation, bradypnea, decreased bowel sounds, bradycardia/hypotension/ hypothermia (severe)
Sedative-hypnotic	Sedation, bradypnea, bradycardia/hypotension/ hypothermia (severe)
Sympathomimetic	Mydriasis, agitation, tachycardia, hypertension, diaphoresis, hyperthermia

References: [5–8]

blood gas (ABG) or venous blood gas (VBG) can quantitate this derangement. An ABG or VBG can also identify the primary acid/base disorder, as well as the presence of mixed disorders. A lactate level should be considered, as many toxins cause lactic acidosis. Other toxins may cause renal injury (ethylene glycol, NSAIDs, methotrexate) or are primarily renally excreted (digoxin, lithium), and reduced kidney function may alter management. Electrolyte derangements may be a direct result of a toxin (hypokalemia and theophylline) or secondary to vomiting and diarrhea, caused by a toxin (iron and lithium). Finally, elevated transaminases may be a clue to a late-presenting acetaminophen overdose or represent toxicity from any number of other hepatotoxins. While likely not as critical as a CMP, a complete blood count (CBC) can provide useful information. Hemoglobin is helpful in caustic or iron ingestions, which can cause gastrointestinal hemorrhage and blood loss. In some cases, leukocytosis or leukopenia may be encountered and give clues to the etiologic agent, such as with iron and colchicine, respectively (although colchicine may cause an early leukocytosis). The importance of a blood glucose level has been discussed and will not be examined further. Obtaining a measured osmolality and comparing this to the calculated value for an osmolality gap may indicate a toxic alcohol exposure [3, 4, 6, 8]. There are many ways to calculate an osmolality gap, as well as many pitfalls, and the reader should have experience with this laboratory analysis or seek guidance from a medical toxicologist or poison center. Many poisonings result in rhabdomyolysis, and a creatine phosphokinase should be obtained in these cases [9]. Urine drug screens (UDS) are often ordered in the workup of suspected poisoned patients. UDS should be interpreted with caution for the following reasons. Positive results are often based on drug metabolites, which may remain after clinical effects of the drug have subsided, and thus a positive UDS does not necessarily indicate intoxication; also, the UDS is plagued by many false positives and negatives, and the findings infrequently change management [3, 4, 6, 8].

Some specific drug and other laboratory levels can be obtained in real time to aid in diagnosis and management. Examples include acetaminophen, salicylates, iron, lithium, theophylline, carboxyhemoglobin, methemoglobin, valproic acid, digoxin, and phenobarbital [5, 10]. This is not a comprehensive list. These should not be sent on every undifferentiated patient but should be ordered based on the patient's medication list, history of ingestion, or within the clinical context of the toxidrome or physical exam findings. One possible exception to this rule is acetaminophen levels. Data show a small number of potentially toxic acetaminophen ingestions are found with a routine screening of patients presenting with intentional ingestions [11–13]. Initial acetaminophen poisoning may be asymptomatic or only present with nonspecific findings, making clinical diagnosis difficult, if not impossible. Also, N-acetylcysteine is a highly effective antidote, but its efficacy decreases if the administration is greater than 8 hours out from ingestion [5]. For these reasons, some advocate universal testing of acetaminophen concentrations in all intentional ingestions. The small number of significant ingestions found, however, leads others to argue against routine screening.

Radiographic imaging, although less frequently than laboratory evaluation, can be useful in the poisoned patient as well. A chest X-ray can identify aspiration pneumonitis, a common complication of poisoning [4, 5, 9]. Certain substances (iron, halogenated hydrocarbons, lead, mercury, salicylates) are radiopaque and can be identified on routine abdominal radiographs to help confirm or quantitate exposure [4, 5]. Computed tomography (CT) of the head is helpful in undifferentiated patients with alterations in mental status.

Many toxins cause bradycardia, tachycardia, and various dysrhythmias, as well as changes in intervals such as the QTc, QRS, and variable degrees of heart block [3, 5, 6]. An electrocardiogram is invaluable in identifying life-threatening cardiovascular effects, as well as aiding diagnosis of certain classes of drugs such as beta-blockers, calcium channel blockers, sodium channel blockers, cardiac glycosides, and other cardioactive drugs.

Decontamination

Decontamination is a core tenant of toxicology. The primary route of most toxic exposures is via ingestion [14]. Consequently, techniques for GI decontamination are discussed below. Dermal and ocular exposures do occur, and remediation is still crucial in these cases. Generally, irrigation of skin with saline or slightly soapy water (if the substance is hydrophobic) is adequate. Dry or powdered substances should be brushed off the patient, as dissolution in water may cause burns if the substance is caustic. Ocular exposures should be aggressively irrigated with saline until pH is within the normal range or symptoms improve/resolve.

Activated Charcoal

Activated charcoal (AC) is formed by the burning of variable plant matter to form charcoal. This charcoal is subsequently processed to increase its surface area, forming "activated" charcoal [15]. It is by far the most commonly used method for decontamination of those discussed below [14]. AC is known to adsorb many compounds and decrease the percent systemically absorbed in a time-dependent fashion [16]. It is not recommended for use with ingestion of metals, ions, toxic alcohols, or corrosives secondary to poor binding or increased risk of aspiration [3, 9, 17].

Of the randomized trials comparing AC versus none, which examined clinically meaningful endpoints, none demonstrated a benefit [18, 19]. In one study by Merigian et al. among a subgroup analysis of self-poisoned patients who were ultimately discharged from the emergency department, those who received AC had a shorter length of stay (about 3 hours) versus those who did not [20]. There was no statistically significant difference between AC versus none among all admitted patients, however [20]. Numerous other studies and reports of AC use in poisoning exist. These have been well reviewed by Chyka et al. and will not be discussed here.

There are many potential reasons (small sample size, exclusion of significantly ill patients, the inclusion of patients with delayed presentation) why these studies did not show any benefit for AC. Despite this, AC is still recommended, owing to its ability to reduce absorption, its relative safety, and theoretical benefit. AC is recommended when potentially toxic substances have been ingested within the last hour [15]. Some substances may have delayed absorption in overdose (salicylates or anti-muscarinic compounds). These and sustained- or extended-release preparations of drugs may benefit from more delayed administration of AC [21]. Optimal dosing is dependent on the specific substance, but adults are typically administered 50–100 g of AC. Classically, the major concern with the administration of AC is aspiration leading to a pneumonitis. As such, AC is contraindicated in those without an intact airway (seizing or patients with CNS depression) or who are expected to vomit from their specific ingestion. Forced administration to an awake but noncompliant patient is likely to have an unfavorable risk/benefit ratio. Patients with gastrointestinal perforation or hemorrhage should also not receive AC [15].

Whole-Bowel Irrigation (WBI)

Administration of large amounts of polyethylene glycol electrolyte solution (PEG-ES) can be used to clear the gastrointestinal (GI) tract of ingested substances. This clearance ultimately can reduce drug absorption and at least theoretically be of benefit in the poisoned patient [22]. PEG-ES is used, as it does not cause clinically significant fluid or electrolyte shifts [23]. A single study has shown the benefit of WBI on clinically relevant endpoints. Patients receiving WBI had a decreased odds ratio (OR) for developing seizures (all from venlafaxine overdose) versus those without any decontamination, although the OR did cross one. WBI and AC combined were superior to either alone, also suggesting a benefit to WBI [24]. Multiple, randomized volunteer studies have been performed, looking at pharmacokinetic data. Interpretation of this data is difficult. Some studies showed statistically significant decreased absorption [25–27], whereas others did not [28, 29], and another did not compare WBI to a control [21]. Another study of WBI in venlafaxine overdose showed a benefit of AC and WBI compared to AC alone. WBI used alone did not result in a reduction of absorbed dose, however [30]. Multiple case reports of WBI with PEG-ES have been published; many of these are reviewed in a position statement on WBI by the American Academy of Clinical Toxicology and European Association of Poison Centres. Conclusions are difficult to draw, owing to the nature of case reports. The reader is referred to the position statement for a synopsis of these reports and their citations [22].

Indications for WBI include ingestions of sustained-release preparations, large ingestions of substances not adsorbed to charcoal, iron, and for body stuffers/packers [22].

In adults, the goal is to administer 1–2 liters of PEG-ES an hour until the patient passes clear rectal effluent. In children, 500–1000 milliliters an hour is recommended [22]. In compliant patients, this may be from typical oral ingestion (although the total amount ingested is often below the goal) or via a nasogastric (NG) tube in intubated patients. An NG tube can undoubtedly be forcefully inserted into a noncompliant patient for WBI. However, the risk–benefit ratio may not be in favor of this and should be assessed on a case-by-case basis within the clinical context. Contraindications include bowel obstruction/perforation/hemorrhage, ileus, or an unprotected airway [22].

Gastric Lavage and Syrup of Ipecac

Neither gastric lavage nor induced emesis with syrup of ipecac is routinely recommended, and they will not be reviewed further here [31, 32].

Elimination

Even after a substance has been absorbed into the systemic circulation, techniques exist to increase its rate of elimination, depending on the specific agent involved. Increasing the rate of elimination of toxic compounds can reduce the time of exposure and total body burden of a toxic substance. Whether to institute enhanced elimination techniques depends on the inherent toxicity of the specific drug or chemical involved, dose ingested (or however otherwise exposed), existence and efficacy of specific antidotes, and endogenous methods of elimination and their integrity. Common methods to increase elimination are discussed below.

Extracorporeal Elimination

Multiple methods for the extracorporeal elimination of foreign and endogenous substances exist. These include but are not limited to intermittent hemodialysis (HD), hemoperfusion (HP), and various methods of continuous renal replacement therapy (CRRT). Hemodialysis is by far the most frequently employed technique [14, 33]. Other techniques include exchange transfusion, liver dialysis, and plasmapheresis, but these are rare and will not be reviewed here [14, 34]. In general, substances that are amenable to extracorporeal removal are of small size, have low protein binding, and a small volume of distribution (V_d) [34–36]. In HD, solutes are eliminated through a semipermeable membrane from the blood. These membranes have certain size pores through which the solute must be eliminated. This limits which solutes, or toxins, can be effectively removed in this manner [34]. The specifics of the size have changed as technology advances [33, 37]. The pore size of filters used in CRRT is larger than in HD, and to some extent, larger molecules may be removed via this methodology [34, 35, 38]. Another benefit is its use in hemodynamically unstable patients. These benefits are tempered by its slower clearance of drugs [35]. In HP, blood is forced through a column (charcoal or resin), which adsorbs drugs and toxins. This technique allows for the elimination of larger compounds, as well, but is limited by availability and an increased rate of complications [34, 35, 39, 40]. In addition, as alluded to above, advancements in HD have negated some of the benefits of HP versus HD [33, 37].

Protein-bound substances are often too large for effective extracorporeal removal [37]. In some cases (Valproic acid), protein binding becomes saturated at high doses and the amount of free drug becomes large enough to make extracorporeal removal beneficial [34].

The V_d describes the relative partitioning of various compounds into water and fat. As the vasculature (a major water compartment) is the location of extracorporeal removal, substances that distribute more to the water compartment are more amenable to extracorporeal removal [37]. Compounds with a V_d less than 1 liter per kilogram are considered amenable to extracorporeal removal [35]. Substances with a higher V_d have greater distribution into fat and are not available for extracorporeal removal.

Other pros and cons of these methods exist but will not be reviewed here. The decision of when and which technique to use should be made in conjunction with a nephrologist.

Examples of more commonly dialyzed substances include lithium, metformin, salicylates, toxic alcohols, and valproic acid [33, 35]. This is not a comprehensive list. Determination of the utility of extracorporeal techniques for other specific substances should be made with the aid of toxicologists, the local poison center, and nephrologists.

Multidose Activated Charcoal

Rather than limiting absorption, as with single-dose activated charcoal (SDAC), multidose activated charcoal (MDAC) is used to increase the elimination of certain substances. It entails the administration of at least two doses of AC (in practice, often many more). A study by Mckinnon et al. helps to explain how MDAC works. Mckinnon et al. showed that AC could increase the clearance and decrease the half-life of intravenously (IV) administered theophylline. As the theophylline was given IV, there is obviously no drug in the GI tract for the AC to bind. As theophylline has some biliary excretion, there is the possibility that AC may bind some theophylline excreted in the bile, preventing its reabsorption and accounting for the above findings. Mckinnon addressed this in his study via biliary drainage (in human and animal subjects), which interrupted the enterohepatic recirculation of theophylline. Thus, any increase in theophylline clearance would be from some other route. Mckinnon found only very small amounts of the administered dose of theophylline (less than 2%) in the bile. This is too small of an amount to explain the increased clearance and decreased half-life of theophylline with AC. Rather, the thought is that the AC interrupts what is called the enteroenteric recirculation of drugs. In the same study, McKinnon demonstrated that theophylline given IV resulted in the presence of theophylline in jejunal aspirate. The thought is that drugs will diffuse down their concentration gradient out of the circulation into the GI tract. In the presence of AC, this diffused drug is bound, preventing later reabsorption but also maintaining a favorable gradient for continued diffusion of a toxin into the GI tract for more binding to AC [41]. Other studies have shown similar results [42, 43].

Unlike with SDAC, there are some randomized studies showing benefit in clinically meaningful endpoints in patients treated with MDAC versus not. One study by Brahmi et al. found a statistically significant decrease, with respect to MDAC vs. SDAC, in length of coma, mechanical ventilation, and stay for patients presenting with carbamazepine poisoning [44]. Another study analyzed the benefit of MDAC in yellow oleander poisoning. The control population received sterile water, rather than MDAC, and both groups received SDAC and gastric lavage. Statistically significant decreases in mortality, intensive-care-unit admissions, need for digoxin-specific antibodies, cardiac pacing, presence of life-threatening arrhythmias, and mean dose of atropine given were found [35]. In contrast, a study by Eddleston et al. found no benefit to MDAC vs. SDAC vs. no decontamination with respect to mortality [19].

Current guidelines recommend the use of MDAC for life-threatening ingestions of carbamazepine, dapsone, phenobarbital, quinine, and theophylline. These recommendations were based on the review of multiple animal, volunteer, and case reports/series. MDAC can increase the clearance of digoxin, but given its large V_d and other effective treatment modalities (mainly digoxin-specific antibodies), it is not currently recommended [45]. Contraindications are the same as those for SDAC.

Urinary Alkalinization

Urinary alkalinization is the administration of IV sodium bicarbonate to alkalinize the urine and thereby increase the excretion of certain substances. An alkaline, or high pH, environment will favor the charged form of acidic substances. This charged state reduces passive reabsorption through the hydrophobic cell membrane of kidney tubule endothelial cells. This is sometimes referred to as ion trapping. The substance in question must have some significant renal elimination for this treatment to work. Increasing renal elimination for a drug with minimal-to-small renal elimination is unlikely to offer any clinical or even theoretical benefit.

Urinary alkalinization has been examined with respect to various compounds, as reviewed by Proudfoot et al. [10]. Of these compounds, the more commonly encountered include phenobarbital, methotrexate, and salicylates. Current guidelines recommend the use of urinary alkalinization as first-line therapy for salicylate toxicity in those not meeting indications for extracorporeal elimination. Although urinary alkalinization does significantly increase the elimination of phenobarbital, it is not recommended as first-line due to the superior effectiveness of MDAC [10, 46]. Similarly, urinary alkalinization has been shown to increase the clearance of methotrexate, but these studies were case reports, series, or had no controls, making it difficult to draw concrete conclusions [47–51]. As such, urinary alkalinization cannot be recommended as first-line treatment for methotrexate poisoning [10].

Definitive Management

Supportive care, much of which will have been addressed in the initial stabilization of the ABCs, is often adequate to support patients through their poisoning. Certain drugs and toxins, however, have specific antidotes which should be administered with the guidance of a medical toxicologist or local poison center. Please see Table 4.2 for a

Table 4.2 Antidotes

Toxin	Antidote
Acetaminophen	N-acetylcysteine
Anti-muscarinic compounds	Physostigmine
Benzodiazepines	Flumazenil
Beta blockers	Glucagon
Cardiac glycosides	Digoxin Specific Antibodies
Cyanide	Hydroxocobalamin
Isoniazid	Pyridoxine
Methemoglobinemia	Methylene blue
Opioids	Naloxone
Organophosphates	Atropine, pralidoxime
Sulfonylureas	Octreotide
Toxic alcohols (ethylene glycol, methanol, propylene glycol)	Fomepizole

References: [5, 6, 9]

list of the more commonly used antidotes. Some patients may be assessed, treated, and ultimately cleared from a medical perspective, but it is important to involve psychiatry in the care of patients presenting with intentional ingestions or exposures.

Conclusion

- Poisoning is a significant cause of mortality in the United States.
- Initial stabilization focuses on the ABCs.
- Toxidromes can help identify an etiologic poison.
- Decontamination and elimination techniques should be considered.
- Supportive care is often adequate, but various antidotes exist for select poisonings.

References

1. Xu JQ, Murphy SL, Kochane KD, Arias E. Mortality in the United States, 2015. NCHS data brief, no. 267. Hyattsville, MD: National Center for Health Statistics; 2016.
2. Mohammad A, Branicki F, Abu-Zidan FM. Educational and clinical impact of advanced trauma life support (ATLS) courses: systematic review. World J Surg. 2014;38:322–9.
3. Boyle JS, Bechtel LK, Holstege CP. Management of the critically poisoned patient. Scand J Trauma Resusc Emerg Med. 2009;17:29.
4. Eldridge DL, Dobson T, Brady W, Holstege CP. Utilizing diagnostic investigations in the poisoned patient. Med Clin N Am. 2005a;89:1079–105.
5. Gupta S, Taneja V. Poisoned child: emergency room management. Indian J Pediatr. 2003a;70(Suppl 1):S2–8.
6. Holstege CP, Dobmeier SG, Bechtel LK. Critical care toxicology. Emerg Med Clin North Am. 2008;25:715–39.
7. Mofenson HC, Greensher J. The unknown poison. Pediatrics. 1974;54(3):336–42.
8. Lam SW, Engebretsen KM, Bauer SR. Toxicology today: what you need to know now. J Pharm Pract. 2011;24(2):174–88.
9. Coulson JM, Thompson JP. Investigation and management of the poisoned patient. Clin Med (Lond). 2008;8(1):89–91.
10. Proudfoot AT, Krenzelok EP, Brent J, Vale JA. Position paper on urine alkalinization. J Toxicol Clin Toxicol. 2004;42(1):1–26.
11. Ashbourne JF, Olson KR, Khayam-Bashi H. Value of rapid screening for acetaminophen in all patients with intentional drug overdose. Ann Emerg Med. 1989;18(10):1035–8.
12. Dargan PI, Ladhani S, Jones AL. Measuring plasma paracetamol concentrations in all patients with drug overdose or altered consciousness: does it change outcome? Emerg Med J. 2001;18(3):178–82.
13. Sporer KA, Khayam-Bashi H. Acetaminophen and salicylate serum levels in patients with suicidal ingestion or altered mental status. Am J Emerg Med. 1996;14(5):443–6.
14. Mowry JB, Spyker DA, Brooks DE, Zimmerman A, Schauben JL. 2015 Annual Report of the American Association of Poison Control Centers' National Poison Data System (NPDS): 33rd Annual Report. Clin Toxicol (Phila). 2016;54(10):924–1109.
15. Chyka PA, Seger D. Position statement: single-dose activated charcoal. Clin Toxicol. 2005;43:61–87.
16. Isbister GK, Kumar VV. Indications for single-dose activated charcoal administration in acute overdose. Curr Opin Crit Care. 2011;17:351–7.
17. Olsen KM, Ma FH, Ackerman BH, Stall RE. Low-volume whole bowel irrigation and salicylate absorption: a comparison with ipecac-charcoal. Pharmacotherapy. 1993;13:229–32.
18. Cooper GM, Le Couteur DG, Richardson D, Buckley NA. A randomized clinical trial of activated charcoal for the routine management of oral drug overdose. QJM. 2005;98(9):655–60.
19. Eddleston M, Juszczak E, Buckley NA, Senarathna L, Mohamed F, Dissanayake W, Hittarage A, Azher S, Jeganathan K, Jayamanne S, Sheriff MR, Warrell DA, Ox-Col Poisoning Study collaborators. Multiple-dose activated charcoal in acute self-poisoning: a randomised controlled trial. Lancet. 2008;371(9612):579–87.
20. Merigian KS, Blaho KE. Single-dose oral activated charcoal in the treatment of the self-poisoned patient: a prospective, randomized, controlled trial. Am J Ther. 2002;9(4):301–8.
21. Olson KR. Activated charcoal for acute poisoning: one toxicologist's journey. J Med Toxicol. 2010;6(2):190–8.
22. Tenenbein M. Position statement: whole bowel irrigation. American Academy of Clinical Toxicology; European Association of Poisons Centres and Clinical Toxicologists. J Toxicol Clin Toxicol. 1997;35:753–62.
23. Davis GR, Santa Ana CA, Morawski SG, Fordtran JS. Development of a lavage solution associated with minimal water and electrolyte absorption or secretion. Gastroenterology. 1980;78:991–5.
24. Kumar VV, Isbister GK, Duffull SB. The effect of decontamination procedures on the pharmacodynamics of venlafaxine in overdose. Br J Clin Pharmacol. 2011;72(1):125–32.
25. Kirshenbaum LA, Mathews SC, Sitar DS, Tenenbein M. Whole-bowel irrigation versus activated charcoal in sorbitol for the ingestion of modified-release pharmaceuticals. Clin Pharmacol Ther. 1989;46:264–71.

26. Smith SW, Ling LJ, Halstenson C. Whole-bowel irrigation as a treatment for acute lithium overdose. Ann Emerg Med. 1991;20:536–9.
27. Tenenbein M, Cohen S, Sitar DS. Whole bowel irrigation as a decontamination procedure after acute drug overdose. Arch Intern Med. 1987;147:905–7.
28. Ly BT, Schneir AB, Clark RF. Effect of whole bowel irrigation on the pharmacokinetics of an acetaminophen formulation and progression of radiopaque markers through the gastrointestinal tract. Ann Emerg Med. 2004;43(2):189–95.
29. Rosenberg PJ, Livingstone DJ, McLellan BA. Effect of whole-bowel irrigation on the antidotal efficacy of oral activated charcoal. Ann Emerg Med. 1988;17:681–3.
30. Kumar VV, Oscarsson S, Friberg LE, Isbister GK, Hackett LP, Duffull SB. The effect of decontamination procedures on the pharmacokinetics of venlafaxine in overdose. Clin Pharmacol Ther. 2009;86(4):403–10.
31. Benson BE, Hoppu K, Troutman WG, Bedry R, Erdman A, Hojer J, Megarbane B, Thanacoody R, Caravati EM. American Academy of Clinical Toxicology; European Associations of Poisons Centres and Clinical Toxicologists. Clin Toxicol (Phila). 2013;51(3):140–6.
32. Krenzelok EP, McGuigan M, Lheur P. Position statement: ipecac syrup. American Academy of Clinical Toxicology; European Association of Poisons Centres and Clinical Toxicologists. J Toxicol Clin Toxicol. 1997;35(7):699–709.
33. Holubek WJ, Hoffman RS, Goldfarb DS, Nelson LS. Use of hemodialysis and hemoperfusion in poisoned patients. Kidney Int. 2008;74(10):1327–34.
34. Ghannoum M, Gosselin S. Enhanced poison elimination in critical care. Adv Chronic Kidney Dis. 2013;20(1):94–101.
35. De Pont AC. Extracorporeal treatment of intoxications. Curr Opin Crit Care. 2007;13(6):668–73.
36. Winchester JF, Harbord NB. Intoxications amenable to extracorporeal removal. Adv Chronic Kidney Dis. 2011;18(3):167–71.
37. Ghannoum M, Nolin TD, Lavergne V, Hoffman RS. Blood purification in toxicology: nephrology's ugly duckling. Adv Chronic Kidney Dis. 2011;18(3):160–6.
38. Tyagi PK, Winchester JF, Feinfeld DA. Extracorporeal removal of toxins. Kidney Int. 2008;74(10):1231–3.
39. Gil HW, Kim SJ, Yang JO, Lee EY, Hong SY. Clinical outcome of hemoperfusion in poisoned patients. Blood Purif. 2010;30:84–8.
40. Shannon MW. Comparative efficacy of hemodialysis and hemoperfusion in severe theophylline intoxication. Acad Emerg Med. 1997;4:674–8.
41. Mckinnon RS, Desmond PV, Harman PJ, Kamm M, Ghabrial H, Martin CJ, Mashford ML. Studies on the mechanisms of action of activated charcoal on theophylline pharmacokinetics. J Pharm Pharmacol. 1987;39(7):522–5.
42. Berlinger WG, Spector R, Goldberg MJ, Johnson GF, Quee CK, Berg MJ. Enhancement of theophylline clearance by oral activated charcoal. Clin Pharmacol Ther. 1983;33(3):351–4.
43. Wakabayashi Y, Maruyama S, Hachimura K, Ohwada T. Activated charcoal interrupts enteroenteric circulation of phenobarbital. J Toxicol Clin Toxicol. 1994;32(4):419–24.
44. Brahmi N, Kouraichi N, Thabet H, Amamou M. Influence of activated charcoal on the pharmacokinetics and the clinical features of carbamazepine poisoning. Am J Emerg Med. 2006;24(4):440–3.
45. Vale JA, Krenzelok EP, Barceloux GD. Position statement and practice guidelines on the use of multi-dose activated charcoal in the treatment of acute poisoning. American Academy of Clinical Toxicology; European Association of Poisons Centres and Clinical Toxicologists. J Toxicol Clin Toxicol. 1999;37:731–51.
46. Frenia ML, Schauben JL, Wears RL, Karlix JL, Tucker CA, Kunisaki TA. Multiple-dose activated charcoal compared to urinary alkalinization for the enhancement of phenobarbital elimination. J Toxicol Clin Toxicol. 1996;34:169–75.
47. Christensen ML, Rivera GK, Crom WR, Hancock ML, Evans WE. Effect of hydration on methotrexate plasma concentrations in children with acute lymphocytic leukemia. J Clin Oncol. 1988;6:797–801.
48. Grimes DJ, Bowles MR, Buttsworth JA, Thomson DB, Ravenscroft PJ, Nixon PJ, Whiting RF, Pond SM. Survival after unexpected high serum methotrexate concentrations in a patient with osteogenic sarcoma. Drug Saf. 1990;5:447–54.
49. Haviv YS, Gillis S. Forced diuresis and high dosage folinic acid for the treatment of severe methotrexate toxicity. Clin Drug Investig. 2000;19:79–81.
50. Sand TE, Jacobsen S. Effect of urine pH and flow on renal clearance of methotrexate. Eur J Clin Pharmacol. 1981;19:453–6.
51. Tsavaris N, Karabelis A, Vonorta P, Karvounis N, Papagrigoriou D, Tsoutsos E, Halvidi-Kozatsani D, Koutsiouba-Kazakou P, Kosmidis P. Intravenous urine alkalinization in high dose methotrexate (HDMTX) treatment: a short communication. Rev Clin Pharmacol Pharmacokinet. 1991;5:107–9.

5 Drug Intoxication in the Emergency Department

Jagoda Pasic and Margaret A. Cashman

Introduction

Substance use is highly prevalent among patients presenting to emergency departments (EDs). According to the Substance Abuse and Mental Health Services Administration (SAMHSA) Drug Abuse Warning Network report, in 2011, there were approximately 2.5 million drug-abuse-related ED visits nationwide [1]. Twenty-five percent of the total drug-related ED visits involved illicit drugs, and 28% involved pharmaceuticals. The most common illegal drugs of abuse were cocaine, marijuana, and heroin. Between 2004 and 2011, the most massive pharmaceutical increase was recorded for oxycodone (220%) [1] (Fig. 5.1).

Approximately one in eight visits to EDs in the United States involves mental and substance-use disorders [2]. Between 2007 and 2011, the rate of ED visits related to mental and substance-use disorders increased by over 15% [3]. The majority of drug-related ED visits were made by patients 21 years and older (81%). The rates for cocaine use are the highest among individuals aged 45–54 and for heroin in the age group 35–44. Race/ethnic differences in substance use are described best as in the DAWN 2011 report: White individuals preferentially used heroin and methamphetamine, compared with Black individuals (4.6 times and 8.5 times, respectively), while Black individuals preferentially used cocaine, compared with White individuals (1.2 times) [4].

Existing studies typically address substance use in global terms and rarely elaborate on whether a patient presented to an ED in a state of intoxication or withdrawal. According to one study, 32% of patients came into the psychiatric emergency service (PES) in a state of acute alcohol or drug intoxication, and 17% had a primary diagnosis of substance abuse or dependence [5]. This study also reported that these patients consumed considerable time and resources, as 64% of the patients were suicidal and 26% were hospitalized.

Psychiatric Comorbidity

Substance use complicates the differential diagnosis of the ED patient, as the effects of drugs can mimic a variety of psychiatric syndromes. For example, in a patient who presents with psychotic

J. Pasic (✉) · M. A. Cashman
Department of Psychiatry and Behavioral Sciences, University of Washington School of Medicine, Seattle, WA, USA
e-mail: jpasic@uw.edu

L. S. Zun et al. (eds.), *Behavioral Emergencies for Healthcare Providers*, https://doi.org/10.1007/978-3-030-52520-0_5

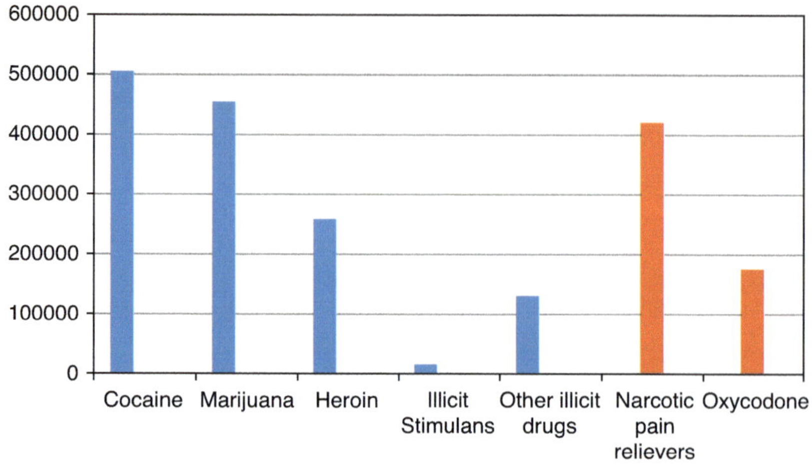

Fig. 5.1 Drug-related emergency department visits: 2011. (Source: 2011 SAMHSA Drug Abuse Warning Network (DAWN) [1] (*2011 was the last year that the DAWN report was generated))

symptoms and who recently has used an illicit drug, often it is unclear whether the psychosis is a direct consequence of a substance or whether the patient has a primary psychotic disorder that coincides with drug use. One study that addressed this issue reported that in as many as 25% of patients who presented with psychotic symptoms, the PES clinicians attributed psychotic symptoms to a primary psychotic disorder that later was determined to be a substance-induced psychosis. The potential consequences of misdiagnosing psychosis in ED or PES are severalfold: unnecessary hospitalization, inappropriate use of antipsychotics, lack of appropriate follow-up, and inattention to substance-use treatment [6]. The literature on first-episode psychosis indicates a high association with substance-use disorders (SUDs). Approximately one-half of first-episode patients have a history of cannabis abuse or dependence, and one-third have a current cannabis-use disorder [7].

Substance use is highly prevalent among patients with psychiatric disorders, and drug or alcohol use often contributes to frequent ED visits. Patients with comorbid psychiatric and SUD have up to 5.6 times greater use of ED services [8].

Alcohol and substance-use disorders are associated with suicide risk [9]. Individuals with a SUD are about six times more likely to report a lifetime suicide attempt than those without a substance-use disorder. One study found particularly high suicidality among cocaine users who presented to an urban PES [10]. Another study evaluated the relationship of alcohol and drug use and severity of suicidality in patients who were admitted through an urban PES to an acute psychiatric inpatient unit. In the most severely suicidal group, 56% had substance use or dependence [11]. Particularly vulnerable groups for the effects of alcohol and substances include youth (ages 12–17), and veterans. A recent study showed that veterans with a substance-use disorder are approximately 2.3 times more likely to die by suicide than those who are not substance users. Concerning specific SUDs, the suicide rate associated with sedative use was the highest (4.7 times greater), followed by amphetamine (2.6×) and opioid (2.4×) use [12]. The astounding finding in this study is that women had 11 times higher likelihood of dying from suicide associated with sedative-hypnotics than men (hazard ratio 11.4 vs. 4.7).

There is an active link between depression and suicidality in individuals with comorbid mood and substance-use disorders [13]. The National Epidemiologic Survey on Alcohol and Related Conditions (NESARC), an extensive national study conducted among adults in the US, found that among individuals with an anxiety disorder, almost 15% had SUD. Similarly, among individuals with an SUD, nearly 18% had alcohol use disorder [14]. The effects of comorbid alcohol and SUD on premature death were found to be the highest among individuals with bipolar disorder [15].

The current conventions in diagnosing a comorbid psychiatric disorder and a substance-use disorder are as follows:

1. Do not list "substance-induced psychosis" or "substance-induced mood disorder" as additional diagnoses when the substance use exacerbates the symptoms of an already established psychiatric disorder. Only list the substance-use disorder and the psychiatric disorder that was worsened.
2. Examine and contrast the onset of psychiatric symptoms with the beginning of substance use, as well as examining whether symptoms seem to persist to a robust degree even when the patient is abstinent from the substance, in determining whether to attribute a psychiatric syndrome to the substance use.
3. Most substances of abuse are associated with syndromes that persist even with prolonged abstinence.

Medical Comorbidity

Chronic drug and alcohol use significantly increases the likelihood that a person will use an ED for medical treatment [16]. Chronic substance use has deleterious effects on the general health of drug users. For example, injection heroin users are more vulnerable to HIV, hepatitis B and C, abscess formation at injection sites, avascular necrosis of the bone, endocarditis, and renal insufficiency. Cocaine use is associated with stroke, acute myocardial infarction, dysrhythmias, aortic dissection, seizures, and respiratory problems. Methamphetamine use is associated with acute renal failure due to rhabdomyolysis.

Service Utilization

Substance-use disorders are highly prevalent among patients presenting in the ED. The 2007 Nationwide Emergency Department Sample (NEDS) shows that 12.5% of all ED visits involved diagnoses related to mental health and substance-use disorders. Of all mental health and substance-use disorders (SUDs), 64% were for mental health disorders alone, 24% were for substance-use disorders alone, and 12% were for co-occurring disorders [2]. Between 2006 and 2013, the population rate of ED visits involving SUDs increased by 37% [17].

Unintentional poisoning from opiate prescription drugs is a rising problem. According to the CDC, opioid overdose deaths in the US have quadrupled from 8050 in 1999 to 33,091 in 2015. The deaths were initially driven by prescription opioid misuse and more recently by heroin and other illicit opioid use. In the period from 2010 to 2015, heroin overdose deaths also quadrupled from 3036 to 12,989. A sharp increase in the supply of heroin and illicitly manufactured fentanyl is considered to be contributing to increased deaths [18] (see more in ref. [28, 29, 30]).

Brief Interventions

The ED provides a unique opportunity to engage patients about their drug use. Clinical reports for screening, brief intervention, and referral to treatment (SBIRT) instituted by SAMHSA in the EDs across the US initially reported a reduction in illicit drug and alcohol abuse 12 months after the screening [19]. However, a recently published benefit–cost analysis indicates that this intervention did not result in any significant impact on total economic benefit from SBIRT [20].

Drugs of Abuse and Intoxication

Alcohol Prevalence and Community Impact

Alcohol intoxication is the most prevalent of the substance intoxications encountered in the ED. The estimated total number of ED visits attributable to alcohol from 1992 through 2000 was 68.6 million (65.6–71.7 million), which averages to 7.6 million alcohol-related ED visits per year. Alcohol-related visits accounted for 8% of the total 866.5 million ED visits from 1992 through 2000 [21].

According to the CDC's Alcohol-Related Disease Impact (ARDI) tool for 2006–2010, excessive drinking led annually to 88,000 deaths and 2.5 million years of life lost [22]. Excessive alcohol use is accounted for 1 in 10 deaths among working-age adults in the United States [23].

Alcohol is highly prevalent among individuals with mood and anxiety disorders. According to the results from the National Epidemiological Survey on Alcohol and Related Disorders, of individuals who presented to treatment for alcohol use disorder, 41% had independent (comorbid) mood disorder, and 33% had an independent anxiety disorder. The authors of this study argue that treatment for a mood or anxiety disorder should not be withheld from those with alcohol or drug use in stable remission on the assumption that most of these disorders are due to intoxication or withdrawal [24].

Binge drinking (defined as intake of at least five drinks on one occasion for men and at least four drinks on one occasion for women) and heavy drinking (defined as daily intake of more than two drinks for men and more than one drink for women) are considered excessive drinking [23]. Binge drinking, the most common form of excessive alcohol consumption, usually results in acute intoxication and is responsible for over half of the deaths and three-quarters of the economic costs of excessive drinking. Binge drinking can be harmful without the drinker being alcohol-dependent. In fact, the majority of binge drinkers are not alcohol-dependent.

Compared with patients presenting to primary care settings, ED patients are more likely to be drinking alcohol to an excessive and harmful level [25]. Underage drinking (ages 12–20) is a significant factor in ED visits: Between 2010 and 2013, an estimated 656,827 alcohol-misuse-related ED visits were made by patients aged 12–20. Alcohol-only visits accounted for 80% of all underage alcohol-misuse-related visits [26].

Management

When a patient presents with suspected alcohol intoxication as part of the clinical presentation, it makes sense to check the BAL (blood alcohol level) early in the evaluation process. If the patient refuses a blood draw, a urine alcohol level is a less accurate but modestly useful method of estimating blood alcohol. The breath alcohol level appears to be less reliable as serum blood alcohol increases, so it is probably unsuitable for ED use [27]. It is essential to ask the patient when he or she last drank. A person who drank a significant amount just before entering the ED may have sequestered alcohol in the stomach, and the BAL will continue to rise as he or she absorbs the bolus. It is also important to ask the patient about any illicit drug use and how recently the substance was used. Note that a highly tolerant individual can appear only modestly impaired at a BAL that would render an alcohol-naïve individual unconscious.

Blood alcohol levels will decline at a rate determined by such factors as liver volume, liver health, ethnicity, gender, and patient tolerance to alcohol. Nontolerant individuals metabolize more slowly than alcohol-tolerant individuals, and women metabolize more slowly than men if their level of tolerance is equal. Individuals with the impaired hepatic function will metabolize more slowly. A rate of 0.015–0.02 g/dL per hour is a fair estimate overall of nontolerant individuals' capacity for metabolizing alcohol. A tolerant individual may metabolize at a rate closer to 0.04 g/dL per hour. Knowing the likely rate, one can estimate how long it will take before the patient is ready to be seen for a mental health interview. Emergency physicians and psychiatrists take varying approaches to the timing of a mental health interview for the patient intoxicated with alcohol. No single standard exists, but the patient should, at a minimum, be clinically assessable. Some follow more objective BAL cutoffs that correlate with established legal limits for driving, which vary by state. In some instances (e.g., for legal purposes), a BAL of 0 may be needed before the interview is completed.

Intoxicated patients may be brought to the ED for assessment after expressing suicidal or homicidal impulses and intent, causing a disturbance in the community, or having been found in a state of unconsciousness. The mental health exam should be completed once the patient is decisional. Suicidal or homicidal ideation may be disavowed once the patient is sober. If the patient continues to endorse suicidal or homicidal ideation after sobering, the patient should be assessed and managed accordingly.

Physical findings in the chronically overdrinking individual include conjunctival injection, abnormal skin vascularization evident on face and neck, tongue tremor, hand tremor, and hepatomegaly. Laboratory findings may consist of high mean red cell volume (MCV) on the complete blood count, elevated serum aspartate aminotransferase (AST), and elevated serum gamma-glutamyl transferase (GGT). The serum carbohydrate-deficient transferrin (CDT) assay is also sensitive to heavy drinking and is not affected by the comorbid liver disease.

If the patient shows up-gaze paresis, along with confusion, one should be concerned mainly with acute thiamine-deficiency-associated Wernicke's encephalopathy. In such a situation, thiamine should be administered immediately (100 mg IV or IM) and supplemented daily with oral 100-mg doses for at least 3 days. One needs to keep in mind that high utilizers of the ED services due to alcohol intoxication may end up receiving multiple doses of thiamine and exhibit signs of thiamine intoxication, such as dysrhythmia, hypotension, headache, weakness, and seizures.

One should also keep in mind the possibility for an alcohol-intoxicated patient to have suffered a traumatic brain injury, typically from falling, before arriving at the ED. The resulting confusion could be mistaken for simple intoxication. Alcoholic psychosis may recur during subsequent episodes of alcohol intoxication. If the patient experiences a subacute or chronic psychosis, management with antipsychotic medication is indicated. The assessment and management of alcohol withdrawal state in the ED are covered elsewhere in this text.

The ED is a critical platform for engaging alcohol-affected patients. Patients should be offered follow-up in the community, including non-hospital-based detoxification, though in most states these resources are limited. As noted above, the SBIRT program has shown limited cost impact.

Opioids

Unless opioid intoxication occurs in the context of accidental or intentional overdose, patients rarely come to the ED in a state of opioid intoxication per se. Opioid abusers, however, are more likely to seek ED services in the state of opioid withdrawal. Individuals who abuse opioids receive medical attention because of medical complications of drug use, withdrawal, or overdose. Opioid intoxication is suspected when a patient has pupillary constriction and symptoms of slurred speech, drowsiness, and impaired attention and memory. Opioid overdose is a medical emergency, and patients with the triad of classic symptoms (pinpoint pupils, respiratory depression, and altered sensorium/coma) warrant emergency administration of naloxone, which can be administered intravenously, intramuscularly, or subcutaneously. The usual initial dose is 0.4–2 mg. If the desired degree of counteraction and improvement in respiratory function is not obtained, it may be repeated at 2–3-minute intervals. One should be cautioned that abrupt reversal can result in elevated blood pressure, tachycardia, tremulousness, seizure, and, in rare events, cardiac arrest. Opioid withdrawal, in contrast, is rarely fatal, but the comfort of the patient may be helped by the appropriate use of an opiate withdrawal regimen.

Prescription opiate use has become increasingly prevalent among patients presenting in EDs, and the most commonly abused drugs include hydromorphone (Dilaudid), hydrocodone (in Vicodin/Norco), oxycodone (Oxycontin and in Percocet), and oxymorphone (Opana), though methadone also is commonly abused. In recent years, two opioid trends have emerged that are particularly menacing: (1) increasingly prevalent fentanyl and fentanyl analogs flooding the drug market from illicit sources and leading to what is termed an epidemic of opioid-related overdose deaths [28, 29] and (2) the appearance of an array of synthetic opioids, such as U-47700, nicknamed "Pink" [30]. Additionally, a potent opioid, carfentanil, is appearing in some street mixtures with heroin and other drugs. This is a drug used for sedation or general anesthesia in large animals, such as elephants, and is not meant for human use [31]. In the last several years, especially after the FDA approval of naloxone intranasal spray for reversal of heroin overdose in 2015, EDs across the country have been distributing naloxone to patients identified at risk for opioid overdose [32]. There is an increasing awareness that the distribution of naloxone kits to laypersons who might witness an opioid overdose can help reduce opioid overdose mortality [33]. This action undoubtedly is a complex matter raising some controversies, including a concern that readily available naltrexone for laypersons may increase opiate addiction [34]. Additionally, ED-initiated buprenorphine for opioid dependence with continuation in primary care was found to increase engagement in addiction treatment and reduce illicit opioid use at 30 days, compared to referral only or a brief intervention with referral [35]. A subsequent study replicated the short-term benefit of ED-initiated buprenorphine at 2 months but showed no difference in addiction treatment engagement at 6 and 12 months [36].

Sedative-Hypnotics

Benzodiazepines

Benzodiazepines are sedative, hypnotic, and anxiolytic agents that are typically referred to by drug uses as "downers." According to the Drug Abuse Warning Network (DAWN) report, drug-related ED visits involving benzodiazepines increased by 124% from 2004 to 2011, and alprazolam (Xanax) and clonazepam (Klonopin) were the most frequently reported as the drugs of abuse [1]. While opioids are most often associated with accidental overdose, benzodiazepines are the most commonly ingested prescription medications in suicide attempts. The symptoms of benzodiazepine intoxication are similar to alcohol intoxication, and they include an altered level of consciousness, drowsiness, confusion, impaired judgment, slow and slurred speech, incoordination, and ataxia. Severe intoxication/overdose can lead to coma, respiratory depression, and death. Benzodiazepine overdose patients are typically managed in EDs with supportive care such as maintenance of adequate ventilation and hydration. In contrast to the role in iatrogenic oversedation, caution is advised regarding the utility of flumazenil, the benzodiazepine antidote, in a chronic user, as it may precipitate severe withdrawal symptoms, including seizures.

Of particular concern is when benzodiazepines are used in combination with substances like opioid pain relievers or alcohol. According to the DAWN report, over a 7-year period (2005–2011), 32% of hospital emergency department visits involving benzodiazepines resulted in severe medical outcomes such as hospitalization (or in rare cases, death). The risk of a severe outcome was 44% for the visits involving the use of benzodiazepines in combination with opioid pain relievers. Similarly, 44% of ED visits associated with the combined use of benzodiazepines and alcohol resulted in serious adverse medical outcomes [37]. Benzodiazepine withdrawal is a serious medical emergency due to the risk of seizures, peripheral nervous system and electrolyte instability (due to profuse diaphoresis), and acute anxiety syndrome with restlessness and insomnia. Patients with acute anxiety due to benzodiazepine withdrawal are often seen and managed in the psychiatric emergency service.

Barbiturates

Barbiturates are used to treat various seizure disorders. They are classified based on their duration of action: ultra-short-acting, short-acting, intermediate-acting, and long-acting. Barbiturate intoxication causes central nervous system (CNS) depression symptoms that are similar to alcohol and benzodiazepine intoxication, including nystagmus, vertigo, slurred speech, lethargy, confusion, ataxia, and respiratory depression. Severe overdose may result in coma, shock, apnea, and hypothermia. In combination with alcohol or other CNS depressants, barbiturates have additive CNS and respiratory depression effects.

Barbiturate withdrawal is life-threatening, with signs and symptoms developing within

24 hours. Patients may present to the ED with insomnia, restlessness, and severe anxiety.

Gamma-Hydroxybutyrate (GHB)

GHB is known as a dietary supplement that gained popularity as a club drug in the late 1990s and early 2000s. Sporadically, GHB is a drug of abuse leading to an ED visit. GHB, also referred to as "liquid ecstasy," is a potent CNS depressant, and the effects of intoxication are a profound alteration of mental status and respiratory depression, with periods of apnea. Deaths have been reported with severe GHB intoxication [38]. GHB discontinuation can lead to a significant withdrawal syndrome that is similar to sedative-hypnotic and alcohol withdrawal. With appropriate management, most patients fully recover within 6 hours. Nevertheless, the challenge lies in the recognition and detection of GHB, because routine toxicology screening does not detect this substance [39].

Stimulants

Cocaine

As noted above, cocaine is the most common illegal substance that leads to ED visits, which in 2011 accounted for 162 visits per 100,000 [1]. Cocaine is a stimulant with powerful effects on the central and peripheral nervous system that acts by blocking the reuptake of dopamine, norepinephrine, and serotonin. It also modulates the endogenous opiate system. Cocaine intoxication leads to some physical signs and symptoms, such as hypertension, tachycardia, chest pain, myocardial infarction (MI), mydriasis, diaphoresis, delirium, stroke, and seizures. Acute cocaine intoxication may present with anxiety; agitation; paranoia; hallucinations; feelings of increased energy, alertness, and intense euphoria; and decreased tiredness, appetite, and sleep.

Cocaine may be smoked (crack-cocaine), insufflated (snorted), injected, and orally ingested (cocaine salt). The onset, peak, and duration of cocaine's effects vary depending on the route of administration. The fastest absorption and the peak effect are after inhalation. Repeated cocaine users may use it as frequently as every 10 minutes, may binge with it for as long as 7 days, and may use as much as 10 grams per day.

Chest pain due to cardiac ischemia is the most frequent cocaine-related medical event for which patients seek treatment in inner-city EDs [40]. The most frequently occurring cardiac complications of cocaine are syncope, angina pectoris, and MI. In some instances, the outcome is acute cardiac death. The typical patient with cardiac-related MI is a young man without cardiovascular risk factors other than smoking. The relative risk of MI is elevated 24 times within 60 minutes after cocaine use, and the incidence of MI is about 6% [41]. There have been recent reports of fever and severe agranulocytosis associated with cocaine that had been adulterated with levamisole [42].

Psychiatric symptoms are prominent in cocaine intoxication and account for about 30% of cocaine-related presentations, compared to 16% and 17% for cardiopulmonary and neurologic symptoms, respectively. Suicidal intent was the most common psychiatric reason for presentation [43]. Psychiatric manifestations of cocaine intoxication include anxiety, agitation, euphoria, and intense paranoia. Because of overlapping psychiatric manifestations of cocaine intoxication and bipolar mania, differentiation between the two can be challenging in the ED. One should keep in mind the following: SUD are commonly comorbid in patients with bipolar affective disorder, and substance abuse often is a manifestation of the core criteria of mania, specifically excessive involvement in activities with a high potential for painful consequences. Manic episodes can frequently be triggered by insomnia due to stimulant abuse. These factors are often exacerbated by the elevated rates of noncompliance with medication in patients abusing substances, which in turn render patients vulnerable to decompensation [44].

Depression and suicidal thoughts often accompany acute cocaine withdrawal. Excessive tearfulness has been described as a distinct sign of cocaine-induced depression in patients presenting in a busy urban PES [45]. A typical patient with cocaine-related psychiatric symptoms presents to the ED in the early morning hours after a binge in a state of high adrenergic dysregulation, dysphoric and suicidal, with injected conjunctiva, asking for food and promptly falling asleep. Disposition of such patients may be a challenge due to their suicidality [44]. The treatment of cocaine intoxication is determined by the presenting symptoms. Chest pain warrants a medical workup for cardiovascular complications. Such patients often receive hydration and benzodiazepine or other sedating agents to reduce anxiety and blunt surges in blood pressure and heart rate. It is worth noting that beta-blockers should be avoided in cocaine-associated MI because of theoretical concerns of unopposed alpha-adrenergic stimulation. In patients who are severely agitated or intensely paranoid, treatment with oral or intramuscular antipsychotic medication may be indicated.

Methamphetamine

In the early 2000s, there was a nationwide methamphetamine epidemic. In some localities, ED visits involving methamphetamine declined by 2006. However, since 2007 the rates of methamphetamine have increased again. According to DAWN 2011 report, ED visits involving methamphetamine accounted for 4% of all drug-related ED visits [46]. The majority (62%) of these ED visits involved other drugs. Injecting methamphetamine along with heroin ("meth-ball") has risen rapidly in some localities, as noted in Denver in a recent epidemiological study [47].

Like cocaine, methamphetamine exerts powerful stimulant effects on the brain, but the results last longer than after cocaine use, giving rise to more noticeable medical and psychiatric symptoms. Methamphetamine intoxication can lead to serious medical consequences, including hypertension, arrhythmias, MI, stroke, acute renal failure due to rhabdomyolysis, seizure, delirium, and death. People who inject methamphetamine are at increased risk of contracting infectious diseases such as HIV and hepatitis B and C. Methamphetamine use can also alter judgment and decision-making, leading to risky behaviors such as unprotected sex, which also increases the risk for sexually transmitted infection. Psychiatric consequences include psychosis, mania-like symptoms, severe agitation, and violence. Psychosis is the most common presenting symptom (80%) in methamphetamine-intoxicated patients who are seen in PES. These patients were most often Caucasians (75%) referred by police with an extended duration of stay in the ED [48]. By clinical observation, patients most often present in a state that has been described by the term "tweaking," which involves a state of high arousal, agitation, and uncontrollable movements, with prominent dysphoria, hallucinations, and paranoia (Table 5.1).

Due to their extreme agitation, patients with methamphetamine intoxication are often treated with sedating agents (benzodiazepines), alone or in combination with antipsychotic agents. There are regional differences that dictate the utilization of physical restraints and involuntary administration of medications in methamphetamine-intoxicated patients. However, it is essential to keep in mind that such patients are highly distressed and are likely to accept medications voluntarily, mainly if the medication is offered in a rapidly dissolvable form [48]. As in treating cocaine-intoxicated patients in the ED, methamphetamine-intoxicated patients may need

Table 5.1 Methamphetamine: effects and duration of euphoria by route of administration

Route	Onset	Peak effect (min)	Duration (hrs)
Smoking	Within seconds	1–5	20
Snorting	Within seconds	3–5	12
Intravenous	Within seconds	1–3	12
Oral	10 min	15–20	12

intravenous rehydration to correct electrolyte imbalance and acute renal insufficiency.

MDMA (3,4-Methylenedioxymetham phetamine)

MDMA—also known as "Ecstasy" or, more recently, "Molly"—is similar to both the stimulant amphetamine and the hallucinogen mescaline. Ecstasy is known as a club drug, and typically, it is used by young individuals in parties, raves, and clubs. Ecstasy/Molly is a powerful indirect releaser of serotonin and a moderate releaser of dopamine. Regarded by most users as a harmless substance, the acute effects of MDMA intoxication are an increase in energy and a sense of empathy. Its psychiatric effects include blunting of the senses, confusion, lack of judgment, depression, anxiety, anger, paranoia, hallucinations, and aggression.

Ecstasy intoxication can lead to serious medical complications such as hypertension, tachycardia, rhabdomyolysis with acute renal failure, and hyperthermia. One should keep in mind that some MDMA users believe that they can avoid hyperthermia by drinking large amounts of water, which puts them at risk of hyponatremia from diuresis and marked increase in free water intake.

Ecstasy users may present in a hyperactive delirious state. Molly—slang for "molecular"—refers to the pure crystal powder form of MDMA. Usually purchased in capsules, Molly has become more popular in the past few years. Users may be seeking out Molly to avoid the additives, such as caffeine, methamphetamine, and other harmful substances that are commonly found in in Ecstasy pills. News stories have reported Molly capsules containing harmful substances that include synthetic cathinones. The effects of Molly can last from 3 to 6 hours [49]. ED staff must be alert to addressing serotonin syndrome, which can be precipitated by the patient's concurrent use of stimulant drugs. Most standard urine drug screen tests have low sensitivity for MDMA, so the Ecstasy level needs to be quite high to show a positive test.

"Bath Salts"

Recently, there has been increased attention to a new generation of designer drugs, the so-called "bath salts." The Drug Abuse Warning Network (DAWN) first detected a measurable number of emergency department (ED) visits involving bath salts in 2011 [50]. Bath salts were named in 22,904 visits, or about 1% of all drug-related ED visits. One-third of these visits involved bath salts only, and two-thirds involved other drugs.

Bath salt products were sold legally online as "legal highs" under a variety of names such as "Ivory Wave," "White Lightning," and "Vanilla Sky," but in 2011, the Drug Enforcement Agency (DEA) declared bath salts to be a controlled substance. The use of such products has led to an increasing number of ED visits and overdoses throughout the country. These products contain amphetamine-like substances such as methylenedioxypyrovalerone, mephedrone, and methylone [51]. However, to keep ahead of the game with the law, bath salt developers are persistently coming up with new substitute compounds [52]. These drugs are chemically similar to amphetamines, cocaine, and MDMA, and the effects are more potent to the brain. Ingesting or snorting bath salts can cause arrhythmias, chest pain, MI, hypertension, hyperthermia, seizure, stroke, aggressive and violent behavior, hallucinations, paranoia and delusions, excited delirium, and, in extreme cases, death. Bath salts are rapidly absorbed after oral ingestion, with intoxication peaking at 1.5 hours and lasting for 3–4 hours. Patients who are intoxicated on bath salts may require physical restraints and high doses of sedatives because of the risk of harming themselves or others. Treatment includes hydration to address emerging rhabdomyolysis and benzodiazepines to control seizures [53].

ADHD Stimulant Medications

Several CNS stimulants are used for the treatment of the attention-deficit/hyperactivity disorder (ADHD), including methylphenidate (e.g., Ritalin, Concerta), amphetamine-dextroamphetamine (e.g., Adderall), dexmethylphenidate (e.g., Focalin), and dextroamphetamine (e.g., Dexedrine). ADHD stimulant medications can also be misused to suppress appetite, enhance alertness, or cause feelings of euphoria. The primary abusers are young individuals (<25 years of age) who obtain the drug from a friend or a classmate. Other abusers may purchase it from a fraudulent prescription or by doctor shopping. According to DAWN, the number of ED visits involving ADHD stimulant medications increased between 2005 and 2010 from 13,379 to 31,244 visits [54]. The number of ED visits involving ADHD stimulant medications increased significantly for adults aged 18 or older. Acute intoxication with a substance such as methylphenidate results in symptoms similar to those seen with cocaine, including euphoria, delirium, confusion, paranoia, and hallucinations. Additional symptoms may include extreme anger, threats, or aggressive behavior.

Hallucinogens and Dissociative Agents

Phencyclidine (PCP)

Since phencyclidine entered the market in 1957 as a dissociative anesthetic, it has become a significant drug of abuse, due to its psychotropic effects. The estimated number of PCP-related ED visits increased more than 400% between 2005 and 2011 (from 14,825 to 75,538 visits). The most substantial increase in PCP-related ED visits was seen among patients aged 25–34. It is smoked (usually in a mix with marijuana) or, less often, ingested orally. Low doses cause an acute confusional state with excited delirium lasting several hours; stimulant effects predominate. More massive doses cause nystagmus, muscle rigidity, ataxia, stereotyped movements, hypertension, hypersalivation, sweating, amnesia, and an agitated psychosis. The psychotic state induced by phencyclidine is so similar to that of schizophrenia that intermittent administration of phencyclidine has become a standard pharmacological model for schizophrenia in the laboratory. The increase in ED visits involving PCP is of particular concern because it is reputed to be the most dangerous among hallucinogens for causing violent behavior [55].

Unfortunately, PCP is relatively easy and inexpensive to manufacture illicitly. Marijuana has replaced alcohol as the most common secondary substance of abuse in phencyclidine abusers who present for medical attention.

The PCP user is managed conservatively in the ED by keeping the patient physically safe and providing reduced stimulation. An early check for emerging rhabdomyolysis is advisable, and hydration should be maintained.

Ketamine

Ketamine—or the street-named "K," "Special K," "KitKat," or "Vitamin K"—is a powerful dissociative anesthetic that produces similar effects to phencyclidine but with a shorter duration. The common presenting complaints include prominent anxiety, chest pain, and palpitations, and typical findings include confusion, amnesia, mydriasis, bidirectional nystagmus, tachycardia, rigidity, seizures, and usually short-lived hallucinations. The most common complication of ketamine intoxication is severe agitation and rhabdomyolysis. Symptoms are typically short-lived, and patients most often are discharged within 5 hours of presentation [56]. Ketamine intoxication is managed with benzodiazepines to mitigate the anxiety and agitation. Lorazepam, 1–2 mg orally or IV, is the mainstay of treatment. Of note, in recent years, ketamine IM has been used by emergency medical response teams across the country for prehospital sedation of violent and agitated patients and excited delirium [57].

Lysergic Acid (LSD)

LSD is not a standard drug of abuse. However, its damage is prevalent among high school students. According to the DAWN 2011 report, there were 4819 LSD-related visits. These visits were primarily made by young individuals, aged 18–24 [1].

Typically, it is ingested in pill form or dissolved on a piece of paper. The signs and symptoms of intoxication develop within an hour after ingestion and include tachycardia, hypertension, hyperthermia, dilated pupils, distorted perception of time, and depersonalization. LSD is associated with the unique sensory misperception called "synesthesia," whereby colors are heard and noises are seen. These symptoms usually clear 8–12 hours after ingestion, though feelings of numbness may last for several days [58].

ED presentations typically include manifestations of intense anxiety, such as a panic attack ("bad trip"), and can be managed with reassurance and, in some instances, lorazepam or diazepam. Other presenting symptoms include delirium with hallucinations, delusions, and paranoia. Occasionally, a patient may present to the ED with ongoing psychotic symptoms, long after the drug was eliminated from the system, or with the spontaneous recurrence of drug effects, known as "flashbacks." While death from an overdose of LSD is rare, ingestion of high doses carries a significantly higher risk of death due to convulsions, hyperthermia, and cardiovascular collapse.

Phenethylamines (such as mescaline from the peyote cactus, 2C synthetic products (2C-I ("Smiles"), 2C-B ("Nexus"), 2C-E, and 2C-T-7 ("7-up," "Blue Mystic")), psilocybin/psilocin (the psychoactive ingredient in psilocybin mushrooms), and Salvia divinorum) are also hallucinogens. The frequency of use is not well known, since ED visits for intoxication are uncommon. The effects of intoxication are similar to LSD [59].

Dextromethorphan

Dextromethorphan (DXM) is a cough suppressant that is found in many over-the-counter cough and cold preparations, such as Coricidin, Nyquil, and Robitussin. Some popular street names for DXM include "Tripple C," "Candy," "Dex," "Robo," "Rojo," and "Tussin." According to DAWN reports, DXM accounts for about 1% of all drug-related ED visits. However, the significance of DXM misuse is that 50% of such ED visits are made by youth, aged 12–20 years. Structurally related to the opiate receptor antagonist codeine, its metabolite dextrorphan exhibits serotonergic activity and inhibits NMDA receptors. Its unique mechanism of action results in psychotropic effects that are similar to ketamine and phencyclidine. Neurobehavioral effects of DXM typically begin from 30 to 60 minutes after the ingestion and may persist for up to 6 hours. DXM intoxication leads to a combination of euphoric, stimulant dissociative, and sedative effects, and neurological signs such as ataxia, dystonia mydriasis, nystagmus, and coma. It also causes nausea and vomiting, diaphoresis, hypertension, tachycardia, and respiratory depression. In rare instances, DXM has been associated with the development of serotonin syndrome. To address these dangers, the American Association of Poison Control Centers has developed practice guidelines for the management of DXM poisoning/intoxication [60].

Inhalants

Inhalants and inhalant use disorders recently were the subject of a comprehensive review by Howard et al. [61]. Inhalants are substances that produce a psychoactive effect when their vapors are inhaled, and are rarely abused by any other means. These substances include aerosols (containing propellants and solvents), gases (e.g., nitrous oxide), volatile solvents (liquids that vaporize at room temperatures, such as correction fluid, paint thinner, dry-cleaning fluids, and glues), and nitrites. Everyday household products often are a source for the first three types of inhalants. This makes the inhalants a particular problem among early- to mid-adolescents, who may not have easy access to other substances of abuse [62]. The first three types of inhalants act directly on the central nervous system.

The fourth type of inhalant, the nitrites (e.g., amyl nitrite, isobutyl nitrite), are abused by adults and older teens, for the most part, with a goal of enhancing the sexual experience. Unlike the first three types of inhalant, nitrites relax the muscle and dilate blood vessels. Known as "poppers" or "snappers," abuse of nitrites is linked to unsafe sexual practices, increasing the risk of contracting and spreading hepatitis and HIV.

Inhalants enter the bloodstream rapidly and produce intoxication effects within seconds of inhalation. The short-term effects may include initial euphoria, dizziness, impaired coordination, slurred speech, loss of inhibition, hallucinations, and delusions. Users often deal with the short duration of intoxication by repeatedly inhaling, which can lead to a decreased level of consciousness and death. After repetitive use within the span of a few minutes, an inhalant user may be drowsy for several hours. A headache often accompanies repetitive inhalation. Many common inhalants (butane, propane, Freon, trichloroethylene, amyl nitrite, butyl nitrite) are linked to "sudden sniffing death syndrome." Chronic abuse of volatile solvents can lead to demyelination and clinical syndromes resembling multiple sclerosis. Such neurologic functions as movement, vision, hearing, and cognition can be affected. In the worst cases, dementia is the result. Hepatotoxicity, cardiomyopathy, impaired immune function, and lung and kidney damage all can result from inhalant abuse. In earlier stages, such a loss may be partially or even wholly reversible. There are concerns about prenatal exposure to inhalants as well [63].

Cannabinoids

The increasing medicalization of marijuana has thrown a new wrinkle into our understanding of the costs and benefits of marijuana use. It has been described that medicalization typically for severe pain or severe nausea and vomiting associated with chemotherapy often encourages regular use [64]. Such steady use can tip the balance so that what might have been a relatively minor contributor to psychiatric problems becomes more substantial. In some patients, for example, increased marijuana use can be associated with increased impulsivity and suicidality, with or without a preexisting depression [65].

The acute effects of marijuana intoxication, such as sedation, failure to consolidate short-term memory, altered sense of time, perceptual changes, decreased coordination, and impaired executive functioning, are commonly seen. There is substantial evidence that patients with schizophrenia who use cannabis experience a more severe course of illness [66]. Patients with recent-onset psychosis who use cannabis regularly have more severe psychotic symptoms and more cognitive disorganization than comparable patients who do not use cannabis [67].

Cannabis dependence is associated with physiological tolerance and a physiological withdrawal syndrome. Symptoms may appear as early as a day after discontinuation and last 1–3 weeks. Withdrawal symptoms include craving, irritability, anger, dysphoric mood, restlessness, insomnia, and diminished appetite. Treatment relies on psychosocial therapies such as motivational interviewing, specific cognitive-behavioral therapy, and contingency management.

Synthetic Cannabinoids

Further complicating our understanding of cannabinoids in the ED, synthetic cannabinoids (e.g., "Spice" products or "K2") are a rapidly emerging class of drugs of abuse [66]. They are chemically similar to marijuana and sometimes are misleadingly called "synthetic marijuana" (or "fake weed"). They are often marketed as safe and legal. Because they act as a full agonist to the THC receptors, they may affect the brain much more powerfully than marijuana.

It was estimated that in 2011 there were 28,531 ED visits related to synthetic cannabinoids [69]. The harmful effects of these products were first reported in the US in 2009. Since then, the drugs have spread throughout the country. Poison centers received 2668 calls about expo-

Table 5.2 Adverse clinical effects of synthetic cannabinoids

Central nervous system	Seizures Agitation Irritability Loss of consciousness Anxiety Confusion Paranoia
Cardiovascular	Tachycardia Hypertension Chest pain Cardiac ischemia
Metabolic	Hypokalemia Hyperglycemia
Gastrointestinal	Nausea Vomiting
Autonomic	Fever Mydriasis
Other	Conjunctivitis

From Seely et al. [68]

sures to these drugs in 2013; 3682 exposures in 2014; and 7794 exposures in 2015 [70]. Adverse effects reported with these synthetic cannabinoids are listed in Table 5.2. To date, at least 10 different plant species are being used in the manufacture of these substances, and the potency, duration of action, and potential for unexpected toxicity are variable as well. These products will not show up on current urine toxicological screens.

Conclusion

Drug intoxication is commonly involved in ED visits, and patients may present with a variety of medical and psychiatric complaints. Drug intoxication complicates clinical presentation and can lead to prolonged ED length-of-stay and deployment of resources (including the use of restraints in severe intoxication syndromes), and creates a challenge for disposition and treatment. Clinicians who work in the ED setting, including nursing staff, social workers, emergency medicine physicians, and psychiatrists, should be familiar with the toxidromes of the conventional drugs of abuse in order to: (1) make an appropriate diagnosis, (2) provide emergency management, including proper psychiatric and substance-use assessment and administration of medications, (3) refer to a short-term treatment that may include detoxification or admission into the hospital, or (4) relate to a longer term treatment in the community.

References

1. Substance Abuse and Mental Health Services Administration, Center for Behavioral Health Statistics and Quality. The DAWN report: highlights of the 2011 drug abuse warning network (DAWN) findings on drug-related emergency department visits. Rockville. Available at https://www.samhsa.gov/data/sites/default/files/DAWN127/DAWN127/sr127-DAWN-highlights.htm. Accessed 15 Sept 2017.
2. Owens PL, Mutter R, Stocks C. Mental health and substance abuse-related emergency department visits among adults, 2007. HCUP Statistical Brief #92. Rockville: U.S. Agency for Healthcare Research and Quality; 2010. Available at http://www.hcup-us.ahrq.gov/reports/statbriefs/sb92.pdf. Accessed 17 Sept 2017.
3. Agency for Healthcare Research and Quality. Chartbook on Care Coordination. Measures of care coordination: preventable emergency department visits. Rockville: Agency for Healthcare Research and Quality; 2015. Available at http://www.ahrq.gov/research/findings/nhqrdr/2014chartbooks/carecoordination/carecoord-measures2.html. Accessed 17 Sept 2017.
4. Substance Abuse and Mental Health Services Administration, Drug Abuse Warning Network, 2011: National Estimates of Drug-Related Emergency Department Visits. HHS Publication No. (SMA) 13-4760, DAWN Series D-39. Rockville: Substance Abuse and Mental Health Services Administration; 2013. Available at http://store.samhsa.gov. Accessed 29 Sept 2017.
5. Breslow RE, Klinger BI, Erickson BJ. Acute intoxication and substance abuse among patients presenting to a psychiatric emergency service. Gen Hosp Psychiatry. 2006;18(3):183–91.
6. Schanzer BM, First MB, Dominquez B, Hosin DS, Caton CIM. Diagnosing psychotic disorders in the emergency department in the context of substance use. Psychiatr Serv. 2006;57(10):1468–73.
7. Wisdom JP, Manuel JI, Drake RE. Substance use disorder among people with first-episode psychosis: a systematic review of course and treatment. Psychiatr Serv. 2011;62:1007–12.

8. Curran GM, Sullivan G, Williams K, Han X, Allee E, Kotria KJ. The association of psychiatric comorbidity and use of the emergency department among persons with substance use disorders: an observational cohort study. BMC Emerg Med. 2008;8:17.
9. Wilcox HC, Conner KR, Caine ED. Association of alcohol and drug use disorders: an empirical review of cohort studies. Drug Alcohol Depend. 2008;76(Suppl):S11–9.
10. Garlow SJ, Purlselle D, D'Orio B. Cocaine use disorders and suicidal ideation. Drug Alcohol Depend. 2003;70:101–4.
11. Ries RK, Yuodelis-Flores C, Roy-Byrne P, Nilssen O, Russo J. Addiction and suicidal behavior in acute psychiatric inpatients. Compr Psychiatry. 2009;50:93–9.
12. Bohnert KM, Ilgen MA, Louzon S, McCarthy JF, Katz IR. Substance use disorders and the risk of suicide mortality among men and women in the US Veterans Health Administration. Addiction. 2017;112:1193–201.
13. Conner KR, Pinquart M, Gamble SA. Meta-analysis of depression and substance use among individuals with alcohol use disorder. J Subst Abuse Treat. 2009;37:127–37.
14. Kessler RC, Chiu WT, Demler O, Merikangas KR, Walters EE. Prevalence, severity, and comorbidity of 12-month DSM-IV disorders in the National Comorbidity Survey Replication. Arch Gen Psychiatry. 2005;62:617–27.
15. Hunt GE, Malhi GS, Cleary M, Man H, Lai X, Sitharthan T. Prevalence of comorbid bipolar and substance use disorders in clinical settings, 1990–2015: systematic review and meta-analysis. J Affect Disord. 2016;206:331–49.
16. McGeary KA, French MT. Illicit drug use and emergency room utilization. Health Serv Res. 2000;35(1):153–69.
17. Weiss AJ, Barrett ML, Heslin KC, Stocks C. Trends in emergency department visits involving mental and substance use disorders, 2006–2013. HCUP Statistical Brief #216. Rockville: Agency for Healthcare Research and Quality; 2016. Available at http://www.hcup-us.ahrq.gov/reports/statbriefs/sb216-Mental-Substance-Use-Disorder-ED-Visit-Trends.pdf. Accessed 17 Sept 2017.
18. O'Donnell JK, Gladden RM, Seth P. Trends in deaths involving heroin and synthetic opioids excluding methadone, and law enforcement drug product reports, by census region—United States, 2006–2015. MMWR Morb Mortal Wkly Rep. 2017;66:897–903. Available at https://doi.org/10.15585/mmwr.mm6634a2. Accessed 17 Sept 2017.
19. D'Onofrio G, Fiellin DA, Pantalon MV, Chawarski MC, Owens PH, Degutis LC, Busch SH, Bernstein LS, O'Conner PG. A brief intervention reduces hazardous and harmful drinking in emergency department patients. Ann Emerg Med. 2012;60(2):181–92. Available at https://doi.org/10.1016/j.annemergmed.2012.02.006. Accessed 17 Sept 2017.
20. Horn BP, Crandall C, Forcehimes A, French M, Bogenschultz M. Benefit-cost analysis of SBIRT interventions for substance using patients in emergency departments. J Subst Abuse Treat. 2017;79:6–11.
21. McDonald AJ, Wang N, Camargo CA. US emergency department visits for alcohol-related diseases and injuries between 1992 and 2000. Arch Intern Med. 2004;164(5):531–7.
22. Centers for Disease Control and Prevention. Morbidity and Mortality Weekly Report. Opioid overdose prevention programs providing naloxone to laypersons—United States, 2014. Available at http://www.cdc.gov/mmwr/preview/mmwrhtml/mm6423a2.htm. Accessed 30 Sept 2015.
23. Stahre M, Roeber J, Kanny D, Brewer RD, Zhang X. Contribution of excessive alcohol consumption to deaths and years of potential life lost in the United States. Prev Chronic Dis. 2014;11:130293. https://doi.org/10.5888/pcd11.130293.
24. Grant BF, Stinson FS, Dawson DA, Chou SP, Dufour MC, Compton W, Pickering RP, Kaplan K. Prevalence and co-occurrence of substance use disorders and independent mood and anxiety disorders: results from the national epidemiologic survey on alcohol and related conditions. Arch Gen Psychiatry. 2004;61(8):807–16.
25. Cherpitel CJ. Drinking patterns and problems: a comparison of primary care with the emergency room. Subst Abus. 1999;20:85–95.
26. Naeger S. Emergency department visits involving underage alcohol misuse: 2010 to 2013. In: The CBHSQ report. Rockville: Substance Abuse and Mental Health Services Administration (US); 2013. 2017 May 16. Available at https://www.ncbi.nlm.nih.gov/books/NBK436366/. Accessed 23 Sept 2017.
27. Currier GW, Trenton AJ, Walsh PG. Innovations: emergency psychiatry: relative accuracy of breath and serum alcohol readings in the psychiatric emergency service. Psychiatr Serv. 2006;57:34–6.
28. Macmadu A, Carroll JJ, Hadland SE, Green TC, Marshall BD. Prevalence and correlates of fentanyl-contaminated heroin exposure among young adults who use prescription opioids non-medically. Addict Behav. 2017;68:35–8.
29. United States Drug Enforcement Administration. Counterfeit prescription pills containing fentanyls: a global threat. 28 July 2016.
30. United States Drug Enforcement Administration. DEA temporarily bans synthetic opioid U-47700 ("Pink"), linked to nearly 50 deaths. Accessed 23 Sept 2017.
31. United States Drug Enforcement Administration. DEA issues nationwide warning on carfentanil. Accessed 23 Sept 2017.
32. Samuels EA, Hope J, Papp J, Whiteside L, Raja AS, Bernstein E. Naloxone distribution strategies needed in emergency departments. ACEP Now. 2016 March. Available at http://www.acepnow.com/article/naloxone-distribution-strategies-needed-in-emergency-departments/. Accessed 26 Sept 2017.
33. Wheeler E, Jones TS, Gilbert MK, Davidson PJ. Opioid overdose prevention programs providing naloxone to laypersons—United States, 2014. MMWR. 2015;64:23.

34. Marco CA, Jesus JE, Geiderman JM, Baker EF. Naloxone distribution to patients in emergency department raises controversy. ACEP Now. 2016 June. Available at http://www.acepnow.com/article/naloxone-distribution-patients-emergency-department-raises-controversy/. Accessed 26 Sept 2017.
35. D'Onofrio G, O'Connor PG, Pantalon MV, Chawarski MC, Busch SH, Owens PH, Bernstein SL, Fiellin DA. Emergency department-initiated buprenorphine/naloxone treatment for opioid dependence: a randomized clinical trial. JAMA. 2015;28;313(16):1636–44.
36. D'Onofrio G, Chawarski MC, O'Connor PG, Pantalon MV, Busch SH, Owens PH, Hawk K, Bernstein SL, Fiellin DA. Emergency department-initiated buprenorphine for opioid dependence with continuation in primary care: outcomes during and after intervention. J Gen Intern Med. 2017;32(6):660–6.
37. Substance Abuse and Mental Health Services Administration, Center for Behavioral Health Statistics and Quality. The DAWN report: benzodiazepines in combination with opioid pain relievers or alcohol: greater risk of more serious ED visit outcomes. Rockville; 2014. Available at https://www.samhsa.gov/data/sites/default/files/DAWN-SR192-BenzoCombos-2014/DAWN-SR192-BenzoCombos-2014.pdf. Accessed 27 Sept 2017.
38. Galicia M, Nogue S, Miro O. Liquid ecstasy intoxication: clinical features of 505 consecutive emergency department patients. Emerg Med J. 2011;28:462–6.
39. Mason PE, Kerns WP. GAMMA hydroxybutyric acid (GHB) intoxication. Acad Emerg Med. 2002;9(7):730–9.
40. Wryobeck JM, Walton MA, Curran GM, Massey LS, Booth BM. Complexities of cocaine users presenting to the emergency department with chest pain: interactions between depression symptoms, alcohol, and race. J Addict Med. 2007;4:213–21.
41. Vroegop MP, Franssen EJ, van den Voort PHJ, van den Berg TN, Langeweg RJ, Kramers C. The emergency care of cocaine intoxications. Neth J Med. 2009;67(4):122–6.
42. Zhu NY, Legatt DF, Turner AR. Agranulocytosis after consumption of cocaine adulterated with levamisole. Ann Intern Med. 2009;150(4):287–9.
43. Rich JA, Singer DE. Cocaine-related symptoms in patients presenting to an urban emergency department. Ann Emerg Med. 1991;20(6):616–21.
44. Pasic J, Zarkowski P, Nordstrom K, Wilson MP. Psychiatric emergencies for clinicians: emergency department management of cocaine-related presentations. J Emerg Med. 2017. pii: S0736-4679(17)30365-7. https://doi.org/10.1016/j.jemermed.2017.04.023. Epub ahead of print.
45. Zarkowski P, Pasic J, Russo J, Roy-Byrne P. Excessive tears: a diagnostic sign for cocaine-induced mood disorder? Compr Psychiatry. 2007;48:252–6.
46. Substance Abuse and Mental Health Services Administration, Center for Behavioral Health Statistics and Quality. The DAWN report: emergency department visits involving methamphetamine: 2007 to 2011. Rockville; 2014. Available at https://www.samhsa.gov/...EDVisitsMeth.../DAWN-SR167-EDVisitsMeth-2014.htm. Accessed 24 Sept 2017.
47. Al-Tayyib A, Koester S, Langegger S, Raville L. Heroin and methamphetamine injection: an emerging drug use pattern. Subst Use Misuse. 2017:1–8. https://doi.org/10.1080/10826084.2016.1271432. Epub ahead of print. Accessed 25 Mar 2017.
48. Pasic J, Russo J, Ries R, Roy-Byrne P. Methamphetamine users presenting to psychiatric emergency services: a case-control study. Am J Drug Alcohol Abuse. 2007;33:675–86.
49. NIDA. MDMA (Ecstasy/Molly). National Institute on Drug Abuse. 2016 Oct. 12. Available at https://www.drugabuse.gov/publications/drugfacts/mdma-ecstasy-molly. Accessed 26 Sept 2017.
50. Substance Abuse and Mental Health Services Administration, Center for Behavioral Health Statistics and Quality. 2013 Sept. 17. The DAWN report: "Bath Salts" were involved in over 20,000 drug-related emergency department visits in 2011. Rockville, MD. Accessed 26 Sept 2017.
51. NIDA. Synthetic cathinones ("Bath Salts"). National Institute on Drug Abuse website. 2016 Jan. 6. Available at https://www.drugabuse.gov/publications/drugfacts/synthetic-cathinones-bath-salts. Accessed 26 Sept 2017.
52. Gunderson EW, Kirkpatrick MG, Willing LM, Holstege CP. Substituted cathinone products: a new trend in "bath salts" and other designer stimulant drug use. J Addict Med. 2013;7(3):153–62.
53. Ross EA, Watson M, Goldberger B. "Bath Salts" intoxication. N Engl J Med. 2011;365:967–8.
54. Substance Abuse and Mental Health Services Administration, Center for Behavioral Health Statistics and Quality. The DAWN report: emergency department visits involving attention deficit/hyperactivity disorder stimulant medications. Rockville; 2013. Accessed 26 Sept 2017.
55. Substance Abuse and Mental Health Services Administration, Center for Behavioral Health Statistics and Quality. The DAWN report: emergency department visits involving phencyclidine (PCP). Rockville; 2013. Available at https://www.samhsa.gov/data/sites/default/files/DAWN143/DAWN143/sr143-emergency-phencyclidine-2013.pdf. Accessed 27 Sept 2017.
56. Hoffman RJ. Ketamine poisoning. In: Basow DS, editor. UpToDate. Waltham. Available at https://www.uptodate.com/contents/ketamine-poisoning. Accessed 11 Aug 2018.
57. Scheppke KA, Braghiroli J, Shalaby M, Chait R. Prehospital use of IM ketamine for sedation of violent and agitated patients. West J Emerg Med. 2014;15(7):736–41.
58. Passie T, Halpern JH, Stichtenoth DO, Emrich HM, Hintzen A. The pharmacology of lysergic acid diethylamide: a review. CNS Neurosci Ther. 2008;14(4):295–314.
59. Delgado J, Traub ST, Gayzel J. Intoxication from LSD and other common hallucinogens. In: UpToDate. Aug. 2017. Last update Sept 20, 2017. Available at http://

www.uptodate.com/contents/intoxication-from-lsd-and-other-common-hallucinogens. Accessed 29 Sept 2017.

60. Chyka PA, Erdman AR, Manoguerra AS, Christianson G, Booze LL, Nelson LS, Woolf AD, Cobaugh DJ, Caravati EM, Scharman EJ, Troutman WG, American Association of Poison Control Centers. Dextromethorphan poisoning: an evidence-based consensus guideline for out-of-hospital management. Clin Toxicol (Phila). 2007;45:662–77.
61. Howard MO, Bowen SE, Garlan EL, Perron BE, Vaughn MG. Inhalant use and inhalant use disorders in the United States. Addict Sci Clin Pract. 2011;6(1):18–31.
62. Garland EL, Howard MO, Vaughn MG, Perron BE. Volatile substance misuse in the United States. Subst Use Misuse. 2011;46(Suppl. 1):8–20.
63. Bowen SE. Two serious and challenging medical complications associated with volatile substance misuse: sudden sniffing death and fetal solvent syndrome. Subst Use Misuse. 2011;46(Suppl. 1):68–72.
64. Nussbaum A, Thurstone C, Binswanger I. Medical marijuana use and suicide attempt in a patient with major depressive disorder. Am J Psychiatry. 2011;168(8):778–81.
65. Pedersen W. Does cannabis use lead to depression and suicidal behaviors? A populations-based longitudinal study. Acta Psychiatr Scand. 2008;118:395–403.
66. Foti DJ, Kotov R, Guey LT, Bromet EJ. Cannabis use and the course of schizophrenia: 10-year follow-up after first hospitalization. Am J Psychiatry. 2010;167:987–93.
67. Grech A, Van Os J, Jones PB, Lewis SW, Murray RM. Cannabis use and outcome of recent onset psychosis. Eur Psychiatry. 2005;20:349–53.
68. Seely KA, Prather PL, James LP, Moran JH. Marijuana-based drugs: innovative therapeutics or designer drugs of abuse? Mol Interv. 2011;11(1):36–51.
69. NIDA. Synthetic cannabinoids. 2015 Nov. 9. Available at https://www.drugabuse.gov/publications/drugfacts/synthetic-cannabinoids. Accessed 29 Sept 2017.
70. Intoxication from LSD and other common hallucinogens. Poison Control Centers, AAPCC. Last update August 31, 2017. Available at http://www.aapcc.org/alerts/synthetic-cannabinoids/. Accessed 29 Sept 2017.

Part III

Psychiatric Illnesses

6 Co-occurring Substance-Use Disorder in the Emergency Department

Scott A. Simpson and Julie Taub

Introduction

All healthcare professionals working in emergency settings will encounter patients with substance-use disorders. Sixty-four percent of emergency department (ED) patients have problematic substance use, and more than 10% have a significant use disorder [1, 2]. Over the last decade, the number of ED visits involving substance use has increased by 37% [3]. Half of the trauma visits are associated with alcohol use, and generally the presence of a substance-use disorder is associated with higher ED utilization [4, 5].

In this chapter, we review an approach to the ED patient with a substance-use disorder:

1. Treat and stabilize the acute presentation
2. Assess for the presence of substance use
3. Manage the substance-use disorder as appropriate
4. Arrange appropriate disposition

Figure 6.1 summarizes this approach and the involved clinical steps. Throughout the chapter, we emphasize issues in the treatment of a patient with an alcohol-use disorder, as this presentation is common, and the involved complications are complex and life-threatening.

S. A. Simpson (✉)
Department of Behavioral Health Services, Denver Health & Hospital Authority, Denver, CO, USA
e-mail: scott.simpson@dhha.org

J. Taub
Department of Medicine, Denver Health & Hospital Authority, Denver, CO, USA

The Diagnosis of Substance-Use Disorders

Substance-use disorders comprise a group of problematic symptoms and behaviors resulting from drug or alcohol use that result in functional impairment. The Diagnostic and Statistical Manual, Fifth Edition (DSM-5) describes syndromes for specific substances, although the symptoms are similar regardless of substance used [6]. In general, the more symptoms that are present, the greater the severity of illness:

- Greater use of a substance than intended
- Unsuccessful efforts to control substance use
- Spending time obtaining or using substances, or recovering from their use
- Continued use despite recurrent social problems related to use
- Continued use in hazardous situations
- Reducing important occupational or recreational activities because of use
- Tolerance to the effects of a substance
- Characteristic withdrawal symptoms

L. S. Zun et al. (eds.), *Behavioral Emergencies for Healthcare Providers*,
https://doi.org/10.1007/978-3-030-52520-0_6

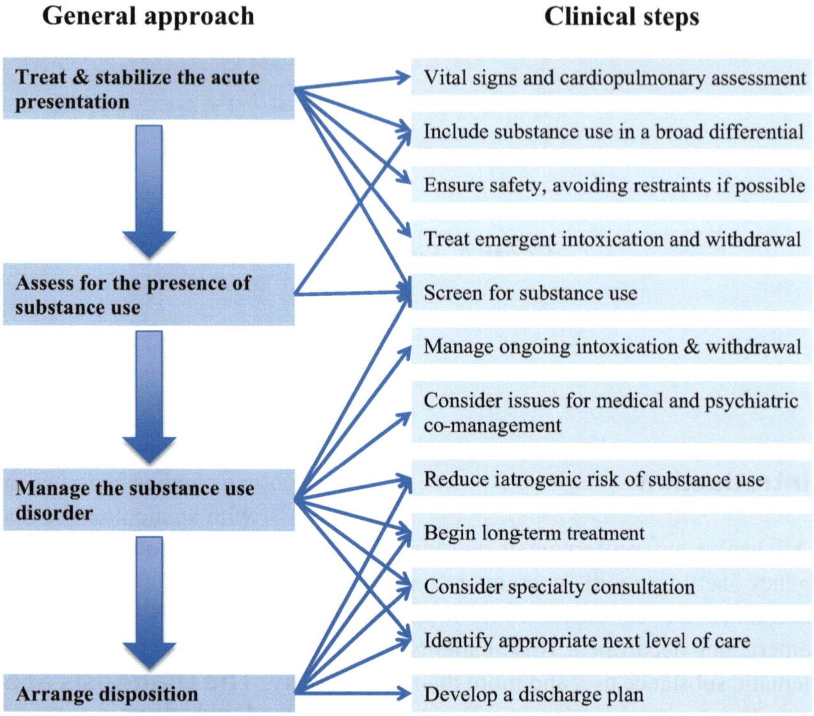

Fig. 6.1 Clinical approach to the ED patient with a substance use disorder

Not all patients who use substances fulfill the criteria for a formal use disorder. Although more than half of Americans are using alcohol in a given month, only about 10% of those have an alcohol-use disorder. About 19% of cannabis users have a cannabis-use disorder, and about 60% of cocaine users have a cocaine-use disorder. Patients may still exhibit risky substance use in the absence of a formal use disorder. For example, almost 40% of young adults have binged on alcohol (had ≥ 5 drinks on the same occasion) in the last month, although most would not fulfill criteria for a DSM-5 use disorder [7].

Treat and Stabilize the Acute Presentation

Substance-use disorders often present in two ways. First, patients present primarily because of the complications related to substance use. For example, a patient intoxicated on alcohol is violent and brought to the ED by the police. Alternatively, patients present for other reasons, and their treatment is complicated by substance use. For example, a patient with pneumonia is at increased risk for mortality because of concurrent alcohol use [8].

Maintain Safety, Stability, and a Broad Differential Diagnosis

As with any medical or behavioral emergency, initial treatment must start with ensuring hemodynamic stability and physical safety. Intravenous (IV) fluids and cardiac monitoring should be initiated as indicated, and the possibility of acute medical illness excluded [9]. Abnormal vital signs may represent the sequelae of substance use, but they may also indicate alternative or concurrent illnesses such as infection. Substance use may be associated with a number of life-threatening presentations:

- Behavioral illness, including agitation, violence, and suicidality.
- Cardiovascular illness, including myocardial infarction or arrhythmias, may occur in the setting of stimulant intoxication and, rarely,

cannabis intoxication. Alcohol withdrawal frequently causes arrhythmias.

- Neurological complications such as intracerebral hemorrhage can occur due to stimulant intoxication. Seizures may occur in the setting of alcohol or benzodiazepine withdrawal. Individuals who smoke are at risk for embolic events. Overdoses may result in a coma.
- Rhabdomyolysis may occur with patients who have been unconscious for prolonged periods or as a result of excited delirium due to stimulant use.
- Dangerous metabolic complications include hyponatremia, hepatic encephalopathy, or thiamine deficiency.

One particularly concerning metabolic complication in patients with severe alcohol-use disorder and malnutrition is beer potomania, in which a hypo-osmolar hyponatremia develops when the kidneys lack sufficient solute to excrete water. In the ED, a patient given just 1 l of IV normal saline may receive sufficient solute (in the form of sodium and chloride) to urinate several liters of fluid and reverse a severe hyponatremia over the course of only a few hours. This rapid reversal puts the patient at risk for central pontine myelinolysis. Thus, IV fluids should be given judiciously and only after evaluating for hyponatremia. A serum osmolality, urine osmolality, and urine sodium should be obtained. If beer potomania is suspected, renal consultation should be considered before administering IV fluids.

Providers must also ensure the safety of the patient and staff. Patients with alcohol and/or stimulant intoxication often arrive at the ED with intense agitation. Emergency medication treatment or physical restraints may be necessary, as described in the related Chap. 24. Also, consider that patients may have received treatment from paramedics prior to ED arrival (see the related Chap. 27).

Treat Emergent Intoxication

The medical implications of intoxication depend on the primary substance involved. Stimulant intoxication induces tachycardia, hyperthermia, and hypertension via its sympathomimetic effects; patients are at risk of myocardial infarction, arrhythmias including QT prolongation, intracerebral hemorrhage, and rhabdomyolysis [10, 11]. Cannabis toxidromes may be of greater intensity and length after the consumption of edible cannabis products [12]. These hyper-adrenergic states contrast with the profile of opioid intoxication, in which patients exhibit bradypnea and hypoactivity. Table 6.1 summarizes several intoxication syndromes and their treatment. See related Chap. 5 on drug intoxication for more guidance on management strategies.

Table 6.1 Clinical features and ED treatment of drug intoxication and withdrawal syndromes

Drug class	Features of intoxication	Treatment of intoxication[a]	Features of withdrawal	Treatment of withdrawal[a]
Alcohol	Belligerence, dysarthria, unsteady gait, smells of alcohol, variable vital signs	Typical antipsychotics, avoid benzodiazepines, may require restraint	Tachycardia, hypertension, diaphoresis, nausea, anxiety, tremor, seizures, psychosis	Benzodiazepines, barbiturates, anticonvulsants
Barbiturates	Bradycardia, hypotension, variable pupillary constriction, comatose	Respiratory support as indicated	Tachycardia, hypertension, diaphoresis, nausea, anxiety, tremor, seizures, psychosis	Benzodiazepines, barbiturates
Benzodiazepines	Vitals often normal, somnolent, comatose	Respiratory support as indicated, generally avoid flumazenil	Tachycardia, hypertension, diaphoresis, nausea, anxiety, tremor, seizures, psychosis	Benzodiazepines, barbiturates

(continued)

Table 6.1 (continued)

Drug class	Features of intoxication	Treatment of intoxication[a]	Features of withdrawal	Treatment of withdrawal[a]
Cannabis	Tachycardia, slowed speech lethargy, injected sclera, psychosis, smells of cannabis	Low-dose benzodiazepine or atypical antipsychotic	Irritability, anxiety, insomnia, decreased sleep, restlessness	Symptomatic treatment
Cocaine	Tachycardia, hypertension, dilated pupils, impulsive, agitation, perspiration, psychosis	Benzodiazepine	Fatigue, unpleasant dreams, irritability, somnolence, increased appetite	Symptomatic treatment
Dissociatives (ketamine, dextromethorphan)	Tachycardia and hypertension, psychomotor retardation	Benzodiazepine	Insomnia	Symptomatic treatment
Hallucinogens	Tachycardia, hypertension, dilated pupils, diaphoresis, impoverished thought process, psychosis, hyponatremia	Benzodiazepine, low stimulation environment	Clinically insignificant, may include fatigue, irritability, anhedonia	Symptomatic treatment
Inhalants	Nystagmus, incoordination, dysarthria, depressed reflexes, tremor, coma	Respiratory support as indicated	Tachycardia, diaphoresis	Symptomatic treatment
Opioids	Bradypnea, poor oxygen saturation, constricted pupils, dysarthria, lethargic	Respiratory support and oxygen as indicated; naloxone	Fever, dilated pupils, piloerection, dysphoria, nausea, muscle aches, diarrhea, fever, yawning	Opioid substitution (methadone or buprenorphine), clonidine, symptomatic treatment
MDMA	Tachycardia and hypertension, dilated pupils, awake, hypersexual	Benzodiazepine, low stimulation environment	Clinically insignificant, may include muscle pain	Symptomatic treatment
Methamphetamine	Tachycardia, hypertension, dilated pupils, agitation, psychosis, affective instability, leukocytosis	Benzodiazepine, atypical antipsychotic, may require restraint	Fatigue, unpleasant dreams, irritability, somnolence, increased appetite, diarrhea	Symptomatic treatment
PCP	Tachycardia, hypertension, dilated pupils, vertical nystagmus, hyperacusis, agitation, psychosis, belligerence	Benzodiazepine, antipsychotics, may require restraint	Somnolence, anxiety, diaphoresis	Symptomatic treatment

[a]All patients should receive supportive treatment including intravenous fluids, oxygen, and possible cardiac monitoring

Treat Emergent Withdrawal

Withdrawal syndromes may also require immediate treatment. As with toxidromes, the particular withdrawal syndrome reflects the substance of choice and may be indistinguishable from other psychiatric or medical illnesses. Table 6.1 summarizes some withdrawal syndromes and their treatment.

It is most important to recognize alcohol, benzodiazepine, or barbiturate withdrawal, as these syndromes may rapidly progress to life-threatening agitation, seizures, and delirium tremens. Moreover, early recognition and treatment of alcohol withdrawal in the ED improve mortality [13]. Risk factors for alcohol withdrawal include a history of withdrawal symptoms, concurrent misuse of benzodiazepines, increased autonomic activity, or a blood alcohol level (BAL) of 200 or greater on presentation [14]. Acute medical or traumatic comorbidities increase the risk of severe withdrawal [15].

ED patients with an alcohol-use disorder often require treatment for withdrawal before their BAL decreases to zero, especially if the patient maintains a BAL above 300. Serious withdrawal can occur before the BAL is zero. Seizures may be the first sign of withdrawal and typically occur within the first few hours—and almost always within 48 hours—of the patient's last drink [16]. For example, a patient who typically maintains a BAL near 400 may seize with an elevated BAL. One-third of patients who experience a seizure will develop delirium tremens [16, 17].

There are three main pharmacologic approaches to treating alcohol withdrawal: front-loading, symptom-triggered, and a standing fixed taper method. Benzodiazepines are the mainstay of alcohol withdrawal treatment [18].

Front-loading involves administering high medication doses early in the course of withdrawal—for example, diazepam 20 mg IV every 5 minutes until the patient is sedated. Benzodiazepines with a quick onset of action and long half-life are ideal for front-loading, as they rapidly control symptoms and can self-taper over time [19]. Patients can be dosed in the presence of symptoms or the level of sedation (e.g., until their Richmond Agitation-Sedation Scale score is −1 or −2) [20]. Front-loading phenobarbitol decreases the risk of an intensive care unit admission and, later, more aggressive medication treatment [21]. Lorazepam drips—which are sometimes confused with front-loading, but rather are given over longer periods of time—should be avoided due to the risk of excessive sedation and prolonged lengths of stay.

Symptom-triggered benzodiazepine regimens provide safe, comfortable withdrawal, although they have limitations. Symptom scales must be administered by an experienced nurse or clinician, and patients must be able to appropriately answer questions. Some patients might score points for reasons other than alcohol withdrawal (e.g., due to anxiety from a primary psychiatric disorder) and thereby receive excessive medication. Patients who cannot be reliably assessed with a symptom-triggered scale should be treated with the fixed tapering regimen or front-loading approach.

Assess for the Presence of Substance Use

The assessment of substance use often begins with the provider's initial approach to the patient, when acute intoxication or withdrawal is part of a broad differential diagnosis. Less commonly considered are the implications of comorbid substance when treating other illnesses. Yet, the most common reason for patients with substance use to present to the ED is common illness [22]. Nonintoxicated ED trauma patients screen positive for substance-use disorders up to 46% of the time [23]. Providers should have little to no threshold to screen patients for substance-use disorders. Patients with frequent ED utilization, accidents or traumas, and substance-related presentations may particularly benefit from screening, as these conditions correlate with problematic substance use.

All patients with psychiatric symptoms should be screened for substance-use disorders. Many toxidromes induce psychiatric symptoms, including hallucinations, delusions, disorientation, and impaired consciousness. Acute psychiatric symptoms alone are insufficient to differentiate among etiologies, due to primary mental illness, delirium, or substance-induced conditions [24]. Additional history, laboratory testing, collateral information, or prolonged observation may be necessary for an accurate diagnosis.

Screening for substance use can begin with only a single question. The National Institute on Drug Abuse (NIDA) Quick Screen begins with an initial inquiry as to whether the patient has used illegal drugs, prescription drugs for nonmedical reasons, tobacco, or alcohol excessively (≥5 drinks/day for men or 4 for women) in the past year [25]. A response of "yes" merits further evaluation, perhaps using the Alcohol, Smoking, and Substance Involvement Screening Test (ASSIST) or Alcohol Use Disorders Identification Test (AUDIT) [26]. Another screening approach is the Drug Abuse Screening Test Modified for ED (DAST-ED), which incorporates brief questions for all substances [9]. In general, screening for greater frequency of use is more likely to identify patients with significant substance-use disorders (greater specificity) at the cost of missing some patients who may benefit from treatment (less sensitivity) [27].

Toxicology testing offers minimal diagnostic value when evaluating substance-use disorders and is unlikely to alter disposition decisions from the ED [28, 29]. Instead, the use of screeners and a clinical history are more valuable for diagnosis. Acute clinical signs, including vitals and physical examination findings, help identify acute intoxication or withdrawal. Toxicology testing in the ED is most helpful when the patient's mental status precludes a reliable history or the diagnosis is unclear.

Manage the Substance-Use Disorder

Once the patient has sobered and the presence of a substance-use disorder ascertained, providers will need to manage the use disorder in the setting of ongoing medical illness and provide appropriate treatment for the use disorder.

Manage Ongoing Withdrawal

Most withdrawal syndromes are not life-threatening, but they do complicate treatment and disposition from the ED. For example, patients with methamphetamine withdrawal experience intense dysphoria and psychomotor retardation such that they may be unable to provide a history, participate in treatment decisions, or discharge safely.

Opioid withdrawal is uncomfortable—so much so that these patients are more likely to leave the hospital prior to the completion of treatment [30]. Patients may benefit from the administration of methadone or buprenorphine to prevent detoxification while hospitalized. Patients who withdraw will be at increased risk for overdosing after hospital discharge, due to their decreased tolerance; maintaining tolerance with opioid substitution reduces this risk.

Consider Issues for Medical Management

Emergency providers must consider the impact of substance-use disorders on treatment plans for other medical conditions. For example, patients with opioid-use disorders and significant tolerance will require higher opioid doses for pain control; patients with sedative–hypnotic use are at risk for respiratory depression when administered opioids. The presence of an alcohol-use disorder may increase the risk of in-hospital mortality for conditions commonly seen in the ED, including pneumonia and orthopedic injuries [8, 31]. Substance use is a risk factor for early hospital discharge [30, 32, 33], and early discharge correlates with a greater 30-day mortality risk [34].

Pathology related to substance use must be considered when delivering treatment. For example, patients with an alcohol-use disorder are often deficient in thiamine and may develop an iatrogenic Wernicke's encephalopathy if given IV glucose prior to thiamine replenishment. Beer potomania should be considered in patients with hyponatremia who have an alcohol-use disorder. And alcohol use incurs significant liver toxicity that alters drug metabolism.

Consider Issues for Psychiatric Management

Substance-use disorders and other psychiatric illnesses are syndemic—co-occurring and exacerbating one another. The presence of a psychiatric disorder is a risk factor for the development of a substance-use disorder, and around half of illicit drug users have a psychiatric diagnosis besides their use disorder [2]. Among patients with severe mental illness, more than 20% have a substance-use disorder, which is associated with higher rates of hospitalization, suicide, and violence [35]. Some substance-use disorders are primarily restricted to the mentally ill, as with anticholinergic drugs among patients with schizophrenia [36].

In the ED, the presence of the comorbid substance and other psychiatric illness makes diagnosis challenging. In general, the quality of presenting symptoms is insufficient to discern whether psychiatric symptoms are substance-induced. Comorbid diagnosis also makes disposition difficult, as many substance treatment facilities cannot manage other psychiatric illnesses. Patients with behavioral dyscontrol or other psychiatric illness may require a higher level of care for detoxification. (See section "Arrange Appropriate Disposition.")

Reduce Iatrogenic Risk of Substance Use

The rise of opioid-related deaths has brought scrutiny to prescription practices in the ED. More than 40% of opioid prescriptions from the ED are likely to be misused [37]. Patients receiving larger opioid prescriptions from ED providers are more likely to transition to long-term opioid use than similar patients receiving lower doses [38]. Particular patterns of drug-seeking behavior—for example, requests for early refills or demanding behaviors—have not proven to be reliable in identifying the risk of misuse [39]. Risk factors for aberrant opioid use include a history of use disorders, a history of sexual abuse, and certain psychiatric illnesses including schizophrenia, attention-deficit/hyperactivity disorder, depression, and obsessive-compulsive disorder [40].

Benzodiazepine prescriptions should be avoided on ED discharge. Benzodiazepine misuse is frequently associated with emergency department visits [41]. Although providers often feel the urge to prescribe these medications for anxious patients, benzodiazepines are contraindicated for many types of anxiety, including post-traumatic stress—a condition for which these medications are not only unhelpful but also increase the risk of substance use [42]. Benzodiazepine prescriptions are also associated with self-harm after ED discharge [43]. ED providers should only consider bridging prescriptions after discussion with the patient's primary provider. Patients with risk of mild or moderate alcohol withdrawal syndromes on discharge may benefit from a prescription for carbamazepine, gabapentin, or another nonbenzodiazepine regimen [44].

All clinicians should review a patient's history in a prescription-monitoring database before prescribing opioids or benzodiazepines. Clinicians should be aware of local rules governing opioid prescribing. Many states and health systems have implemented policies governing ED prescriptions [45, 46].

Begin Long-Term Treatment

Effective interventions for substance-use disorder in the ED help patients achieve sobriety and reduce ED recidivism. Although many ED providers will deliver these interventions on their own, a dedicated consultant or substance-use specialist may provide additional support for the identification and treatment of use disorders. One model for providing this care is screening, brief intervention, and referral for treatment (SBIRT), described in the inset.

Motivational interviewing (MI) is a brief counseling method designed to explore a patient's ambivalence about behavior change and emphasize the patient's motivation for positive change [47]. MI interventions no longer than 10–15 minutes can reduce substance use, and MI appears even more effective when reiterated [48, 49]. MI may be combined with other treatment modalities, including problem-solving therapy and directed feedback to enhance treatment efficacy [50, 51].

Growing evidence speaks to the efficacy of initiating pharmacotherapy for relapse prevention in the ED. For example, a randomized trial demonstrated that initiating buprenorphine in the ED for opioid-dependent patients improved rates of treatment adherence after 30 days to 78%, compared to 37–45% for patients in non-medication control groups [52]. In another trial, a multimodal pharmacotherapy and MI intervention for smoking cessation delivered in the ED achieved abstinence rates of 12%, compared to 5% of controls [53]. Gabapentin and opioid antagonists reduce heavy alcohol consumption [54, 55].

Screening, Brief Intervention, and Referral for Treatment (SBIRT)

SBIRT is a public health approach designed to identify and treat patients with substance-use disorders in clinical settings [56]. SBIRT has been widely adopted in EDs and recommended by the American College of Surgeons for Level I Trauma Centers. The SBIRT model typically starts with a standardized screening program comprised of a patient's self-report or a clinician's referral. A trained SBIRT counselor then conducts a brief intervention most often comprised of motivational interviewing. Finally, appropriate treatment referrals are provided.

SBIRT programs have demonstrated the prominence of substance-use disorders in the ED and how the ED visit is a teachable moment to engage patients in treatment. The expertise provided by embedded SBIRT teams increases the capacity of trauma centers to address substance-use disorders, and SBIRT provides a platform to initiate novel treatments for relapse prevention [57]. Published data suggest that for every $1 spent on SBIRT in the ED, $3.81 is saved—a savings of several hundred dollars per patient per month—although other analyses are less conclusive [23, 58, 59].

There are several challenges to implementing SBIRT. Reimbursement rates have traditionally been poor [56]. Although SBIRT appears helpful for patients with mild or even moderate use disorders, there is less evidence of efficacy in severe use disorders [59, 60]. It remains unclear what populations are most likely to benefit [27].

Arrange Appropriate Disposition

After a substance-use disorder has been diagnosed and treatment initiated, the ED clinician must arrange a suitable disposition. Successfully connecting patients to outpatient care after their ED visit reduces future substance use, hospitalizations, and ED recidivism [61].

Patients with substance-use disorders often have multiple medical, psychiatric, and social needs complicating disposition. The American Society of Addiction Medicine (ASAM) placement criteria help guide disposition for patients with substance-use disorders [62]. Considerations for disposition include the risk of withdrawal, the existence of medical or psychiatric conditions, the patient's readiness to change, the potential for relapse, and psychosocial needs. For example, a patient at low risk of withdrawal, with stable chronic medical illness and a supportive social network, is often appropriate for outpatient referral and a 12-step program (e.g., Alcoholics Anonymous). On the other hand, hospitalization is typically indicated for alcohol and benzodiazepine withdrawal syndromes occurring in the presence of comorbid medical illness [63]. Between those levels of care exist intensive outpatient programs, "social detoxification" programs, sober living environments, and other recovery programs, depending on locale. An ED clinician should be familiar with local treatment resources.

Consult Mental Health in the ED if Necessary

Suicide and violence risk should be assessed in all patients with substance-use disorders. Particularly when co-occurring with mental illness, substance use confers considerable risk for self-harm and suicide [54, 64]. Patients considered to be at elevated risk for self-harm or violence merit mental health consultation, if available.

Other indications for mental health consultation depend on local resources and the ED clinician's facility with psychiatric care. In general, patients with co-occurring substance use and mental illness may benefit from diagnostic clarification by a psychiatrist or mental health specialist. These patients are often challenging to treat. For example, a patient with intense anxiety and a history of substance misuse who is requesting benzodiazepines is more likely to benefit from alternative pharmacotherapy or brief psychotherapy in the ED. Or a patient with a severe substance-use disorder who is not interested in stopping may benefit from an SBIRT consult for motivational interviewing and disposition recommendations according to the ASAM placement criteria.

Develop a Discharge Plan

Most patients with substance-use disorders in the ED will be discharged home. The risk of iatrogenic harm from prescription medication should be managed using the strategies described in this chapter. ED clinicians should also screen for suicide and violence risk; patients and family should be advised to remove firearms from the home and secure dangerous medications [65]. Arranging an appointment for the patient prior to discharge—rather than providing only a phone number—improves the probability of successful follow-up [66, 67].

For patients who are not yet ready to quit using substances, clinicians should consider offering a peer-based recovery resource, such as the local hotline or website for Alcoholics Anonymous (www.aa.org) or SMART Recovery (www.smartrecovery.org). In the United States, the Suicide Prevention Lifeline number (800-273-8255(TALK)) can be provided to patients and families not only for emergencies but also as a resource for identifying substance treatment in the future.

Conclusion

Many ED clinicians feel frustrated treating patients with substance-use disorders, particularly when patients present repeatedly to the ED. These patients share their providers' frustration: Substance-use disorders are deadly diseases that bring patients to the ED and complicate the treatment of other conditions. Good treatment is difficult to access and sometimes of limited efficacy.

Fortunately, ED providers can help patients achieve sobriety, avoid relapse, and live longer. Emergency providers are in a unique position to ascertain substance use among patients who infrequently encounter other healthcare providers and, in a moment, when they may be particularly open to change [2]. An awareness of the risks of substance use helps clinicians practice more safely and effectively. As the science of addiction medicine grows, health care professionals in the ED will play an increasingly vital role in treating substance-use disorders.

References

1. Sanjuan PM, Rice SL, Witkiewitz K, Mandler RN, Crandall C, Bogenschutz MP. Alcohol, tobacco, and drug use among emergency department patients. Drug Alcohol Depend. 2014;138:32–8.
2. Wu LT, Gersing KR, Swartz MS, Burchett B, Li TK, Blazer DG. Using electronic health records data to assess comorbidities of substance use and psychiatric diagnoses and treatment settings among adults. J Psychiatr Res. 2013;47(4):555–63.
3. Trends in emergency department visits involving mental and substance use disorders, 2006–2013. Rockville, MD: Agency for Healthcare Research and Quality. 2016. Updated December 6, 2016. Available at https://www.hcup-us.ahrq.gov/reports/statbriefs/sb216-Mental-Substance-Use-Disorder-ED-Visit-Trends.jsp. Accessed 17 Aug 2017.
4. Strezsak V, Baird J, Lee CS, Mello MJ. Cross-sectional study of risky substance use by injured emergency department patients. West J Emerg Med. 2017;18(3):345–8.
5. Vu F, Daeppen JB, Hugli O, Iglesias K, Stucki S, Paroz S, et al. Screening of mental health and substance users in frequent users of a general Swiss emergency department. BMC Emerg Med. 2015;15:27.
6. American Psychiatric Association. Diagnostic and statistical manual of mental disorders: DSM-V. 5th ed. Arlington, VA: American Psychiatric Association; 2013.
7. Substance Abuse and Mental Health Services Administration. Behavioral health trends in the United States: results from the 2014 National Survey on Drug Use and Health. Rockville: National Institutes of Health. 2015. Updated September 2015. Available at https://www.samhsa.gov/data/sites/default/files/NSDUH-FRR1-2014/NSDUH-FRR1-2014.pdf. Accessed 21 Aug 2017.
8. Gili-Miner M, Lopez-Mendez J, Bejar-Prado L, Ramirez-Ramirez G, Vilches-Arenas A, Sala-Turrens J. Alcohol use disorders and community-acquired pneumococcal pneumonia: associated mortality, pro-

longed hospital stay and increased hospital spending. Arch Bronconeumol. 2015;51(11):564–70.
9. Howes DS, Sanders AN. Management of the emergency department patient with co-occurring substance abuse disorder. In: Zun L, Chepenik LG, Mallory MN, editors. Behavioral emergencies for the emergency physician. Cambridge, UK: Cambridge University Press; 2013. p. 150–63.
10. Vroegop MP, Franssen EJ, van der Voort PH, van den Berg TN, Langeweg RJ, Kramers C. The emergency care of cocaine intoxications. Neth J Med. 2009;67(4):122–6.
11. Bazmi E, Mousavi F, Giahchin L, Mokhtari T, Behnoush B. Cardiovascular complications of acute amphetamine abuse: cross-sectional study. Sultan Qaboos Univ Med J. 2017;17(1):e31–e7.
12. Bui QM, Simpson S, Nordstrom K. Psychiatric and medical management of marijuana intoxication in the emergency department. West J Emerg Med. 2015;16(3):414–7.
13. Khan A, Levy P, DeHorn S, Miller W, Compton S. Predictors of mortality in patients with delirium tremens. Acad Emerg Med. 2008;15(8):788–90.
14. Maldonado JR, Sher Y, Das S, Hills-Evans K, Frenklach A, Lolak S, et al. Prospective validation study of the prediction of alcohol withdrawal severity scale (PAWSS) in medically ill inpatients: a new scale for the prediction of complicated alcohol withdrawal syndrome. Alcohol Alcohol. 2015;50(5):509–18.
15. Foy A, March S, Drinkwater V. Use of an objective clinical scale in the assessment and management of alcohol withdrawal in a large general hospital. Alcohol Clin Exp Res. 1988;12(3):360–4.
16. Victor M, Brausch C. The role of abstinence in the genesis of alcoholic epilepsy. Epilepsia. 1967;8(1):1–20.
17. Victor M, Adams RD. The effect of alcohol on the nervous system. Res Publ Assoc Res Nerv Ment Dis. 1953;32:526–73.
18. Mayo-Smith MF, Beecher LH, Fischer TL, Gorelick DA, Guillaume JL, Hill A, et al. Management of alcohol withdrawal delirium. An evidence-based practice guideline. Arch Intern Med. 2004;164(13):1405–12.
19. Gold JA, Rimal B, Nolan A, Nelson LS. A strategy of escalating doses of benzodiazepines and phenobarbital administration reduces the need for mechanical ventilation in delirium tremens. Crit Care Med. 2007;35(3):724–30.
20. Sessler CN, Gosnell MS, Grap MJ, Brophy GM, O'Neal PV, Keane KA, et al. The Richmond Agitation-Sedation Scale: validity and reliability in adult intensive care unit patients. Am J Respir Crit Care Med. 2002;166(10):1338–44.
21. Rosenson J, Clements C, Simon B, Vieaux J, Graffman S, Vahidnia F, et al. Phenobarbital for acute alcohol withdrawal: a prospective randomized double-blind placebo-controlled study. J Emerg Med. 2013;44(3):592–8.
22. Espi Martinez F, Nieto Munuera J, Noguera Velasco JA, Espi FF. Detecting substance abuse in the emergency department: a 10-year comparative study. ISRN Emerg Med. 2013;2013:7.
23. Gentilello LM, Ebel BE, Wickizer TM, Salkever DS, Rivara FP. Alcohol interventions for trauma patients treated in emergency departments and hospitals: a cost benefit analysis. Ann Surg. 2005;241(4):541–50.
24. Medhus S, Mordal J, Holm B, Morland J, Bramness JG. A comparison of symptoms and drug use between patients with methamphetamine associated psychoses and patients diagnosed with schizophrenia in two acute psychiatric wards. Psychiatry Res. 2013;206(1):17–21.
25. National Institute on Drug Abuse. The NIDA quick screen 2012. Updated March 1, 2012. Available at https://www.drugabuse.gov/publications/resource-guide-screening-drug-use-in-general-medical-settings/nida-quick-screen. Accessed 21 Aug 2017.
26. Saunders JB, Aasland OG, Babor TF, de la Fuente JR, Grant M. Development of the alcohol use disorders identification test (AUDIT): WHO Collaborative Project on early detection of persons with harmful alcohol consumption—II. Addiction. 1993;88(6):791–804.
27. Merchant RC, Liu T, Baird JR. Variations in substance use prevalence estimates and need for interventions among adult emergency department patients based on different screening strategies using the ASSIST. West J Emerg Med. 2016;17(3):302–14.
28. Kroll DS, Smallwood J, Chang G. Drug screens for psychiatric patients in the emergency department: evaluation and recommendations. Psychosomatics. 2013;54(1):60–6.
29. Wilson MP, Nordstrom K, Anderson EL, Ng AT, Zun LS, Peltzer-Jones JM, et al. American Association for Emergency Psychiatry Task Force on medical clearance of adult psychiatric patients. Part II: controversies over medical assessment, consensus recommendations. West J Emerg Med. 2017;18(4):640–6.
30. Ti L, Milloy MJ, Buxton J, McNeil R, Dobrer S, Hayashi K, et al. Factors associated with leaving hospital against medical advice among people who use illicit drugs in Vancouver, Canada. PLoS One. 2015;10(10):e0141594.
31. Gili-Miner M, Bejar-Prado L, Gili-Ortiz E, Ramirez-Ramirez G, Lopez-Mendez J, Lopez-Millan JM, et al. Alcohol use disorders among surgical patients: unplanned 30-days readmissions, length of hospital stay, excessive costs and mortality. Drug Alcohol Depend. 2014;137:55–61.
32. Lee CA, Cho JP, Choi SC, Kim HH, Park JO. Patients who leave the emergency department against medical advice. Clin Exp Emerg Med. 2016;3(2):88–94.
33. Anis AH, Sun H, Guh DP, Palepu A, Schechter MT, O'Shaughnessy MV. Leaving hospital against medical advice among HIV-positive patients. CMAJ. 2002;167(6):633–7.
34. Yong TY, Fok JS, Hakendorf P, Ben-Tovim D, Thompson CH, Li JY. Characteristics and outcomes

of discharges against medical advice among hospitalised patients. Intern Med J. 2013;43(7):798–802.
35. Buckley PF. Prevalence and consequences of the dual diagnosis of substance abuse and severe mental illness. J Clin Psychiatry. 2006;67(Suppl. 7):5–9.
36. Wells BG, Marken PA, Rickman LA, Brown CS, Hamann G, Grimmig J. Characterizing anticholinergic abuse in community mental health. J Clin Psychopharmacol. 1989;9(6):431–5.
37. Lyapustina T, Castillo R, Omaki E, Shields W, McDonald E, Rothman R, et al. The contribution of the emergency department to opioid pain reliever misuse and diversion: a critical review. Pain Pract. 2017;17(8):1097–104.
38. Barnett ML, Olenski AR, Jena AB. Opioid-prescribing patterns of emergency physicians and risk of long-term use. N Engl J Med. 2017;376(7):663–73.
39. Grover CA, Elder JW, Close RJ, Curry SM. How frequently are "classic" drug-seeking behaviors used by drug-seeking patients in the emergency department? West J Emerg Med. 2012;13(5):416–21.
40. Webster LR, Webster RM. Predicting aberrant behaviors in opioid-treated patients: preliminary validation of the opioid risk tool. Pain Med. 2005;6(6):432–42.
41. Bachhuber MA, Maughan BC, Mitra N, Feingold J, Starrels JL. Prescription monitoring programs and emergency department visits involving benzodiazepine misuse: early evidence from 11 United States metropolitan areas. Int J Drug Policy. 2016;28:120–3.
42. Department of Veterans Affairs, Department of Defense. VA/DOD clinical practice guideline for the management of posttraumatic stress disorder and acute stress disorder: clinician summary. Washington, DC. 2017. Updated June 2017. Available at https://www.healthquality.va.gov/guidelines/MH/ptsd/VADoDPTSDCPGClinicianSummaryFinal.pdf. Accessed 21 Aug 2017.
43. Cooper J, Kapur N, Dunning J, Guthrie E, Appleby L, Mackway-Jones K. A clinical tool for assessing risk after self-harm. Ann Emerg Med. 2006;48(4):459–66.
44. Maldonado JR. Novel algorithms for the prophylaxis and management of alcohol withdrawal syndromes-beyond benzodiazepines. Crit Care Clin. 2017;33(3):559–99.
45. Broida RI, Gronowski T, Kalnow AF, Little AG, Lloyd CM. State emergency department opioid guidelines: current status. West J Emerg Med. 2017;18(3):340–4.
46. Osborn SR, Yu J, Williams B, Vasilyadis M, Blackmore CC. Changes in provider prescribing patterns after implementation of an emergency department prescription opioid policy. J Emerg Med. 2017;52(4):538–46.
47. Miller WR, Rollnick S. Motivational interviewing: helping people change. 3rd ed. New York, NY: Guilford Press; 2013.
48. Rubak S, Sandbaek A, Lauritzen T, Christensen B. Motivational interviewing: a systematic review and meta-analysis. Br J Gen Pract. 2005;55(513):305–12.
49. Kohler S, Hofmann A. Can motivational interviewing in emergency care reduce alcohol consumption in young people? A systematic review and meta-analysis. Alcohol Alcohol. 2015;50(2):107–17.
50. Sorsdahl K, Stein DJ, Corrigall J, Cuijpers P, Smits N, Naledi T, et al. The efficacy of a blended motivational interviewing and problem solving therapy intervention to reduce substance use among patients presenting for emergency services in South Africa: a randomized controlled trial. Subst Abuse Treat Prev Policy. 2015;10(1):46.
51. Blow FC, Walton MA, Bohnert ASB, Ignacio RV, Chermack S, Cunningham RM, et al. A randomized controlled trial of brief interventions to reduce drug use among adults in a low-income urban emergency department: the HealthiER You study. Addiction. 2017;112(8):1395–405.
52. D'Onofrio G, O'Connor PG, Pantalon MV, Chawarski MC, Busch SH, Owens PH, et al. Emergency department-initiated buprenorphine/naloxone treatment for opioid dependence: a randomized clinical trial. JAMA. 2015;313(16):1636–44.
53. Bernstein SL, D'Onofrio G, Rosner J, O'Malley S, Makuch R, Busch S, et al. Successful tobacco dependence treatment in low-income emergency department patients: a randomized trial. Ann Emerg Med. 2015;66(2):140–7.
54. Jarosz J, Miernik K, Wachal M, Walczak J, Krumpl G. Naltrexone (50 mg) plus psychotherapy in alcohol-dependent patients: a meta-analysis of randomized controlled trials. Am J Drug Alcohol Abuse. 2013;39(3):144–60.
55. Anton RF, Myrick H, Wright TM, Latham PK, Baros AM, Waid LR, et al. Gabapentin combined with naltrexone for the treatment of alcohol dependence. Am J Psychiatry. 2011;168(7):709–17.
56. Agerwala SM, McCance-Katz EF. Integrating screening, brief intervention, and referral to treatment (SBIRT) into clinical practice settings: a brief review. J Psychoactive Drugs. 2012;44(4):307–17.
57. Bernstein SL, D'Onofrio G. Screening, treatment initiation, and referral for substance use disorders. Addict Sci Clin Pract. 2017;12(1):18.
58. Estee S, Wickizer T, He L, Shah MF, Mancuso D. Evaluation of the Washington state screening, brief intervention, and referral to treatment project: cost outcomes for Medicaid patients screened in hospital emergency departments. Med Care. 2010;48(1):18–24.
59. Horn BP, Crandall C, Forcehimes A, French MT, Bogenschutz M. Benefit-cost analysis of SBIRT interventions for substance using patients in emergency departments. J Subst Abuse Treat. 2017;79:6–11.
60. Glass JE, Hamilton AM, Powell BJ, Perron BE, Brown RT, Ilgen MA. Specialty substance use disorder services following brief alcohol intervention: a meta-analysis of randomized controlled trials. Addiction. 2015;110(9):1404–15.
61. Neighbors CJ, Zywiak WH, Stout RL, Hoffmann NG. Psychobehavioral risk factors, substance treat-

ment engagement and clinical outcomes as predictors of emergency department use and medical hospitalization. J Stud Alcohol. 2005;66(2):295–304.
62. Mee-Lee D, American Society of Addiction Medicine. The ASAM criteria: treatment for addictive, substance-related, co-occurring conditions. 3rd ed. Chevy Chase, MD: American Society of Addiction Medicine; 2013.
63. Simpson SA, Wilson MP, Nordstrom K. Psychiatric emergencies for clinicians: emergency department management of alcohol withdrawal. J Emerg Med. 2016;51(3):269–73.
64. Ostergaard MLD, Nordentoft M, Hjorthoj C. Associations between substance use disorders and suicide or suicide attempts in people with mental illness: a Danish nation-wide, prospective, register-based study of patients diagnosed with schizophrenia, bipolar disorder, unipolar depression or personality disorder. Addiction. 2017;112(7):1250–9.
65. Nordentoft M, Erlangsen A, Madsen T. Removing firearms from the home after attempted suicide can be life saving. Am J Psychiatry. 2017;174(8):721–2.
66. Magnusson AR, Hedges JR, Vanko M, McCarten K, Moorhead JC. Follow-up compliance after emergency department evaluation. Ann Emerg Med. 1993;22(3):560–7.
67. Kyriacou DN, Handel D, Stein AC, Nelson RR. BRIEF REPORT: factors affecting outpatient follow-up compliance of emergency department patients. J Gen Intern Med. 2005;20(10):938–42.

7 Depression in the Emergency Department

David Hoyer

Introduction

Depression is an increasingly common disease worldwide. Depressive disorders were the largest contributor to nonfatal health loss globally in 2015 [1]. In that year, over 16 million adults suffered from the disease in the United States [2]. Depression is even more common in emergency department (ED) patients: 22–42% of patients fulfill criteria for major depression [3–5].

The American Board of Emergency Medicine identifies depression as "Emergent" in importance for clinicians to identify in patients, given its implications for treatment and prognosis [6]. The United States Preventive Services Task Force recommends routine screening for depression in adults, and the American Heart Association has recommended routine screening for depression in patients with heart disease [7, 8]. Depression is associated with worse physical health outcomes, ED recidivism, and poor patient satisfaction [9–14]. The treatment of depression results in fewer ED visits, provides greater patient satisfaction, and alleviates somatic manifestations that may otherwise result in further workup and testing [15]. Moreover, the ED clinician who detects depression "can prevent patients from decompensation into an acute psychiatric emergency" [15].

Although the stigma of mental illness has been lessening in recent years, both patients and clinicians often remain reticent to discuss depression—resulting in underdiagnosis, undertreatment [3], and increased health care costs [16, 17]. In this environment, the ED visit provides an excellent opportunity to diagnose and treat patients with undiagnosed mental illness [18]. This chapter describes the identification and treatment of patients with depression in the emergency department through a typical case example.

Case Example

Mrs. Smith is a 52-year-old female brought to the ED by her daughter for chest pain that lasted 4 hours after awakening the patient at midnight, and went away en route to the hospital. Her vital signs are unremarkable on arrival. Dr. Jones, the emergency physician, receives the report from the nurse and pushes the portable electronic medical record station in to see the patient, who appears to be in no apparent distress. Mrs. Smith is a pleasant patient who relates that her pain was substernal but otherwise cannot provide a detailed description of her pain. She does share that her

The original version of this chapter was previously published without open access. A correction to this chapter is available at https://doi.org/10.1007/978-3-030-52520-0_48

D. Hoyer (✉)
First Choice ER, First Texas Hospital,
Houston, TX, USA

L. S. Zun et al. (eds.), *Behavioral Emergencies for Healthcare Providers*,
https://doi.org/10.1007/978-3-030-52520-0_7

pain was not worsened by anything and was not alleviated by an antacid pill. "Maybe," Mrs. Smith says, she felt "a little" short of breath.

At this point, Mrs. Smith's daughter interjects that her mother has been visiting for the past week and hasn't been "her usual self," and that she brought the patient in to make sure she "is not having a heart attack." Dr. Jones records a past history notable only for hypertension treated with hydrochlorothiazide "for years." The personal/social history reveals occasional alcohol ("a glass of wine with dinner"), no smoking or drug use, and "a lot of stress" in the past 3 months since her husband told her that he wanted a divorce. Mrs. Smith went to see her primary care physician (PCP) a month ago about difficulty sleeping and was given "some pills" that "knocked me out," and she thus stopped taking them. The physical exam is unremarkable except for a flat, intermittently tearful, affect.

Concerned for depression in this patient, Dr. Jones does a brief mental status exam (MSE), which reveals no hallucinations or delusions, but does reveal that Mrs. Smith has been feeling "down" or depressed nearly every day for at least the past couple of months. Dr. Jones wonders about a diagnosis of depression and plans to revisit this diagnosis. Immediately, he orders an electrocardiogram (EKG), chest x-ray, complete blood count (CBC), chemistry profile, troponin, D-dimer, and bilateral blood pressures to exclude life-threatening cardiopulmonary conditions.

Identifying Depression in Emergency Department Patients

The chief complaint of depressed patients is rarely "depression." As in this case, the depressed patient's ED visit is often prompted by a somatic complaint such as chest pain, epigastric pain, neck pain/headache, or panic that may or may not be related to underlying depression [19]. The astute clinician can recognize clues in the history and physical exam, identifying a patient who is possibly suffering from depression—for example, somatic complaints that are often multiple and without medical etiology; vague reasons for coming to the ED; a past or family history of depression or bipolar disorder; and a personal/social history of having been under "stress" recently. A good history should also detect recent medication changes that might explain the patient's presenting symptoms. Signs in the physical exam include a flat, anxious, or tearful affect. The presence of these clues should prompt a brief MSE to be performed. At a minimum, the MSE should include asking about the symptoms of psychosis (such as delusions and hallucinations) and a brief assessment of mood, which can be completed at the end of the patient evaluation, as depression is a diagnosis of exclusion [20].

The diagnosis of major depression is defined by the American Psychiatric Association's Diagnostic and Statistical Manual of Mental Disorders (DSM) [21]. The DSM-V requires that a majority of the nine criteria described in Table 7.1 be present nearly every day for at least 2 weeks and include either loss of interest in activities or depressed mood. For a loss of interest in activities, patients often admit they no longer enjoy doing things that used to interest them. Sleep disturbance is common in depression and can involve difficulty falling asleep, frequent awakening, or hypersomnia. Appetite change may be either an increase or a decrease from baseline. Depressed mood can be subjectively reported by the patient or an observation by oth-

Table 7.1 DSM-V criteria for major depressive episode [21]

Major depression requires that five (or more) of the following nine symptoms be present nearly every day for 2 weeks and significantly impairing. One symptom must be either depressed mood or loss of interest in activities:
1. Depressed mood
2. Loss of interest in activities
3. Appetite change
4. Insomnia or hypersomnia
5. Psychomotor agitation or slowing
6. Decreased energy
7. Sense of worthlessness or guilt
8. Concentration difficulties
9. Thoughts of death or suicidal ideation
These symptoms may be reported by the patient or by others

ers, such as family members [22]. Difficulty concentrating can manifest as mental fatigability or as indecisiveness noted by others. Decreased activity and loss of energy usually accompany a loss of interest in activities. Guilt may be prominent in patients who become depressed following a life change such as divorce or death of a loved one. It is vital to identify the presence of recurrent suicidal thoughts, a suicide plan, or a recent suicide attempt; for an approach to the evaluation of suicidality, see the related chapter on Chap. 8.

To ease remembering the DSM-V criteria in a busy ED, clinicians may use the mnemonic "In SAD CAGES," which is described in Table 7.2 [5]. "In SAD CAGES" not only encompasses the nine DSM-V criteria but also describes the disease in question and takes at most 2 minutes at the bedside with the patient.

The optimal time to screen for depression is after the initial ED workup based on the chief complaint. Especially after a negative workup, patients are often receptive to considering depression as an explanation for their symptoms. This discussion may easily be started with a straightforward question: "Do you think you might be depressed?" Patients find this question nonthreatening and nonjudgmental; the patient's answer will help the clinician understand the patient's openness to a psychiatric diagnosis. Most patients are grateful to have a diagnosis that explains symptoms they have been having for weeks, months, or even years. When the patient admits to a full spectrum of depressive symptoms, the diagnosis is usually easy to make and does not require further laboratory evaluation [24].

Table 7.2 "In SAD CAGES," a screening tool for depression in the ED [23]

In SAD CAGES
In – Loss of interest in activities
S – Sleep disturbance
A – Appetite change
D – Depressed mood
C – Concentration impairment
A – Activity level change
G – Guilt
E – Energy decrease
S – Suicidal ideation

Instructions: Score 1 point for each symptom present. 5–6 points suggest mild depression; 7–8 points suggest moderate depression; 9 points suggest severe depression and should prompt an in-depth suicide risk assessment

Case, Continued

An hour later, Dr. Jones reviews the patient's laboratory results, which are all unremarkable. A quick calculation reveals Mrs. Smith's HEART score to be 2, or "low probability" of a major cardiac event. Dr. Jones then discusses the results with the patient and daughter, who decline further observation and testing. The final emergent condition on Dr. Jones's differential is major depression. Dr. Jones asks if Mrs. Smith thinks she might be depressed. Mrs. Smith tears up and says, "I've been wondering about that myself." Dr. Jones spends a minute to complete "In SAD CAGES," to which the patient and daughter answer "yes" to all criteria except being suicidal, which Mrs. Smith confides is "against my religion."

Treating Depression in Emergency Department Patients

Once depression has been identified, a discussion of treatment options can begin. Exercise and routine physical activity are an effective treatment, particularly for milder cases of depression (five or six positive "In SAD CAGES" symptoms) [25]. One recommended regimen is 1 hour of structured exercise, three times per week for at least 10–14 weeks [26].

ED clinicians should consider initiating pharmacotherapy for patients who have moderate depression (seven or eight positive "In SAD CAGES" symptoms) or prefer medications to nonpharmacologic treatments like exercise [20, 22, 27]. A large body of literature supports the superiority of selective serotonin reuptake inhibitors (SSRIs) compared with placebo in the treatment of depression [28]. Sertraline, starting at 50 mg orally per day, or citalopram, starting at 20 mg orally per day, are safe, effective, and have favorable side effect profiles [29, 30]. No dosage adjustment is typically necessary for older adults [31]. Patients may see symptomatic improvement in the first week on medication [32], but it may take weeks for the complete resolution of depression [20].

Follow up should occur in 1–2 weeks after ED discharge [20]. At that point, patients with persistent symptoms may also consider adding psychotherapy [28]. Psychotherapy—in particular, evidence-based, time-limited therapies like cognitive behavioral therapy—helps patients recognize and reframe negative thinking. Other treatments may be considered for subtypes of depression, such as light therapy for seasonal depression [28]. Patients who are discharged should receive educational instructions about their disease, their medications, and return precautions that include mention of suicidal thinking.

Indications for a psychiatric consult and consideration of hospital admission for a patient include suicidality or a history of bipolar disorder [20]. Also, consider a consultation for depression in adolescents through age 24, as 2% of adolescents experience an increase in suicidal thinking after starting treatment [20]. For more information on the indications for psychiatric admission, see the related Chap. 20 on when to admit psychiatric patients.

Case, Conclusion

Mrs. Smith expressed gratitude for a diagnosis to explain her recent suffering. Since she has been exercising the past month and has at least moderate depression (eight of nine criteria), a discussion about medication prompts a request for a prescription antidepressant from the patient and daughter. Dr. Jones discharges Mrs. Smith with a prescription for citalopram, 20 mg by mouth daily for 30 days with no refills. Dr. Jones tells Mrs. Smith that she might need to take citalopram for a few months, but fortunately, it is available as an inexpensive $4-per-month generic medication at stores like Walmart. Mrs. Smith also receives teaching about depression and the need to follow up with her PCP in 1–2 weeks. She is advised to return to the ED if she has medication side effects or suicidal thoughts; the family is also provided the number for the National Suicide Prevention Lifeline, 800-273-8255(TALK). Mrs. Smith and her daughter leave the ED with new optimism, and they promise to recommend Dr. Jones and this ED to others.

Conclusion

Depression is a common reason for presentations to emergency departments. Depression should be identified by the ED clinician, who is in a position to initiate treatment and refer the patient for definitive care. With astute identification and evidence-based treatment of depression, ED clinicians can reduce physical and emotional suffering, ED recidivism, and health care costs, while improving patients' satisfaction with care.

References

1. Friedrich MJ. Depression is the leading cause of disability around the world. JAMA. 2017;317(15):1517.
2. Mohamed S, Johnson GR, Chen P, et al.; VAST-D Investigators. Effect of antidepressant switching vs. augmentation on remission among patients with major depressive disorder unresponsive to antidepressant treatment: the VAST-D randomized clinical trial. JAMA. 2017;318(2):132–45.
3. Abar B, Hong S, Aaserude E, Holub A, DeRienzo V. Access to care and depression among emergency department patients. J Emerg Med. 2017;53(1):30–7.
4. Boudreaux ED, Clark S, Camargo CA. Mood disorder screening among adult emergency department patients: a multicenter study of prevalence, associations and interest in treatment. Gen Hosp Psychiatry. 2008;30:4–13.
5. Hoyer D, David E. Screening for depression in emergency department patients. J Emerg Med. 2012;43(5):786–9.
6. Counselman FL, Babu K, Edens MA, Gorgas DL, Hobgood C, Marco CA, et al.; for the 2016 EM Model Review Task Force, Beeson MS, Keehbauch JN, for the American Board of Emergency Medicine. The 2016 model of the clinical practice of emergency medicine. J Emerg Med. 2017 March 25;pii:S0736-4679(17)30108-7. https://doi.org/10.1016/j.jemermed.2017.01.040. Epub ahead of print.

7. Siu AL, Bibbins-Domingo K, Grossman DC, et al. Screening for depression in adults: US preventive services task force recommendation statement. JAMA. 2016;315(4):380–7.
8. Lichtman JH, Bigger JT Jr, Blumenthal JA, et al; American Heart Association Prevention Committee of the Council on Cardiovascular Nursing, American Heart Association Council on Clinical Cardiology, American Heart Association Council on Epidemiology and Prevention, American Heart Association Interdisciplinary Council on Quality of Care and Outcomes Research, American Psychiatric Association. Depression and coronary heart disease: recommendations for screening, referral and treatment: a science advisory. Circulation. 2008;118(17):1768–75.
9. Hailpern S, Calderon Y, Ghosh R, Haughey M. The association between hemoglobin A1c and depression in an inner city diabetic population. Acad Emerg Med. 2007;14:S134.
10. Lora A, Simpson N, Freed M, Milzman D. Impact of depressive illness on emergency department recidivism: a new approach to the "frequent flyer". Ann Emerg Med. 2004;44(4):S23.
11. Brickman K, Bahl R, Marcinkowski NF, Akpunonu P. ED patients with prolonged complaints and repeat ED visits have an increased risk of depression. West J Emerg Med. 2016;17(5):613–6.
12. Agency for Healthcare Research and Quality. Emergency department patients and visitors are most interested in education about stress and depression: research activities. Rockville; 2011. p. 369. Available at http://www.ahrq.gov/news/newletters/research-activities/may11/0511RA4.html.
13. Pailler ME, Cronholm PF, Barg FK, Wintersteen MB, Diamond GS, Fein JA. Patients' and caregivers' beliefs about depression screening and referral in the emergency department. Pediatr Emerg Care. 2009;25:721–7.
14. Orlando MS, Rothman RE, Woodfield A, Gauvey-Kern M, Peterson S, Miller T, et al. Public health information delivery in the emergency department: analysis of a Kiosk-based program. J Emerg Med. 2016;50(2):223–7.
15. Bode A, Jackson JS. The current emergency medicine residency curriculum: missing psychiatry. Am J Emerg Med. 2017; https://doi.org/10.1016/j.ajem.2017.05.017.
16. Emanuel EJ. How can the United States spend its health care dollars better? JAMA. 2016;316(24):2604–6.
17. Wise-Harris D, Pauly D, Kahan D, Tan de Bibiana J, Hwang SW, Stergiopoulos V. "Hospital was the only option": experiences of frequent ED users in mental health. Adm Policy Ment Health Ment Health Serv Res. 2017;44(3):405–12.
18. Downey LV, Zun LS, Burke T. Undiagnosed mental illness in the emergency department. J Emerg Med. 2012;43(5):876–82.
19. Chang B, Gitlin DF, Patel R. The depressed patient and suicidal patient in the emergency department: evidence-based management and treatment strategies. Emerg Med Pract. 2011;13(9):1–23.
20. Florman J. Depression. In: Schaider JJ, Barkin RM, Hayden SR, Wolfe RE, Barkin AZ, Shayne P, Rosen P, editors. Rosen & Barkin's 5-minute emergency medicine consult. 5th ed. Philadelphia: Wolters Kluwer; 2015. p. 302–3.
21. American Psychiatric Association. Diagnostic and statistical manual of mental disorders. 5th ed (DSM-V). Arlington: American Psychiatric Association; 2013.
22. Edwards CD, Glick R. Depression. In: Glick RL, Berlin JS, Fishkind AB, Zeller SL, editors. Emergency psychiatry: principles and practice. Philadelphia: Lippincott Williams & Wilkins; 2008. p. 175–87.
23. Rund DA. Behavioral disorders: clinical features. In: Tintinalli JE, Kelen GD, Stapczynski JS, editors. Emergency medicine: a comprehensive study guide. 6th ed. Irving, TX: American College of Emergency Physicians; 2004. p. 1810.
24. Zun L. Behavioral disorders: diagnostic criteria. In: Tintinalli JE, Stapczynski JS, Cline DM, Ma OJ, Cydulka RK, Meckler GD, editors. Tintinalli's emergency medicine: a comprehensive study guide. 7th ed. New York: McGraw-Hill; 2011. p. 1946–50.
25. Cooney GM, Dwan K, Greig CA, et al. Exercise for depression. Cochrane Database Syst Rev. 2013;9(9):CD004366.
26. National Institute for Health and Clinical Excellence. Depression: the treatment and management of depression in adults (update). Available at http://www.nice.org.uk/guidance/CG90. Accessed 21 July 2017.
27. Hoyer D. Depression and suicidality in emergency department patients. EMedHome. 2015.
28. American Psychiatric Association. Practice guideline for the treatment of patients with major depressive disorder. 3rd ed. Arlington: American Psychiatric Association; 2010.
29. Reefhuis J, Devine O, Friedman JM, Louik C, Honein MA. Specific SSRIs and birth defects: bayesian analysis to interpret new data in the context of previous reports. BMJ. 2015;351:h3190.
30. Cipriani A, Furukawa TA, Salanti G, Geddes JR, Higgins JPT, Churchill R. Comparative efficacy and acceptability of 12 new-generation antidepressants: a multiple-treatments meta-analysis. Lancet. 2009;373(9665):746–58.
31. Kok RM, Reynolds CF. Management of depression in older adults: a review. JAMA. 2017;317(20):2114–22.
32. Taylor MJ, Freemantle N, Geddes JR, Bhagwagar Z. Early onset of selective serotonin reuptake inhibitor antidepressant action: systematic review and meta-analysis. Arch Gen Psychiatry. 2006;63:1217–23.

8 Discharge of the Emergency Patient with Risk Factors for Suicide: Psychiatric and Legal Perspectives

Jon S. Berlin and Susan Stefan

Introduction: Emergency Psychiatry

Over the last 30 years, the psychiatric approach to individuals in the emergency setting with suicidal ideation and risk factors for suicide has undergone a paradigm shift, from one favoring triage and hospitalization to one favoring treatment and hospital diversion. In the best hands, the goal has always been to collaborate with the patient in resolving the crisis and selecting the most appropriate level of care. But this new emphasis has taken over, evolving from a best practice into the standard of care.

In part, this evolution has been facilitated by a growing range of nonhospital disposition options, including those listed in Table 8.1.

At the same time, the availability and perceived desirability of hospitalization have decreased. Far from always being the gold standard for the psychiatric crisis, hospitalization sometimes exacerbates a crisis by confirming an individual's perceptions of helplessness and inability to cope. Regional differences in criteria for acute hospitalization continue to exist, and out of financial necessity, public-sector mental health has embraced hospital diversion more aggressively than either private or Veterans Affairs systems. But if a general psychiatrist of the 1980s were transported to the present, today's practice landscape would be almost unrecognizable.

It is a striking about-face, driven by a mixture of science, patient empowerment, economic policy, and social change. Elements of this mixture include improved differentiation between acute and subacute risk; innovations in crisis and outpatient treatment technique; a stronger emphasis on patient-centered care, with an overall healthier acceptance of risk; less irrational fear about medicolegal liability; managed care's redefinition of medical necessity; severe cuts in hospital beds; surging numbers of mental health referrals to emergency departments (EDs); patient reports of

Table 8.1 Nonhospital options for psychiatric care

Psychiatric emergency service (PES)
Community-based crisis house or center
In-home crisis services with a case manager, family, peers, or others
Partial hospitalization
Intensive outpatient (IOP)
Assertive community treatment teams (ACT or PACT)
Peer-run alternative crisis setting
Strategic acceptance of treatment refusal or no treatment (cf. the case of Mr. E. in Chap. 3) [1]

J. S. Berlin (✉)
Department of Psychiatry and Behavioral Medicine, Department of Emergency Medicine, Medical College of Wisconsin, Wauwatosa, WI, USA

S. Stefan
Rutland, MA, USA

L. S. Zun et al. (eds.), *Behavioral Emergencies for Healthcare Providers*,
https://doi.org/10.1007/978-3-030-52520-0_8

disappointing experiences with inpatient psychiatric treatment [2]; and an increased appreciation of the potential negative effects of involuntary hospitalization, such as increased stigma, exacerbated patient helplessness, and damaged therapeutic alliance [3].

Many psychiatric emergency service (PES) units combine these contemporary thoughts and practices in offering interventions, lasting from a few hours to a day or two. The PES model achieves hospital diversion rates around 70% [4, 5]. Such a safety net for temporary psychiatric regression enables outpatient and subacute care practitioners to manage sicker patients in the outpatient setting. Unfortunately, a PES is rarely available to emergency medicine (EM) practitioners. This chapter applies clinical principles from that setting to the general medical ED.

The Challenge for Emergency Medicine

EM practitioners must often manage psychiatric emergencies with limited training and access to consulting services. A recent report on ED presentations from 2006 to 2014 indicates a fourfold increase in patients with suicidal ideation and a 44% increase in psychiatric cases [6]. EM staff has had increased external demands placed on their performance as well. In response to reports of suicides during hospitalization [7] and soon after an ED visit [8], the Joint Commission has set new standards for hospitals to identify and care for the suicidal patient [7]. This expectation is giving rise to routine screening of all psychiatric patients for suicidal risk in the ED and the hospital and, therefore, potential identification of even more patients with suicidal risk factors in need of evaluation and referral.

EM physicians, in particular, want an efficient, empirically validated tool or scale for suicide screening and suicide evaluation. The need is for a screening tool with very high sensitivity and specificity that would facilitate rapid disposition without causing the admission of false positives or the discharge of false negatives. Boudreaux et al. report some success [9], but successful screening remains very much a work in progress. The Suicide Prevention and Resource Center has created a screening tool that tries to distinguish when an individual needs a psychiatric evaluation before being discharged [10]. However, screening tools rely on patients' self-reports of suicidal ideation, and self-reports may be unreliable [11] unless elicited by a skilled evaluator [12]. In fact, people both underreport and overreport suicidal thoughts for a variety of complex reasons [13, 14].

Standardized instruments for in-depth suicide assessment do not fare much better than screening tools. A recent comprehensive literature review concluded that while these instruments may contribute something to the overall clinical picture, none have enough scientific validity to give them independent value [15].

Despite the seriousness of suicide from a public health perspective, the incidence of suicide is very low. Statistics from the Centers for Disease Control and Prevention indicate that 99.5% of people with suicidal ideation do not kill themselves [16]. From a practical standpoint, picking out the truly high-risk person can be like finding a needle in a haystack.

Suicide Risk Assessment and Management

Risk assessment is a key component of the overall psychiatric assessment. It is a repeating, four-part process that involves: (1) gathering data relevant to risk (mental status, risk factors, and protective factors); (2) synthesizing and interpreting the data; (3) intervening therapeutically; and (4) documenting the process, including one's clinical decision-making. Screening can be thought of as a first, brief cycle of these components. Further, all evaluation schemes, such as the popular Suicide Assessment Five-Step Evaluation and Triage (SAFE-T) [17], follow this conceptual outline. The Collaborative Assessment and Management of Suicidality (CAMS) model also uses this framework and has been adapted to the emergency department setting [18].

The four component activities may and should occur simultaneously. For example, evaluations are most productive when patients collaborate, and cooperation is usually best obtained when patients are approached as an equal possibly needing some help, rather than as a "specimen of pathology being examined" [19]. There are also times that suicidal behavior is so emergent that immediate intervention is called for. In both scenarios, risk assessment and risk management are inseparable; thus, these terms are merely shorthand for a hybrid process.

Risk assessment in the emergency setting is often brief. Emergency practitioners typically truncate the psychiatric examination to focus on its most salient elements. These will vary depending on the case but must include the interview, the mental status exam, history of present illness, collateral history, past history of dangerousness, and an attempt to answer the question, Why now? Instruments that help to gather and synthesize data (e.g., empirically validated risk factors and protective factors) may be useful adjuncts to clinical judgment. The analogous field of violence risk assessment has termed the combination of the two approaches "Structured Professional Judgment" and now considers it to be best practice.

A consensus of opinion does not exist as to whether to conclude the assessment with an estimate of the level of risk. SAFE-T suggests deciding among three levels of risk: high, moderate, or low. The American Psychiatric Association Practice Guideline for Patients with Suicidal Behaviors describes four degrees of suicide risk [20]. One of us (JB) working in an established PES found that experienced emergency psychiatrists achieved more than a modicum of interrater reliability stratifying risk into five degrees: minimal-to-none, low, moderate, high, and imminent. When patients living with elevated risk are asked to rate their own risk, they often spontaneously use a scale of 1–10. Although some practitioners avoid documenting an explicit risk summary, it seems to us that a conclusion about risk is nevertheless being made and determining disposition. And if such an important opinion is being rendered, it should be stated.

Concepts and Guidelines

Suicide assessment remains both an art and a science. But emergency psychiatric practice has coalesced around a set of concepts and guidelines that is medicolegally safe and clinically sound.

1. *Collaborate with Patient*

   Collaborate with the patient and trustworthy significant others in selecting the most appropriate level of care. Consider all outpatient and subacute options. Little else but a note is needed when the parties involved reliably engage with one another and reach a shared, logical conclusion.
2. *Assess and Stratify Risk*
   (a) Perform the risk assessment and stratify short-term risk at a minimum into low, moderate, or high (cf. Kemp, SAFE-T). Key domains of information to review are support system, dangerous ideas and behaviors, engagement in treatment, clinical risk factors, and life stressors.
   (b) Consider use of rating scales and screening and assessment tools as adjuncts to clinical assessment, while acknowledging their limitations (cf. Crisis Triage Rating Scale, Bengelsdorf et al. [21]).
3. *Treat*
   (a) Triage as necessary, but also treat [22]. The goal of emergency psychiatric care is to turn an acute patient into an outpatient (adapted from Sederer) [23]. Initiate or carry out this process to its conclusion. Include targeted treatments aimed at suicidality (cf. CAMS [18]).
   (b) Repeat cycles of intervention and reassessment for suicide risk. Emergency work is an iterative process, and suicidal states are dynamic: They may improve or worsen in a short period of time. Do not assume that a risk assessment performed 8 hours ago is still valid.
   (c) For discharges, facilitate a good transition to, and ongoing partnership with, appropriately intensive and timely outpatient services. The higher risk the discharge, the better the aftercare needs to be.

Attempt to restrict or limit access to lethal means until the crisis has passed.

4. *Set a High Bar for Hospitalization*
   (a) Set a high bar for hospitalization and a higher bar for involuntary hospitalization. Inpatient treatment is not for most patients with risk factors, but for some it remains a crucial endpoint on the care continuum. Consider admission for: (i) high, short-term risk for serious harm [20]; (ii) failure or inadequacy of the most intensive community-based crisis services; and (iii) new onset of severe mental illness, when risk potential, underlying diagnosis, and receptivity/responsiveness to treatment are largely unknown. (For more thoughts on when to hospitalize, see Chap. 20).
   (b) Develop an appropriately high degree of risk tolerance for low, moderate, and chronically high risk. Understanding the difference between ongoing chronic risk and acute risk is crucial. "Sometimes the acceptance of a chronic risk of suicide is the price of outpatient treatment …" [24].
5. *Medicolegal Risk Management*

   Documentation and consultation are the two pillars of medicolegal risk management [25].
   (a) When in doubt, obtain a consultation. Sometimes, a curbside consult may be sufficient.
   (b) Document one's attention to protective factors, risk factors, risk mitigation, consults, and clinical decision-making (see the Columbia-Suicide Severity Rating Scale (C-SSRC)/SAFE-T combination form [26] or Appendix 1: Berlin-Stefan form—Brief Documentation of Release).
   (c) Foster a good doctor–patient relationship with patient and family.
6. *Avoid Excessive Risk Tolerance*

Be on guard for excessive risk tolerance and nonadmission driven by bed shortages, cost capitation, or other factors, an overcorrection more likely to occur at present in PESs than EDs. Hospitalization should never be the default, but is sometimes the most appropriate choice.

Clinical Correlations

The greatest pitfall seen in ED practice today is excessive fear of considering discharge for a patient with suicide risk factors, even when the risk is remote and mitigating measures are readily available.

Case Example 1: Low Risk

Mr. A. was a schoolteacher brought into the ED by his wife for a citalopram refill. She was concerned about his being low-key at a party that evening. He confessed to making the mistake of going off his antidepressant. Neither of them regarded the situation as an emergency, but his psychiatrist was on vacation, and they decided to visit a local ED for a refill.

On exam, Mr. A. presented as likable and relaxed. He acknowledged some down moods recently and admitted to a remote history of non-dangerous, fleeting suicidal thoughts, but he believably denied any suicidal ideation in the past 3 years or any hospitalization. He was committed to his family and work. He had no problems with sleep, high anxiety, or emotional turmoil. He had no family history of suicide. Wife corroborated his history. The physician promised discharge and left to retrieve his prescription pad. Instead, he called the police to have Mr. A. forcibly taken to the local PES without explanation.

Discussion

The ED physician's information gathering was excellent, but his medical decision-making was outdated. At a minimum, he should have told Mr. A. that he needed a psychiatric consult and regretted that there was only one way to obtain it. However, when used unnecessarily, coercive intervention is humiliating, stigmatizing, and wasteful of resources. It may also prevent future help-seeking. Much better would have been to call the PES psychiatrist for a telephone consult. He would have been told something like this:

> This is a very low-risk case. I'm hearing two risk factors—remote history of suicidal ideation and possible early recurrence of a clinical depression—

and an abundance of protective factors: good support system, absence of serious suicidal thoughts or behavior past or present, willingness to accept professional help, a history of good response to treatment, an absence of acute clinical risk factors such as severe anxiety, insomnia, or despair, and a coherent story, which the wife corroborates. Just to be on the safe side, you ought to ask about substance abuse, firearms, and major life stressors. I'll see him if you really want me to, but bottom line: If you think he and his wife are telling the truth, I don't need to—you can let him go. Just document this consultation and use my name. (The consultant might also have asked what was making the doctor uneasy about discharge.)

In the absence of specialty consultation, the EM physician's use of risk or depression screening tools would have corroborated Mr. A.'s low suicide risk. By any measure, he would have scored as safe to discharge. His Crisis Triage Rating Scale score would have been a perfect 15, his Patient Health Questionnaire-9 (PHQ-9) would have put him in the minimal depression group, his Columbia Suicide Severity Rating Scale would have been 0 out of 6 positive responses indicating suicide concern [26], and his believable absence of suicidal ideation would not even warrant use of the Suicide Prevention Resource Center's second-step screening tool [10]. Under the American Psychiatric Association's guidelines for selecting a treatment setting for patients at risk for suicide, this man's risk is too low even to make the low end of the chart [20].

What about the legal perspective? Haven't individuals judged to be low risk gone on to kill themselves?

Yes, but … No one believes that clinicians can predict or always prevent suicide with any degree of certainty. They are held to a standard of care that expects them to assess and manage risk as well as possible under real-world conditions [14, 25, 27].

Liability is based on whether or not the practitioner conducts an appropriate and careful assessment of risk, which he clearly did in this case. Suicide cases are disfavored and rarely taken by malpractice lawyers [14, 27]. Lawyers require more than a bad outcome to take a case. They look for a gasp-worthy narrative of neglect or indifference to the patient's circumstances.

Examples of malpractice-worthy cases include patients held involuntarily with literally no face-to-face evaluation at all [28–30]; individuals with extremely recent and lethal suicide attempts who wanted to be hospitalized being turned away [31]; strip-searching a woman in the presence of male security guards with no cause to believe she had contraband [30, 32]; soliciting psychiatric specialists' advice and then ignoring it; failing to take into account the detailed information of credible family members; failing to read available records or to consult with readily available community treaters; and basing clinical decisions on nonclinical factors, such as insurance status.

A carefully done evaluation and thoughtful weighing of risk factors rarely bring litigation, even when the outcome is tragic. Many states have immunized the decisions of ED professionals to admit or discharge from liability if the evaluation is done professionally and according to the applicable commitment statute [30, 31, 33].

Documentation is essential in obviating medicolegal risk, but is also time-consuming. The authors developed a checklist called the Brief Documentation of Release and Mitigation of Risk (BDR) to supplement the charting on an elevated-risk patient deemed appropriate for release (or nondetention). It is a public domain tool regularly requested at conference presentations and published here for the first time.

ED clinicians can also take steps interpersonally to reduce their legal risk. In the remote likelihood of a bad outcome, patients and families can always retaliate, but fostering and maintaining a good working relationship with them reduces the risk of retaliatory malpractice lawsuits [25]. One of us (SS) has successfully represented a number of individuals who were initially only looking for an acknowledgment of error and an apology from a hospital, but who decided to sue because their complaints were met with defensive hostility. Doctors who are perceived as distant, cold, and uncaring are sued more often than those who are perceived as genuinely caring, regardless of the nature of the medical error involved [14]. One study showed a higher rate of being sued when the physician's voice tone scores high for perceived dominance [34].

Case 2: Moderate and Chronic Risk

Ms. B. was a 45-year-old woman with a schizoaffective disorder and posttraumatic stress who presented to the ED requesting hospitalization for overwhelming thoughts of taking an overdose. She had also forgotten to take her psychotropic medication, which resulted in an increase in her self-denigrating auditory hallucinations. She had a history of suicide attempts and helpful psychiatric hospitalizations. The physician agreed with her self-assessment and wrote the order to proceed with admission.

Unfortunately, there were no open psychiatric beds anywhere in the city. Ms. B. agreed to wait in the ED overnight and take her usual medicines. However, when there were no beds available the next day, either, she requested to be released. This placed her EM physician in a quandary. There was no mental health consultation available, and he wondered if Ms. B. should be placed on a mental health hold and detained until a bed opened up, or would this only make her worse? Luckily, he decided to reevaluate the patient and obtain a collateral history.

Ms. B. readily engaged in conversation and smiled. Her mood was somewhat depressed but not hopeless. She believed that restarting her medication and staying in a safe place overnight had helped. On a scale of 1–10, the usual degree of suicidal ideation that she lived with on an outpatient basis was in the 3–7 range. It had increased to a 9 when she sought admission yesterday and was now back down to a 5. When asked, Ms. B. also disclosed the acute precipitant for her current trouble: Her stepfather who had molested her as a child had just been released from prison, triggering flashbacks and dissociation.

The doctor still wondered whether she might be downplaying her suicidal thinking in order to be released. She gladly gave him her case manager's cell phone number. The case manager corroborated all of Ms. B.'s history, noting that she was a reliable historian and rarely minimized symptoms. If anything, Ms. B. was too quick to retreat to the safety of the hospital. She lived in supported housing for people with mental illness. She had a psychiatrist, nurse, case manager, therapist, and peer support specialist.

The doctor's reevaluation was that an acute exacerbation of an ongoing illness and increased risk had subsided. Ms. B. was now subacute and no longer a high, short-term risk for serious harm to self or others. She had a good support system, no imminent suicidal thoughts or behaviors, engagement in treatment, partial relief of her most acute symptoms, and the ability to talk about her life stressors. Her deciding against hospitalization was positive, and involuntary treatment was contraindicated. She was discharged back to her group home and the care of her assertive community treatment (ACT) team.

Discussion

Discharging a chronically suicidal patient with moderate risk to return to treatment in the community was a new concept to the EM physician in Case 2, but there are classic writings on the subject [3, 35]. In his own mind, this doctor compared it to releasing patients with hard-to-control diabetes or hypertension, and high but nonemergent blood sugars or blood pressures.

A number of articles from different disciplines are suggesting that treatment in the ED is a crucial component of ED response to individuals with suicidality [36], and recent developments suggest that it may be legally required under the Emergency Medical Treatment and Labor Act (EMTALA) for psychiatric patients who are seriously suicidal [37].

Most of the concepts and guidelines above informed Ms. B.'s clinical management. There is one additional practice tip from a legal standpoint: Documentation should not only attempt to justify the discharge, it should also clearly delineate the risk factors—the triggering release of the stepfather, the suicidal ideation, and past hospitalizations—and the ways Ms. B's wraparound supports would mitigate those risks. Documentation of the decision-making process, based on the knowledge reasonably available to the ED professional at the time, including consultation with the case manager who knew Ms. B well, serves as a protection from liability in the event that, unbeknownst to the ED staff, those community supports somehow fail the patient.

Exaggerated or Feigned Risk

There are other clinical scenarios of suicide risk that can safely proceed from an ED or PES to nonhospital management. For example, EM practitioners and psychiatric trainees are often challenged by the individual who exaggerates or feigns suicidal risk in order to obtain hospitalization [13, 38]. (See Chap. 14, "Malingering and Factitious Disorders in the Emergency Department.") Briefly, we note that for patients not well known to the emergency service, an extended stay in the emergency setting may permit a more definitive assessment. Given time, patients may confide in a staff member and become less contentious when approached in a consistent, nonpunitive, therapeutic manner. In addition to attempts at engagement and identifying something to treat, consultation, referrals, risk tolerance, and documentation of clinical decision-making are all key. In the final analysis, it is perfectly acceptable to discharge a person threatening suicide if one's careful assessment is that, based on all available information, the threat is not credible. However, practitioners should be prepared to contain explosive reactions in the malingering patient and negative feelings in themselves (e.g., indignation, fear, and self-doubt) at the point that the patient's request for admission is denied.

Conclusion

At present, the Joint Commission goal of preventing suicides through better screening in the emergency setting [7] may be more aspirational than realistic. Moreover, without adequate preparation, this goal might inadvertently encourage reflexive, counterproductive treatments such as unwarranted involuntary hospitalization. However, there are multiple more realistic opportunities for improving care. Current trends in psychiatry and jurisprudence are guiding us toward positive, effective, less restrictive approaches for patients with suicide risk. In situations when patients cannot believably describe their own risk—unlike Mr. A. and Ms. B. who could—this chapter hopefully provides a framework for nuanced, evidence-based management of suicide risk in contemporary emergency settings.

Appendix 1: Brief Documentation of Release and Mitigation of Risk

It is usually appropriate to treat individuals outside the hospital who are not acutely dangerous, but who do have some risk factors for harm to self or others [1–12]. This form is a synopsis of key protective and risk factors, mitigation of risk, and clinical decision-making. It is designed to augment individualized documentation and be a reminder of steps to decrease risk. It is not an interview or assessment tool. **(Note: Collaterals, consults, referrals, and warnings are particularly important to document.)**

I. Protective Factors

Mental Status and Response to Intervention

☐ Believably reports no overpowering urge to hurt self or others

☐ Not feeling like such a burden to others that death would be a relief to them

☐ Can maintain or regain composure while talking about the acute precipitants

☐ Acknowledges and is motivated to cope with life stressors

☐ Engages constructively with treatment staff

☐ Convincingly states reasons for living: ☐ Responsibility to children ☐ Belief system ☐ Looking forward to: Click here to enter text. ☐ Other: Click here to enter text.

☐ Would not want one's dangerous behavior to hurt others

☐ Shows interest in treatment outside of the hospital

☐ Symptoms known to be risk factors diminish during intervention (e.g., anxiety, agitation, insomnia, despair, rage, unbearable psychosis, intoxication, suicidal/homicidal ideation)

☐ Makes progress resolving the crisis

☐ Can look back on successfully handling a similar crisis in the past

Dangerousness

☐ Aborted attempt to hurt self or others on own/called for help

☐ Suicide attempt or assault did not seriously endanger health

☐ Suicide attempt involved significant availability of rescue

☐ Did not rehearse attempt or make preparation for death

☐ Dangerous action was designed to achieve something other than serious injury or death

☐ Contingent suicidality: Appears to be exaggerating suicidal thoughts for secondary gain [9]

☐ **Collateral history corroborates impression of safety OR: Collateral is: ☐ Unavailable ☐ Inessential in this case ☐ Unreliable**

☐ Limited past history of serious harm to self or others

Support Network

☐ Has a good alliance with outpatient clinician ☐ Values current job or school

☐ Has interested and available family and/or friends ☐ Observed to respond positively to them

Other: Click here to enter text.

II. Risk Factors

Mental Status and Response to Intervention

☐ Express some thoughts of hurting self or others but with ambivalence

☐ Despair, rage, psychosis, insomnia, or emotional turmoil: treated enough for release, but recurrence always possible

☐ Minimizes problems in life and with oneself ☐ Unable to identify or talk about the acute precipitants

Dangerousness [5]

☐ Harm to self or others required medical treatment in ER or hospital

☐ Past history of doing harm to self or others ☐ Recently/Being discharged from psychiatric hospital or observation unit

☐ Family history of or recent exposure to suicide ☐ Problem with substance abuse

☐ Access to weapons

☐ Presence of chronic, disabling medical illness, especially with poor prognosis

☐ CNS trauma, signs, symptoms such as cognitive loss of executive function

Support Network

☐ Limited availability of interested family, friends, or other supports

☐ Shows little or no interest in professional help (not due to anger at involuntary detention)

Other: Click here to enter text.

III. Mitigation of Risk and Aftercare Plan

☐ **Weapons or other means of harm (e.g., medications)** ☐ Recommended securing ☐ Secured

☐ **Cautioned individual to avoid alcohol or illicit drugs until crisis is resolved**

☐ **Discussed risk factors and explained the importance of continuing treatment**

☐ **Referred for appropriate, nonhospital level of care:** ☐ Partial hospitalization ☐ Community-based crisis facility ☐ Staying with supportive friends or family ☐ Scheduled follow-up phone call, mobile team visit, or other correspondence ☐ Other: Click here to enter text.

☐ **Discussed exactly what actions to take if symptoms and risk occur**

Safety plan includes: ☐ Using personal crisis plan ☐ Call crisis line, warm line, or other emergency support ☐ Return to this facility ☐ Go to psychiatric hospital ☐ Other: Click here to enter text.

☐ **Consulted with:** ☐ Colleague ☐ Supervisor ☐ Attending ☐ Psychiatrist ☐ Medical Director ☐ Patient's own treatment professional ☐ Patient's future treatment professional

☐ Treated acute symptoms to the point where they are not high-risk factors

☐ Arranged for safe amount of appropriate medication ☐ Helped individual begin to mitigate conflict or crisis in his/her life ☐ Educated significant others and enlisted their understanding and support ☐ Inessential in this case

Other: Click here to enter text.

IV. Clinical Decision-Making

☐ **Protective factors are more compelling than risk factors**

☐ **Patient judged not to be a high short-term risk for causing serious harm or death to self or others**

☐ Patient collaborated in disposition planning and prefers nonhospital treatment

☐ Patient declines hospitalization, and the risks of coercive care (damaged therapeutic alliance, interference with work and relationships, increased stigma) outweigh the benefits (increased immediate safety, more concentrated evaluation and treatment, more data to support decision to release)

☐ Abuse history: a risk factor, but weighed carefully … also associated with minor self-harm [13] and a tendency to experience involuntary interventions as traumatic.

☐ Chronic self-destructive potential is not responding to hospitalization; acceptance of chronic risk is the price of outpatient treatment [8, 10]

☐ Hospitalization might worsen a problem with dependency

☐ Contingent suicidality: Patients who threaten suicide if discharged are typically not high risk [9]

☐ In unguarded moments, patient does not appear to be in as much crisis as he or she reports

☐ Patient self-assessment is out of proportion to observations for ____ hours by multiple, trained observers

____

Evaluator—Print Name

____

Signature

____

Date & Time

Appendix 1 References:

1. Jacobs D, et al. Practice guideline for the assessment and treatment of patients with suicidal behaviors. American Psychiatric Publishing Inc.; 2003. p. 52–5.
2. Bengelsdorf H, et al. A crisis triage rating scale: brief dispositional assessment of patients at risk for hospitalization. J Nerv Ment Dis. 1984;172:424–30. Lippincott Wilkins.
3. Currier G. Hospital-based psychiatric emergency services. In: Textbook of hospital psychiatry. American Psychiatric Publishing Inc.; 2009. p. 311–8.
4. Fleischmann A, et al. Effectiveness of brief intervention and contact for suicide attempters: a randomized controlled trial in five countries. WHO Bulletin. 2008;86(9).
5. Gelenberg AJ, et al. Practice guideline for the treatment of patients with major depressive disorder. Supp to Am J Psychiatry. 2010;167(10).
6. Shea SC. The practical art of suicide assessment. Hoboken, NJ: John Wiley & Sons, Inc.; 2002.
7. Mackinnon RA, et al. The psychiatric interview in clinical practice. 2nd ed. American Psychiatric Publishing Inc.; 2009.
8. Paris J. Half in love with easeful death: the meaning of chronic suicidality in borderline personality disorder. Harv Rev Psychiatry. 2004;12(1):42–8.
9. Lambert MT. Seven-year outcomes of patients evaluated for suicidality. Psychiatr Serv. 2002;53:92–4.
10. Kernberg O. Severe personality disorders. Yale University Press; 1984. p. 261–3.
11. Glick, et al. Emergency psychiatry: principles & practice. Lippincott Williams & Wilkins; 2008.
12. Stefan S. Emergency department treatment of the psychiatric patient. Oxford University Press; 2006. p. 65–72.
13. Harned MS, et al. Impact of co-occurring posttraumatic stress disorder on suicidal women with borderline personality disorder. Am J Psychiatry. 2010;167:1210–7.
14. Meloy JR. Violence risk and threat assessment. Specialized Training Services. 2000.

Coauthors of this form (BDR-MOR): Jon S. Berlin, MD, and Susan Stefan, Esq. Draft 9, October 2010; Draft 13, November 12, 2017.

References

1. Berlin J. Chapter 3: The modern emergency psychiatry interview. In: Zun L, Nordstrom K, Wilson MP, editors. Behavioral emergencies for healthcare providers. Cham: Springer; 2020.
2. Stefan S. Emergency department treatment of the psychiatric patient: policy issues and legal requirements. New York: Oxford University Press; 2006.

3. Paris J. Half in love with death: managing the chronically suicidal patient. New York: Routledge; 2006.
4. Zeller S. "emPATH Units" as a Solution for Psychiatric Emergency Department Boarding. Psychiatry Ad. 2017 Sept 7. Available at http://www.psychiatryadvisor.com/practice-management/empath-mental-health-crisis-management-emergency-department-setting/article/687420/.
5. Zeller S, Calma N, Stone A. Effects of a dedicated regional psychiatric emergency service on boarding of psychiatric patients in area emergency departments. West J Emerg Med. 2014;15(1):1–6.
6. Moore BJ, Stocks C, Owens PL. Trends in emergency department visits, 2006–2014. Statistical Brief #227. Healthcare Cost and Utilization Project (HCUP). Rockville, MD: Agency for Healthcare Research and Quality. September 2017. Available at www.hcup-us.ahrq.gov/reports/statbriefs/sb227-Emergency-Department-Visit-Trends.jsp?utm_source=ahrq&utm_medium=en1&utm_term=&utm_content=1&utm_campaign=ahrq_en10_17_2017. Accessed 30 Oct 2017.
7. Joint Commission. Detecting and treating suicide ideation in all settings. Sentinel Event Alert #56. 2016. Available at https://www.jointcommission.org/sea_issue_56/.
8. Knesper DJ; American Association of Suicidology, Suicide Prevention Resource Center. Continuity of care for suicide prevention and research: suicide attempts and suicide deaths subsequent to discharge from the emergency department or psychiatry inpatient unit. Newton, MA: Education Development Center, Inc.; 2010.
9. Boudreaux ED, Camargo CA Jr, Arias SA, Sullivan AF, Allen MH, Goldstein AB, Manton AP, Espinola JA, Miller IW. Improving suicide risk screening and detection in the emergency department. Am J Prev Med. 2016;50(4):445–53.
10. Caring for adult patients with suicide risk: a consensus guide for emergency departments: quick guide for clinicians. Suicide Prevention Resource Center (SPRC). 2013. Available at http://www.sprc.org/sites/default/files/EDGuide_quickversion.pdf.
11. Berman AL. Risk factors proximate to suicide and suicide assessment in the context of denied suicidal ideation. Suicide Life Threat Behav. 2018;48(3): 340–52.
12. Shea SC. The practical art of suicide assessment. Hoboken, NJ: John Wiley & Sons, Inc.; 2002.
13. Lambert MT. Seven-year outcomes of patients evaluated for suicidality. Psychiatr Serv. 2002;53:92–4.
14. Stefan S. Rational suicide, irrational laws: suicide law and policy. New York: Oxford University Press; 2016.
15. Franklin JC, Ribeiro JD, Fox KR, Bentley K, et al. Risk factors for suicidal thoughts and behaviors: a meta-analysis of 50 years of research. Psychol Bull. 2017;143:187–232.
16. Center for Disease Control, National Center for Injury Prevention and Control, Violence Prevention Division. Preventing suicide: a technical package of policies, programs and practices. 2017.
17. SAFE-T: Suicide Assessment Five-Step Evaluation and Triage for Mental Health Professionals. Conceived by Douglas Jacobs, MD, and developed as a collaboration between Screening for Mental Health, Inc. and the Suicide Prevention Resource Center Available at https://www.integration.samhsa.gov/images/res/SAFE_T.pdf. Accessed 31 Oct 2017.
18. Jobes D. Managing suicidal risk: a collaborative approach. 2nd ed. New York: The Guilford Press; 2016.
19. MacKinnon RA, Michels R. The psychiatric interview in clinical practice. Philadelphia, PA: WB Saunders Co.; 1971. p. 6–7.
20. Jacobs DG, et al. American Psychiatric Association Practice Guideline for the assessment and treatment of patients with suicidal behaviors. 2003. p. 52–5.
21. Benglesdorf H, Levy LE, Emerson RL, Barile FA. A crisis triage rating scale. Brief dispositional assessment of patients at risk for hospitalization. J Nerv Ment Dis. 1984;172(7):424–30.
22. Allen MH. Definitive treatment in the psychiatric emergency service. Psychiatry Q. 1996;67:247–62.
23. Sederer LI. Inpatient psychiatry: diagnosis and treatment. 3rd Sub Edition. Baltimore: Lippincott Williams & Wilkins; 1991.
24. Kernberg OF. Severe personality disorders: psychotherapeutic strategies. Binghamton, N.Y: Vail-Ballou Press; 1984. p. 261.
25. Gutheil TG. Liability issues and liability prevention in suicide. In: Jacobs DG, editors. The Harvard Medical School guide to suicide assessment and interventions. San Francisco: Jossey-Bass, Inc. 1999, p. 561–78.
26. Columbia Suicide Severity Rating Scale/SAFE-T combined form. Available at http://cssrs.columbia.edu/wp-content/uploads/SAFE-T-Protocol-w-C-SSRS-embedded-recent.docx. Accessed 31 Oct 2017.
27. Risenhoover CC. The suicide lawyers: exposing lethal secrets. Avinger, TX: Simpson PC; 2004.
28. Marion v. LaFargue, 2004 U.S. Dist. LEXIS 2601. S.D.N.Y. Feb. 23, 2004.
29. Barker v. Netcare, 147 Ohio App. 3d 1. 2001.
30. Clifford v. Maine General Medical Center, 91 A3d 567. Me. 2014.
31. Binkley v. Allina Health System, 877 NW2d 547. 2016.
32. Sampson v. Beth Israel Deaconess Medical Center, No. 1:06-cv-10973-DPW. D. Mass. filed June 2006.
33. Williams v. Peninsula Regional Medical Center, 440 Md. 573. 2014.
34. Ambady N, LaPlante D, Nguyen T, Rosenthal R, Chaumeton N, Levinson W. Surgeon's tone of voice: a clue to malpractice history. Surgery. 2002;132(1): 5–9.

35. Dawson D, MacMillan H. Relationship management of the borderline patient: from understanding to treatment. New York: Routledge; 1993.
36. Kondrat DC, Teater B. Solution-focused therapy in an emergency room setting: increasing hope in persons presenting with suicidal ideation. Journal of Social Work. 2012;12(1):3–15.
37. Office of the Inspector General, Center for Medicare and Medicaid Services, Department of Health and Human Services. Settlement Agreement with AnMed Health. June 2, 2017. (On file with authors).
38. Adetunji BA, Basil B, Mathews M, Williams A, et al. Detection and management of malingering in a clinical setting. Prim Psychiatry. 2006;13(1):61–9.

9 Somatic Symptom and Related Disorders in the Emergency Department

Divy Ravindranath

Introduction

Somatic symptom and related disorders exist at the intersection between psychiatric disease and medical disease. Patients with these conditions present with bodily symptoms or concerns about having a disease. As such, they are more commonly encountered in general medical settings like the emergency department (ED) than in psychiatric environments like the acute mental health ward. Indeed, patients with somatization disorders use more primary care, emergency, and hospital resources even when controlling for other medical and psychiatric comorbidities [1]. However, psychiatric pathology drives their healthcare utilization.

The *Diagnostic and Statistical Manual (Fifth Edition)* (DSM-V) chapter on somatic symptom and related disorders represents a major update to the DSM-IV-TR chapter on somatoform disorders. This diagnosis group includes somatic symptom disorder, illness anxiety disorder, conversion disorder, and psychological factors affecting medical illness. The diagnostic criteria are described in Table 9.1 and discussed in this chapter. Factitious disorder is also included in this group and reviewed separately in Chap. 14, "Malingering and Factitious Disorder in the Emergency Department."

Differential Diagnosis

Case Example 1

Mr. Y. is a 68-year-old man with a history of generalized anxiety disorder and panic disorder who presents to the ED with chest pain. The pain is present at low intensity nearly all of the time but does worsen from time to time. There has been no pattern to the exacerbations. There are no associated symptoms, like nausea, diaphoresis, or radiation of the pain to the neck or left arm. He is worried that the pain is coming from his heart.

He suffered a heart attack a few years ago and had an automatic implantable cardioverter-defibrillator (AICD) placed. About 6 months after the heart attack, the AICD fired due to a run of ventricular fibrillation, saving Mr. Y.'s life. Since that time, however, Mr. Y. has had chest pain and a mental preoccupation with having another AICD firing. Reassurance that the pain is not cardiac in origin does not diminish the pain or worry that the chest pain may represent another cardiac event. The initial event happened when Mr. Y. was eating dinner—spaghetti with meat sauce and a diet soda. He has avoided these foods

D. Ravindranath (✉)
Department of Psychiatry, Palo Alto Veterans Affairs Health Care System, Palo Alto, CA, USA
e-mail: divy.ravindranath@va.gov

L. S. Zun et al. (eds.), *Behavioral Emergencies for Healthcare Providers*,
https://doi.org/10.1007/978-3-030-52520-0_9

Table 9.1 Diagnostic criteria [2]

Diagnosis	Criteria
Somatic symptom disorder	Patient has somatic symptoms of clinical significance Patient has excessive thoughts, feelings, or behaviors related to the somatic symptoms, with disproportionate thoughts about the seriousness of the symptoms, high levels of anxiety about health, and/or excess time/energy devoted to these symptoms Symptoms persist for more than 6 months
Illness anxiety disorder	Patient has worry about having a serious illness Somatic symptoms are absent or mild, such that preoccupation with the illness is excessive or disproportionate Patient has high levels of health anxiety Patient either performs excess health-related behaviors or avoids health-related behaviors Condition lasts at least 6 months
Conversion disorder (functional neurologic symptom disorder)	Patient has alteration in motor or sensory function Clinical findings are incompatible with recognized neurologic or medical conditions The symptom or functional deficit causes significant impairment or distress
Psychological factors affecting other medical conditions	The patient has a medical condition Psychological or behavioral factors adversely affect the medical condition via exacerbation of the medical condition, interfere with treatment of the medical condition, serve as a health risk for the individual, and/or influence the underlying pathophysiology of the medical condition

ever since. He also avoids physical activity around the house and hobbies he used to enjoy, like golf, worrying that these will induce an attack.

Case Example 2

P. is a 12-year-old boy with a history of epilepsy that has been well managed with two antiepileptic drugs. He is brought to the emergency department by his parents for further evaluation and management after an attack that lasted 12 minutes. The patient has not had a seizure for almost 2 years, but his seizures have returned in the context of his parents' divorce. Now, the seizures are of a slightly different semiology than those before he was stabilized on medications. Instead of falling to the floor, he now seems to lower himself to the floor. His eyes are clenched closed during the attacks. He has had no urinary incontinence nor tongue biting. He also remembers some of what is said during the attacks.

These presentations will be familiar to ED clinicians. In these cases, the patient presents to the ED with symptoms of concern, though with peculiar features inconsistent with somatic pathology. Regardless, the first step in working through the differential diagnosis is to assess for somatic pathology that could produce the symptoms of concern.

Once somatic pathology has been considered and the need for medical hospitalization excluded, it is important to note that somatic symptoms and worries about the presence of physical illness are found in a variety of psychiatric conditions. For example, a patient with panic disorder can experience panic attacks that include chest pain, palpitations, shortness of breath, dizziness, diplopia, auditory distortions, and so on. A patient with major depression may experience fatigue, sleep disturbance, poor appetite, and problems with concentration and memory. A patient with a psychotic disorder may experience somatic hallucinations or carry a delusion that their organs are diseased. As such, clinicians should consider common psychiatric illnesses like depression, generalized anxiety disorder, posttraumatic stress disorder, or schizophrenia. In the ED, the clinician should also consider the presence of suicidal or violent ideation or an inability to care for oneself that may require psychiatric hospitalization.

(See Chap. 20, "When to Admit the Psychiatric Patient.")

Somatic symptom and related disorders are considered last among this psychiatric differential. Somatic symptom, illness anxiety disorders, and psychological factors affecting other medical conditions are considered if the symptoms or worries present are neither fully explained by a medical condition nor by another psychiatric condition. Conversion disorder can exist in the presence of another psychiatric illness.

Somatic Symptom and Related Disorders Diagnostic Group

Somatic Symptom Disorder

Somatic symptom disorder represents an excessive concern about the experience of one or more somatic symptoms out of proportion to the known seriousness of the medical condition underlying the symptom. Somatic symptom disorder may coexist with a diagnosed medical condition. The key is that the worry about the condition is out of proportion to the somatic pathology identified. Social or functional impairment in somatic symptom disorder arises because of the concern, anxiety, or worry about the symptom(s), leading to maladaptive behaviors. Case 1 has features of somatic disorder in that Mr. Y. worries about his pain and engages in avoidance of foods and activities that probably are not causes of worsening chest pain.

Illness Anxiety Disorder

Illness anxiety disorder represents mental preoccupation with having a serious medical illness, resulting in either excessive health-related behaviors (like checking for the disease) or maladaptive medical avoidance. Physical symptoms are either absent or mild. Social and functional impairment arises because of the preoccupation with the illness. The patient in Case 1 also has features of illness anxiety disorder in that Mr. Y. is worried about having a cardiac event (e.g., acute coronary syndrome or discharge of his AICD) and presents to the ED as part of his checking behavior.

Conversion Disorder

Conversion disorder (also known as functional neurologic symptom disorder) involves an alteration of neurologic functioning that is incompatible with known neurologic or medical conditions. Patients with conversion disorder tend to have dissociative qualities, such that they may present without worry about even catastrophic neurologic dysfunction. This feature can help distinguish this condition from a somatic symptom disorder featuring worries about neurologic symptoms or illness anxiety disorder featuring worries about a neurologic syndrome. Case 2 illustrates conversion disorder in a patient who presents with symptoms concerning for a seizure, though with multiple features that are inconsistent with an epileptic event. Partial dissociation is demonstrated by the patient's partial memory of events happening during his spells.

The evaluation of conversion disorder primarily focuses on neurologic conditions that can produce symptoms similar to those experienced by the patient. Thus, a comprehensive neurologic assessment is critical when conversion disorder is suspected. Table 9.2 lists a number of validated neurologic exam findings and studies that are not compatible with known neurologic conditions and, therefore, suggests the presence of conversion disorder.

Conversion disorder cases in the ED can be particularly vexing because the presentation is often dramatic and reflective of a serious neurologic condition for which immediate action is needed, like a stroke or seizure. For example, patients with conversion disorder mimicking seizures, also known as psychogenic nonepileptic spells, can present in nonepileptic psychogenic status [5]. Of note, one study found that patients whose "seizures" are recalcitrant to high-dose benzodiazepines and who have a venous port system are more likely to present with psychogenic status rather than status epilepticus [6].

Table 9.2 Selected validated exam and study findings to establish conversion disorder [3, 4]

Neurologic symptom	Exam/study finding suggesting conversion disorder
Motor	Hoover sign: paretic leg moves when testing hip flexion for contralateral leg Abductor sign: leg that is paretic under active hip abduction exerts resistance to examiner forced adduction Abductor finger sign: finger abduction against examiner resistance for 2 minutes in functional hand reveals synkinetic abduction finger movement in contralateral/paretic hand Spinal injury test: with patient supine, leg flexed at knee holds position against gravity despite report of paresis Collapsing/give-away weakness: limb collapses under minimal pressure or normal strength suddenly gives way Co-contraction: contraction agonist and antagonist muscle groups to keep limb in fixed position during exam Motor inconsistency: muscle that has two functions (e.g., hip flexion and knee extension) can perform one function but not the other
Sensory	Midline splitting: sensation goes from present to absent exactly at midline Splitting of vibration: sensation is different on left vs. right side of bones that cross midline (e.g., sternum or frontal bone) Nonanatomic sensory loss: sensation does not fit known dermatomes Inconsistent or changing pattern of sensory loss
Gait	Dragging monoplegic gait: leg is dragged instead of performing circumduction Chair test: patient is able to propel a wheeled chair despite reports of not being able to walk
Seizure	Spell semiology Long duration Gradual onset Fluctuating course Side-to-side head or body movements Eyes closed during episode Memory recall Absence of postictal confusion Exam findings/provocative testing Low ictal and postictal heart rate Resistance to noxious stimuli (e.g., forcing open eyes to test corneal reflex) Resolution of spell with noxious stimuli (e.g., foul smell or pressure to nail bed) Voluntary saccades followed by deviation away from examiner when head is turned Resolution of the spell with instruction/reassurance from examiner Lab studies Normal postictal lactate Normal postictal prolactin Normal intraictal video EEG (gold standard)

Psychological Factors Affecting Other Medical Conditions

This diagnosis reflects the notion that individuals may engage in behaviors that are contrary to medical treatment goals. The maladaptive behaviors can be as broad as treatment nonadherence and dietary indiscretion or as narrow as anxiety exacerbating shortness of breath. The critical difference between this diagnosis and others within the diagnostic group is that the psychological factors generate social and functional impairment by adversely affecting a medical condition. If the psychological factors in question are better explained by a psychiatric diagnosis outside of this group, like major depressive disorder, then the diagnosis of psychological factors affecting other medical conditions is excluded.

Therapeutic Three-Step Approach

Each of these diagnoses shares the characteristic that psychological factors interdigitate with and sometimes exacerbate physical symptoms.

Patients present to the ED seeking redress for what they consider to be a physical (or somatic) emergency, whereas psychological factors are at the core of their pathology. ED providers, however, are obligated to ensure that there are no emergencies present in every patient who presents to the ED. As such, patients with somatic symptom and related disorders who present to the ED often gain themselves the "million-dollar workup," resulting in expense for the hospital system and increased wait times for others in the ED, often only to get the answer that there is nothing wrong with them.

Here, we present a three-step clinical approach to address patients with somatic symptom and related disorders [7–9].

The first clinical step to consider is to limit the workup to only that which is absolutely needed to rule out a somatic emergency. In the prototypic cases presented above, psychiatric illness is comorbid with physical illness, and the symptoms present may merit the use of multiple consultants, extensive serum and radiographic testing, and/or admission to the hospital to ensure that the presenting concern does not represent a somatic emergency. The pursuit of this full workup when the likelihood of a positive result seems low exposes the patient to iatrogenic risk, as well as psychological reinforcement that significant somatic pathology exists. The extent of necessary workup always entails clinical judgment. However, each clinician should have a threshold at which to say that the ED workup carries more risk than benefit and defer further evaluation to an outpatient setting. One study in a primary care setting found that somatic illness is not often missed in patients with medically unexplained somatic symptoms [10].

Each of the diagnoses discussed in this chapter has positive diagnostic criteria developed so as to exclude the need to exclude all possible somatic pathologies that may present with the symptoms in question. Even conversion disorder can be established prospectively in the ED [11] and without the need for an extensive workup. Establishing a psychosomatic diagnosis may also lead to a reduction in the use of emergency resources to address what is not an emergency. In one prospective study, diagnosis of psychogenic nonepileptic spells led to a 51% reduction in ED use for neurologic symptoms [12], and a second study found a 91% reduction in ED use among patients after a diagnosis of psychogenic nonepileptic spells [13].

The second clinical step is to attempt to move the patient's focus away from their physical complaints. Patients often think about their body and mind as two separate and distinct objects, and think that a physical symptom necessarily means that the pathology is in the body, rather than the mind. Discussion about the neurologic basis for mental experiences may help the patient accept that the body influences the mind, and vice versa. Moving the conversation from a mutually exclusive paradigm of body versus mind invites the patient to consider a role for mental health treatment. This conversation needs to happen in a very supportive fashion. Patients with chronic somatic symptom and related disorders have all too often left medical encounters hearing, "There is nothing wrong with you," or, "It is all in your head." However, their suffering is real, and they want a plan to resolve the suffering. ED clinicians should validate patients' distress to ensure that the patient does not feel rejected by the health system or feel their suffering is being minimized.

The third clinical step is to feel confident in referring or retreating. If the patient accepts a mental health referral, then the clinician should facilitate connection with treatment. This would be a reasonable time to involve a psychiatrist for an independent (psychiatrist and patient) or joint (psychiatrist, medical or neurology consultant, and patient) consultation. Treatments for somatic symptom and related disorders are typically longer term, so the main goal of the consulting psychiatrist is to build motivation for outpatient follow-up. If the patient holds to the notion that what they are experiencing is a somatic concern, then the ED provider can retreat, knowing that serious somatic emergencies have been ruled out and the patient can safely leave the ED. A primary care provider can reattempt this conversation and referral to mental health at a later time.

Of the four somatic symptom disorders discussed above, conversion disorder carries the greatest risk of impaired insight into the condition and, therefore, provides the greatest challenge in terms of moving the conversation from the somatic to the psychosomatic. Patients with somatic symptom disorder, illness anxiety disorder, and psychological factors affecting other medical conditions tend to maintain awareness that mental factors may be affecting the course of their physical illness and thus may be more willing to accept the involvement of mental health professionals, if only as adjuncts to their somatic evaluation and treatment. All the same, receiving the diagnosis of conversion disorder and treatment early in the illness course correlates with improved clinical outcomes [14, 15]. This correlation highlights the importance of moving the treatment conversation toward the psychosomatic as early as possible, even in the ED.

Patients with conversion disorder may also still warrant hospitalization. Even if the patient accepts that their condition has roots in mental illness, they may not have sufficient recovery in function to allow discharge. For example, a patient with lower extremity paralysis due to conversion disorder may be unable to ambulate or transfer to a toilet or wheelchair. A patient in this category may be considered gravely disabled by their psychiatric illness, depending on local laws and practice patterns. Whether the patient is admitted to the psychiatry hospital or to a general medical floor depends on the local availability of nursing services and treatment capacity. For example, a psychiatric specialty hospital may not have access to seizure pads, machines to lift the patient in and out of bed, equipment to prevent pressure sores, or physical therapy expertise. At the same time, the medical hospital may not have access to the mental health expertise needed to push the patient toward full recovery. Successful disposition requires a collaborative decision among multiple services with the patient's best interests in mind.

Longer Term Treatment

Evidence on the definitive treatment of somatic symptom and related disorders is thin. However, there is literature to support structured treatment modalities and medications from a primary care or specialty environment. Patients with a somatic symptom or illness anxiety disorders benefit from frequent structured primary care visits to address worries and initiate testing as needed. Such patients also benefit from cognitive–behavioral therapy and tricyclic antidepressants or selective serotonin reuptake inhibitors [16].

Patients with conversion disorder are often diagnosed and treated in a neurology specialty environment. Such patients benefit from weaning off unnecessary medications, like antiepileptic medications, and initiation of cognitive–behavioral therapy and/or selective serotonin reuptake inhibitors. Interestingly, patients with motor-symptom conversion disorder may benefit from referral to physical therapy to help them regain function. Other treatment modalities that have been studied include transcutaneous electrical nerve stimulation (TENS), transcranial magnetic stimulation (TMS), biofeedback, and sedation [17, 18].

Conclusions

Somatic symptom and related disorders represent a set of conditions where somatic symptoms are the focus of concern, whereas the pathology lies more in the mind. When patients with these conditions present to the ED, the primary concern is to exclude psychiatric or somatic emergencies and thereafter defer the remainder of the workup to the outpatient setting. ED providers should take advantage of the opportunity to help the patient to consider the possibility of mental pathology and consider consultation with a mental health provider.

References

1. Barsky AJ, Orav EJ, Bates DW. Somatization increases medical utilization and costs independent of psychiatric and medical comorbidity. Arch Gen Psychiatry. 2005;62(8):903–10.
2. American Psychiatric Association. Diagnostic and statistical manual of mental disorders. 5th ed. Arlington, VA: American Psychiatric Association; 2013. p. 309–28.

3. Daum C, Hubschmid M, Aybek S. The value of "positive" clinical signs for weakness, sensory and gait disorders in conversion disorder: a systematic and narrative review. J Neurol Neurosurg Psychiatry. 2014;85(2):180–90.
4. Siket MS, Merchant RC. Psychogenic seizures: a review and description of pitfalls in their acute diagnosis and management in the emergency department. Emerg Med Clin North Am. 2011;29(1):73–81.
5. Dworetzky BA, Weisholtz DS, Perez DL, Baslet G. A clinically oriented perspective on psychogenic nonepileptic seizure-related emergencies. Clin EEG Neurosci. 2015;46(1):26–33.
6. Holtkamp M, Othman J, Buchheim K, Meierkord H. Diagnosis of psychogenic nonepileptic status epilepticus in the emergency setting. Neurology. 2006;66(11):1727–9.
7. Schecker NH. Childhood conversion reactions in the emergency department: part I—Diagnostic and management approaches within a biopsychosocial framework. Pediatr Emerg Care. 1987;3(3):202–8.
8. Cottencin O. Conversion disorders: psychiatric and psychotherapeutic aspects. Neurophysiol Clin. 2014;44(4):405–10.
9. Stephenson DT, Price JR. Medically unexplained physical symptoms in emergency medicine. Emerg Med J. 2006;23(8):595–600.
10. Skovenborg EL, Schröder A. Is physical disease missed in patients with medically unexplained symptoms? A long-term follow-up of 120 patients diagnosed with bodily distress syndrome. Gen Hosp Psychiatry. 2014;36(1):38–45.
11. de Gusmão CM, Guerriero RM, Bernson-Leung ME, Pier D, Ibeziako PI, Bujoreanu S, et al. Functional neurological symptom disorders in a pediatric emergency room: diagnostic accuracy, features, and outcome. Pediatr Neurol. 2014;51(2):233–8.
12. Jirsch JD, Ahmed SN, Maximova K, Gross DW. Recognition of psychogenic nonepileptic seizures diminishes acute care utilization. Epilepsy Behav. 2011;22(2):304–7.
13. Razvi S, Mulhern S, Duncan R. Newly diagnosed psychogenic nonepileptic seizures: health care demand prior to and following diagnosis at a first seizure clinic. Epilepsy Behav. 2012;23(1):7–9.
14. Couprie W, Wijdicks EF, Rooijmans HG, van Gijn J. Outcome in conversion disorder: a follow-up study. J Neurol Neurosurg Psychiatry. 1995;58(6):750–2.
15. Pehlivantürk B, Unal F. Conversion disorder in children and adolescents: a 4-year follow-up study. J Psychosom Res. 2002;52(4):187–91.
16. Kurlansik SL, Maffei MS. Somatic symptom disorder. Am Fam Physician. 2016;93(1):49–54.
17. Lehn A, Gelauff J, Hoeritzauer I, Ludwig L, McWhirter L, Williams S, et al. Functional neurological disorders: mechanisms and treatment. J Neurol. 2016;263(3):611–20.
18. Perez DL, LaFrance WC. Nonepileptic seizures: an updated review. CNS Spectr. 2016;21(3):239–46.

10 The Patient with Anxiety Disorders in the Emergency Department

Naomi A. Schmelzer

Introduction

> Panic. You open your mouth. Open it so wide your jaws creak. You order your lungs to draw air, NOW, you need air, need it NOW. But your airways ignore you. They collapse, tighten, squeeze, and suddenly you're breathing through a drinking straw. Your mouth closes and your lips purse and all you can manage is a croak. Your hands wriggle and shake. Somewhere a dam has cracked open and a flood of cold sweat spills, drenches your body. You want to scream. You would if you could. But you have to breathe to scream. Panic. (Khaled Hosseini, The Kite Runner)

Anxiety is a common presentation in the emergency department, as well as across medical settings. It contributes to the human emotional experience, and its presence is not always detrimental or pathological. When symptoms of anxiety become overwhelming, disruptive, or disabling, they may prompt patients (or others on their behalf) to seek treatment. Approximately one-fifth of patients presenting with mental health concerns to the emergency department are given an anxiety disorder diagnosis. This is not surprising given that anxiety disorders affect up to a quarter of the general population during their lifetime and are even more prevalent in the medically ill [1, 2].

The symptom of anxiety can represent a broad range of etiologies, from primary anxiety disorders to a variety of medical conditions. Because core features of anxiety disorders are somatic in nature, there is much overlap in clinical presentations between anxiety disorders and other medical conditions. Patients may come to the ED seeking help for a known anxiety disorder, for first-time symptoms of anxiety, or for related symptoms. Encounters with medical settings, in particular the emergency room, may also provoke secondary anxiety unrelated to the initial complaint.

The first step in providing care is to recognize anxiety in the patient. In one study, a quarter of patients presenting with chest pain met criteria for panic disorder, though 98% of these identified cases went unrecognized [3], demonstrating that anxiety can often be a hidden contributor. In the emergency department, the clinician must first determine the underlying cause of the anxiety, especially ruling out any life-threatening causes and considering common diagnoses such as anxiety disorders. This will guide the plan for acute management, providing treatment, and disposition decisions that are comprehensive, safe, and appropriate for the condition [4].

N. A. Schmelzer (✉)
Department of Psychiatry, Brigham and Women's Faulkner Hospital, Harvard Medical School, Boston, MA, USA
e-mail: nschmelzer@bwh.harvard.edu

L. S. Zun et al. (eds.), *Behavioral Emergencies for Healthcare Providers*,
https://doi.org/10.1007/978-3-030-52520-0_10

The Experience of Anxiety

Anxiety is a tense inner state, a feeling of heightened emotional arousal that is often accompanied by physical symptoms such as palpitations or chest discomfort, shortness of breath, muscle tension, gastrointestinal discomforts such as nausea and vomiting or diarrhea, tingling or weakness, or tremulousness. As Rickels described it, anxiety is an "experience of intense dread and foreboding, conceptualized as internally derived and unrelated to an external threat" [5].

Anxiety symptoms can have an impact that extends beyond the emergency room visit. They can lead to disability, increased use of health-care services, diminished quality of life, and impaired social and occupational functioning. They can also impact how a patient experiences other conditions, such as pain [6], even when anxiety is not the major complaint. Addressing secondary anxiety as part of a visit may assist in the treatment of comorbid conditions.

Emergency departments can be chaotic environments where patients are faced with uncertainty about medical tests and diagnosis, and unknown clinicians are providing care. By nature, the visit is likely unplanned and represents an unanticipated crisis. There may be pain or distressing physical symptoms. Patients may be crowded into small areas, facing tests in enclosed or tight spaces (such as an MRI), or separated from their loved ones. The patient may have concerns about how the visit will impact finances and social or occupational functioning in the short or long term. These conditions may precipitate anxiety, especially in individuals already vulnerable.

Differential Diagnosis of Anxiety

The presence of anxiety in the ED may fall into one of the following groups [4]:

- The response to a stressful event
- A primary anxiety disorder
- A medical illness or substance use disorder
- An anxiety disorder with other comorbid medical or psychiatric disorder

After recognizing that anxiety is present, the task is to determine the underlying etiology. While anxiety disorders are common in the emergency room, it is important to remember that many medical disorders, including life-threatening conditions, can mimic anxiety states.

Primary Anxiety Disorders

While fear or anxiety can occur on a spectrum of severity, anxiety disorders are considered when the symptoms lead to significant distress or functional impairment. Freud described anxiety in terms of apprehension, either a chronic state of anxious expectation or coming into consciousness suddenly as anxiety attacks, associated with somatic symptoms [5]. These concepts have persisted in psychiatry, with the anxious expectation now known as the excessive worry associated with generalized anxiety disorder and anxiety attacks referred to as "panic attacks." The structuring of anxiety disorders has gone through diagnostic revisions in each subsequent DSM version since the first edition. From the Diagnostic and Statistical Manual of Mental Disorders, Fifth Edition [7], generalized anxiety disorder and panic disorder are commonly seen in the emergency room and will be the focus of this chapter.

Generalized anxiety disorder (GAD) is characterized by excessive worry occurring for at least 6 months and associated somatic features including restlessness, fatigue, difficulty concentrating, irritability, muscle tension, and sleep disturbance [7]. It is frequently comorbid with other psychiatric or physical conditions such as depression, substance use disorders, or heart disease and has a lifetime prevalence of approximately 5% [8]. GAD has a chronic course that fluctuates over time, typically beginning in adulthood, and can lead to significant disability [9].

Panic disorder is characterized by recurrent panic attacks, episodes of intense fear and hyperarousal associated with palpitations or rapid heart rate, sweating, trembling, paresthesia, feeling short of breath or the sensation of choking, feeling detached from oneself or the environment, and a fear of loss of control or of dying. These symptoms typically peak within a few minutes and can come on suddenly or in the setting of more persistent worry. Patients may fear or anticipate having another panic attack or be concerned about social, employment, or health implications. Panic disorder occurs with a lifetime prevalence in the US between 1.6% and 3.5% [10–12]. Typical onset is the third decade of life, but symptoms may begin in childhood. Symptoms have a chronic course but can improve with treatment.

Studies show that panic disorder has been present in two-thirds of patients who present to the ED with medically unexplained chest pain and that repeated visits to the ED were higher for patients who screened positive for panic disorder [13]. It is common for patients to revisit the ED with recurring panic attacks even after receiving a diagnosis; one study demonstrated that up to one-third of patients returned within a week after their first panic attack episode for the same symptoms [14].

While acute stress disorder and adjustment disorder with anxiety now fall under the Trauma- and Stressor-Related Disorders section of the DSM-5 [7], they also should be included in the differential diagnosis for anxiety, particularly in the ED setting. Adjustment disorder, defined as emotional or behavioral symptoms occurring in response to an identified stressor, is commonly found among those with medical illness. Both these conditions can follow an acutely stressful or traumatic life event and bring patients to the ED, particularly those with limited resources to seek care elsewhere.

Medical Disorders

A variety of medical conditions can produce anxious states, including cardiovascular, respiratory, endocrine, metabolic, and neurological diseases. Additionally, substance withdrawal or intoxication states, medication side effects, or toxidromes can also mimic anxiety disorders. The presentation of anxiety in older adults, the absence of a psychosocial trigger or event, or other clinically concerning or atypical signs may indicate a medical cause. (See Table 10.1)

Despite the interest, research remains mixed regarding the differentiation of acute coronary syndrome from an anxiety attack based on clinical signs and symptoms alone. There are few differences in symptoms, coronary artery disease risk factors, or cardiac history, and additional screening tools are often needed in this population. Symptoms such as palpitations, chest pain, and shortness of breath should be considered significant for cardiac diseases (including acute coronary syndrome (ACS) or dysrhythmias) or pulmonary diseases (including pulmonary embolism, asthma, or COPD exacerbation) [4]. In one study of patients with panic disorder in the ED, 44% had a history of CAD, 80% had atypical chest pain, and 75% were discharged with noncardiac pain diagnosis [3]. For a patient with unexplained chest pain, it may be helpful to

Table 10.1 Differential diagnosis of acute anxiety, medical etiologies

Cardiovascular: CAD, myocardial infarction CHF Mitral valve prolapse Dysrhythmias	*Metabolic:* Hypokalemia Hypophosphatemia Vitamin B12 deficiency Acidosis
Respiratory: Pulmonary embolism COPD exacerbation Asthma exacerbation	*Hematologic:* Anemia Porphyria
Endocrine: Hypoglycemia Hyperthyroidism Parathyroid disorders Pheochromocytoma Adrenal gland dysfunction	*Substances:* Stimulant intoxication (cocaine, amphetamines) PCP LSD Excessive caffeine Cannabis, synthetic cannabis Withdrawal from alcohol or benzodiazepines Dextromethorphan
Neurologic: Delirium Parkinson's disease Multiple sclerosis Huntington's disease Post-concussive syndrome Migraine Seizures	*Medication side effects:* Anticholinergic medications Corticosteroids Neuroleptics (akathisia) Psychostimulants Bronchodilators SSRI—initiation or discontinuation SSRI—serotonin syndrome OTC cold and cough medications Antivirals

screen for the presence of anxiety disorders and the need for an additional mental health evaluation.

Evaluation

For patients presenting with anxiety, the first approach to the patient should be to ensure safety, including assessment for suicidal thoughts, and to consider monitoring for immediate life-threatening events. This may include vital sign monitoring or other acute interventions such as oxygen. As mentioned earlier, the ED is a chaotic environment: loud, bright, and unpredictable and full of unknown persons and uncertainty. Providing a less stimulating environment, such as a psychiatric treatment room if available, may alleviate this contribution to the patient's distress. The physician should approach the anxious patient in a calm, empathic manner while proceeding with the assessment. For those patients who are also agitated, it should be addressed promptly when recognized with verbal de-escalation as a first-line approach; physical or chemical restraints should be avoided, if possible.

Once acute needs are addressed, the initial evaluation should begin with the presenting complaint, including the course, duration, and severity of symptoms, as well as their impact on daily life. The patient should be asked about recent behavioral changes, stressful life events, substance use (including caffeine), and other associated symptoms. A history should include medical and psychiatric illness, recent medication changes, use of over-the-counter medications and supplements, a psychiatric and physical review of systems, and family history. Some suggested questions to ask during the interview have been included here (see Table 10.2). Family or friends can also provide collateral information that is necessary to the evaluation. Following this, a thorough physical exam should be done in all patients.

The initial evaluation and physical examination findings should guide the next steps regarding laboratory testing and other studies. After a thorough history and physical, a young, healthy patient with normal exam findings and few cardiac risk factors presenting with typical anxiety symptoms may not require additional tests. An older patient or one with medical comorbidities may require additional testing to determine the cause of the symptoms.

Table 10.2 Anxiety: taking a history

Are you frequently tense or irritable, or do you have trouble sleeping [9]?
Are you feeling worried, tense, or anxious most of the time [9]?
Are you distressed by anxiety or worry? [8]
Does anxiety interfere with your work or ability to function at home?
Do you have episodes in which you experience any of the following: palpitations, shortness of breath, chest pain, dizziness, nausea, tingling? [8]
Do these episodes recur?
Do you experience episodes of anxiety where you feel out of control or like you are going to die?
Have you changed your behavior because of these episodes? [8]
Do you fear leaving home? Being on a bus? Being in a crowd? [8]
Has there been any recent stress or big event taking place?
Have you experienced any recent changes in your behavior or the way you think, or have there been any recent changes in your environment?

The specific laboratory tests should be determined by the presenting complaint and associated findings, although generally recommended tests include the following: complete blood count, electrolytes, glucose level, blood urea nitrogen/creatinine ratio, toxicology screen, alcohol blood level, and thyroid-stimulating hormone. An electrocardiogram (EKG) is also recommended for patients with cardiac symptoms. Additional testing should be guided by symptoms and may include, for example, cardiac enzymes for patients with chest pain, an EEG for patients with suspected seizures, and a chest radiograph for patients with respiratory symptoms.

For any organic causes, the underlying medical disorder should be addressed, and this may need to occur prior to completion of the assessment, depending on urgency. Patients with suspected akathisia may be given pharmacologic treatment such as beta-blockers or benzodiazepines. Patients may begin to manifest worsening withdrawal states during the course of the ED visit and require initiation of pharmacologic regimens before their condition progresses, such as administering a longer-acting benzodiazepine to those in alcohol withdrawal. When acute medical disorders have been excluded and anxiety disorder is the differential diagnosis, the emergency physician should then focus on establishing a treatment plan with the patient.

Treatment in the Emergency Room

Anxiety disorders may present with a diverse range of symptoms, but they all share the common feature that the patient is coming to the ED to relieve the distressing feeling of inner tension and seeking out a sense of security or calm. From that point, treatment goals for ED care can be established. Patients should be told of the diagnosis and provided education about the nature of the disorder, what can be expected (such as physical changes) during a panic attack or disease course, and their treatment options.

In the emergency room, benzodiazepines can provide immediate symptomatic improvement, as they are rapid-acting and well tolerated, and can be given in as-needed (PRN) dosing. They can also be continued for short periods on an outpatient basis to address anxiety while other medications, such as SSRIs, are being titrated or as needed for anxiety attacks. The disadvantages to benzodiazepine use include concern for sedating effects, physiologic dependence, withdrawal effects, not being as effective for treatment of comorbid disorders such as depression, and abuse potential. Additionally, use of benzodiazepines in the acute phase may diminish a sense of agency over panic symptoms, which may make recovery with psychotherapy more challenging in the long term. Rarely, upon discharge, a short course of benzodiazepines (one to two times a day for up to 7 days) may be indicated in the case of an acute stress reaction.

Antidepressants, such as selective serotonin reuptake inhibitors (SSRIs), are the first line and generally considered the primary treatment for anxiety disorders. SSRIs, in particular, are generally well tolerated and have been shown to be effective, with a favorable safety profile and a broad spectrum of efficacy for comorbid conditions [10]. They also have a low potential for abuse. The disadvantage is that these are not efficacious for immediate symptom relief, and improvement is not generally seen for a few weeks after initiation of therapy. There may be some therapeutic benefit to initiating an SSRI in the ED, though patients should have a follow-up with a primary care doctor or psychiatrist upon discharge. These should be initiated at a low dose and titrated up slowly to avoid exacerbating symptoms. Monoamine oxidase inhibitors and tricyclic antidepressants have a long history of use with anxiety disorders and can be efficacious but are less common due to their adverse side effect profiles and medication interactions.

There have been some newer studies on the use of antipsychotic medications such as quetiapine for anxiety, though this would not be the first line and is generally indicated for severe and persistent anxiety or symptoms related to organic illness, such as anxiety caused by steroids or delirium [15]. Some physicians favor the use of hydroxyzine, due to its lower abuse potential, though there are no controlled studies on its use in panic disorder. Other options include beta-blockers, which have been found to ease panic attack symptoms (including tremulousness and palpitations), though these should be used more cautiously in patients with COPD. Other anxiolytics like buspirone have some efficacy for the management of GAD, though less with panic disorder. It has a favorable side effect and dependency profile, though slow onset of action, and is tolerated well in the medically ill and elderly. This medication has limited use on an as-needed basis in ED setting. Gabapentin has been increasingly prescribed for anxiety in the outpatient setting but has little evidence for as-needed use for acute anxiety in the ED.

There are several psychotherapeutic interventions that can be initiated in the emergency department as an adjunct or alternative to medication. These approaches include supportive therapy, cognitive behavioral therapy, counseling, and crisis intervention. A physician should not underestimate the therapeutic value of an empathic encounter in which supportive listening, information about treatment choices, and a plan for next steps are provided. A patient's family or friends can be included in the educational and treatment plan discussion (with the patient's consent). In particular, in the case of an acute stress reaction from a traumatic event, reuniting a patient with their loved ones during or shortly after a crisis may be paramount and the essential first step in treatment.

Cognitive behavioral therapy has been shown to be efficacious in the treatment of anxiety disorders, and some CBT techniques can be modified for use in the ED. One approach is muscle relaxation techniques, which involve teaching the patient to release tension in muscle groups throughout the body until the subjective feeling of anxiety is reduced. Breathing retraining is a CBT approach for panic attacks, involving a focus on deep, slow breathing. Both of these exercises can be introduced in the ED, continued in the outpatient setting, and practiced at home.

The ED physician, in conjunction with the patient, should determine a treatment plan for aftercare. Physicians should be familiar with referral resources in their area. Rarely do patients presenting with anxiety have symptoms to a severe degree that require inpatient psychiatric treatment, and these patients should meet a threshold of grave disability or pose a threat to themselves or others. They typically have impaired coping mechanisms and poor social supports, as well as other comorbid conditions. The majority of patients with anxiety disorders can be discharged with referral for psychiatric outpatient follow-up, such as to a community psychiatrist, therapist, or another mental health resource. If available, for those with more distressing symptoms, a partial hospital program may be considered.

Conclusion

Anxiety disorders are prevalent in the population and commonly seen in the emergency department. Familiarity with recognizing anxiety disorders and their associated physical symptoms will help emergency clinicians provide initial evaluation, stabilization, and targeted interventions, including medication, psychotherapy, and education. Patient anxiety can be alleviated by taking steps to reducing environmental stimuli, establishing a trusting rapport and maintaining a calm presence, addressing the underlying etiology of the anxiety, and providing initial treatment, as well as a plan for outpatient care.

Acknowledgment I want to acknowledge the contributions of the co-authors of the earlier version of this chapter (Felder ML and Perry MA) from the first edition of this book for setting the foundation of this chapter.

References

1. Mago R, Gomez JP, Gupta N, Kunhel EJ. Anxiety in medically ill patients. Curr Psychiatry Rep. 2006;8(3):228–33.
2. Smith RP, Larkin GL, Southwick SM. Trends in U.S. emergency department visits for anxiety-related mental health conditions, 1992–2001. J Clin Psychiatry. 2008;69(2):286–94.
3. Fleet RP, Dupuis G, Marchand A, Burelle D, Arsenault A, Beitman BD. Panic disorder in emergency department chest pain patients: prevalence, comorbidity, suicidal ideation, and physician recognition. Am J Med. 1996;101(4):371–80.
4. Felder ML, Perry MA. The patient with anxiety disorders in the emergency department. In: Zun LS, Chepenik LG, MNS M, editors. Behavioral emergencies for the emergency physician. Cambridge: Cambridge University Press; 2013. p. 76–82.
5. Rickels K, Rynn MA. What is generalized anxiety disorder? J Clin Psychiatry. 2001;62 Suppl 11:4–12; discussion 3–4.
6. Craven P, Cinar O, Madsen T. Patient anxiety may influence the efficacy of ED pain management. Am J Emerg Med. 2013;31(2):313–8. Epub Sept. 13, 2012.
7. American Psychiatric Association. DSM-5 task force: diagnostic and statistical manual of mental disorders: DSM-5. 5th ed. Washington, D.C.: American Psychiatric Association; 2013.
8. Dugue M, Neugroschl J. Anxiety disorders. Helping patients regain stability and calm. Geriatrics. 2002;57(8):27–31.
9. Ballenger JC, Davidson JR, Lecrubier Y, Nutt DJ, Borkovec TD, Rickels K, et al. Consensus statement on generalized anxiety disorder from the International Consensus Group on Depression and Anxiety. J Clin Psychiatry. 2001;62 Suppl 11:53–8.
10. Pollack MH, Marzol PC. Panic: course, complications and treatment of panic disorder. J Psychopharmacol. 2000;14(2 Suppl 1):S25–30.

11. Marzol PC, Pollack MH. New developments in panic disorder. Curr Psychiatry Rep. 2000;2(4):353–7.
12. Zun LS. Panic disorder: diagnosis and treatment in emergency medicine. Ann Emerg Med. 1997;30(1):92–6.
13. Zane RD, McAfee AT, Sherburne S, Billeter G, Barsky A. Panic disorder and emergency services utilization. Acad Emerg Med. 2003;10(10):1065–9.
14. Buccelletti F, Ojetti V, Merra G, Carroccia A, Marsiliani D, Mangiola F, et al. Recurrent use of the emergency department in patients with anxiety disorder. Eur Rev Med Pharmacol Sci. 2013;17 Suppl 1:100–6.
15. Raster MJ, Wise TN, Cai J. Anxiety and anxiety disorders in medical settings. In: Stein D, Hollander E, editors. Textbook of anxiety disorders. 1st ed. Washington, D.C.: American Psychiatric Association Publishing; 2002.

11 Post-traumatic Stress Disorder in the Emergency Department

Anna K. McDowell and Scott A. Simpson

Introduction

More than 70% of people experience trauma during their lives, and many individuals experience multiple traumatic events [1]. Trauma affects an individual's life through altered interpersonal relationships, cognitive distortions, and emotional arousal. A significant minority of individuals experiencing trauma will develop post-traumatic stress disorder (PTSD). Emergency department (ED) clinicians must be able to identify PTSD and patients at risk for its development and initiate treatment when appropriate.

Prevalence

Rates of PTSD are higher in the United States and Canada than in other countries. Lifetime prevalence of PTSD ranges from 6% to 9% of the general adult population in North America [2, 3]. Elsewhere, the prevalence is generally around 1–2% [4, 5]. This difference is likely attributable to cultural influences on post-traumatic phenomena, such as how individuals are expected to respond to trauma, how symptoms manifest, and how communities support trauma survivors [6].

Screening in the ED

No clinical guidelines recommend routine screening for PTSD in the emergency setting, and only 7% of level I and II trauma centers conduct such screening [7]. Likely, the prevalence of PTSD among ED patients is high: In one study of trauma patients, 25% screen positive for PTSD [8]. Self-report scales such as the PTSD Checklist and Screening Tool for Early Predictors of Post-traumatic Stress Disorder appear valid and feasible to administer in the emergency setting [9, 10].

Etiology

At an individual level, there are pre-, post-, and trauma-specific risk factors that affect one's likelihood of developing PTSD. Pre-trauma risk factors include female gender, younger age at trauma, minority status, lower education level, prior history of trauma, history of childhood adversity, history of psychiatric illness, childhood abuse, and history of psychiatric illness in the family [11]. Post-trauma risk factors include

A. K. McDowell
Department of Mental Health, Rocky Mountain Regional VA Medical Center, Aurora, CO, USA

S. A. Simpson (✉)
Department of Behavioral Health Services, Denver Health & Hospital Authority, Denver, CO, USA
e-mail: scott.simpson@dhha.org

L. S. Zun et al. (eds.), *Behavioral Emergencies for Healthcare Providers*,
https://doi.org/10.1007/978-3-030-52520-0_11

higher severity of physical problems [12], traumatic brain injury [13], perceived fear of death during the traumatic event [14], heart rate greater than 95 beats per minute at first presentation to ED following the traumatic event [15], and a high level of pain following the traumatic event [16]. The nature of the trauma also increases an individual's risk for PTSD: The highest risk of PTSD is incurred by rape, after which 19% of survivors report PTSD. This rate is higher than after a car accident (2.6%) or physical assault (2.5%) [1]. Trauma as the result of medical problems—consider myocardial infarction, stroke [17], intensive care unit stay [18], or pain [16]—also poses a risk for PTSD.

To make a diagnosis of PTSD, the Diagnostic and Statistical Manual, Fifth Edition (DSM-5), requires that the patient directly experience or witness death, serious injury, or sexual assault [19]. Patients may also develop PTSD from learning about traumatic events that occurred to close family members or friends or from repeated, extreme exposures to details of traumatic experiences, such as with first responders repeatedly encountering life-threatening situations.

Prevention

ED clinicians who encounter patients after a traumatic event should be reassured that even without intervention, many patients will recover well [20]. In the ED, providers should assure medical stability and then proceed to ensure the patient that they are in a safe place. Orient the patient to members of the team, where they are, and what has happened. The ED team should immediately help the patient connect with supportive friends and family. Providers may also identify and support the patient's positive coping skills, for example, by calling a chaplain for a religious patient.

Patients who arrive acutely agitated and anxious may benefit from behavioral interventions such as sensory tools (e.g., weighted blankets) or a supportive presence (e.g., a sitter or family member at the bedside). Some patients may be so escalated that they benefit from low doses of a benzodiazepine or sedating antihistamine, such as hydroxyzine. However, early pharmacologic interventions will not prevent the development of PTSD [21]. Beta-blockers, though initially thought to be effective to this end, have insufficient evidence to be recommended [22]. Similarly, benzodiazepines have not been found to have a beneficial effect in preventing the development of PTSD [23].

Many clinicians and laypersons receive Mental Health First Aid (MHFA), a training paradigm for assisting patients who present in a mental health crisis, including immediately after a trauma [24]. MHFA incorporates these psychological techniques in teaching to assess for immediate suicide or violence risk, listen nonjudgmentally, and encourage the patient to seek help via personal networks or professional mental health care. MHFA helps learners feel more comfortable and confident in their approach to patients in crisis; however, the benefit for recipients of MHFA is less proven [25, 26].

Diagnosis

A diagnosis of PTSD is predicated on exposure to an actual or threatened traumatic event. PTSD comprises a constellation of impairing symptoms that begin thereafter and persist for longer than 1 month. The core symptoms of PTSD may be categorized as intrusive, avoidant, distortions of thought and mood, or hypervigilance [19]. The diagnostic criteria and symptoms of PTSD are summarized in Table 11.1.

Intrusive symptoms of PTSD are characterized by unwanted, recurrent thoughts or reactions related to the traumatic event. These might be memories or distressing thoughts precipitated by exposure to an event or situation reminiscent of the trauma. Nightmares of traumatic experiences are common, and patients may present with complaints of poor sleep or daytime fatigue. Patients may have dissociative reactions during which they feel past traumatic events are happening. They might also have psychological or physiological reactions when exposed to stimuli that

Table 11.1 DSM-5 symptoms of post-traumatic stress disorder (PTSD) [19]

Exposure to actual or threatened death, injury, or sexual violence
Symptoms persist for >1 month, cause impairment, and include examples across symptom cluster:

Symptom cluster	Examples
Intrusive symptoms (≥1 symptom)	Unwanted thoughts Nightmares Flashbacks
Avoidance symptoms (≥1)	Avoiding places or situations associated with trauma
Negative thoughts and mood (≥2)	Overgeneralized fear Guilt
Hyperarousal (≥2)	Exaggerated startle response Recklessness Changes in concentration or sleep

remind them of past events. When patients insightfully describe and attribute these intrusive thoughts to a prior trauma, the diagnosis of PTSD is straightforward. In the absence of a clear description of thoughts, intrusive symptoms may appear similar to disorders of sleep, anxiety, depression, or substance use—either primarily psychiatric or secondary to a medical condition.

Avoidant symptoms are actions undertaken by the patient to avoid intrusive symptoms. For example, some patients may avoid the neighborhood where they were assaulted or change their commute to avoid the street scene of a car accident (if not stop driving altogether). Patients may avoid certain persons or situations, including medical procedures. When these decisions rise to the level of causing impairment in the patient's life, PTSD should be considered. These symptoms may also reflect anxiety disorders, including obsessive-compulsive disorder or simple phobias. Patients who have begun avoiding social contact may have schizoid or avoidant personality disorders, negative symptoms of psychosis, or depression. When social avoidance occurs among formerly social, older patients, changes in cognition (e.g., delirium) should be considered.

Patients with PTSD experience negative alterations of cognition or mood. Cognitive distortions include fears about others and the world around them—for example, that people are not to be trusted and that the world is a dangerous place. They may feel continually scared, angry, or guilty—including about surviving a terrible experience when others did not. Patients may have difficulty voicing positive emotions and instead continually feel detached from others and disinterested in activities. Most of these symptoms are similar to those experienced by depressed patients, although cognitive distortions of PTSD are more likely to relate to external threats rather than, as in major depression, personal inadequacy and a sense of burdensomeness.

Hypervigilance is characterized by irritability and hyperarousal. Patients may startle easily or be continually "scanning" their environment for threats. Patients may situate themselves in a way so that they cannot be surprised, for example, by sitting with their back to the corner of a room, facing the door. This edginess may progress to reckless behaviors or easy anger. Sleep and concentration may be impaired. Once calm, patients with PTSD can often verbalize the sequence of thoughts, fears, and responses that lead to outbursts. Patients who describe premeditated violence or gross disrespect for others are more likely to have an antisocial personality disorder. Other diagnoses that cause hypervigilance and concentration impairment include attention deficit/hyperactivity disorder, panic disorders, psychosis, or medical causes of hyperarousal, such as hyperthyroidism or interictal mood disorders.

A diagnosis of PTSD requires symptoms across all these categories, resulting in a tremendous heterogeneity of presentations: There are 636,120 diagnostic symptom combinations based on DSM-5 [27], and these combinations do not include the more nuanced effects of trauma on survivors' interpersonal and emotional functioning that may not fulfill diagnostic criteria. Fortunately, the diagnosis need not be difficult to make. Clinicians can often identify PTSD by maintaining a suspicion for the diagnosis, identifying a traumatic event, and recognizing the presences of symptoms across all symptom clusters. Many other diagnoses affect single symptom clusters; fewer induce impairment across all areas.

PTSD Complicating Treatment

Preexisting symptoms of PTSD may complicate patients' care and should be considered as a possible contributor to the ED presentation. For example, patients with PTSD have high rates of substance use disorders [28]; one study found that approximately 20% of persons with PTSD had used substances in trying to mitigate PTSD symptoms [29]. As discussed, patients with PTSD might be extremely anxious or on edge, perhaps seeming even paranoid. These patients often voice concerns about being harmed or treated unfairly by providers. Such maladaptive reactions may become more pronounced in stressful situations, including re-traumatization or being in an emergent medical situation. Other patients may appear overly detached or removed from the situation; they may express indifference to treatment or medical outcomes. When under duress, patients may experience dissociative episodes or flashbacks when they act or feel as though they are in a different, unreal situation. Regardless of whether the patient presents to be extremely reactive or dissociated, providers should aim to reorient and de-escalate the patient before proceeding to more complex discussions of treatment planning and disposition.

Given the variability in how patients with PTSD might present to the ED, emergency clinicians should strive to incorporate principles of trauma-informed care. Briefly, trauma-informed care is a model of care that recognizes the impact of trauma on a patient's life. Trauma-informed interventions are designed to help patients feel connected, informed, and hopeful for recovery, acknowledge the connection between previous trauma and current symptoms, and empower the autonomy of the traumatized individual [30].

Treatment

The primary role of the ED clinician is to ensure immediate medical and psychiatric safety. If the diagnosis of PTSD is made, referrals for further treatment may be considered. The first-line and most effective treatments for PTSD are psychotherapies [31]. When available, early trauma-focused cognitive behavioral therapy (CBT) within vivo and imaginal exposure exercises decreases the likelihood that a patient will develop PTSD [21, 32]. Features of trauma-focused CBT include validating the patient's response to trauma, enhancing the patient's expectation that they will recover, and examining the patient's core beliefs relating to the trauma. Briefly, exposure exercises consist of the patient gradually becoming desensitized to the traumatic event via repeated exposure to their trauma narrative.

Pharmacotherapy

Serotonergic agents, including SSRIs and SNRIs, are first-line medications for the treatment of PTSD [33]. These agents should generally be prescribed concurrently with an evidence-based psychotherapy. The ED clinician may consider prescribing a serotonergic agent on discharge if follow-up is clearly in place and the receiving provider is in agreement. Evidence for atypical antipsychotics is limited, with quetiapine [32] or risperidone [34] suggested primarily. Prazosin is helpful for PTSD-related nightmares and sleep [35]. Benzodiazepines are contraindicated, given their potential for abuse and interference with the process of exposure therapies [36]. Under no circumstances should benzodiazepines be prescribed for PTSD symptoms, including poor sleep, upon ED discharge.

Long-Term Treatment

Individual, manualized trauma-focused psychotherapy is the best treatment for PTSD, superior even to medications [31]. Although ED clinicians do not provide these treatments, understanding the therapeutic approach is helpful for briefer interactions with patients. Clinicians should recognize the complications of treatments, which may precipitate an ED visit. Moreover, ED clinicians should be sufficiently familiar to answer basic questions from patients and families.

Visiting the ED for PTSD symptoms is correlated with a patient's greater willingness to engage in PTSD psychotherapy [37]. Prolonged Exposure, Cognitive Processing Therapy, and Eye Movement Desensitization and Reprocessing are the most widely investigated modalities.

Prolonged Exposure (PE) involves the patient reexperiencing the traumatic event via imaginal and experiential exercises [38]. In the process of doing this, patients experience an acute increase in anxiety. Then, and most importantly, anxiety decreases as the previous traumatic experience does not actually recur. By reexposing patients repeatedly in a highly structured manner under the guidance of a therapist, patients grow deconditioned to the traumatic stimulus, and PTSD symptoms decrease. When patients begin treatment, it is not unusual that they experience a generalized increase in mood or anxiety symptoms, including panic attacks that may prompt an ED visit.

In Cognitive Processing Therapy (CPT), the patient writes an impact statement that details the patient's beliefs about the traumatic event [39]. The therapist and patient work together to identify connections among the patient's thoughts, feelings, and behaviors. CPT can also include an exposure component in which the patient writes a detailed narrative of the traumatic experience. The patient reads this narrative to the therapist with the goal of elucidating and adjusting the patient's maladaptive beliefs about the trauma. This process is quite difficult for the patient, and some patients may seek alternative referrals to treatment via the ED in order to avoid the difficult, anxiety-provoking work of a trauma narrative. An appropriate response to this avoidance is to reinforce the importance of therapy and alerting the mental health provider to the patient's visit.

Eye Movement Desensitization and Reprocessing (EMDR) features exposure and visual engagement by the therapist [40]. While in session, the patient imagines the traumatic experience and focuses on the cognitive and physiological symptoms experienced. Meanwhile, the therapist moves two fingers through the patient's visual field while the patient watches. This reimagining in the presence of a distracting stimulus is repeated as the patient's anxiety decreases. Eventually, the patient is able to replace a negative thought associated with the trauma, such as "I'll never get over this," with a more plausible thought: "I am strong and have made it through." Like other trauma-focused therapies, patients often experience increased anxiety when starting treatment.

These psychotherapies are manualized, time-limited, and administered with a strict therapeutic frame. These therapies are generally conducted over 12 to 16 weeks; treatment is intense, efficient, and designed to mitigate resistance to discussing the traumatic episode. Encouraging a patient to talk about the trauma without a specific therapeutic plan is reckless and detrimental.

Conclusion

Though unlikely to be the primary complaint prompting ED presentation, PTSD may influence the patient's behavior and interactions with the ED clinician. The ED diagnosis of PTSD is helpful to understanding the patient's interactions in the ED while also excluding alternative diagnoses and making the first steps toward definitive outpatient psychotherapy and pharmacological management.

References

1. Kessler RC, Aguilar-Gaxiola S, Alonso J, Benjet C, Bromet EJ, Cardoso G, et al. Trauma and PTSD in the WHO world mental health surveys. Eur J Psychotraumatol. 2017;8(sup5):1353383.
2. Kessler RC, Berglund P, Demler O, Jin R, Merikangas KR, Walters EE. Lifetime prevalence and age-of-onset distributions of DSM-IV disorders in the National Comorbidity Survey Replication. Arch Gen Psychiatry. 2005;62(6):593–602.
3. Van Ameringen M, Mancini C, Patterson B, Boyle MH. Post-traumatic stress disorder in Canada. CNS Neurosci Ther. 2008;14(3):171–81.
4. Solimine S, Takeshita J, Goebert D, Lee J, Schultz B, Guerrero M, et al. Characteristics of patients with constant observers. Psychosomatics. 2018;59(1):67–74.
5. Creamer M, Burgess P, McFarlane AC. Post-traumatic stress disorder: findings from the Australian National

Survey of Mental Health and Well-being. Psychol Med. 2001;31(7):1237–47.
6. Kroll J. Posttraumatic symptoms and the complexity of responses to trauma. JAMA. 2003;290(5):667–70.
7. Love J, Zatzick D. Screening and intervention for comorbid substance disorders, PTSD, depression, suicide: a trauma center survey. Psychiatr Serv. 2014;65(7):918–23.
8. Zatzick D, Donovan D, Dunn C, Russo J, Wang J, Jurkovich G, et al. Substance use and posttraumatic stress disorder symptoms in trauma center patients receiving mandated alcohol screening and brief intervention. J Subst Abus Treat. 2012;43(4):410–7.
9. van Meijel EP, Gigengack MR, Verlinden E, Opmeer BC, Heij HA, Goslings JC, et al. Predicting posttraumatic stress disorder in children and parents following accidental child injury: evaluation of the Screening Tool for Early Predictors of Post-traumatic Stress Disorder (STEPP). BMC Psychiatry. 2015;15:113.
10. Ward-Begnoche WL, Aitken ME, Liggin R, Mullins SH, Kassam-Adams N, Marks A, et al. Emergency department screening for risk for post-traumatic stress disorder among injured children. Inj Prev. 2006;12(5):323–6.
11. Brewin CR, Andrews B, Valentine JD. Meta-analysis of risk factors for posttraumatic stress disorder in trauma-exposed adults. J Consult Clin Psychol. 2000;68(5):748–66.
12. Grieger TA, Cozza SJ, Ursano RJ, Hoge C, Martinez PE, Engel CC, et al. Posttraumatic stress disorder and depression in battle-injured soldiers. Am J Psychiatry. 2006;163(10):1777–83; quiz 860.
13. Hoge CW, McGurk D, Thomas JL, Cox AL, Engel CC, Castro CA. Mild traumatic brain injury in U.S. Soldiers returning from Iraq. N Engl J Med. 2008;358(5):453–63.
14. Holbrook TL, Hoyt DB, Stein MB, Sieber WJ. Perceived threat to life predicts posttraumatic stress disorder after major trauma: risk factors and functional outcome. J Trauma. 2001;51(2):287–92; discussion 92–3.
15. Zatzick DF, Russo J, Pitman RK, Rivara F, Jurkovich G, Roy-Byrne P. Reevaluating the association between emergency department heart rate and the development of posttraumatic stress disorder: a public health approach. Biol Psychiatry. 2005;57(1):91–5.
16. Norman SB, Stein MB, Dimsdale JE, Hoyt DB. Pain in the aftermath of trauma is a risk factor for post-traumatic stress disorder. Psychol Med. 2008;38(4):533–42.
17. Edmondson D, Richardson S, Falzon L, Davidson KW, Mills MA, Neria Y. Posttraumatic stress disorder prevalence and risk of recurrence in acute coronary syndrome patients: a meta-analytic review. PLoS One. 2012;7(6):e38915.
18. Davydow DS, Gifford JM, Desai SV, Needham DM, Bienvenu OJ. Posttraumatic stress disorder in general intensive care unit survivors: a systematic review. Gen Hosp Psychiatry. 2008;30(5):421–34.
19. American Psychiatric Association. Diagnostic and statistical manual of mental disorders: DSM-5. 5th ed. Arlington: American Psychiatric Association; 2013.
20. Bryant RA. Acute stress disorder as a predictor of posttraumatic stress disorder: a systematic review. J Clin Psychiatry. 2011;72(2):233–9.
21. Ursano RJ, Bell C, Eth S, Friedman M, Norwood A, Pfefferbaum B, et al. Practice guideline for the treatment of patients with acute stress disorder and posttraumatic stress disorder. Am J Psychiatry. 2004;161(11 Suppl):3–31.
22. Steenen SA, van Wijk AJ, van der Heijden GJ, van Westrhenen R, de Lange J, de Jongh A. Propranolol for the treatment of anxiety disorders: systematic review and meta-analysis. J Psychopharmacol. 2016;30(2):128–39.
23. Gelpin E, Bonne O, Peri T, Brandes D, Shalev AY. Treatment of recent trauma survivors with benzodiazepines: a prospective study. J Clin Psychiatry. 1996;57(9):390–4.
24. Kitchener BA, Jorm AF. Mental Health First Aid: an international programme for early intervention. Early Interv Psychiatry. 2008;2(1):55–61.
25. Booth A, Scantlebury A, Hughes-Morley A, Mitchell N, Wright K, Scott W, et al. Mental health training programmes for non-mental health trained professionals coming into contact with people with mental ill health: a systematic review of effectiveness. BMC Psychiatry. 2017;17(1):196.
26. Wong EC, Collins RL, Cerully JL. Reviewing the evidence base for mental health first aid: is there support for its use with key target populations in California? Rand Health Q. 2015;5(1):19.
27. Galatzer-Levy IR, Bryant RA. 636,120 ways to have posttraumatic stress disorder. Perspect Psychol Sci. 2013;8(6):651–62.
28. Kessler RC, Sonnega A, Bromet E, Hughes M, Nelson CB. Posttraumatic stress disorder in the National Comorbidity Survey. Arch Gen Psychiatry. 1995;52(12):1048–60.
29. Leeies M, Pagura J, Sareen J, Bolton JM. The use of alcohol and drugs to self-medicate symptoms of posttraumatic stress disorder. Depress Anxiety. 2010;27(8):731–6.
30. Muskett C. Trauma-informed care in inpatient mental health settings: a review of the literature. Int J Ment Health Nurs. 2014;23(1):51–9.
31. Department of Veterans Affairs, Department of Defense. VA/DOD clinical practice guideline for the management of posttraumatic stress disorder and acute stress disorder: clinician summary. Washington, D.C.: Department of Veterans Affairs, Department of Defense; 2017. Updated June 2017. Available at https://www.healthquality.va.gov/guidelines/MH/ptsd/VADoDPTSDCPGClinicianSummaryFinal.pdf. Accessed on 21 Aug 2017.
32. Rothbaum BO, Kearns MC, Price M, Malcoun E, Davis M, Ressler KJ, et al. Early intervention may prevent the development of posttraumatic stress disorder: a randomized pilot civilian study with

modified prolonged exposure. Biol Psychiatry. 2012;72(11):957–63.
33. Stein DJ, Ipser JC, Seedat S. Pharmacotherapy for post traumatic stress disorder (PTSD). Cochrane Database Syst Rev. 2006;(1):CD002795.
34. Padala PR, Madison J, Monnahan M, Marcil W, Price P, Ramaswamy S, et al. Risperidone monotherapy for post-traumatic stress disorder related to sexual assault and domestic abuse in women. Int Clin Psychopharmacol. 2006;21(5):275–80.
35. Singh B, Hughes AJ, Mehta G, Erwin PJ, Parsaik AK. Efficacy of prazosin in posttraumatic stress disorder: a systematic review and meta-analysis. Prim Care Companion CNS Disord. 2016;18(4).
36. Rothbaum BO, Price M, Jovanovic T, Norrholm SD, Gerardi M, Dunlop B, et al. A randomized, double-blind evaluation of D-cycloserine or alprazolam combined with virtual reality exposure therapy for posttraumatic stress disorder in Iraq and Afghanistan War veterans. Am J Psychiatry. 2014;171(6):640–8.
37. Buchholz KR, Bohnert KM, Pfeiffer PN, Valenstein M, Ganoczy D, Anderson RE, et al. Reengagement in PTSD psychotherapy: a case-control study. Gen Hosp Psychiatry. 2017;48:20–4.
38. Foa EB, Hembree EA, Rothbaum BO. Prolonged exposure therapy for PTSD: emotional processing of traumatic experiences: therapist guide. Oxford and New York: Oxford University Press; 2007.
39. Resick PA, Monson CM, Chard KM. Cognitive processing therapy for PTSD: a comprehensive manual. New York: Guilford Press; 2017.
40. Shapiro F. Eye movement desensitization: a new treatment for post-traumatic stress disorder. J Behav Ther Exp Psychiatry. 1989;20(3):211–7.

Psychosis in the Emergency Department

12

Abigail Dahan

Introduction

Psychotic symptoms are common. The lifetime incidence of psychotic symptoms in the United States is as high as 10% [1]. These symptoms include hearing voices (auditory hallucinations), visual hallucinations, experiencing mind control, or paranoia. People with psychosis present to the emergency department (ED) for reasons both related and unrelated to their psychosis.

In this chapter, I review the elements of the ED evaluation of the patient with psychotic symptoms:

1. Evaluating agitation and safety
2. Identifying and exploring psychotic symptoms
3. Understanding the etiology of psychotic symptoms: Are they primary, as in schizophrenia, or secondary, as in medical illnesses or intoxication?
4. Performing a screening medical evaluation for patients with known primary psychotic illness who may have untreated medical problems
5. Assessing the patient's acute risk of danger to himself or others due to his psychosis
6. Discharging the patient with psychosis

This evaluation determines the level of medical or psychiatric treatment warranted. As hospitalization is often not indicated, I review interventions in the ED to improve the patient's course of illness in the community. This discussion is organized around brief case examples to highlight key points in the emergency evaluation of the patient with psychosis.

Evaluating Agitation and Safety

If the patient is agitated, agitation must be addressed immediately as it poses a danger to the patient, ED staff, and other patients. If the patient cannot be verbally de-escalated, medication administration will be required to decrease his level of dangerousness, and mechanical restraints may be applied. During the first minutes of the evaluation, the presence of delirium, intoxication, and medical illnesses must be assessed. Patients who received medications may be too sedated to fully participate in the evaluation; however, evaluation of the initial cause of agitation should be actively pursued.

A. Dahan (✉)
Department of Psychiatry, Bellevue Hospital, New York, NY, USA
e-mail: Abigail.Dahan@nyumc.org

L. S. Zun et al. (eds.), *Behavioral Emergencies for Healthcare Providers*,
https://doi.org/10.1007/978-3-030-52520-0_12

Case Example 1: "He's a Runner!"

Chief Complaint (CC): Emotionally Disturbed Person. An approximately 30-year-old man registered as "Unknown, Male" is brought to the hospital by ambulance after he was seen running down the center of a highway. When he was approached by emergency services, he waved a large Bible at them and screamed "Rocks a socks a rocks a socks a!" and then began to bark. On arrival, he was not responsive to attempts at verbal redirection to stop pacing rapidly, barking, and posturing in a fighting stance. He received intramuscular (IM) medication to decrease his level of agitation and became comfortably sedated but unable to engage in a meaningful interview.

It is imperative to remember that psychosis is not the only possible cause of acute agitation, even in a patient with a known severe mental illness. Agitation is commonly caused by delirium, intoxication, psychosis, mania, severe personality disorder, or disinhibition related to intellectual disability or brain injury. Patients with known psychotic illness may present as agitated due to exacerbation of their psychosis or due to another cause. (See references [2–5] for further discussion of the management of acute agitation, verbal de-escalation techniques, and restraint and seclusion.)

Identifying and Exploring Psychotic Symptoms

ED clinicians must identify symptoms of psychosis, as well as negative symptoms of schizophrenia, which will be notable for either their presence or absence during the evaluation of the person with psychosis. Key symptoms of psychosis include delusions, hallucinations, disorganization of thought, and disorganization of motor behavior (including catatonia).

Delusions

Delusions are beliefs that are firmly held despite contradicting evidence; if someone is unable to entertain the thought that their expressed belief could be wrong, it has risen from a firmly held belief into a delusion [6]. Delusions may include the belief that others are following you and trying to harm you (paranoid delusions), belief that someone knows your thoughts or is trying to extract thoughts from your head, belief that an outside force is putting thoughts into your head or trying to control your mind, or belief that innocuous stimuli in the environment hold specific personal meaning (delusions of reference). Grandiose and erotomanic delusions are more commonly seen in the patient with mania with psychotic features. The delusional belief that an outside force or person can control one's mind or body is often very frightening to the patient as it erodes the expectation of personal privacy and agency.

It is imperative to both elicit the presence or absence of delusions, as well as to explore their meaning. Many patients may not spontaneously divulge delusional beliefs. The evaluation of delusions should encompass a discussion of what this belief means to the person because the patient's response is central to risk assessment. For example, when assessing paranoid delusions, the examiner should ask whether the patient knows who is persecuting him and why, how the patient could identify the believed persecutor, and what the patient would do if he had interaction with the believed persecutor. The clinician should understand the patient's behaviors in response to the delusion, such as remaining inside, leaving the house, leaving curtains drawn, changing walking or driving routes, or taking precautions regarding what food is eaten. In the case of delusions of control, it is also important to inquire about the degree to which the patient feels that he can resist such outside influence/control and whether he has ever been in a situation where he was unable to resist such control [7–9]. After engaging with the patient in a discussion of his beliefs, the clinician will have a sufficient understanding of the patient's responses to make an informed assessment of his risk for dangerousness to himself or others.

Hallucinations

Hallucinations are perceptual experiences that occur without outside stimuli. The person may have such perceptual experiences within any of the five senses. Hallucinations are a symptom but are not specific to a diagnosis. Auditory hallucinations are the most common form of hallucination in schizophrenia. Common auditory hallucinations include hearing people mocking, threatening, or egging them onto action [6]. Visual hallucinations will be experienced at some point by more than 20% of people with schizophrenia [10] and are common symptoms in delirium [11]. Olfactory and gustatory hallucinations are seen in patients with seizures, brain tumors, or a primary psychotic illness. Tactile hallucinations, especially formication (the sensation of bugs crawling on the skin), are commonly associated with cocaine and amphetamine intoxication.

The assessment of hallucinations is not a binary assessment, and it is inadequate to indicate only whether or not the person is experiencing hallucinations. It is necessary to explore the person's (1) emotional response to the hallucinations, (2) insight into the experience as hallucinatory, and (3) understanding of the content of the hallucination. The assessment of hallucinations includes both the subjective report and objective evidence. For example, the objective evaluation may include whether the patient displays affect incongruous to his situation or appears to be actively responding to internal stimuli [9]. The patient's responses, both emotional and cognitive, to the hallucination are what will inform the clinician's risk assessment.

Disorganization of Thought

Disorganization of thought is an objective psychotic symptom. It refers not to the content of the thoughts but to the way in which a person's thoughts are strung together. Does one thought logically lead to the next? Is the next thought only obliquely related to the last thought? Are the thoughts not connected in any way, and do they appear to be unrelated [6]? In the first case example, the patient displayed clang associations when he said, "Rocks a socks a rocks a socks a"; the only relationship between these words is their sound. This verbalization is a dramatic example of thought disorganization. Less dramatically, patients with tangential thought process initially appear to have thoughts that are logically connected but then veer off tangentially in a manner that ultimately completely obscures meaningful communication. For example, when the examiner asks, "What brings you here today?," the patient replies, "I was walking down the street when a policeman stopped me, just stopped me like you stop a train in its tracks, like a train that was traveling from California to New York, and, well, it arrived in Penn Station and just stopped." Even an attentive clinician may feel confused by the patient's verbal responses: The clinician's feeling of confusion is an important clue, suggesting the patient's disorganization of thought.

Disorganization of Behavior

Disorganization of behavior is another objective psychotic symptom. Examples of this symptom include odd behavior such as posturing like an animal, miming, displaying psychomotor agitation, purposeless movements, or extreme negativism (including holding a rigid pose or remaining mute). Catatonia is a form of behavioral disorganization [6]. The patient discussed in the first case example displayed disorganized behavior by his purposeless agitation and bizarre barking.

Negative Symptoms of Schizophrenia

Negative symptoms are defined by decreased expressiveness and amotivation. Expressive deficits include restricted affect and poverty of speech. Loss of motivation encompasses decreased spontaneous motor activity, poor attention to grooming/hygiene, decrease in engagement in work/recreation/leisure, and decreased social engagement [12]. Negative symptoms of schizophrenia contribute significantly to its overall illness burden and morbidity. Recent estimates indicate that one or more negative symptoms are present in nearly 60% of patients with schizophrenia. Antipsychotic medications have limited impact on negative symptoms [13].

Delusions, hallucinations, disorganization of thought, and disorganization of behavior are terms for psychotic symptoms collectively referred to as "positive symptoms." Positive symptoms may be seen in either a primary or secondary psychosis, which will be discussed later in this chapter. Negative symptoms are found primarily in schizophrenia. The presence of prominent negative symptoms can help to narrow the differential diagnosis of a patient's psychosis.

Case Example 2: "She's So Lazy."

"She's talking to herself." A 28-year-old woman is brought to the ED by her husband because he has noticed that she has been talking and laughing to herself for the past month and has had a decline in functioning over the past year. He reports that she stopped going to work months ago for no apparent reason other than "laziness," and he says that she is "so lazy that when I leave for work, she is sitting on the couch, and when I get home, she's still sitting there. She's so lazy that she doesn't even bother to turn on the TV!" The patient is observed quietly talking to herself. When spoken to, she has a long latency of response, and then shakes her head and says, "What?" She then briefly engages with you. She denies having hallucinations, says that she feels "fine," and cannot give any explanation for her behavior or recent lack of engagement or interest. Suddenly, she interrupts speaking with you and turns, whispering under her breath, "Oh, hush! I can handle this without your help!" and then resumes speaking with you. She has no medical problems and does not use drugs or alcohol. Neither the patient nor her husband has any concerns about her harming herself or anyone else.

This woman has both prominent negative symptoms and hallucinations. Psychotic symptoms may be seen in a number of illnesses. Negative symptoms are specific to schizophrenia. This patient's symptoms are consistent with those of schizophrenia, a chronic psychotic illness defined as experiencing at least two out of five symptom clusters for at least 6 months. The major symptom clusters are hallucinations, delusions, disorganization of thought, disorganization of behavior, and negative symptoms [6]. This patient's hallucinations may compel the clinician's attention, but the negative symptoms are more diagnostically specific and may have a greater impact on her functioning.

Understanding the Etiology of Psychotic Symptoms

In the ED, it is imperative to determine whether the patient with psychotic symptoms has psychosis as a result of a primary psychiatric illness or if the symptoms are the result of intoxication or medical illness. Primary psychotic symptoms are due to a mental illness, most likely schizophrenia, schizoaffective disorder, delusional disorder, mania, depression with psychotic features, or schizotypal personality disorder. Secondary psychotic symptoms are due to intoxication or medical illness [6]. Unfortunately, there is no way to distinguish between primary and secondary psychosis on the basis of the presenting psychotic symptoms alone. New-onset psychotic symptoms presenting after age 45 generally warrant evaluation for delirium and a workup for a medical and/or substance-induced cause [14]; late-life onset of primary psychotic illness is rare. For a discussion of the many medical etiologies of psychotic symptoms in the ED, see Chap. 15.

The differential diagnosis for secondary psychotic symptoms is broad. Table 12.1 lists some of the many medical illnesses associated with psychotic symptoms. In the ED, common toxidromes that cause psychosis include:

1. Stimulant drugs
   (a) Cocaine
   (b) Amphetamine
   (c) Methamphetamines
   (d) 3,4-methylenedioxymethamphetamine (MDMA)/ecstasy
   (e) Bath salts

Table 12.1 Medical illnesses that can cause psychotic symptoms

Type of illness	Examples
Infection	Human immunodeficiency virus (HIV) Neurosyphilis Meningitis Cerebral malaria
Endocrine disorders	Thyroid disorder Steroid-producing tumors Pheochromocytoma Insulinomas
Autoimmune disease	Multiple sclerosis Systemic lupus erythematosus [20]
Dementia	Vascular Alzheimer's Lewy body/frontotemporal Huntington's [21] Parkinson's [22]
Brain injury	Trauma Stroke Seizure Tumor Abscess
Cancer	Paraneoplastic syndrome Ovarian teratoma
Encephalopathy	Limbic [23, 24] Uremic Hepatic Wernicke's
Other [25]	Wilson's disease Porphyrias

2. Hallucinogens
   (a) Phencyclidine (PCP)
   (b) Lysergic acid diethylamide (LSD)
3. Cannabinoids
   (a) Marijuana
   (b) Synthetic cannabinoids ("K2," "Spice")
   (c) High doses of dextromethorphan

Drug-induced psychosis typically resolves with the metabolism of acute intoxication but can persist for weeks or months following acute intoxication. Prescribed medications may also cause psychosis. Examples include Parkinson's disease medications (carbidopa-levodopa and amantadine), steroids, anticholinergic medications, stimulants, antihistamines, antibiotics (isoniazid, penicillin, macrolides, and fluoroquinolones), antivirals (acyclovir, efavirenz, and interferon), anticonvulsants, beta-blockers, meperidine, disulfiram, and benzodiazepines. Also consider withdrawal syndromes, including alcohol, benzodiazepines, or baclofen, as possible cause of psychotic symptoms [15].

Toxic exposures are a less common cause of psychotic symptoms. The onset of such symptoms closely follows the exposure. Chemicals that cause psychosis at certain exposure levels include many metals (mercury, lead, and manganese), pesticides (organophosphates [16]), and industrial solvents (carbon disulfide and toluene). Historically, clusters of cases of new-onset psychosis have occurred among rayon industry workers exposed to carbon disulfide, miners with manganese intoxication, and hatters or felt workers with mercury intoxication [17]. More recently, public health measures have been instituted to prevent such occupational exposures, but exposure may occur after accidents or natural disasters disrupt normal safety controls.

Delirium is a common etiology of psychosis in the ED. Unlike patients with schizophrenia, the patient with delirium will have had an acute onset of symptoms, as well as waxing and waning of symptoms. Delirium always causes inattention and typically causes impairment of short-term memory. A patient with delirium may or may not be oriented to person, place, and time [18]. Immediate recognition and treatment of delirium are important as the condition predicts poor outcomes, including increased mortality, institutionalization, prolonged hospitalization, and cognitive impairment [19]. For more on the identification and treatment of delirium, see Chap. 15.

Performing a Screening Medical Evaluation

As with any ED evaluation, vital signs must be evaluated, and the patient examined for acute physical illness or injury. Some patients present with medical complaints that may at first appear to be related to psychosis. Regardless, the patient's medical complaints must be evaluated prior to attributing any symptoms to psychosis. For example, a patient who presents with weakness "because my roommate is blowing toxic chemicals into my window" may demonstrate objective weakness notwithstanding any delusional symptom attribution. The following case example demonstrates the importance of a proper medical evaluation.

Case Example 3: "He's So Stinky."

"My shoulder hurts." A 58-year-old man is brought into the ED by ambulance after he walked up to a stranger, grabbed him, and screamed, "The mission has been compromised!" On arrival to the ED, he tells the triage nurse that he is here because of shoulder pain. He presents as extremely disheveled, malodorous, and wrapped in many layers of clothing. When asked by the ED doctor what brought him in, he responds with a lengthy and illogical diatribe about how "they" nearly got him and how, as an undercover CIA agent, he is on a secret mission to expose a foreign sleeper cell. He grimaces and intermittently moans throughout this interaction. Psychiatry is consulted and recommends admission to inpatient psychiatry for stabilization of psychosis. Only when the patient is changed into hospital pajamas immediately prior to being brought to the psychiatric department is it noticed that he is holding his left arm immobile and there is tenting and blanching of the skin above his left clavicle. This was not observed earlier under the patient's multiple layers of clothes. X-ray reveals a grossly displaced left clavicular fracture that requires surgical intervention.

People with primary psychotic illnesses receive inadequate health care. The socioeconomic disadvantages and decreased ability to function caused by primary psychotic illnesses lead to premature morbidity and mortality. One large study found that people with severe mental illness live, on average, 8.2 years less than the general population, with 95% of these deaths attributable to medical illnesses rather than accidents or injuries [26]. A large meta-analysis showed that people with schizophrenia have a 2.6-fold increase in mortality as compared with age-matched peers in the general population [27]. In the emergency setting, it is necessary to evaluate for untreated medical conditions, paying particular attention to wounds (both recent and chronic), foot care, bug infestation, respiratory illnesses, and untreated (or inadequately treated) sexually transmitted illnesses (including syphilis and HIV). Lab testing and imaging may be needed to clarify the etiology of the patient's psychosis, evaluate for acute medical problems, and obtain baseline levels prior to initiating treatment. Because the psychotic patient may be a poor historian, the ED clinician's close observations and physical examination will provide the clues to understanding the patient's medical stability.

Assessing the Patient's Acute Risk for Danger to Himself or Others

The psychiatric history of present illness will focus primarily on the (1) mode of arrival, (2) precipitating events, and (3) risk factors for dangerousness (to both self and others). The ED physician's role is not only to examine the patient but to evaluate his level of risk. Such evaluation extends beyond what the patient tells you and will include additional information from family, friends, or community treatment providers, as well as information found in the medical record. The standard of care for the ED evaluation includes reaching out to the patient's contacts in the community in order to fully understand the patient's functioning in the community, including overt symptoms of illness or worrisome behavior.

A suicide risk assessment should be completed and documented for all patients with psychosis. Suicide is a very real risk for those with schizophrenia: In the general US population, approximately 13 per 100,000 people complete suicide [28], compared to 5 per 100 people with schizophrenia. This risk is greatest early in the course of the illness [29]. For more information on risk assessment, see Chap. 8.

Among psychotic patients, violence toward other is less common than suicidal actions but nonetheless requires assessment. In the popular imagination, people with psychosis are believed to be at high risk for violence. However, the vast majority of violent acts committed in the United States are done by people who have no psychotic symptoms, and the majority of those who have psychosis do not engage in violence. It is true that the likelihood of committing violence is greater for people with major mental illness than for those without [30, 31]. Violence may be intentional or unintentional. For example, the highly disorganized, agitated patient may accidentally cause another injury by his actions, without specifically intending to harm another. This presentation contrasts with that of a patient who has a linear and coherent thought process and deliberately acts violently toward another. For example, a person who believes that he is about to be killed may harm another in what he perceives to be self-defense. Again, understanding the patient's reaction to delusional thinking is a critical part of the clinical assessment.

The third element of risk assessment, in addition to evaluation for risk for harm to self or others, is a person's ability to care for himself. This self-care is not based on functional ability but, rather, is a reflection of insight into the need for basic hygiene, food, clothing, and shelter. Patients with primary psychotic illness may be so disabled by their illness that they are unable to care for themselves in the community.

Case Example 4: "He's So Dirty."

"I don't know why I'm here." A 45-year-old man was brought into the ED by ambulance after homeless outreach workers called 911. Those workers observed him sleeping on the street and barely changing position for days. On arrival, the patient is calm and generally cooperative with everything that is asked of him. He is observed to have lice and is showered with a pediculicide body wash and shampoo. Afterward, the patient has a paucity of spontaneous speech but does not appear to be responding to internal stimuli. He denies having hallucinations and reports his mood to be "fine." No delusions are elicited on the exam. Lab testing reveals an anemia (hemoglobin 7.2 g/dL), most likely resulting from severe and chronic lice infestation coupled with dietary malnutrition iron deficiency. Psychiatry advises that the patient requires psychiatric hospitalization as he is unable to care for himself (as evidenced by his lice infestation and nutritional deficiency).

While this patient is similar to the patient in case example 2 in that he has prominent negative symptoms, unlike that patient, he cannot care for himself due to the severity of his illness coupled with his lack of social supports. For more on the decision to admit, see Chap. 20.

Discharging the Patient with Psychosis

Most patients with psychosis will be found to be at no acute risk for dangerousness toward themselves or others and will be deemed able to care for themselves. In such instances, the ED clinician must facilitate a discharge plan.

Antipsychotic medication may be started in the ED if local resources allow for close follow-up in the community. Such follow-up can be either with a psychiatrist or with a primary care provider with psychiatric consultation resources. The standard of care for starting antipsychotic medications includes obtaining a baseline metabolic screening, including a body mass index, waist circumference, blood pressure, blood glucose, and lipid panel [32], which may be easier to obtain in the ED than in certain outpatient office settings. A complete blood count and liver function testing may also be helpful. An electrocardiogram should be obtained in any patient with risk factors for QTc prolongation as antipsychotics may increase the QTc. These risk factors include age greater than 65, electrolyte disturbance, known cardiac disease, concomitant use of other medications that increase the risk for prolonged QTc, endocrine or metabolic disorders, or central nervous system injury [33]. Test results should be sent to the community provider on discharge. Additionally, the patient and his family must be educated that psychosocial interventions—together with medication treatment—are key components in the treatment of schizophrenia.

Psychosocial interventions include providing support and education for the patient's family and engaging patient in cognitive-behavioral therapy for psychosis [34]. The ED clinician can set the tone for ongoing treatment by listening to the patient's and family's concerns, providing realistic yet hopeful education about the patient's illness and need for treatment, and helping the patient and his family find ongoing treatment in the community. The patient and his family should be given clear guidelines as to what symptoms should trigger their return to the ED: any acute safety concerns by the patient or his family (even if these concerns are not well verbalized), verbalization of suicidal thoughts, increased agitation, scary displays of inappropriate affect, or verbalization of thoughts to harm others.

Conclusion

Many patients present to the ED with psychotic symptoms—perhaps these symptoms trigger the emergency evaluation or are entirely incidental findings. After managing acute agitation and medical concerns, the ED clinician should formulate an assessment of the most likely etiology of the patient's psychotic symptoms, as well as any other causes that are high in the differential diagnosis and require further evaluation. This assessment enables treatment, risk assessment, and discharge to the least restrictive level of care. When discharging patients, the ED clinician should educate the patient and his family as to symptoms that should trigger return to the ED and the need for ongoing treatment, including both medications and psychosocial treatments. Coordinating with outpatient providers may further improve the patient's prognosis and reduce ED recidivism.

References

1. DeVylder JE, Oh HY, Corcoran CM, Lukens EP. Treatment seeking and unmet need for care among persons reporting psychosis-like experiences. Psychiatr Serv. 2014;65(6):774–80.
2. Wilson MP, Pepper D, Currier GW, Holloman GH, Feifel D. The psychopharmacology of agitation: consensus statement of the American Association for Emergency Psychiatry Project BETA Psychopharmacology Workgroup. West J Emerg Med. 2012;13(1):26–34.
3. Wilson MP. Acute agitation. In: Tintinalli J, editor. Tintinalli's emergency medicine. 9th ed. (In press).
4. Pepper D, Wilson MP. The ethics of agitation: when is an agitated patient decisionally capable? In: Zeller S, Nordstrom K, Wilson MP, editors. The diagnosis and management of agitation. UK: Cambridge Press; 2017.
5. Zeller S, Nordstrom K, Wilson MP, editors. The diagnosis and management of agitation. Cambridge: Cambridge Press; 2017.
6. American Psychiatric Association. Schizophrenia spectrum and other psychotic disorders. In: Diagnostic and statistical manual of mental disorders. 5th ed. Washington, D.C.: American Psychiatric Association; 2013.
7. Bo S, Abu-Akel A, Kongerslev M, Haahr UH, Simonsen E. Risk factors for violence among patients with schizophrenia. Clin Psychol Rev. 2011;31(5):711–26.
8. Swanson JW, Swartz MS, Van Dorn RA, Elbogen EB, Wagner HR, Rosenheck RA, Stroup TS, McEvoy JP, Lieberman JA. A national study of violent behavior in persons with schizophrenia. Arch Gen Psychiatry. 2006;63(5):490–9.
9. Dahan AL, Woodman J. In: Maloy K, editor. A case-based approach to emergency psychiatry. New York: Oxford University Press; 2016. p. 41–50.
10. McCarthy-Jones S, Smailes D, Corvin A, Gill M, Morris DW, Dinan TG, Murphy KC, Anthony ONeill F, Waddington JL, Australian Schizophrenia Research Bank, Donohoe G, Dudley R. Occurrence and co-occurrence of hallucinations by modality in schizophrenia-spectrum disorders. Psychiatry Res. 2017;252:154–60.
11. Webster R, Holroyd S. Prevalence of psychotic symptoms in delirium. Psychosomatics. 2000;41(6):519–22.
12. Messinger JW, Tremeau F, Antonius D, Mendelsohn E, Prudent V, Stanford AD, Malaspina D. Avolition and expressive deficits capture negative symptom phenomenology: implications for DSM-5 and schizophrenia research. Clin Psychol Rev. 2011;31(1):161–8.
13. Bobes J, Arango C, Garcia-Garcia M, Rejas J, CLAMORS Study Collaborative Group. Prevalence of negative symptoms in outpatients with schizophrenia spectrum disorders treated with antipsychotics in routine clinical practice: findings from the CLAMORS study. J Clin Psychiatry. 2010;71(3):280–6.
14. Wilson MP, Nordstrom K, Anderson EL, Ng AT, Zun LS, Peltzer-Jones JM, Allen MH. American Association for Emergency Psychiatry Task Force on medical clearance of adult psychiatric patients. Part II: controversies over medical assessment, and consensus recommendations. West J Emerg Med. 2017;18(4):640–6.
15. Available at http://pdr.net. Accessed September 19, 2017.
16. Singh S, Sharma N. Neurological syndromes following organophosphate poisoning. Neurol India. 2000;48(4):308–13.
17. Kim Y, Kim JW. Toxic encephalopathy. Saf Health Work. 2012;3(4):243–56.

18. Inouye SK, van Dyck CH, Alessi CA, Balkin S, Siegal AP, Horwitz RI. Clarifying confusion: the confusion assessment method. A new method for detection of delirium. Ann Intern Med. 1990;113(12):941–8.
19. Oldham MA, Flanagan NM, Khan A, Boukrina O, Marcantonio ER. Responding to ten common delirium misconceptions with best evidence: an educational review for clinicians. J Neuropsychiatry Clin Neurosci. 2018;30(1):51–7.
20. Benros ME, Eaton WW, Mortensen PB. The epidemiologic evidence linking autoimmune diseases and psychosis. Biol Psychiatry. 2014;75(4):300–6.
21. Correa BB, Xavier M, Guimaraes J. Association of Huntington's disease and schizophrenia-like psychosis in a Huntington's disease pedigree. Clin Pract Epidemiol Ment Health. 2006;2:1.
22. Weintraub D, Hurtig HI. Presentation and management of psychosis in Parkinson's disease and dementia with Lewy bodies. Am J Psychiatry. 2007;164(10):1491–8.
23. Anderson NE, Barber PA. Limbic encephalitis—a review. J Clin Neurosci. 2008;15(9):961–71.
24. Ramanathan S, Mohammad SS, Brilot F, Dale RC. Autoimmune encephalitis: recent updates and emerging challenges. J Clin Neurosci. 2014;21(5):722–30.
25. Freudenreich O. Differential diagnosis of psychotic symptoms: medical "mimics.". Psychiatr Times. 2012;03:56–61.
26. Druss BG, Zhao L, Von Esenwein S, Morrato EH, Marcus SC. Understanding excess mortality in persons with mental illness: 17-year follow up of a nationally representative US survey. Med Care. 2011;49(6):599–604.
27. Saha S, Chant D, McGrath J. A systematic review of mortality in schizophrenia: is the differential mortality gap worsening over time? Arch Gen Psychiatry. 2007;64(10):1123–31.
28. National Center for Health Statistics. Available at https://www.cdc.gov/nchs/fastats/suicide.htm. Accessed 28 Oct 2017.
29. Palmer BA, Pankratz VS, Bostwick JM. The lifetime risk of suicide in schizophrenia: a reexamination. Arch Gen Psychiatry. 2005;62(3):247–53.
30. Link BG, Stueve A, Phelan J. Psychotic symptoms and violent behaviors: probing the components of the "threat/control-override" symptoms. Soc Psychiatry Psychiatr Epidemiol. 1998;33 Suppl 1:S55–60.
31. Douglas KS, Guy LS, Hart SD. Psychosis as a risk factor for violence to others: a meta-analysis. Psychol Bull. 2009;135(5):679–706.
32. American Diabetes Association, American Psychiatric Association, American Association of Clinical Endocrinologists, North American Association for the Study of Obesity. Consensus development conference on antipsychotic drugs and obesity and diabetes. Diabetes Care. 2004;27(2):596–601.
33. Shah AA, Aftab A, Coverdale J. QTc prolongation with antipsychotics: is routine ECG monitoring recommended? J Psychiatr Pract. 2014;20(3):196–206.
34. Norman R, Lecomte T, Addington D, Anderson E. Canadian treatment guidelines on psychosocial treatment of schizophrenia in adults. Can J Psychiatry. 2017;62(9):617–23.

Personality Disorders in the Emergency Department

13

Ashley Curry and Megan Riddle

Introduction

Patients with personality disorders can be challenging to care for in emergency settings. Their poor coping, unstable affect, impulsivity, and interpersonal dysfunction can present unique challenges for health-care professionals. Having a personality disorder negatively affects medical outcomes [1] and increases health-care utilization [2]. In most cases, a personality disorder is suspected when a patient's behavior is unusual, results in conflict, or elicits a strong emotional reaction from providers. Making a formal diagnosis of a personality disorder can be complicated and time-consuming and is generally beyond the scope of emergency care. However, identification of features commonly seen in individuals with personality disorders is helpful for patient care. Even individuals who do not meet full diagnostic criteria may have significant impairment and can benefit from the interventions described in this chapter [3].

A. Curry (✉)
Psychiatric Emergency Services, Denver Health Medical Center, Denver, CO, USA

M. Riddle
Eating Recover Center, Bellevue, WA, USA

Key Features of Personality Disorders

Personality is the collection of thoughts and behaviors that shape how a person views himself and how he interacts with the rest of the world. A personality disorder is defined as an enduring pattern of distorted cognitions, affective dysregulation, and interpersonal conflict that causes significant impairment in daily functioning. Since any person can exhibit maladaptive traits under stress, a personality disorder is only diagnosed in cases of pervasive dysfunction over a period of many years that cannot be explained by another medical or psychiatric condition. Personality disorders can be comorbid with other mental disorders, and multiple observations over time are recommended to make a diagnosis [4]. The need for serial assessments and an in-depth social history typically mean that the diagnosis of personality disorder should be deferred to a less acute setting.

Salient features of the ten personality disorders defined by the Diagnostic and Statistical Manual, Fifth Edition (DSM-5), are described in Table 13.1, along with common behaviors that can interfere with care. Cluster A disorders (paranoid, schizoid, and schizotypal) are classified as odd or eccentric and may be difficult to engage and less likely to voluntarily seek clinical care. Cluster B disorders (antisocial, borderline,

L. S. Zun et al. (eds.), *Behavioral Emergencies for Healthcare Providers*,
https://doi.org/10.1007/978-3-030-52520-0_13

Table 13.1 DSM-5 personality disorders [4, 5]

Classification	Key features	Potential challenges
Cluster A	*Odd, eccentric*	
Paranoid	Suspicious, distrustful	Hostility, unfounded accusations, or assumed malicious intent
Schizoid	Socially distant	Difficult to engage, disinterested
Schizotypal	Strange behaviors and/or magical thinking	Refusing care for bizarre reasons; presentation may look like prodromal psychosis
Cluster B	*Labile, impulsive*	
Antisocial	Disregard/violation of rights of others	Experienced as threatening, charming, or manipulative
Borderline	Interpersonal conflict, unstable self-image, impulsivity	Prone to splitting the team, may engage in self-harm
Histrionic	Dramatic, attention-seeking	Act out to gain attention from team members
Narcissistic	Grandiose, need for admiration, lack of empathy	Belittling team members or questioning status
Cluster C	*Anxious, neurotic*	
Avoidant	Socially inhibited, feelings of inadequacy	Inadequately relay history or avoid asking for clarification
Dependent	Clinging, need to be cared for	Appear to simultaneously seek and reject help
Obsessive-compulsive	Rigid and perfectionistic	Unreasonable or overly particular about care

histrionic, narcissistic) are typically characterized by emotional lability and erratic behavior. Of the three clusters, Cluster B traits are most commonly associated with difficult or disruptive patients in emergency settings. Cluster C disorders (avoidant, dependent, obsessive-compulsive) are described as anxious and fearful and may be experienced by care team members as needy and demanding or obsequious [4].

Epidemiology of Personality Disorders

Prevalence of personality disorder in the general population is estimated at 6–15% [6–10]. Risk factors for personality disorders include low socioeconomic status and being divorced, separated, or widowed [7]. Comorbidity with mood, anxiety, psychotic, and substance use disorders is significant even when controlling for socioeconomic status [7–10]. Personality disorders are associated with significant disability, and patients' life expectancy is nearly two decades shorter than the general population's, due in part to higher rates of tobacco use, other substance use, obesity, metabolic syndrome, cardiovascular disease, and sleep problems [1, 7, 11]. Moreover, the very structure of these individuals' personalities makes it difficult for them to engage with providers and utilize health care effectively, likely contributing to increased morbidity and mortality. Patients with personality disorders (particularly Cluster B) have higher utilization of medical services, including inpatient hospital, imaging, and ED services [2, 12].

Nature and Nurture

Personality disorders arise from an interplay of genetic and environmental factors. Personality disorders are highly heritable, and genetics play a significant role in their development [13–15]. Traumatic events during childhood further exacerbate this risk, and many individuals with personality disorders have experienced trauma and neglect [16–19]. Such trauma induces chronic stress and production of stress hormones that alter physiology and neurodevelopment [17]. For example, neuroimaging of adults with personality disorders shows differences in areas of the brain involved in processing emotions and interpreting social interactions, suggesting that underlying neuronal differences may contribute to difficulty with interpersonal relationships [20–23]. Trauma alters neurotransmitter systems key to regulating emotions, such as serotonin, dopamine, and norepinephrine, and thereby likely contributes to pathology found in personality disorders [17, 24–26].

Differential Diagnosis

Any individual can manifest maladaptive behaviors and interpersonal dysfunction when under stress, so it is important to exclude other medical or psychological problems. Paranoia, neuroticism, psychosis, emotionality, and erratic behavior can be symptoms of a variety of mental and medical disorders. Establishing a time course of symptoms can aid in narrowing the differential. An abrupt or late-life personality change without signs of personality pathology earlier in life is not consistent with a personality disorder. Other causes such as a mood or psychotic disorder, post-traumatic stress disorder, substance use, delirium, or dementia should be investigated. Collateral information from social supports and outpatient providers is indispensable in determining the chronicity of personality changes.

The stressful ED environment can unmask maladaptive personality traits in psychologically tenuous patients. It is not necessary to formally diagnose a personality disorder before considering the impact a patient's personality structure might have on their presentation. Patients who exhibit just one feature of a personality disorder are at increased risk for suicide, hospitalization, and social or occupational dysfunction [3]. In addition, a patient's trauma history has implications for health-care delivery. Being aware of how a history of trauma can affect the way these individuals experience care in the ED can reduce the risk of re-traumatization, improve the patient experience, and decrease potential conflict [27, 28].

Management in the ED

Emergency settings demand that providers quickly establish rapport with patients to gather information and create a treatment plan. Yet rapport can be particularly challenging to establish with patients with personality disorders who have fundamental difficulties with interpersonal relationships. Clinicians often experience feelings of confusion, frustration, or helplessness in reaction to patients with personality disorders. These feelings contribute to stigma toward individuals with personality disorders [11, 29]. Such stigma can negatively impact health-care delivery, even when not conscious on the part of the provider. Unconscious bias impacts not only patient-provider interactions but also diagnosis, treatment decisions, and medical outcomes [30]. Acknowledging these feelings early in the patient encounter enables clinicians to employ behavioral interventions to strengthen their rapport with patients and ultimately improve care [5].

When a patient arrives at the ED with a historical diagnosis of a personality disorder or exhibits the symptoms or behaviors outlined in Table 13.1, the ED clinician should begin considering potential pitfalls in treatment and appropriate management strategies. The following cases highlight common presentations of patients with personality disorders. The cases focus on Cluster B pathology as these traits are most commonly associated with difficult and disruptive patients in the ED. The interventions described are examples of the management approach summarized in Table 13.2.

Case Example 1: A Chronically Suicidal and Self-Harming Patient

A 27-year-old woman with a history of depression presents to the ED with superficial lacerations to her upper arms, saying she wants to die. She shares tearfully that she has just recently broken up with her boyfriend, saying, "He was my whole world. Now I don't know what I'm going to do." The nurse spends a significant amount of time with her, listening and trying to comfort her. When the physician comes to see her, she gushes, "These are the best nurses I've ever had." The physician initially feels a desire to protect and comfort the patient as she is quite distressed. However, a review of her medical record then reveals that she has been to the ED nearly weekly for the past several months with similar complaints; the physician then feels frustrated

Table 13.2 Behavioral management of patients with a personality disorder in the ED

Keep emotions in check	Recognize that these patients elicit strong emotions; be aware of the emotional responses of various team members (positive and negative). Acknowledging your reaction to the patient can help you provide appropriate care. Do not allow your reaction to patient behaviors to overshadow legitimate safety or medical concerns.
Set limits	Identify what boundaries are important to maintain and where there is flexibility; not all battles are worth fighting.
Maintain a consistent message	Communicate within the team so the patient receives a consistent message.
Offer empathy and validation	Acknowledge the real distress these patients experience; listen intently and validate the emotions that can be validated.
Reinforce appropriate behavior	Reinforce collaboration and engagement—this might include talking with the patient or offering comfort items. If safe to do so, disengage when the patient is disruptive. Often, patients get most attention from acting out, which reinforces these behaviors.

that she is abusing the ED and quickly loses his patience with her. He confronts her, saying, "You've been here three times this month. What's different this time?" The patient yells at the physician and refuses to talk with him. The physician exits the room and informs the nurse that he was unable to perform a safety assessment due to the patient's behavior. The nurse is confused because the patient was very pleasant with her.

This patient exhibits emotional dysregulation, non-suicidal self-injury, and a tendency to idealize some persons while devaluing others (splitting). She may meet criteria for borderline personality disorder (Table 13.1), although making a diagnosis requires further history and collateral. Regardless of whether she meets full criteria, behavioral interventions are the first line for management:

- Offer empathy and validation. While the intense emotionality displayed by the patient can feel manipulative, keep in mind that the patient is experiencing genuine distress. Empathy and validation should be offered through careful, active listening, naming emotions, and normalizing feelings. It may be valuable to say something like, "This is a really difficult situation. I can see that you're upset. Does anything help you feel better in these situations?" This response acknowledges the patient's distress while also encouraging her to use positive coping skills.
- Keep emotions in check. Here, frustration on the part of the physician further escalated the situation and interfered with the safety evaluation. Because these patients evoke strong emotional responses, providers need to be aware of their own emotions. Ideally, providers should maintain a positive regard for the patient, but even a neutral stance helps to defuse the situation. If a provider feels that emotions are running too high, taking a step back from the situation allows all parties to cool off.

The patient is eventually able to engage in safety planning and plans for discharge. When the physician returns to sign her out, she states that the social worker promised her a cab ride to her brother's house 1 hour away. The physician angrily confronts the social worker, asking him why he did not update the team on this change to the plan. The social worker said he only offered a bus ticket, is hurt by the accusation, and attempts to avoid the physician for the rest of his shift.

- Maintain a consistent message. In this case, the patient may have misunderstood the social worker or stretched the truth in an attempt to meet her needs. Had the physician not already been upset by this patient's previous behavior, he might have used a different approach to talk with his colleague. This case highlights a tendency of these patients to see individuals as either all good or all bad. This splitting lead to divisions among team members. Lapses in communication both among team members and with the patient can lead to conflict. The solution to this pitfall is to maintain consistent communication among the ED team. Brief all team members on updates to the treatment plan. If concerned about miscommunication, the team might see the patient together to ensure the plan is clearly communicated.

Case Example 2: A Disruptive and Demanding Patient

A 40-year-old male presents to the ED complaining of chest pain. He appears to be in significant distress and is initially appreciative to the staff for their assistance. He makes frequent requests for a private room and a more comfortable bed, and when he is told this is not possible, he is belittling toward staff. When he is asked to provide urine for toxicology, he becomes angry and accuses the team of not taking his complaints seriously and "doing any test they can think of" to increase his hospital bill. He adamantly refuses to provide a urine sample, swears at the nurse, and throws his urinal across the room.

This patient is exhibiting both narcissistic and paranoid traits. He has a sense of entitlement when it comes to his medical care. He becomes angry when he perceives that his concerns are not being appropriately addressed. He is suspicious of doctors and the hospital system. The following interventions are helpful when working with angry or disruptive patients:

- Set limits. This patient's behavior is unsafe, disruptive, and unsettling to providers and may interfere with the care of other patients. Set boundaries and clearly communicate expectations for behavior at the first sign of problems. It is still reasonable to use validation to try to de-escalate the situation and find common ground. However, contingencies for ongoing disruptive behavior should be clearly communicated to the patient and other staff members.
- Reinforce appropriate behaviors. Providers do not need to tolerate abusive language. Request that the patient stop swearing, and if that is ineffective, offer to return later. The offer to return may serve as positive reinforcement: "I can't work with people when they swear at me. If you can stop, I'd like to try to help you now. Otherwise, I'll come back in a little bit when the situation has cooled down." Note that this remark specifically references that "the situation," rather than "the patient," needs to cool down; depersonalizing the episode helps prevent further escalation.

Staff is advocating for the patient's immediate discharge. The physician is considering this until his repeat troponin returns as elevated and a repeat electrocardiogram is concerning for a myocardial infarction.

- Keep emotions in check. The team's reaction to this patient's disruptive behavior overshadowed his initial complaint of chest pain. Although difficult to do, it is the responsibility of emergency providers to look beyond behaviors to provide a thorough medical evaluation. Now that this patient is going to be admitted, a discussion regarding expectations for behavior on the inpatient unit may help to reduce future conflict.

Care Plans

While behavioral interventions form the bedrock of the management and treatment of personality disorders [31], it is difficult to maintain consistency across multiple ED encounters. For frequent ED utilizers, a care plan provides greater uniformity in care [32]. Care plans should be created in collaboration with outpatient providers so that the patient's treatment in the ED is consistent with long-term goals [33]. Plans might include information about when psychiatric hospitalization is beneficial and guidance around disposition and safety planning. ED care plans should include the components described in Table 13.3 in order to decrease disruptive behaviors and reinforce adaptive ones. These plans help ensure the ED visit itself is not reinforcing by providing clini-

Table 13.3 Components of an ED care plan

Recommended behavioral interventions	Description of effective ways to interact with the patient. What helps the patient when distressed? Does the patient have self-harm history in ED?
Medical treatment guidance	Management of chronic medical issues; appropriateness of providing refills from the ED
Medication recommendations	Guidelines regarding use of opiates, benzodiazepines, antipsychotics
Disposition planning	Appropriateness of hospitalization—specific warning signs that merit hospitalization
Safety plan and important contacts	Contact information for outpatient providers Crisis plan, including ways to manage distress once patients leave the ED and important contacts

cians clear, consistent guidelines around specific medications (e.g., benzodiazepines, opiates), and certain comfort measures (e.g., meals). A care plan also creates a reassuring treatment structure for providers who feel overwhelmed or frustrated by these patients.

Pharmacologic Intervention

It is natural to want to offer anxiolytic medication to a patient in distress, out of desire to ease suffering and resolve disruptive behaviors. While medications may be indicated to treat comorbid disorders such as depression, anxiety, and psychosis, there are no FDA-approved medications for personality disorders and no formal guidelines for treating agitation in patients with personality disorders. Patients with personality disorders are frequently prescribed medication, especially benzodiazepines, to address personality traits, but benefits are generally limited [34–36]. Unless toxicity is a concern, outpatient regimens should not be changed in the ED as changes may reinforce more frequent visits without benefit for the patient [35].

In cases of agitation, de-escalation with behavioral techniques should be the focus of the treatment plan. Medication should be reserved for behavior that poses a risk to the patient or staff or significantly interferes with care. First-line medications are benzodiazepines (lorazepam, diazepam) for agitation in the absence of psychosis and second-generation antipsychotics (olanzapine, risperidone, ziprasidone) or haloperidol for agitation associated with psychosis [37]. If medication is administered, the rationale for using medication should be clearly explained to the patient so that the patient does not interpret medication as punitive or a substitute for psychosocial interventions [33].

Safety Assessment and Suicide Risk

Some estimated 9–28% of individuals who complete suicide and 55% of individuals who attempt suicide have a diagnosis of a personality disorder [38]. Borderline personality disorder is most closely associated with suicide attempts; emotional dysregulation, affect lability, and nonsuicidal self-injury are all risk factors for suicide and key diagnostic features of borderline personality disorder. Approximately 50–90% of individuals with borderline personality disorder report engaging in suicidal behavior, and up to 10% complete suicide [39]. It is theorized that frequent self-injury allows individuals to become practiced in suicidal behavior, which decreases fear of suicide and increases understanding of lethality [38]. While most of this chapter, and the literature in general, focuses on suicide risk in Cluster B personality disorders, Cluster A and C individuals are also at increased risk of suicide. The most important factor to consider when assessing risk in these individuals is the severity of comorbid depression [40].

When assessing safety in an individual with a personality disorder, particular attention should be paid to personality traits that could increase the individual's risk for suicide, including emotional dysregulation, interpersonal conflict, impulsivity, anger, and social isolation [38]. Due to poor coping, individuals with personality disorders are at increased risk of suicide following certain adverse life events, such as breakups, financial problems, loss of job, or legal problems [41, 42]. Also consider unique traits that might interfere with assessment of suicide risk. Patients might be unaware of or unable to articulate feelings of grief, shame, or hopelessness. Suicidal ideation may be withheld out of fear of appearing vulnerable, being labeled a "bad" patient, or being involuntarily committed. Odd beliefs about medication or treatment options may lead to unintentional self-harm. Furthermore, an individual may have developed a pattern of self-harming or expressing suicidal ideation to avoid abandonment or escape legal, financial, or housing problems.

Violence Risk

The risk of violent behavior is elevated in patients with personality disorders, particularly those with Cluster B traits [39, 43, 44]. Impulsivity and affect dysregulation, paranoia, and narcissistic injury are all risk factors for violence. High comorbidity of personality disorders with substance use further compounds risk [43]. Antisocial traits are most strongly associated with violence, and a diagnosis of antisocial personality disorder increases an individual's risk of violence independent of any other signs or symptoms [44]. If a patient's violent or threatening behavior is volitional and does not appear to be the result of an underlying mental disorder, staff should consider involving law enforcement and filing criminal charges. If a patient has a history of violence, all providers should be informed of this history prior to interacting with the patient so they can take appropriate safety precautions. Additionally, providers should be familiar with the interpretation of Tarasoff laws in the state in which they practice [45].

Disposition Planning

Developing a treatment plan should include evaluating symptoms and safety, gathering collateral, and coordinating with outpatient providers. Inpatient psychiatric hospitalization is not beneficial to all patients and has not been shown to reduce suicide risk in chronically self-harming patients with personality disorders [37]. When contacted by the ED, outpatient therapists or case managers may share a crisis plan that includes alternatives to hospitalization.

The helplessness the patient exhibits may reinforce the provider's sense of futility when caring for patients who repeatedly self-harm. ED clinicians should consider that each visit to the ED is an opportunity to build and reinforce the patient's adaptive coping skills. Proven methods for risk reduction—including addressing access to lethal means, fostering connectedness to the community, and writing a safety plan—should be employed at every visit. Mobilizing social supports and providing psychoeducation to family and friends on how to reinforce adaptive coping skills help to prevent future visits. For patients without those supports, involving a crisis team or referring the patient to a community clubhouse or drop-in center can create connectedness with the community.

Return precautions should urge patients to seek help again if faced with overwhelming suicidal ideation or aggressive impulses. This advice resembles that given to patients with a chronic medical illness with frequent exacerbations and reduces patients' sense of alienation and rejection [45]. Follow-up telephone calls or postcards after discharge from the ED further reduce subsequent suicidal behavior. If these interventions are not available, leaving a caring message for the patient on the after-visit summary reduces the patient's sense of isolation.

Documentation

Providers may be tempted to document their strong reactions to these patients in the chart. Avoid this error. Pejorative or judgmental rhetoric in the medical chart reflects poorly on the writer and increases the potential for litigation [45]. Documentation should remain descriptive and nonjudgmental; when in doubt, describe patient behaviors, rather than interpreting them. Additionally, it is important to document a rationale for discharge of high-risk individuals. This documentation may include differentiation of acute and chronic risk, the unlikelihood of an inpatient admission modifying a patient's risk, or details of consultation with outpatient providers [46]. Even if a formal care plan is not developed, ED clinicians can aid their colleagues in the future by documenting effective behavioral interventions, the patient's response to medication, details of the safety plan, and important social contacts.

Conclusion

Patients with personality disorders present challenges to the entire treatment team in the ED and require extra time and emotional effort from the team. Providers who feel frustrated or manipulated should keep in mind that these patients are trying their best to feel better in the face of a chronic illness that affects their coping skills and interpersonal functioning. Clinicians should also keep in mind that these patients do get better: over the course of 10 years, patients with personality disorders remit at rates comparable to those with depression [47]. Working with these patients, rather than in opposition to them, helps them obtain the care they need while also decreasing behavioral disruptions in the ED and reducing staff burnout.

References

1. Dixon-Gordon KL, Whalen DJ, Layden BK, Chapman AL. A systematic review of personality disorders and health outcomes. Can Psychol. 2015;56(2):168–90.
2. Keuroghlian AS, Frankenburg FR, Zanarini MC. The relationship of chronic medical illnesses, poor health-related lifestyle choices, and health care utilization to recovery status in borderline patients over a decade of prospective follow-up. J Psychiatr Res. 2013;47(10):1499–506.
3. Zimmerman M, Chelminski I, Young D, Dalrymple K, Martinez J. Does the presence of one feature of borderline personality disorder have clinical significance? Implications for dimensional ratings of personality disorders. J Clin Psychiatry. 2012;73(1):8–12.
4. American Psychiatric Association. DSM-5 task force. Diagnostic and statistical manual of mental disorders: DSM-5. 5th ed. Washington, D.C.: American Psychiatric Association; 2013, p. xliv, 947.
5. Riddle M, Meeks T, Alvarez C, Dubovsky A. When personality is the problem: managing patients with difficult personalities on the acute care unit. J Hosp Med. 2016;11(12):873–8.
6. Lenzenweger MF, Lane MC, Loranger AW, Kessler RC. DSM-IV personality disorders in the National Comorbidity Survey Replication. Biol Psychiatry. 2007;62(6):553–64.
7. Grant BF, Hasin DS, Stinson FS, Dawson DA, Chou SP, Ruan WJ, et al. Prevalence, correlates, and disability of personality disorders in the United States: results from the national epidemiologic survey on alcohol and related conditions. J Clin Psychiatry. 2004;65(7):948–58.
8. Grant BF, Chou SP, Goldstein RB, Huang B, Stinson FS, Saha TD, et al. Prevalence, correlates, disability, and comorbidity of DSM-IV borderline personality disorder: results from the wave 2 National Epidemiologic Survey on alcohol and related conditions. J Clin Psychiatry. 2008;69(4):533–45.
9. Pulay AJ, Stinson FS, Dawson DA, Goldstein RB, Chou SP, Huang B, et al. Prevalence, correlates, disability, and comorbidity of DSM-IV schizotypal personality disorder: results from the wave 2 national epidemiologic survey on alcohol and related conditions. Prim Care Companion J Clin Psychiatry. 2009;11(2):53–67.
10. Stinson FS, Dawson DA, Goldstein RB, Chou SP, Huang B, Smith SM, et al. Prevalence, correlates, disability, and comorbidity of DSM-IV narcissistic personality disorder: results from the wave 2 national epidemiologic survey on alcohol and related conditions. J Clin Psychiatry. 2008;69(7):1033–45.
11. Tyrer P, Reed GM, Crawford MJ. Classification, assessment, prevalence, and effect of personality disorder. Lancet. 2015;385(9969):717–26.
12. Chang G, Weiss AP, Orav EJ, Rauch SL. Predictors of frequent emergency department use among patients with psychiatric illness. Gen Hosp Psychiatry. 2014;36(6):716–20.
13. Gjerde LC, Czajkowski N, Roysamb E, Orstavik RE, Knudsen GP, Ostby K, et al. The heritability of avoidant and dependent personality disorder assessed by personal interview and questionnaire. Acta Psychiatr Scand. 2012;126(6):448–57.
14. Kendler KS, Myers J, Torgersen S, Neale MC, Reichborn-Kjennerud T. The heritability of cluster A personality disorders assessed by both personal interview and questionnaire. Psychol Med. 2007;37(5):655–65.

15. Torgersen S, Myers J, Reichborn-Kjennerud T, Roysamb E, Kubarych TS, Kendler KS. The heritability of cluster B personality disorders assessed both by personal interview and questionnaire. J Pers Disord. 2012;26(6):848–66.
16. Battle CL, Shea MT, Johnson DM, Yen S, Zlotnick C, Zanarini MC, et al. Childhood maltreatment associated with adult personality disorders: findings from the Collaborative Longitudinal Personality Disorders Study. J Pers Disord. 2004;18(2):193–211.
17. De Bellis MD, Zisk A. The biological effects of childhood trauma. Child Adolesc Psychiatr Clin N Am. 2014;23(2):185–222. vii
18. Grover KE, Carpenter LL, Price LH, Gagne GG, Mello AF, Mello MF, et al. The relationship between childhood abuse and adult personality disorder symptoms. J Pers Disord. 2007;21(4):442–7.
19. Johnson JG, Smailes EM, Cohen P, Brown J, Bernstein DP. Associations between four types of childhood neglect and personality disorder symptoms during adolescence and early adulthood: findings of a community-based longitudinal study. J Pers Disord. 2000;14(2):171–87.
20. Boen E, Westlye LT, Elvsashagen T, Hummelen B, Hol PK, Boye B, et al. Regional cortical thinning may be a biological marker for borderline personality disorder. Acta Psychiatr Scand. 2014;130(3):193–204.
21. Liu H, Liao J, Jiang W, Wang W. Changes in low-frequency fluctuations in patients with antisocial personality disorder revealed by resting-state functional MRI. PLoS One. 2014;9(3):e89790.
22. Thoma P, Friedmann C, Suchan B. Empathy and social problem solving in alcohol dependence, mood disorders and selected personality disorders. Neurosci Biobehav Rev. 2013;37(3):448–70.
23. Yang Y, Raine A. Prefrontal structural and functional brain imaging findings in antisocial, violent, and psychopathic individuals: a meta-analysis. Psychiatry Res. 2009;174(2):81–8.
24. Bukh JD, Bock C, Kessing LV. Association between genetic polymorphisms in the serotonergic system and comorbid personality disorders among patients with first-episode depression. J Pers Disord. 2014;28(3):365–78.
25. Checknita D, Maussion G, Labonte B, Comai S, Tremblay RE, Vitaro F, et al. Monoamine oxidase: a gene promoter methylation and transcriptional downregulation in an offender population with antisocial personality disorder. Br J Psychiatry; J Ment Sci. 2015;206(3):216–22.
26. Perez-Rodriguez MM, Weinstein S, New AS, Bevilacqua L, Yuan Q, Zhou Z, et al. Tryptophan-hydroxylase 2 haplotype association with borderline personality disorder and aggression in a sample of patients with personality disorders and healthy controls. J Psychiatr Res. 2010;44(15):1075–81.
27. Isobel S, Edwards C. Using trauma informed care as a nursing model of care in an acute inpatient mental health unit: a practice development process. Int J Ment Health Nurs. 2017;26(1):88–94.
28. Reeves E. A synthesis of the literature on trauma-informed care. Issues Ment Health Nurs. 2015;36(9):698–709.
29. Knaak S, Szeto A, Fitch K, Modgill G, Patten S. Stigma towards borderline personality disorder: effectiveness and generalizability of an anti-stigma program for healthcare providers using a pre-post randomized design. Borderline Personal Disord Emot Dysregul. 2015;2:9.
30. FitzGerald C, Hurst S. Implicit bias in healthcare professionals: a systematic review. BMC Med Ethics. 2017;18(1):19.
31. Bateman AW, Gunderson J, Mulder R. Treatment of personality disorder. Lancet. 2015;385(9969):735–43.
32. Townsend MC. Nursing diagnoses in psychiatric nursing: care plans and psychotropic medications. 8th ed. Philadelphia: F.A. Davis Co.; 2011, p. xxxv, 696.
33. Hong V. Borderline personality disorder in the emergency department: good psychiatric management. Harv Rev Psychiatry. 2016;24(5):357–66.
34. Zanarini MC, Frankenburg FR, Hennen J, Silk KR. Mental health service utilization by borderline personality disorder patients and Axis II comparison subjects followed prospectively for 6 years. J Clin Psychiatry. 2004;65(1):28–36.
35. Zeller SL, Nordstrom K, Wilson MP. The diagnosis and management of agitation. Cambridge, NY: Cambridge University Press; 2017, p. xii, 281.
36. Paton C, Crawford MJ, Bhatti SF, Patel MX, Barnes TR. The use of psychotropic medication in patients with emotionally unstable personality disorder under the care of UK mental health services. J Clin Psychiatry. 2015;76(4):e512–8.
37. Wilson MP, Pepper D, Currier GW, Holloman GH Jr, Feifel D. The psychopharmacology of agitation: consensus statement of the American Association for Emergency Psychiatry project, beta psychopharmacology workgroup. West J Emerg Med. 2012;13(1):26–34.
38. Joiner TE Jr, Brown JS, Wingate LR. The psychology and neurobiology of suicidal behavior. Annu Rev Psychol. 2005;56:287–314.
39. McCloskey MS, Ammerman BA. Suicidal behavior and aggression-related disorders. Curr Opin Psychol. 2017;22:54–8.
40. Zaheer J, Links PS, Liu E. Assessment and emergency management of suicidality in personality disorders. Psychiatr Clin North Am. 2008;31(3):527–43, viii–ix.
41. Blasco-Fontecilla H, Baca-Garcia E, Duberstein P, Perez-Rodriguez MM, Dervic K, Saiz-Ruiz J, et al. An exploratory study of the relationship between diverse life events and specific personality disorders in a sample of suicide attempters. J Pers Disord. 2010;24(6):773–84.
42. Yen S, Pagano ME, Shea MT, Grilo CM, Gunderson JG, Skodol AE, et al. Recent life events preceding suicide attempts in a personality disorder sample: findings from the collaborative longitudinal personality disorders study. J Consult Clin Psychol. 2005;73(1):99–105.

43. Nestor PG. Mental disorder and violence: personality dimensions and clinical features. Am J Psychiatry. 2002;159(12):1973–8.
44. Sands N, Elsom S, Gerdtz M, Khaw D. Mental health-related risk factors for violence: using the evidence to guide mental health triage decision making. J Psychiatr Ment Health Nurs. 2012;19(8):690–701.
45. Zun LS, Chepenik LG, Mallory MNS. Behavioral emergencies for the emergency physician. Cambridge: Cambridge University Press; 2013, p. xiii, 400.
46. Bundy C, Schreiber M, Pascually M. Discharging your patients who display contingency-based suicidality: 6 steps. Curr Psychiatry. 2014;13(1):e1.
47. Gunderson JG, Stout RL, McGlashan TH, Shea MT, Morey LC, Grilo CM, et al. Ten-year course of borderline personality disorder: psychopathology and function from the Collaborative Longitudinal Personality Disorders study. Arch Gen Psychiatry. 2011;68(8):827–37.

14 Malingering and Factitious Disorder in the Emergency Department

Rachel L. Glick

Introduction

In malingering and factitious disorders, the patient pretends to be ill and intentionally causes his or her own symptoms. Physicians, who are trained to trust what patients tell them, have difficulty assessing and treating patients who lie. This chapter will review the diagnosis, assessment, and management of these difficult patients and provide practical advice to the emergency department (ED) clinician.

Somatization is the bodily representation of a psychological need [1]. It is a common way for children to indicate that they need psychological support, such as when a child who is anxious develops a "tummy ache" to avoid school. In older children and adults, somatization is considered a less healthy way to satisfy emotional needs. For patients with somatic symptom disorders, factitious disorders, or malingering, somatization has become dysfunctional, impairing, and pathologic [1].

Malingering and factitious disorder are both forms of somatization in which the patient is aware of producing or feigning his/her symptoms [1]. The patient's awareness is what distinguishes these two disorders from other somatic symptom disorders (see Table 14.1).

R. L. Glick (✉)
Psychiatry, University of Michigan, Ann Arbor, MI, USA
e-mail: rglick@umich.edu

In malingering, the patient is motivated to seek secondary gain by using symptoms to get something or get out of something, such as avoiding jail time by claiming to be suicidal [2]. In factitious disorder, however, the motivation is unconscious—the patient desires to adopt the sick role to fulfill a psychological need, rather than other tangible benefits. This fulfillment represents primary or psychological gain. Primary gain is believed to decrease unconscious stress or anxiety [2]. Table 14.2 compares and contrasts the clinical features of malingering and factitious disorder.

The concept of malingering physical or psychological complaints to one's benefit for tangible gains is a relatively straightforward idea. The patient's desire to take on the sick role for psychological needs is more difficult for many clinicians to understand. Regardless, both disorders challenge ED clinicians, who see their jobs as taking care of "real" patients, not those who do things to themselves or pretend to have symptoms.

Table 14.1 Illness production and patient motivation among somatic disorders

Disorder	Mechanism of illness production	Motivation for illness behavior
Somatoform disorders	Unconscious	Unconscious
Factitious disorder	Conscious	Unconscious
Malingering	Conscious	Conscious

L. S. Zun et al. (eds.), *Behavioral Emergencies for Healthcare Providers*,
https://doi.org/10.1007/978-3-030-52520-0_14

Table 14.2 Clinical features of malingering and factious disorder

Malingering	Factitious disorder
Men > woman	Women > men, except in Munchausen's variant
Substance abuse	Employment/training in medical field
Vague, unverifiable history	Vague, unverifiable history
Refuses tests, treatments, AMA	Not bothered by invasive procedures
Antisocial personality disorder	Borderline personality disorder

Malingering

Case Example

A twenty-two-year-old man comes to the ED complaining of severe pain in his leg. He explains he was in a motorcycle accident a few days prior to this presentation, and although his leg was not broken, it was "bruised and banged up." Nursing staff note that he was walking around the waiting room without a limp until he was aware of being observed, at which time he began limping and wincing in pain upon putting weight on this leg. Examination of his leg reveals some bruises and abrasions on his leg that are healing well. When the physician recommends ibuprofen for the pain, the patient says he knows he "needs Vicodin" because that is all that ever works for his pain. A review of his medical records shows he often comes to the ED requesting narcotics and that he has been given small amounts for various injuries in the past. The physician suspects he is exaggerating his pain to obtain narcotics unnecessarily.

According to DSM-5, malingering is given a v-code designation, suggesting it is not in and of itself a diagnosis. Rather, it is an issue that can be the focus of the clinical encounter [3]. Malingering is defined as "the intentional production of false or grossly exaggerated physical or psychological symptoms, motivated by external incentives such as avoiding military duty, avoiding work, obtaining financial compensation, evading criminal prosecution, or obtaining drugs" [4]. The DSM-5 notes that malingering behavior can be adaptive in some instances, for example, when a prisoner of war feigns illness to avoid torture [4]. Adaptive malingering can be seen in the ED when an abused person feigns illness to get away from their abuser, for example.

There is no gold standard for the diagnosis of malingering. The suspicion of malingering is based on an informed clinical evaluation. The DSM-5 lists some situations in which malingering should be suspected. The ED clinician might consider malingering when there is a discrepancy between the patient's stated level of impairment and the objective findings, or if the patient is uncooperative with the assessment [4]. It is helpful to observe the patient when they do not know they are being observed, to see if the purported impairment persists [5]. Patients facing arrest or being evaluated in forensic settings might use medical complaints to avoid legal or other consequences. Patients who are malingering often have vague, confusing, and unverifiable stories [6]. They often refuse testing.

Other elements of the patient presentation might lead the ED clinician to consider malingering. The physician should pay attention to the patient's affect, as well as his or her degree of cooperativeness and guardedness with the examiner. Patients who are malingering may exaggerate symptoms or appear to be acting, rather than feeling pain or anxiety [7]. Patients might ask specifically for controlled medications and can quickly be labeled "drug-seeking" by nursing staff and physicians. Alternatively, patients might demand letters for work, school, attorneys, court, or other entities to verify that they are ill. They often have comorbid antisocial personality disorder and substance-use disorders [5, 8].

To make a final diagnosis, the clinician must identify the external incentive that is driving malingering behavior and exclude other medical and psychiatric diagnoses. Malingering should be suspected in patients who have clearly evident secondary gain.

The incidence of malingering in the ED setting is unknown, although one small study in an urban ED suggests that 13% of patients presenting with psychiatric complaints were suspected of seeking care for secondary gain [9]. Malingering using psychiatric symptoms appears to be more common in people dealing with the legal system, while physical symptoms are more often associated with financial gain or disability-seeking behavior [3]. The preceding case illustrates a case suspicious for malingering.

Patients with malingering can engage in behaviors that are potentially harmful and lead to true medical emergencies. An example is a homeless man who takes a friend's nitroglycerin and goes to the ED reporting chest pain (and presenting with abnormally low blood pressure) in order to stay in the hospital for a few days. Patients may also feign overdose, as described in a recent report of a patient who claimed to have overdosed on enoxaparin [10].

Factitious Disorder

Case Example

A thirty-four-year-old medical assistant is brought to the ED unconscious and is found to have a blood glucose that is dangerously low. She is revived with intravenous dextrose in water and tells the physician that she has diabetes that has never been well controlled. She states that she has had many episodes of both hypo- and hyperglycemia that have led to hospitalizations. She lives in another city and has never been evaluated at this hospital. Her mother is at her bedside when the physician returns to discuss control of her diabetes. Her mother seems surprised and says that, as far as she knows, her daughter does not have diabetes. The patient then abruptly starts to dress and asks for paperwork to sign out against medical advice.

Factitious disorder is diagnosed, according to DSM-5, when three conditions are met:

- There is intentional production, or feigning, of physical or psychological symptoms.
- The motivation for symptom production is to take on the sick role.
- No external incentives drive the behavior [4].

Case reports of individuals with factitious disorder demonstrate the lengths to which patients will go to take on the sick role [5]. For example, one patient with factitious disorder injected feces under her skin to cause cellulitis, while another manipulated his urethra with a pencil to cause hematuria. Factitious disorder is more common in women than in men, and a preponderance of patients have studied or worked in a medical field [8, 11].

A subcategory of factitious disorder, Munchausen's syndrome—named after the eighteenth-century traveling storyteller, Baron von Munchausen—is characterized by patients who travel widely and tell elaborate tales about their illnesses and treatments. These patients are career medical imposters. This term should be reserved for those with the most severe form of factitious disorder [5], but it is often misused in the lay press and even medical settings to describe all patients with factitious disorder. Interestingly, Munchausen's syndrome is likely more common in men [8].

Finally, emergency providers must be aware of Munchausen's syndrome by proxy. In this rare disorder, a parent or guardian causes a factitious illness in a child. Munchausen's syndrome by proxy is child abuse, and most clinicians are required to report its occurrence to legal authorities.

The patient with factitious disorder is rarely identified as such in the ED setting. Persons with factitious disorder want to be a patient: They are more or less compliant in the ED setting, although their histories may be vague and inconsistent. Patients often produce findings on examination, falsify lab results, or tell stories that lead to appropriate treatment for the illness they are fabricating. Sometimes, they present with complications from treatment of the feigned illness [7]. Case reports describe numerous examples of factitious disorder, ranging from hypoglycemia caused by use of insulin to sepsis due to multiple traumas [12–14].

Some clues help the clinician consider the presence of factitious disorder. Factors suggestive of factitious disorder include multiple hospital admissions, lack of verifiable history, social isolation and few interpersonal connections, early history of serious or chronic illness, multiple scars, failure to respond to typical treatments, and comorbid personality disorder, particularly borderline personality disorder [8].

During the assessment, a patient with factitious disorder might lack concern for his or her serious clinical situation or appear unbothered by the prospect of invasive or painful procedures. Patients might also describe resistance to typical treatments. For example, a young woman reported to have Bartter's syndrome is admitted for bradycardia because of low potassium levels. Yet her potassium levels do not increase with supplementation. The team grows suspicious and orders a furosemide level from a research lab. The results show that the patient is taking a diuretic to lower her potassium, despite the risk of arrhythmia. Again, these presentations are difficult to recognize in the ED, since the patient has become legitimately ill as a result of what he/she has done to him/herself and may well require ongoing hospital care. Typically, extended observation and repeated clinical encounters are required to definitively make the diagnosis.

Management

Patients with malingering and factitious disorder can present with almost any symptom or complaint. The ED physician must first focus on ruling out medical illness and treating any true pathology that is found. Both malingering and factitious disorder are diagnoses of exclusion: The patient must be evaluated for emergent physical or psychological illness before a diagnosis of malingering or factitious disorder is made.

If either malingering or factitious disorder is suspected, attempts should be made to obtain old records and collateral information to inform the diagnosis. Often, patients with these disorders will present at off hours, when they suspect less-seasoned providers will be on duty [5]. They also may travel from ED to ED, such that recording a full history of contacts with the healthcare system is difficult.

Once deception is suspected, the ED clinician can manage these disorders with several tenets in mind: avoid invasive procedures, extensive evaluations, and unnecessary hospital admissions. Appropriate limits must be set around further tests and medications. For example, in the first case example, the patient requests opioids for severe pain but does not have objective findings and appears well when he thinks he is unobserved; he should not be provided opioids. However, patients who have already harmed themselves, such as the patient who has manipulated her skin so that she now has cellulitis, need medical care regardless of the initial cause.

Healthcare professionals must also be aware of their own reactions toward these patients. Common reactions to malingering or factitious patients include anger, frustration, injustice, and a need for vengeance [15]. Clinicians must keep in mind that these patients have psychological needs and simply do not know how to deal with their pain and/or satisfy their needs in more appropriate ways.

In the ED, clinicians may find it more productive to focus on the patient's most pressing needs. When the patient reports a long history of symptoms, why is he or she in the ED now? What does the patient need that has led him/her to seek your help at this particular time? Asking this question allows the provider to ascertain the "real" reason the patient is presenting now, while reducing the strong reactions provoked by the patient's deceptive behaviors. The clinical interaction may then focus on what the patient is requesting and whether you can help with that request. For example, a patient presents to the ED complaining of pain that started with a car accident 2 years ago. He wears a neck brace and insists that he needs X-rays today. There are no objective findings on exam, and X-rays are normal. When the physician questions why he is in the ED now, he explains he needs a doctor to fill out disability forms to take to his new lawyer.

Long-term psychiatric treatment options for both conditions are limited [8]. Nevertheless, psychiatric consultants may assist in the evaluation and management of these patients. The consultant will often help identify risk factors for deceptive disorders in ambiguous cases. Often, the consultant's greatest help is less for the patient directly and more for staff, who are struggling with negative feelings toward the patient.

There is debate in the literature about the wisdom of confronting deceptive patients. Patients who are confronted rarely admit the deception [5]. Patients with both malingering and factitious

Table 14.3 Suggested management of factitious disorder and malingering in the ED

Rule out serious medical illness
Treat injuries or conditions produced by the patient
Review records/get collateral history if possible
Avoid iatrogenic injuries
Set limits
Manage negative feelings toward the patient
Document management and medical decision-making

disorder will often leave the hospital if confronted with medical staff suspicion of their story, as illustrated in the second case example. A better (and more difficult) approach is to give them a face-saving way out of the situation.

ED clinicians should document suspected malingering or factious disorder, albeit carefully. Documentation should honestly summarize findings and reasons for your suspicions. Some legal experts suggest describing the patient's behavior, rather than using the words "malingering" or "manipulative," since both can be seen as pejorative. For example, in the first case example, one might document, "The patient reported severe pain and inability to walk but was observed walking with no limp or apparent discomfort in the waiting area. No opioids were prescribed." Table 14.3 summarizes recommendations for the management of malingering and factitious disorders.

Conclusion

Patients with malingering and factitious disorders present unique challenges to the emergency clinician. In the busy setting of an ED, where patients face life-and-death situations, the presentation of a person who is making him or herself sick or pretending to be sick is extremely frustrating. The clinician should try to put aside any negative feelings toward these patients and remember that these presentations are maladaptive behaviors to meet certain needs. These patients must be evaluated for true medical needs, while providers set appropriate limits and carefully document objective findings and medical decision-making.

References

1. Folks DG, Ford CV, Houcki CA. Somatoform disorders, factitious disorders, and malingering. In: Stoudemire A, editor. Clinical psychiatry for medical students. Third ed. Philadelphia: Lippincott-Raven Publishers; 1998.
2. Hollifield MA. Somatization disorder. In: Sadock BJ, Sadock VA, editors. Kaplan & Sadock's comprehensive textbook of psychiatry. Eighth ed. Philadelphia: Lippincott Williams &Wilkins; 2005.
3. McDermott BE, Feldman MD. Malingering in the medical setting. Psychiatr Clin N Am. 2007;30:645–62.
4. American Psychiatric Association. Diagnostic and statistical manual of mental disorders. Fifth ed. Washington, DC: American Psychiatric Association; 2013.
5. Epstein LA, Stern TA. Factitious disorders and malingering. In: Glick RL, Berlin JS, Fishkind AB, Zeller SL, editors. Emergency psychiatry, principles and practice. Philadelphia: Lippincott Williams & Wilkins; 2008.
6. Schwartz P, Weathers M. The psychotic patient. In: Riba M, Ravindranath D, editors. Clinical manual of emergency psychiatry. Washington, DC: American Psychiatric Publishing, Inc; 2010.
7. Simakhodskyay Z, Haddad F, Quintero M, Ravindranath D, Glick RL. Disposition and resource options. In: Riba M, Ravindranath D, editors. Clinical manual of emergency psychiatry. Washington, DC: American Psychiatric Publishing, Inc; 2010.
8. Smith FA. Factitious disorders and malingering. In: Stern TA, Rosenbaum JF, Fava M, et al., editors. Massachusetts general hospital comprehensive clinical psychiatry. Philadelphia: Mosby Elsevier; 2008.
9. Yates BD, et al. Feigned psychiatric symptoms in the emergency room. Psychiatr Serv. 1996;47(9):998–1000.
10. Caplan JP. Bleeding the system: a case of feigned enoxaparin overdose. Psychosomatics. 2009;50(4):413–5.
11. Krahn LE, Li H, O'Connor MK. Patients who strive to be ill: factitious disorder with physical symptoms. Am J Psy. 2003;160:1163–8.
12. Lazarus A, Kozinn WP. Munchausen's syndrome with hematuria and sepsis: an unusual case. Int J Psychiatry Med. 1991;21(1):113–6.
13. Bretz SW, Richards JR. Munchausen syndrome presenting acutely in the emergency department. J of Emer Med. 2000;18(4):417–20.
14. Hedges BE, Dimsdale JE, Hoyt DB. Munchausen syndrome presenting as recurrent multiple trauma. Psychosomatics. 1995;36(1):60–3.
15. Ekstrom LW. Liars, medicine, and compassion. J Med Philos. 2012;37:159–80.

Part IV

Medical Illnesses in Psychiatric Patients

15 The Patient with Delirium and Dementia in the Emergency Department

Samidha Tripathi, Kristen Baker, and Carly Eastin

Introduction

You are working in the emergency department one night when a young male brings in his agitated brother with a history of schizophrenia, stating, "His schizophrenia is acting up again." You watch as the patient is brought back to a room, intermittently thrashing about the stretcher. You are able to calm him long enough to obtain vital signs and check his glucose, which is shockingly low. The nurse swiftly obtains IV access and gives him dextrose-containing fluids. To the brother's astonishment, the patient's status immediately reverts back to normal. You realize this change in mental status was secondary to delirium caused by hypoglycemia. The patient reports he forgot to eat after taking insulin, causing this predicament. As further diagnostic studies are underway, you learn of an impending case of Alzheimer's dementia found wandering outside the nursing home …

According to DSM-5, dementia and delirium are considered neurocognitive disorders, which represent cognitive decline from a previously attained level of functioning [1]. Since symptoms of delirium, dementia, and primary psychiatric disorders often overlap, this chapter will focus on how to differentiate those with medical illnesses so appropriate treatment is provided.

Delirium

The DSM-V criteria for the diagnosis of delirium consist of a disturbance in attention (ability to focus and sustain attention) and awareness (reduced orientation to the environment) that develops over a short period of time. Delirium tends to fluctuate in severity throughout the day and is associated with an additional cognitive deficit (memory, disorientation, language, or perception) attributable to a medical condition, substance intoxication, or withdrawal. Delirium may be considered hyper- or hypoactive, and the patient may switch between the two states [1].

Patients with hyperactive delirium may present as hypervigilant, restless or agitated, paranoid, and can report perceptual disturbances. The hypoactive form will present as increased lethargy, somnolence, psychomotor retardation, and might often be overlooked by physicians or be mistaken for depression [2–3]. Approximately 10% of older patients in the emergency department present with delirium, which was only

S. Tripathi (✉)
Department of Psychiatry, University of Arkansas for Medical Sciences, Little Rock, AR, USA

K. Baker · C. Eastin
Department of Emergency Medicine, University of Arkansas for Medical Sciences, Little Rock, AR, USA

L. S. Zun et al. (eds.), *Behavioral Emergencies for Healthcare Providers*,
https://doi.org/10.1007/978-3-030-52520-0_15

acknowledged by healthcare providers in 25% of cases [4]. Of those patients admitted to the hospital with known dementia, 46% had superimposed delirium, wherein the recognition of such cause is unknown [5].

Causes of Delirium

The three most prevalent causes of delirium are toxic ingestions or withdrawal, infection, and fluid/electrolyte imbalance, but these are often overlooked in the acute setting [6]. A study in Mississippi found 64 cases of patients admitted to psychiatric facilities who were found to actually have unrecognized medical emergencies. In this case series, the diagnoses most often missed were severe intoxication, drug/alcohol withdrawal/delirium tremens, and prescription drug overdose [6]. An expanded but not all-inclusive list of delirium etiologies can be seen in Table 15.1.

Table 15.1 Causes of delirium

Category	Cause
Emergency	Shock
	Hypoxia
	Hypoglycemia
	Electrolyte/acid–base disturbance
	Thyroid storm
	Hyperthermia/hypothermia
	Delirium tremens
	Toxic alcohol ingestion
	Wernicke's encephalopathy
	Intracranial disturbance (trauma, abscess, etc.)
Medications/drugs	Illicit drugs/alcohol
	Drug and alcohol withdrawal
	Anticholinergic medications/drugs
	Medications in overdose
Neurologic	Seizure/post-ictal state
	Hypertensive encephalopathy
Endocrine	Hyperthyroidism/hypothyroidism
	Diabetes mellitus and DKA/HHS
Metabolic	Hepatic encephalopathy
	Renal failure
Infectious	Encephalitis/meningitis
	Neurosyphilis
	Urinary tract infection
	Pneumonia
	Sepsis

Intoxications

A significant number of the undiagnosed emergencies in the aforementioned study were secondary to drug and alcohol intoxication. In ethanol intoxication (such as beer, wine, or liquor), patients may present with euphoria, emotional lability, and disinhibition. They may appear flushed and diaphoretic, with slurred speech and incoordination. Patients who have consumed toxic alcohol (such as methanol, ethylene glycol, or isopropyl alcohol) may also present with the same symptoms as in ethanol ingestion, bolstering the importance of adequate history. Opiate intoxication presents with pinpoint pupils, nausea, vomiting, decreased respiratory drive, decreased blood pressure associated with lethargy, and, at times, agitation. Benzodiazepine intoxication often results in drowsiness with slurred speech. However, some cases of paradoxical excitation might exhibit hallucinations, hostility, psychosis, delirium, and seizures. Users of synthetic cannabinoids (such as "K2" or "Spice") may present with nausea, burning sensation in their eyes, dilated pupils, hot flushes, diaphoresis, and agitation. Stimulant use like cocaine and methamphetamines can lead to a sympathomimetic response, which is characterized by increased heart rate, blood pressure, and temperature; dilated pupils; psychosis; agitation; and extreme, possibly violent, muscular activity. Similarly, phencyclidine (PCP) intoxication may present with euphoria, auditory hallucinations, and visual distortions, nystagmus, disconnection from reality, and aggression, which may be severe, with "superhuman strength" [7].

Withdrawal

In a similar context, those in withdrawal may also suffer behavioral disturbances. Patients with opiate withdrawal may have dilated pupils, nausea, vomiting, diarrhea, abdominal pain, runny nose, excessive tearing, and insomnia. Opiate withdrawal is unpleasant but not life-threatening. Benzodiazepine withdrawal, however, may be life-threatening. Benzodiazepine withdrawal is characterized by agitation, hallucinations, confusion, tremors, restlessness, and seizures. Likewise, alcohol withdrawal can also be life-threatening. Alcohol withdrawal is characterized by four stages, all of which do not necessarily occur in a single individual. The first stage consists of tremulousness, which begins 6–24 hours after cessation of alcohol and is characterized by high blood pressure, high heart rate, tremor, and a normal mental status. The second stage, or alcoholic hallucinosis, consists of visual hallucinations and formication (tactile hallucinations) with preserved sensorium. The third stage, which typically peaks at 24–48 hours, can present with seizures. The fourth and potentially lethal stage is delirium tremens [7], which occurs after between 24 and 96 hours of abstinence and consists of elevated heart rate, elevated blood pressure, hyperthermia, confusion, hallucinations, agitation, and disorientation. The mortality for delirium tremens may be up to 20%. Ethanol level can still be elevated (greater than 0) during withdrawal [8].

Overdose

Prescription medication overdose can also present as behavioral disturbances. MAOI (monoamine oxidase inhibitor)-related hypertensive crisis can occur as a result of a "cheese reaction" due to consumption of tyramine-rich food. This reaction is characterized by sympathomimetic symptoms, which begin within 30–90 minutes from ingestion. A typical presentation includes headache, elevated blood pressure, elevated heart rate, diaphoresis, and agitation, which may lead to seizures and coma. Carbamazepine in overdose can lead to dizziness, heart conductance disturbances, restlessness, confusion, aggression, drowsiness, and, eventually, coma. Lithium toxicity can lead to potentially lethal outcomes. Acute manifestation includes nausea, vomiting, tremor, agitation, and weakness. Progression of acute toxicity can manifest as confusion, slurred speech, decreased blood pressure, neuromuscular involvement leading to ataxia, renal failure, convulsions, and coma. Anticholinergic toxicity is associated with a wide variety of medications, ranging from tricyclic antidepressants to diphenhydramine use. A mnemonic used to remember the symptoms of anticholinergic toxicity is "Hot as a hare, dry as a bone, blind as a bat, and mad as a hatter," which note the cardinal symptoms of fever, dry skin, dry mucous membranes, dilated pupils, and agitation with altered mental status [7]. Medication overdose and toxicity occur in patients of all ages, and prudent care must be taken to appropriately care for these patients.

Other Important Considerations

Hypoxia or anoxia, temperature fluctuations, electrolyte imbalances such as glycemic shifts, abnormal acid–base status, and hypo or hypernatremia may also contribute to altered mental status and should be investigated further [7].

Infection is another common cause of delirium, particularly in the elderly. Young patients with delirium secondary to infection are more likely to be suffering from meningitis or encephalitis, while elderly patients are more likely to have pneumonia or a urinary tract infection.

Identification and Workup of Delirium

In patients with altered mental status or acute behavioral disturbances, a thorough history and physical examination is the first step in achieving an accurate diagnosis. This examination should place emphasis on identifying underlying medical conditions, like urinary tract infections or recent falls, toxidromes, or medication interactions. There are several key characteristics to further assist in differentiating between a primary psychiatric illness and delirium. Primary psychiatric illness does not cause decreased level of consciousness, abnormal vital signs, or focal neurologic deficits. In other words, unless there is an underlying medical condition or intoxication, the patient should be alert and neurologically intact. And while psychiatric disorders may also include perceptual disturbance like auditory and visual hallucinations, visual or tactile should raise suspicion for a medical etiology [6]. Additionally, new onset of psychosis in older adults should also prompt further workup [7]. Tests to consider in a delirious patient include, but are not limited to, complete blood count, glucose, basic metabolic panel, liver function tests with ammonia level, urinalysis, chest X-ray, lumbar puncture, electrocardiogram, and/or a head CT [7].

Assessment of Delirium

Several instruments for diagnosing and assessing the severity of delirium have been created. The Confusion Assessment Method (CAM) and the Delirium Rating Scale-Revised Edition (DRS-R-98) are both based on DSM criteria and are considered reliable and valid. The CAM is considered to be relatively easy to use and understand. DRS-R-98 is relatively comprehensive and sensitive to change, and so may be useful for monitoring patients over time [9].

Management of Delirium

The management of delirium includes identifying and managing the underlying cause. Measures must be taken to monitor and ensure safety of an agitated patient and staff. Environmental interventions like minimizing noise, fall prevention, proper illumination, limiting use of restraints, cueing, and redirection are an integral part of treatment [10]. Pharmacological intervention may be required in cases of severe agitation to ensure safety of patient and staff. Both typical (haloperidol) and atypical antipsychotics (olanzapine, risperidone, quetiapine, and aripiprazole) have been shown to be equally effective in the treatment of delirium. Atypical antipsychotic use is often preferred, due to lower risk of extra-pyramidal side effects and better tolerability. These are typically offered in oral formulations, with olanzapine being the only parenteral option available in intramuscular form. Finally, acutely delirious patients should be admitted for stabilization until the delirium resolves [11–12].

Dementia

The DSM-5 defines dementia, now known as major neurocognitive disorder, as cognitive decline with impairment in cognitive performance that may affect independence [1]. Several subtypes of dementia can lead to alterations in a patient's personality and emotional control causing irritability and disinhibition.

As compared to delirium, dementia is insidious in onset, with a clear sensorium and no alterations in attention. Each type varies in age of onset, progression, and features, and can manifest behavioral disturbances [13–14]. Table 15.2 below summarizes several subtypes of dementia with their age of onset, progression, and features.

Several studies have shown that patients with previously diagnosed psychiatric disorders are at increased risk of developing dementia. Delirium also accelerates cognitive decline in dementia [15–16]. In 2015, investigators in Denmark revealed that patients with schizophrenia had an almost two-fold increased risk of dementia, particularly in patients less than 65 years old [17]. Another Denmark study showed that the risk of dementia increases with the number of episodes of depression and bipolar disorder that lead to admission. The study calculated that the rate of dementia increased 13% with every depressive episode requiring admission, and 6% with every bipolar episode leading to admission [18]. Furthermore, in patients diagnosed with depressive "pseudo-dementia," when cognition and function could be entirely restored to normal if depression was adequately treated, approximately 40% ultimately developed dementia. With the above in mind, it is prudent to monitor the cognition of patients with psychiatric disorders, as dysfunction may not be minor or temporary [19].

Table 15.2 Types of dementia

Type of dementia	Age of onset	Onset and progression	Cognitive features	Behavioral features
Alzheimer's	Early: 40s–50s; late: 70s–80s	Insidious and gradual	Decline in memory	Depression, apathy, irritability, agitation, combativeness, wandering
Frontotemporal	20s–80s; 50s most often	Insidious and gradual	Decline in executive function; spares learning/memory and motor function	Disinhibition, apathy, loss of inertia, compulsive, hyperorality
Lewy body	50s–80s	Insidious and gradual	Fluctuating decline in executive function	Visual hallucinations, delusions, Parkinson's, and REM sleep behavior disorder features
Vascular	Variable	Variable	Decline in executive function	Variable
Traumatic brain injury	Variable	Presents immediately	Variable	Loss of emotional control, personality changes, suspicion, irritability, aggression
HIV	Variable	Variable with fluctuant course	Variable	Loss of emotional control, irritability
Prion	Variable	Insidious and rapid	Variable	Problems with appetite, anxiety and sleeping
Parkinson's	50s–80s	Insidious and gradual	Variable	Apathy, depression, anxiety, hallucinations, delusions, personality changes, REM disorder
Huntington's	30s–40s	Insidious and gradual	Variable	Depression, apathy, irritability, OCD symptoms, disinhibition, impulsivity, impaired insight

Workup of Dementia

An accurate and detailed history is essential to diagnosis of dementia. Onset of symptoms, progression, and level of functional impairment are important considerations during assessments. Evaluation to identify potentially reversible causes like vitamin deficiency can proceed simultaneously [20].

Evaluating cognitive dysfunction requires involvement of family or other independent observers (not just the patient). Cognitive abilities should be screened and documented using the Folstein Mini-Mental State Examination (MMSE). A maximum of 30 points can be awarded based on responses that evaluate orientation, registration, attention, calculation, and visuospatial domains [21]. Typically, a score of 24 or less is considered suggestive of dementia, with a sensitivity and specificity of 87% and 82%, respectively. Limitations of the MMSE include few pure recall items and a relatively low sensitivity to early or mild cognitive impairment (MCI), particularly in highly educated individuals. It is also not sensitive to frontal lobe dysfunction. The Mini-Cog is a time-efficient and clinically efficient bedside measure with similar sensitivity and specificity for dementia. The test includes three-word recall and clock drawing test [22].

The Montreal Cognitive Assessment Battery (MoCA) was developed for the assessment of MCI and includes expanded assessments of visuospatial and executive function. It has excellent sensitivity for MCI (90%) compared to a clinical evaluation in a memory clinic [23]. It is now gaining popularity, as it is freely available and can be administered easily at the bedside. It is available in multiple languages, including both a version for the visually impaired and a telephone version.

A complete physical and neurological examination is necessary to identify comorbid medical illnesses that maybe affecting cognition. Apraxia, focal deficits, gait abnormality, and pyramidal or extrapyramidal motor deficits can suggest neurological etiology. Laboratory testing should be considered to identify potentially reversible conditions that may mimic dementia. Common tests include complete blood counts (CBC), chemistry panels, erythrocyte sedimentation rate, thyroid function tests (thyroid-stimulating hormone, or TSH, and free thyroxine, or FT4), a vitamin B12 level, a thiamine level, and a syphilis screening [20].

Brain imaging (magnetic resonance imaging (MRI) or computed tomography (CT)) is recommended for all patients to identify structural, demyelinating, inflammatory, or vascular etiologies. There is no consensus guideline recommending one imaging modality over the other [24].

Management of Dementia

The best way to manage behavioral disturbances in dementia depends on the severity of the symptoms. Reversible causes like delirium, pain, comorbid medical illness, medications, and environmental factors must be addressed. In patients with mild–moderate disturbances, nonpharmacological approaches like cognitive training, exercise, family training, or environmental training should be the primary intervention [25].

Cholinergic deficiency contributes to the neuropsychiatric symptoms of Alzheimer's disease, and cholinomimetic therapies such as cholinesterase inhibitors (donepezil, rivastigmine, galantamine) are being utilized for treatment as well [26]. Low-dose atypical antipsychotics can be considered for management of agitation and behavioral disturbances, though literature supporting its use is limited. Antidepressants and anxiolytics can help with depression and anxiety. Lastly, in those with mania-like symptoms and aggression, mood stabilizers and/or atypical antipsychotics should be used. Prior to initiating medications, environmental factors should be adjusted whenever possible. Loneliness may be treated by interaction with those with positive relationships with the patient, videotapes of family members, and contact with animals. Boredom is best alleviated with both structured and unstructured stimulation, including but not limited to music and items with which to play, such as aprons with buttons. Patients with a need to wander should be encouraged to walk in sheltered gardens. Those who need to hoard should be provided bags and safe areas where they may "shop" for their treasures, after which they may be restored to their rightful owners [27].

As the population continues to age, there are increasing numbers of elderly patients with psychiatric disorders and dementia, leading to the formation of a geriatric psychiatry unit. These have become a key part of treatment, as patients with dementia are particularly vulnerable in acute hospitals to environmental change and communication difficulties. Some of the key characteristics of joint geriatric/psychiatric wards are joint medical care by geriatricians and psychiatrists, securing the home environment to facilitate rehabilitation and maintain independence, patient-centered care, dedicated multidisciplinary team and continuity of care, good community links to facilitate safe discharge, and specialized training of staff to manage behavioral problems without recourse to physical or pharmacological restraint. These wards have many potential advantages in hospital care of the frail and elderly, and are being evaluated for clinical and cost-effectiveness worldwide [28].

Patients presenting with behavioral disturbances may have these changes secondary to delirium and dementia. As discussed above, delirium is acute in onset and is characterized by a disturbance in consciousness with a change in cognition, while dementia is more gradual in onset and is characterized by intellectual impairment that may interfere with functioning. Care must be taken to ensure patients with neurocognitive disorders are accurately diagnosed and cared for to ensure the best outcomes.

References

1. American Psychiatric Association. Diagnostic and Statistical Manual of Mental Disorders (DSM-5®): American Psychiatric Pub; 2013.
2. Fong TG, Davis D, Growdon ME, Albuquerque A, Inouye SK. The interface between delirium and dementia in elderly adults. Lancet Neurol. 2015;14(8):823–32.
3. Fong TG, Tulebaev SR, Inouye SK. Delirium in elderly adults: diagnosis, prevention and treatment. Nat Rev Neurol. 2009;5(4):210–20.
4. Tamune H, Yasugi D. How can we identify patients with delirium in the emergency department?: a review of available screening and diagnostic tools. Am J Emerg Med. 2017;35(9):1332–4.
5. Reynish EL, Hapca SM, De Souza N, Cvoro V, Donnan PT, Guthrie B. Epidemiology and outcomes of people with dementia, delirium, and unspecified cognitive impairment in the general hospital: prospective cohort study of 10,014 admissions. BMC Med. 2017;15(1):140.
6. Reeves RR, Pendarvis EJ, Kimble R. Unrecognized medical emergencies admitted to psychiatric units. Am J Emerg Med. 2000;18(4):390–3.
7. Wolfson AB, Cloutier RL, Hendey GW, Ling LJ, Schaider JJ, Rosen CL. Harwood-Nuss's clinical practice of emergency medicine: Lippincott Williams & Wilkins; 2014.
8. Rabinowitz T. Delirium: an important (but often unrecognized) clinical syndrome. Curr Psychiatry Rep. 2002;4(3):202–8.
9. Grover S. Assessment scales for delirium: a review. World J Psychiatry. 2012;2(4):58.
10. American Psychiatric Association. Practice guideline for the treatment of patients with delirium: Amer Psychiatric Pub Incorporated; 1999.
11. Grassi L, Caraceni A, Mitchell AJ, Nanni MG, Berardi MA, Caruso R, et al. Management of delirium in palliative care: a review. Curr Psychiatry Rep. 2015;17(3):550.
12. Odiari EA, Sekhon N, Han JY, David EH. Stabilizing and managing patients with altered mental status and delirium. Emerg Med Clin North Am. 2015;33(4):753–64.
13. Hendry K, Hill E, Quinn TJ, Evans J, Stott DJ. Single screening questions for cognitive impairment in older people: a systematic review. Age Ageing. 2015;44(2):322–6.
14. Meyers J, Stein S. The psychiatric interview in the emergency department. Emerg Med Clin North Am. 2000;18(2):173–83.
15. Davis DHJ, Muniz-Terrera G, Keage HAD, Stephan BCM, Fleming J, Ince PG, et al. Association of delirium with cognitive decline in late life: a neuropathologic study of 3 population-based cohort studies. JAMA Psychiat. 2017;74(3):244–51.
16. Fong TG, Jones RN, Shi P, Marcantonio ER, Yap L, Rudolph JL, et al. Delirium accelerates cognitive decline in Alzheimer disease. Neurology. 2009;72(18):1570–5.
17. Ribe AR, Laursen TM, Charles M, Katon W, Fenger-Grøn M, Davydow D, et al. Long-term risk of dementia in persons with schizophrenia: a Danish population-based cohort study. JAMA Psychiat. 2015;72(11):1095–101.
18. Kessing LV, Andersen PK. Does the risk of developing dementia increase with the number of episodes in patients with depressive disorder and in patients with bipolar disorder? J Neurol Neurosurg Psychiatry. 2004;75(12):1662–6.
19. da Silva J, Gonçalves-Pereira M, Xavier M, Mukaetova-Ladinska EB. Affective disorders and risk of developing dementia: systematic review. Br J Psychiatry. 2013;202(3):177–86.
20. Adelman AM, Daly MP. Initial evaluation of the patient with suspected dementia. Am Fam Physician. 2005;71(9):1745–50.
21. Folstein MF, Folstein SE, McHugh PR. "Mini-mental state." a practical method for grading the cognitive state of patients for the clinician. J Psychiatr Res. 1975;12(3):189–98.
22. Borson S, Scanlan JM, Chen P, Ganguli M. The mini-cog as a screen for dementia: validation in a population-based sample. J Am Geriatr Soc. 2003;51(10):1451–4.
23. Nasreddine ZS, Phillips NA, Bédirian V, Charbonneau S, Whitehead V, Collin I, et al. The Montreal Cognitive Assessment, MoCA: a brief screening tool for mild cognitive impairment. J Am Geriatr Soc. 2005;53(4):695–9.
24. Knopman DS, DeKosky ST, Cummings JL, Chui H, Corey-Bloom J, Relkin N, et al. Practice parameter: diagnosis of dementia (an evidence-based review). Report of the Quality Standards Subcommittee of the American Academy of Neurology. Neurology. 2001;56(9):1143–53.
25. Jensen L, Padilla R. Effectiveness of environment-based interventions that address behavior, perception, and falls in people with Alzheimer's disease and related major neurocognitive disorders: a systematic review. Am J Occup Ther. 2017;71(5): 7105180030p1–7105180030p10.
26. Cummings JL, Back C. The cholinergic hypothesis of neuropsychiatric symptoms in Alzheimer's disease. Am J Geriatr Psychiatry. 1998;6(2 Suppl 1):S64–78.
27. Desai AK, Grossberg GT. Recognition and management of behavioral disturbances in dementia. Prim care companion. J Clin Psychiatry. 2001;3(3):93–109.
28. George J, Adamson J, Woodford H. Joint geriatric and psychiatric wards: a review of the literature. Age Ageing. 2011;40(5):543–8.

Excited Delirium Syndrome: Diagnosis and Treatment

16

Michael P. Wilson and Gary M. Vilke

Introduction

Excited delirium syndrome (ExDS) is a specific type of agitation in which individuals typically present in an extremely violent and uncontrollable manner. The actual existence of ExDS, which is not currently listed in the APA Diagnostic and Statistical Manual (DSM), has been criticized by some as having been "invented" to classify and ultimately justify deaths that occur in highly agitated individuals during police arrest and restraint. Many researchers, however, believe that ExDS has a long history and has been described using various terms over the past two centuries. Although ExDS does not always result in death, it does carry relatively high mortality compared to other acute behavioral emergencies. Similar to delirium generally, ExDS is a behavioral manifestation of a medical emergency. Knowledge of this condition is therefore significant for individuals who take care of patients in the acute setting, both in and out of the hospital. This includes law enforcement officers, emergency medical system (EMS) providers, critical care psychiatrists, and emergency physicians.

Forensic pathologists and medical examiners have generally applied the term "Excited Delirium" retrospectively to describe findings in a subgroup of patients with delirium who died suddenly while in police custody [1]. Patients with ExDS, due to their extreme aggressiveness, bizarre behaviors, and violent tendencies, have therefore traditionally first been encountered by law enforcement and prehospital personnel. As these patients are often transported to an emergency department (ED), they are also cared for by emergency medicine clinicians.

Excited delirium syndrome, also previously called agitated delirium, has defied a natural unifying definition. There are no specific biologic tests or imaging studies that can be used to make the diagnosis, but like other medical syndromes, ExDS is a specific clinical presentation with a host of common features. The more features present, the more likely the diagnosis [2]. ExDS is generally defined as altered mental status due to delirium, combined with severe excitement or aggressiveness, in which other medical etiologies have been excluded. This severe agitation often attracts the attention of law enforcement, due to the sometimes bizarre and aggressive public presentations of individuals with ExDS. Although other signs and symptoms are variable, most

M. P. Wilson (✉)
Department of Emergency Medicine, University of Arkansas for Medical Sciences, Little Rock, AR, USA
e-mail: mpwilso1@outlook.com

G. M. Vilke
Department of Emergency Medicine, University of California Health Sciences, San Diego, CA, USA

L. S. Zun et al. (eds.), *Behavioral Emergencies for Healthcare Providers*,
https://doi.org/10.1007/978-3-030-52520-0_16

experts agree that ExDS patients typically display several of the following [1, 2]:

- Imperviousness to significant pain
- Rapid breathing
- Sweating
- Extreme agitation
- Constant or near constant physical activity
- Elevated temperature/hot to the touch
- Lack of response to verbal commands by police
- Lack of fatiguing
- Unusual or superhuman strength
- Inappropriate clothing for the environment and/or
- Keening (unintelligible animal-like noises)

Tolerance to pain is an almost universal feature, displayed by nearly every patient with ExDS. As is implied in the syndrome's name, these patients also generally have an acute cognitive impairment, with a waxing and waning course. Thus, they have a true delirium. This combination of the above-noted signs and symptoms is particularly lethal, with a mortality rate as high as 11% based on limited epidemiologic data [3].

History

ExDS is felt by most experts to be related to Bell's mania, a clinical presentation that was first described in the medical literature in the mid-1800s. In 1849, Dr. Luther Bell, the superintendent of the McLean Asylum of the Insane in Somerville, Massachusetts, described 40 cases of a unique clinical condition that seemed "scarcely suited for the cares of an institution for the insane" [4]. Instead, continued Bell, "his physiognomy and articulation are rather those of fever and delirium." This syndrome had a high mortality rate, with nearly 75% of cases ending in death. Bell's initial report was followed by several subsequent similar reports. A 1934 review by Kraines noted several patients who had a "syndrome of sudden onset, with over-activity, great excitement, sleeplessness, apparent delirium, and distorted ideas; without any clear evidence of a definite toxic infectious factor" [5]. Kraines also noted that a standardized nomenclature for this syndrome did not yet exist, and at that time, similar cases were described in the medical literature from across the country, as well as in Europe, variously referred to as Bell's mania, acute delirious mania, delirium grave, acute delirium, specific febrile delirium, acute psychotic furors, or collapse delirium.

The descriptions of ExDS-like presentations by Bell and Kraines in the late 1800s and early 1900s were noted in the medical literature mainly as case reports, until the 1950s when the introduction and increased utilization of antipsychotics like chlorpromazine became more common in psychiatric facilities for the treatment of acutely agitated patients. As agitated psychotic individuals were more aggressively treated with pharmacologic therapy, the reporting of the ExDS-like deaths essentially disappeared from the medical literature. With effective treatment to interrupt the progressively worsening delirium and excitation, mortality from this condition, which was nearly 75% when first described, was reduced dramatically.

In the 1980s, reports of an ExDS-like syndrome started to reappear in the medical literature. Unlike previous reports, which concerned patients in psychiatric facilities, these new cases were being reported by medical examiners from autopsy findings. Also novel was the fact that these cases appeared to be in young men without a previous psychiatric illness, in association with recreational cocaine use. The first use of the term "Excited Delirium" was in a 1985 report by Wetli and Fishbain, who described seven cases of an agitated delirium in association with illicit drug use [6]. While all cases in this series were eventually fatal, deaths in these individuals differed from a typical cocaine overdose in two significant ways. First, extreme agitation and aggressive behavior preceded the deaths, even though postmortem levels of cocaine were more typical of recreational use than overdose. Second, unlike death from a typical cocaine overdose, none of these seven patients had preterminal seizures. Wetli and Fishbain warned of the potential for sudden death in conjunction with this "Excited

Delirium" syndrome, and this term is now preferred in the medical literature.

Despite the many descriptions of ExDS since the time of Bell, some civil rights advocates have claimed that the syndrome was invented by police and lawyers to absolve them of guilt for sudden deaths that occurred while placing and maintaining individuals in police custody. However, in 2004, the National Association of Medical Examiners published a position paper that recognized the existence of an excited delirium syndrome as a medical diagnosis for the first time and rejected the idea that deaths were caused by restraint or TASER use [7–10]. In 2009, the American College of Emergency Physicians published a white paper report, also recognizing the existence of the syndrome [1], and some review papers and a textbook have since been written on the topic to improve the understanding of and provide education about this syndrome [11–19]. With the additional research in the field, there is currently a greater awareness and knowledge that ExDS is a distinct type of medical emergency with potentially lethal consequences.

Diagnosis and Etiology

Diagnosis of ExDS is often challenging, as many causes and clinical features of ExDS overlap with other disease states. Stimulant intoxication, hypoglycemia, thyroid storm, seizures, or head injury, for instance, can cause agitation and aggression similar to ExDS [20]. If there is a medical condition or diagnosis that is responsible for the symptoms consistent with ExDS, then the patient does not have ExDS. ExDS is, therefore, a diagnosis of exclusion.

The exact etiology of ExDS is unknown. Some basic science and epidemiologic investigations have implicated sympathomimetic agents like cocaine, methamphetamine, or phencyclidine (PCP), as well as untreated or undertreated mental illness, especially schizophrenia and bipolar disorder [14–17, 21]. Currently, the majority of reported cases of ExDS are associated with stimulant drug use, although cases of ExDS still occur in psychiatric patients who are untreated or have abruptly discontinued their medications [1, 21–33].

In cases in which illicit stimulants are involved, the presentation is often abrupt and does not involve increased or elevated levels of the drug. Reports demonstrate typical recreational patterns of use. However, postmortem examinations of the brain of chronic cocaine patients have demonstrated a characteristic down-regulation of dopamine transporters in the ventral striatum, which is normally strongly innervated by dopaminergic neurons [34, 35]. This allows dopamine to persist in the synapses and suggests that excessive dopamine transmission, particularly in the striatum, may play a role in the clinical presentation of ExDS. Associated and novel alternative mechanisms and pathways are also being explored as potential contributing features of the clinical presentation [36–39].

Regardless of the exact pathophysiologic cause, ExDS is a true medical emergency. All ExDS patients will require emergency medical care for stabilization and treatment. Many current efforts have focused on training prehospital personnel and police to recognize the signs and symptoms of this syndrome. The rest of this chapter will focus on evaluation and treatment considerations.

Initial Approach and Workup

As noted above, many different medical conditions can cause a clinical presentation that is similar to ExDS. Stimulant intoxication, hypoglycemia, thyroid storm, seizures, head injury, serotonin syndrome, heatstroke, pheochromocytoma, and neuroleptic malignant syndrome all may present similarly, and several psychiatric conditions may also overlap with ExDS, including substance intoxication, paranoid-type schizophrenia, severe mania, or any of the anger disorders. Recognition of a severely agitated patient is typically not difficult. Rather, the main challenge revolves around initiating management and protecting the safety of providers. Patients with ExDS should be approached the same way that all patients with agitation are approached: cautiously. Whether in the prehospital environment or the hospital, providers must keep their safety in mind.

Current expert guidelines on the management of agitated patients recommend verbal de-escalation as the first step when possible [39, 40]. By definition, ExDS patients respond poorly to verbal cues, including police redirection. Consequently, by the time most of these patients are encountered by medical providers, this initial preferred approach has already failed. Though the verbal de-escalation will typically have minimal to no effect on the ExDS patient, the continued verbal communication may be calming to other nearby patients and staff during the use of restraint. This should ideally be performed by a single individual, who communicates expectations and give commands in a firm but calming tone. If possible, an effort should be made to reduce excessive environmental stimuli. In the prehospital environment, this is challenging, given the inherent chaos in an uncontrolled setting and myriad environmental stimuli from bystanders, family, police dogs, lights, sirens, and additional responding officers. Environmental stimuli can be problematic for physically gaining control of the patient. Although there is little formal scientific evidence on this point, a patient who is experiencing a catecholamine surge from ExDS typically does not respond to pain-compliance techniques. Thus, the amount of force needed will correspondingly be greater; use of greater force increases the possibility of injury to both patients and providers.

Related chapters on de-escalation, restraint, and seclusion, and rapid treatment for agitated patients elsewhere in this text merit review. In the prehospital setting, the basic principles used by law enforcement to control a patient in ExDS revolve around rapid physical restraint, minimization of the patient's exertional activity, and safety for all. The use of a TASER electronic control device (ECD) is felt by many experts to be preferable to the more traditional physical wrestling and grappling for control, since fighting and heavy physical exertion with repeated flexion and extension of the large muscle groups have a more deleterious effect on a patient's acid-base status by way of increased lactic acid production [40–43]. Incapacitating an individual first with a TASER ECD, then rapidly gaining physical control of the arms and legs will reduce the muscle activity of the large muscle groups, thus reducing the amount of lactic acid that is being produced, as well as the amount of oxygen being consumed. Throughout, the patient's airway should be carefully protected during any forceful maneuver, and respiratory status carefully monitored both during and after restraint. The purpose of this chapter is not to define police practices, but rather to bring attention to the fact that patients with ExDS are violent and dangerous, and will need physical control before medical assessment and therapy can safely begin.

Treatment Options for ExDS

Once the patient is restrained, rapid medical assessment can begin [44]. Law enforcement officers and prehospital medical providers are typically not expected to diagnose the cause of an acute behavioral disturbance. Instead, prehospital personnel should recognize the clinical syndrome of ExDS as a medical emergency and rapidly initiate therapeutic interventions within their scope of practice. Medical conditions and psychiatric diagnoses are entertained by the emergency physicians and consultants, usually with the help of laboratory and radiographic imaging, before making the final concluding diagnosis of ExDS.

Though not mandatory, certain tests are more frequently ordered on patients presenting with signs and symptoms consistent with ExDS. These include diagnostic EKG, electrolytes and renal function, creatinine kinase levels, cardiac markers, and TSH. Lactate levels are almost uniformly elevated and typically do not affect the need for treatment and resuscitation. If history indicates recent drug use, a drug "binge," or significant struggle, the laboratory studies above may be more prudent.

In choosing treatment options, providers should focus on identifying the most likely cause of the agitation [45]. Expert consensus guidelines for treatment of agitation generally recognize three classes of medications for the initial calming of agitated patients: benzodiazepines, first-generation antipsychotics (FGA), and second-generation antipsychotics (SGA). Experts in the field of ExDS often include dissociative agents such as ketamine as the fourth class of medication, particularly in the extreme agitation seen in ExDS. Extremely agitated trauma patients, especially those who have suffered blunt trauma or in whom there is a high suspicion of head injury, should be sedated, paralyzed, and intubated to protect the airway while additional diagnostic workup proceeds. Once the patient is calmed, other treatment modalities are generally used for supportive care.

The decision of when initially to use each of the classes of antipsychotic medication is not always clear. In general, expert consensus guidelines recommend that providers treat the underlying cause of the agitation, if it is known [45]. In many cases, the cause of agitated delirium may not be known before the need for pharmacological intervention, and so benzodiazepines are typically recommended as a first-line treatment. This may be especially useful in ExDS, as the majority of cases are associated with sympathomimetic illicit drug use [1]. If the patient is known to have a behavioral disorder and the likely ExDS symptomatology is due to medication noncompliance, antipsychotic medications can be used primarily or as adjunctive therapy with benzodiazepines.

Benzodiazepines

Benzodiazepines as a class bind to inhibitory γ-aminobutyric acid (GABA) receptors in the human brain. Drugs in this class include lorazepam, diazepam, and midazolam, which are injectable benzodiazepines widely available to prehospital and hospital personnel. As these medications cause sedation, they are accommodating in the management of ExDS patients. This is especially true if the source of the agitation is thought to be secondary to stimulant drug use, in which case benzodiazepines are the drug of choice.

Benzodiazepines are most often administered parenterally by intramuscular (IM), intravenous (IV), or intraosseous (IO) routes, although intranasal (IN) formulations also exist for midazolam. Serial doses may be required for sedation, and the doses of benzodiazepines typically are much higher in ExDS patients than those needed for anxious or mildly agitated persons. On the contrary, benzodiazepines may work relatively slowly if given IM (for instance, an onset of 1–5 minutes for midazolam). Also, potential side effects include oversedation, respiratory depression, and hypotension. Although the ExDS patient population is typically hyperstimulated, the clinical course can fluctuate, and the potential for sedative side effects exists. Ongoing cardiopulmonary monitoring may be indicated, and supportive care is easily managed in the ED setting, if needed.

First-Generation Antipsychotics

Conventional, or first-generation antipsychotics (FGA), are an older class of medications often used for calming. The butyrophenone class, which includes both haloperidol and droperidol, is the most widely used in US emergency departments [20]. These agents are thought to produce calming by inhibiting dopamine transmission in the brain. As butyrophenones are structurally similar to GABA, they may additionally interact with GABA receptors at higher doses [46].

Haloperidol and droperidol generally bind tightly to dopamine receptors, which is associated with significant side effects [20]. Both haloperidol and droperidol can lengthen the QT portion of the cardiac cycle and have been associated with sudden death. Since sudden death is a feature of ExDS and some ExDS deaths have been associated with ventricular dysrhythmias, it is wise to be cautious when administering these medications, especially repeated doses. In particular, if long QT syndrome is suspected based either on history or concomitant medications, these medications should be avoided, if possible. Of further note, when haloperidol or droperidol are administered, injections are generally given IM for both safety and efficacy in the physically agitated patient. The Food and Drug Administration (FDA) has required warnings for both of these medications when administered intravenously. Cardiac arrhythmias can result from the higher doses that are typically required in ExDS patients. Lower doses may be most effective when given as part of a combination therapy, such as a benzodiazepine. If given intravenously, cardiac monitoring should be performed when possible, but can be challenging in patients who are sweaty and combative, as cardiac monitoring in this population usually results in an artifact on the monitor.

A final additional reason for caution with the use of FGAs is hyperthermia. ExDS patients often have elevated temperatures, and there is some theoretical concern that this condition may result from dopamine disorders similar to those with the neuroleptic malignant syndrome. If so, dopamine antagonists like the FGAs may better be avoided if possible. In practice, however, this is rarely seen and may be more of a theoretical concern.

Second-Generation Antipsychotics

Second-generation antipsychotics available in an injectable form include both olanzapine and ziprasidone. Both of these agents bind more tightly to receptor types other than dopamine and so have fewer cardiac and movement-related side effects than FGAs. Both ziprasidone and olanzapine are equally as effective as haloperidol alone for calming [47, 48]. Unlike FGAs, however, there is limited evidence about the use of SGAs in combination with benzodiazepines. Several retrospective reviews have not noted any significant vital sign abnormalities with the combination of SGAs with benzodiazepines, unless the patient is significantly intoxicated with alcohol [49–52]. In these cases, haloperidol or haloperidol with benzodiazepines may be a safer choice.

Ketamine

Ketamine is an older medication that is structurally related to PCP. It is a dissociative anesthetic that binds N-methyl-D-aspartate (NMDA) receptor and may be given IM or IV. Ketamine rapidly causes a dissociative state, with preservation of airway reflexes [53]. Given its rapid onset of action, preservation of airway reflexes, and wide therapeutic range of dosing, ketamine is an attractive agent for use in ExDS. However, there have been some concerns raised about its use. First, there was initial theoretical concern about ketamine's ability to worsen preexisting hypertension and tachycardia. Second, ketamine has been associated with side effects such as increased oral secretions and laryngospasm. Finally, ketamine use prehospital has been associated with increased intubation. Regarding the first two concerns, growing clinical evidence, which includes several case reports and case series, have not demonstrated evidence of harm with the use of ketamine [54–59]. Increased rates of intubation may be partly explainable by the fact that patients typically present with low Glasgow Coma Scale (GCS) scores, combined with a history of aggressive behavior and altercation. These patients may, therefore, be intubated for low GCS until a trauma workup is complete. When a similar population of patients was treated with ketamine in an ED by physicians, the intubation rate was zero [60].

Initial Combination Therapy

To increase calming, many clinicians commonly pair benzodiazepines with antipsychotics, especially FGAs. In a 1997 study, Battaglia and colleagues published the largest emergency department investigation of haloperidol and lorazepam [61]. This study compared three different medications: haloperidol alone, lorazepam alone, and haloperidol combined with lorazepam. The researchers noted that side effects from haloperidol were reduced when this medication was combined with a benzodiazepine like lorazepam. Despite this study, two separate Cochrane reviews have found no evidence for the combination of haloperidol and benzodiazepines [62, 63]. Other randomized studies, however, had noted the reduction in side effects when haloperidol was combined with an anticholinergic such as promethazine [20]. Consequently, the use of promethazine may be reasonable if the QT is not prolonged.

Other reports have described using ketamine for initial therapy, followed by benzodiazepines once the patient was calm enough for IV access [60]. These agents are felt to have synergistic effects, and the use of benzodiazepines may help prevent emergence phenomena.

Other Treatment Modalities

The goal of calming with any class of medication, whether antipsychotics, benzodiazepines, ketamine, or a combination, is to prevent harm to the patient or staff, and to facilitate an examination, assessment, and emergency treatment of the patient [44]. This therapeutic approach should occur with all patients exhibiting signs and symptoms of ExDS, even if the final diagnosis changes after the ensuing workup. As with all ED patients with delirium, the underlying medical explanation is investigated, usually including reexamination, review of medical records, laboratory studies, and neuroimaging. Hypoglycemia can present as an agitated adrenergic state and is immediately reversible when recognized with a bedside blood-glucose-level check. Other identified medical conditions are treated as indicated. When a medical or psychiatric disorder is thought to be the etiology of the delirium and agitation, then the diagnosis of ExDS is no longer applicable. When no correctable etiology is identified, the diagnosis of ExDS is presumed. After adequate sedation, appropriate therapeutic measures include intravenous fluids, consideration for sodium bicarbonate, and cooling when necessary.

Intravenous Fluids

Patients with ExDS are commonly hyperthermic. When coupled with agitated and aggressive behavior, patients generally have a significant amount of insensible water loss. As such, most have some degree of dehydration. Also, aggressive behavior and typically violent struggles predispose patients to the development of rhabdomyolysis. Once safely permitted, intravenous fluid administration proceeds, unless otherwise contraindicated by underlying medical conditions. If vascular access is needed urgently, interosseous (IO) access is an option. IO access may also be safer, since it is often easier to restrain a limb for this procedure, which does not require precise vein cannulation.

Sodium Bicarbonate

As with most other treatments, routine use of intravenous sodium bicarbonate has not been evaluated for the treatment of metabolic acidosis in ExDS. Violent struggles cause a lactic acidosis that is associated with electrolyte abnormalities, which subsequently predispose the patient to the development of ventricular arrhythmias. Use of sodium bicarbonate in other conditions with lactic acidosis, however, has not shown benefit and may counterintuitively worsen the clinical picture by causing intracellular acidification [64].

Cooling

Hyperthermia is present in many patients with ExDS and can often be assessed clinically with a tactile temperature instead of a core temperature measurement, if this is not available. Profuse sweating may be evident. Patients who are suffering significant or presumed hyperthermia should be cooled aggressively as soon as is practical. Some experts have noted that substantial hyperthermia in the face of ExDS is a predictor of increased mortality, though definitive epidemiologic data is currently lacking [1].

Although often difficult to cool a patient in the prehospital arena, both cooled intravenous fluids and ice packs to the neck, groin, or axillae may be used to initiate the temperature-lowering process. If not already undressed, all ExDS patients should be disrobed. In the emergency department, other techniques such as evaporative cooling with misting across bare skin or utilizing fans, commercial cooling blankets, and ice water immersion are effective. Patients with significant temperature elevations should be cooled by more than one method. When feasible, continuous core temperature measurements are ideal so as not to overshoot normothermia. Although some researchers have likened the dopamine dysfunction in ExDS to the neuroleptic malignant syndrome, there has been no work evaluating the use of dantrolene in these patients. Typical management of hyperthermia is, therefore, more similar to heatstroke or heat-illness protocols.

Conclusions

Although once controversial, ExDS is now accepted as a unique clinical syndrome with a long history, albeit by various names, in the medical literature. Although ExDS is not universally fatal as was initially thought, about one in 10 patients will nonetheless progress to sudden cardiac death. Mechanisms responsible for this mortality are not fully understood, and although some associations have been made, the risk factors for sudden death in ExDS have not been identified.

Although there is much to be learned about the pathophysiology of ExDS, most experts agree that early interventions by police, EMS, and emergency department personnel are essential and can impact survival in many patients. In a patient with ExDS, timely treatment is needed to save lives from this disease. Treatment includes both providing physical restraint and chemical sedation as quickly and safely as possible, and in initiating medical stabilization and evaluation to exclude underlying causes. In the event of sudden death, careful observations by law enforcement and health care providers will assist medical examiners in making accurate determinations of ExDS.

References

1. ACEP Excited Delirium Task Force. White Paper Report on Excited Delirium Syndrome; 2009. Available at https://www.acep.org/uploadedFiles/ACEP/Practice_Resources/disater_and_EMS/EMS_resources/ACEP%20Excited%20Delirium%20White%20Paper%20final%20form.pdf. Accessed on 1 Oct 2017.
2. Hall C, Butler C, Kader A, et al. Police use of force, injuries and death: prospective evaluation of outcomes for all police use of force/restraint including conducted energy weapons in a large Canadian city. Acad Emerg Med. 2009;16(4):S198–9.
3. Stratton SJ, Rogers C, Brickett K, Gruzinski G. Factors associated with sudden death of individuals requiring restraint for excited delirium. Am J Emerg Med. 2001;19:187–91.
4. Bell L. On a form of disease resembling some advanced stages of mania and fever, but so contradistinguished from any ordinarily observed or described combination of symptoms, as to render it probable that it may be an overlooked and hitherto unrecorded malady. Am J Insanity. 1849;6:97–127.
5. Kraines SH. Bell's mania. Am J Psychiatry. 1934;91:29–40.
6. Wetli CV, Fishbain DA. Cocaine-induced psychosis and sudden death in recreational cocaine users. J Forensic Sci. 1985;30(3):873–80.
7. Reay DT, Fligner CL, Stilwell AD, et al. Positional asphyxia during law enforcement transport. Am J Forensic Med Pathol. 1992;13(2):90–7.
8. O'Halloran RL, Lewman LV. Restraint asphyxiation in excited delirium. Am J Forensic Med Pathol. 1993;14(4):289–95.
9. Zipes DP. Sudden cardiac arrest and death following application of shocks from a TASER electronic control device. Circulation. 2012;125(20):2417–22. Epub e2012 Apr 30. Erratum in: Circulation. 2013;127(23):e839. Circulation. 2012;126(2):e27.
10. Stephens BG, Jentzen JM, Karch S, Wetli CV, Mash DC. National Association of Medical Examiners position paper on the certification of cocaine-related deaths. Am J Forens Med Sci. 2004;25(1):11–3.
11. DiMaio TG, DiMaio VJM. Excited delirium syndrome cause of death and prevention. 1st ed. Boca Raton, FL: Taylor & Francis Group; 2006. p. 1–60.
12. Grant JR, Southall PE, Mealey J, Scott SR, Fowler DR. Excited delirium deaths in custody past and present. Am J Forensic Med Pathol. 2009;30:1–5.
13. Otahbuchi M, Cevik C, Bagdure S, Nugent K. Excited delirium, restraints, and unexpected death: a review of pathogenesis. Am J Forensic Med Pathol. 2010;31(2):1–6.
14. Takeuchi A, Ahern TL, Henderson SO. Excited delirium. West J Emerg Med. 2011;XII(1):77–83.
15. Vilke GM, DeBard ML, Chan TC, et al. Excited Delirium Syndrome (ExDS): defining based on a review of the literature. J Emerg Med. 2012;43(5):897–905.
16. Gerold KB, Gibbons ME, Fisette RE Jr, et al. Review, clinical update, and practice guidelines for excited delirium syndrome. J Spec Oper Med. 2015;15(1):62–9.
17. Gill JR. The syndrome of excited delirium. Forensic Sci Med Pathol. 2014;10(2):223–8.
18. Vilke GM, Payne-James J, Karsch SB. Excited Delirium Syndrome (ExDS): redefining an old diagnosis. J Forens Legal Med. 2012;19:7–11.
19. Vilke GM, Bozeman WP, Dawes DM, et al. Excited delirium syndrome (ExDS): treatment options and considerations. J Forensic Legal Med. 2012;19(3):117–21.

20. Vilke GM, Wilson MP. Agitation: what every emergency physician should know. EM Rep. 2009;30(19):1–8.
21. Penders TM. The syndrome of excited delirium following use of "bath salts". J Clin Psychiatry. 2013;74(5):518.
22. Escobedo LG, Ruttenber AJ, Agocs MM, Anda RF, Wetli CV. Emerging patterns of cocaine use and the epidemic of cocaine overdose deaths in Dade County, Florida. Arch Pathol Lab Med. 1991;115(9):900–5.
23. Ruttenber AJ, Sweeney PA, Mendlein JM, Wetli CV. Preliminary findings of an epidemiologic study of cocaine-related deaths, Dade County, Florida, 1978–85. NIDA Res Monogr. 1991;110:95–112.
24. Mirchandani HG, Rorke LB, Sekula-Perlman A, Hood IC. Cocaine-induced agitated delirium, forceful struggle, and minor head injury: a further definition of sudden death during restraint. Am J Forensic Med Pathol. 1994;15(2):95–9.
25. Wetli CV, Mash D, Karch SB. Cocaine-associated agitated delirium and the neuroleptic malignant syndrome. Am J Emerg Med. 1996;14:425–8.
26. Hick JL, Smith SW, Lynch MT. Metabolic acidosis in restraint-associated cardiac arrest: a case series. Acad Emerg Med. 1999;6(3):239–43.
27. Ruttenber AJ, McAnally HB, Wetli CV. Cocaine-associated rhabdomyolysis and excited delirium: different stages of the same syndrome. Am J Forensic Med Pathol. 1999;20(2):120–7.
28. Allam S, Noble JS. Cocaine-excited delirium and severe acidosis. Anesthesia. 2001;56(4):385–6.
29. Gruszecki AC, McGwin G, Robinson A, Davis GG. Unexplained sudden death and the likelihood of drug abuse. J Forensic Sci. 2005;50(2):1–4.
30. Bunai Y, Akaza K, Jiang WX, Nagai A. Fatal hyperthermia associated with excited delirium during an arrest. Leg Med (Tokyo). 2008;10(6):306–9.
31. Maher PJ, Walsh M, Burns T, Strote J. Prehospital resuscitation of a man with excited delirium and cardiopulmonary arrest. CJEM. 2014;16(1):80–3.
32. Plush T, Shakespeare W, Jacobs D, Ladi L, Sethi S, Gasperino J. Cocaine-induced agitated delirium: a case report and review. J Intensive Care Med. 2015;30(1):49–57.
33. Kodikara S, Cunningham K, Pollanen MS. "Excited delirium syndrome": is it a cause of death? Leg Med (Tokyo). 2012;14(5):252–4.
34. Mash DC, Duque L, Pablo J, et al. Brain biomarkers for identifying excited delirium as a cause of sudden death. Forensic Sci Int. 2009;190(1–3):e13–9.
35. Mash DC. Biochemical brain markers in excited delirium deaths. In: Kroll MW, Ho JD, editors. TASER conducted electrical weapons: physiology, pathology, and law. New York, NY: Springer; 2009. p. 365–77.
36. Johnson MM, David JA, Michelhaugh SK, et al. Increased heat shock protein 70 gene expression in the brains of cocaine-related fatalities may be reflective of postdrug survival and intervention rather than excited delirium. J Forensic Sci. 2012;57(6):1519–23.
37. Schiavone S, Riezzo I, Turillazzi E, et al. Involvement of the NADPH oxidase NOX2-derived brain oxidative stress in an unusual fatal case of cocaine-related neurotoxicity associated with excited delirium syndrome. J Clin Psychopharmacol. 2016;36(5):513–7.
38. Schiavone S, Neri M, Mhillaj E, et al. The role of the NADPH oxidase derived brain oxidative stress in the cocaine-related death associated with excited delirium: a literature review. Toxicol Lett. 2016;258:29–35.
39. Richmond JS, Berlin JS, Fishkind A, et al. Verbal de-escalation of the agitated patient: consensus statement of the American Association for Emergency Psychiatry Project BETA De-escalation Workgroup. West J Emerg Med. 2012;13(1):17–25.
40. Wilson MP, Zeller SL. Reconsidering psychiatry in the emergency department. J Emerg Med. 2012;43(5):771–2.
41. Ho JD, Dawes DM, Nelson RS, et al. Acidosis and catecholamine evaluation following simulated law enforcement "Use of force" Encounters. Acad Emerg Med. 2010;12:E60–E6.
42. Ho JD, Dawes DM, Cole JB, et al. Lactate and pH evaluation in exhausted humans with prolonged TASER® X26 exposure or continued exertion. Forensic Sci Int. 2009;190:80–6.
43. Ho JD, Dawes DM, Bultman LL, et al. Prolonged TASER® use on exhausted humans does not worsen markers of acidosis. Am J Emerg Med. 2009;27:413–8.
44. Nordstrom K, Zun LS, Wilson MP, et al. Medical evaluation and triage of the agitated patient: consensus statement of the American Association for Emergency Psychiatry Project BETA Medical Evaluation Workgroup. West J Emerg Med. 2012;13(1):3–10.
45. Wilson MP, Pepper D, Currier GW, Holloman GH, Feifel D. The psychopharmacology of agitation: consensus statement of the American Association for Emergency Psychiatry Project BETA Psychopharmacology Workgroup. West J Emerg Med. 2012;13(1):26–34.
46. Richards JR, Schneir AB. Droperidol in the emergency department: is it safe? J Emerg Med. 2001;24(4):441–7.
47. Zeller SL, Rhoades R. Systematic reviews of assessment measures and pharmacologic treatments for agitation. Clin Ther. 2010;32:403–25.
48. Citrome L. Comparison of intramuscular ziprasidone, olanzapine, or aripiprazole for agitation: a quantitative review of efficacy and safety. J Clin Psychiatry. 2007;68:1876–85.
49. Wilson MP, MacDonald K, Vilke GM, Ronquillo L, Feifel D. Use of intramuscular ziprasidone by ED clinicians and its effect on vital signs. National Behavioral Emergencies Conference, December 1–2, 2011; Las Vegas, Nevada.
50. Wilson MP, MacDonald KS, Vilke GM, Feifel D. A comparison of the safety of olanzapine and haloperidol in combination with benzodiazepines in emergency department patients with acute agitation. J Emerg Med. 2012;43(5):790–7.

51. Wilson MP, MacDonald KS, Vilke GM, Feifel D. Potential complications of combining intramuscular olanzapine with benzodiazepines in agitated emergency department patients. J Emerg Med. 2012;43(5):889–96.
52. Macdonald K, Wilson MP, Minassian A, et al. A retrospective analysis of intramuscular haloperidol and intramuscular olanzapine in the treatment of agitation in drug- and alcohol-using patients. Gen Hosp Psychiatry. 2010;32(4):443–5.
53. Green SM, Roback MG, Kennedy RM, et al. Clinical practice guideline for emergency department ketamine dissociative sedation: 2011 update. Ann Emerg Med. 2011;57(5):449–61.
54. Burnett AM, Watters BJ, Barringer KW, et al. Laryngospasm and hypoxia after intramuscular administration of ketamine to a patient in excited delirium. Prehosp Emerg Care. 2012;16(3):412–4.
55. Roberts JR, Geeting GK. Intramuscular ketamine for the rapid tranquilization of the uncontrollable, violent, and dangerous adult patient. J Trauma. 2001;51:1008–10.
56. Hick JL, Ho JD. Ketamine chemical restraint to facilitate rescue of a combative "jumper". Prehosp Emerg Care. 2005;9(1):85–9.
57. Cole JB, Klein LR, Nystrom PC, et al. A prospective study of ketamine as primary therapy for prehospital profound agitation. Am J Emerg Med. 2017;36(5):789–96.
58. Scaggs TR, Glass DM, Hutchcraft MG, et al. Prehospital ketamine is a safe and effective treatment for excited delirium in a community hospital based EMS system. Prehosp Disaster Med. 2016;31(5):563–9.
59. Scheppke KA, Braghiroli J, Shalaby M, et al. Prehospital use of i.m. ketamine for sedation of violent and agitated patients. West J Emerg Med. 2014;15(7):736–41.
60. Hopper AB, Vilke GM, Castillo EM, Campillo A, Davie T, Wilson MP. Ketamine use for acute agitation in the emergency department. J Emerg Med. 2015;48(6):712–9.
61. Battaglia J, Moss S, Rush J, et al. Haloperidol, lorazepam, or both for psychotic agitation? A multicenter, prospective, double-blind, emergency department study. Am J Emerg Med. 1997;15(4):335–40.
62. Powney MJ, Adams CE, Jones H. Haloperidol for psychosis-induced aggression or agitation (rapid tranquillisation). Cochrane Database Syst Rev. 2012;11(11):CD009377.
63. Ostinelli EG, Brooke-Powney MJ, Li X, Adams CE. Haloperidol for psychosis-induced aggression or agitation (rapid tranquillisation). Cochrane Database Syst Rev. 2017;7:CD009377.
64. Kraut JA, Madias NE. Lactic acidosis. N Engl J Med. 2014;371(24):2309–19.

Medical Illness in Psychiatric Disease

17

Victor G. Stiebel and Barbara Nightingale

Introduction: Comorbidity Incidence/Prevalence

Comorbidity is a noun that describes the simultaneous presence of two chronic diseases or conditions in a patient. It is a given that medical illness is common in psychiatric patients and that psychiatric pathology is common in medical conditions. In the following pages, we will attempt to provide a clinical approach to concomitant conditions, rather than a laundry list of diagnoses.

The National Survey on Drug Use and Health estimates that in 2015, 18% of the adult population of the United States suffered from a mental health disorder within the past year [1]. Those diagnosed with any medical condition constitute 58%. In this area of overlap, 68% of adults with mental disorders have some medical condition, and 29% of those with medical conditions have a mental disorder.

The number of physical symptoms reported during a primary care office visit has been shown to strongly correlate with the likelihood of a psychiatric disorder, ranging from 2% to almost 60% [2]. Lipowski [3] was one of the first to identify that between 30% and 60% of medical inpatients will suffer from some psychiatric condition. Within the emergency department, mental health and substance problems account for one in eight visits, and patients with these problems are more than twice as likely to be hospitalized [4, 5]. Unfortunately, these diagnoses are frequently missed by the emergency department (ED) physician for a variety of reasons, including time constraints, lack of training, limited resources, and overall acuity level of other patients [6].

Emergency physicians are experts at evaluation based on complex thought processes, including pattern recognition, laboratory testing, and heuristic strategies to rule out worst-case scenarios. However, these methods, which are inherently imperfect, allow bias to enter our thought processes. In the setting of a patient with both medical and psychiatric diagnoses, this can have catastrophic results. Medical diagnoses and psychiatric conditions do not occur in a vacuum and are often interrelated, and one will frequently impact adversely on the other. Additionally, psychosocial factors can add an exponential degree of complexity to a clinical situation. An open mind and avoidance of early diagnostic closure are vital.

V. G. Stiebel (✉)
Department of Emergency Medicine, University of West Virginia, Morgantown, WV, USA

B. Nightingale
Department of Family Medicine and Psychiatry, University of Pittsburgh Medical Center, Pittsburgh, PA, USA

L. S. Zun et al. (eds.), *Behavioral Emergencies for Healthcare Providers*,
https://doi.org/10.1007/978-3-030-52520-0_17

Duality of Approach

The initial evaluation of the medically ill patient with an unexplained symptom in a medical setting tends to focus on medical diagnoses. The initial evaluation of a mentally ill patient with unexplained symptoms in a mental health setting will tend to focus on psychopathology. When this same medical patient is seen in a psychiatric clinic, or vice versa, there can be a tendency to early diagnostic closure, eliminating potential alternative diagnoses, again with potentially catastrophic results. This artificial dichotomy of "either medical or psychiatric" can result in an evaluation that will be heavily influenced by which part of the clinical picture is being brought into focus first.

The basic problem is that patients and clinical conditions do not exist independently. We noted earlier that between 30% and 60% of medical patients seen in a primary care setting would have a psychosocial diagnosis [3]. It is also known that patients with psychiatric diagnoses have an overall morbidity and mortality rate significantly higher than that of matched controls [7, 8]. The SADHART [9] studies looked at antidepressant use following myocardial infarction and found that mortality doubled over 6.7 years, compared with controls in patients who had not been treated with antidepressants, regardless of whether the patient had depression or not. A recent review in JAMA noted that depression was associated with a significantly increased risk of stroke [10]. Takutsubo cardiomyopathy, or "broken heart syndrome," has been described as acute ventricular dysfunction following acute emotional distress [11]. Finally, a 2017 study of 24,000 patients found that a depression diagnosis at any time following a coronary artery disease diagnosis was associated with a twofold higher risk of death [12].

A dualistic approach would conceptualize comorbid medical and psychiatric conditions as a diagnostic continuum that must be approached from multiple views with both a very high degree of suspicion and a holistic approach to the patient. "Primary" disorders typically refer to classical psychiatric disorders such as mania and schizophrenia. "Secondary" usually refers to conditions due to other medical conditions, drugs/alcohol, or medications. Evaluation of preexisting and comorbid psychiatric conditions and their treatments, which can have a profound impact on the patient's medical evaluation, differential diagnosis, and treatment plan, should quickly follow stabilization of the emergency condition. During the next tier of the investigation, one can begin to evaluate potential comorbidities in developing the differential diagnosis and management plan. In almost all cases, a new psychiatric diagnosis is one of exclusion in the emergency setting.

With this approach in mind, cause-and-effect consideration must be given to a mental health patient with worsening physical symptoms being the result of deterioration in their underlying psychiatric condition. One example would be the anxious or somatic patient presenting with chest pain. A very slow, subdued depressed patient may have a fever. Another example might be a chronic schizophrenic who presents with muscle stiffness and a low blood count. However, these same clinical scenarios could represent a case of angina, sepsis, or neuroleptic malignant syndrome. Since patients may not know the specifics of their condition, and medication lists may be unavailable or incorrect, one is reminded of the need to collaborate with mental health providers, just as one would with a primary care physician.

Risk Factor Assessment

Assessing risk factors for medical illness in patients with psychiatric disorders is essential but often overlooked. There is increased use of harmful substances, exposure to unhealthy environments, side effects from medications used to treat psychiatric disorders, and a lack of resources, which all contribute to higher risk of medical comorbidities. A "supervised" living situation may translate to a guard at the front door or trained staff that monitor medications and hygiene. Meals can range from well-balanced and nutritious to high carbohydrate and fatty. Screening for abuse and dependence of common substances is essential; however, routine drug screens do not typically screen for synthetic opioids. Although there has been much discussion about obtaining "routine" psychiatric laboratory studies, the current emergency visit may be the only time that the psychiatric patient is seen by a non-mental-health medical provider. Ordering a chest x-ray or EKG may not even be possible on some mental health units. A brief questioning of financial resources can help guide medication usage to lower cost options.

Clinical Syndromes: Depression

Depressed patients tend to be quiet and withdrawn, and can easily be forgotten in the back areas of a busy emergency department. Major depressive disorder is estimated to have a lifetime prevalence of 28% [13], but is as high as 30% in the ED [14]. Virtually all medical conditions are associated with some depressive complaints, with diabetes, heart and lung disease, and arthritis being most common. Not all these patients are suffering from a major depressive disorder, however. Patients are often being faced with catastrophic life changes, including physical appearance, pain, isolation, financial uncertainty, and changed relationships. Being sad and demoralized can be a normal and expectable consequence of medical illness in these situations. Detection and management of suicidality are paramount in the emergency department. Given that the incidence of suicide is rising and that the majority of individuals who die by suicide see a health-care provider within the year before death, the Joint Commission's National Patient Safety Goal of suicide prevention includes screening for suicide, conducting a suicide risk assessment, and providing suicide prevention treatment for all patients presenting to the emergency department with a psychiatric symptom [15].

One of the difficulties in making a diagnosis of depression in the medically ill is that there is an exceptional amount of symptom overlap, that is, the duality that recurs during this discussion. Schwab [16] in 1965 suggested that psychological symptoms of depression are often experienced by medically ill patients, even though they may not be suffering from the clinical entity that is called depression. The DSM-V criteria for major depression include at least 2 weeks of low mood or loss of interest in activities, in addition to other somatic symptoms including a change in appetite, sleep, energy, or psychomotor disturbances, and feelings of worthlessness [17]. A patient, boarded in the emergency department for 18 hours, not eating, sleep deprived, and scared, will likely positively endorse symptoms about energy, appetite, worry, and fear. This will only be magnified after time in an ICU setting. If a proper history is not sought, an incorrect diagnosis could result. To assist in the appropriate detection of depressive symptoms, proper screening tools, diagnostic aids, and appropriate workup for depression can be found elsewhere in this book.

Clinical Syndrome: Chronic Obstructive Lung Disease

Chronic obstructive pulmonary disease (COPD), usually as an end result of smoking, is a frequent finding in psychiatric patients. COPD can also be a primary cause of anxiety and depression. Major depression and anxiety may be as high as 44% in patients with COPD [18], and COPD now affects some 24 million Americans [19]. Common treatments for asthma and COPD include steroids and beta-agonists, both of which can worsen depression and anxiety. Mortality is also significantly higher in these comorbidly ill patients [20]. COPD patients by definition suffer from respiratory difficulties that increase the work of breathing. The essential feature of generalized anxiety disorder is "excessive worry," but trouble concentrating, fatigue, and trouble sleeping are symptoms common to depression as well. In the emergency setting with an anxious dyspneic patient, making a determination of excessive worry is problematic, and establishing that depressive symptoms are not related to the medical illness is challenging. These patients do in fact suffer from fatigue that comes from the physical effort of breathing, anxiety from the fear of suffocation, and they often have difficulty with sleep due to positioning, continuous positive airway pressure (CPAP) machines, and medications. Social factors such as not being able to leave the house, loneliness, concern over self-image, and being dependent on oxygen also contribute to the overall disease picture. Treatment for these patients should focus first on optimizing their respiratory status. Continuous oxygen therapy, even at baseline levels of only 90%, can be beneficial. Occasional use of benzodiazepines, even on a long-term basis, can be very useful for the emergent control of breakthrough anxiety, and their use should not be avoided. Routine use, however, can pose challenges due to sedation and tolerance. Use of low-dose tricyclic antidepressants such as nortriptyline (10 mg three times a day) can be very effective. The use of low-dose antipsychotic medication has a place in the treatment armamentarium, but their potential side effect profile should be considered in the risk–benefit analysis. COPD patients suffering from anxiety-spectrum disorders may benefit from psychological interventions such as cognitive behavior therapy, group support, and relaxation training. However, a recent Cochrane review did not find significant long-term improvement [21].

Clinical Syndrome: Cardiovascular Disease

Cardiovascular disease remains one of the leading causes of death and overall morbidity in the United States. It has long been known that there was a strong relationship between depression and heart disease. Stress, "Type A" personality types, and unhealthy lifestyle choices have been the cardiac risk factors identified. Acute cardiac events can trigger stress reactions, fear, sleep–wake-cycle interruptions, loss of previous social status, pain, and disability. Very quickly, this complex duality can result in isolation, sedentary lifestyles, dependency, obesity, worsening depression, and deterioration in cardiac status. Depression has consistently been found in almost 20% of patients with cardiovascular disease [22]. Fleet [23] found, however, that 25% of their sample of chest pain patients had an undiagnosed panic disorder. Frasure-Smith [24] in 1993 first confirmed that depression increased mortality following acute myocardial infarction (MI) by a factor of three. A 2003 study found that heart patients coincidentally treated with selective serotonin reuptake inhibitors (SSRI) had fewer deaths or recurrent MI [25]. This was later shown to be due to their effect on platelet aggregation [26]. The SADHART studies noted earlier provide further justification for the prudent clinician maintaining an open mind toward the duality of comorbid illnesses.

The evaluation of these patients should begin with a thorough medical evaluation. A standard evaluation, including EKG and cardiac enzymes, is an important starting point if the pain is thought to be cardiac in origin. While carefully ruling out organic pathology, it may not be unreasonable to consult with psychiatry early in the course of admission. Aggressive treatment of anxiety and despondency, even if only with short-acting benzodiazepines, could bring significant relief to this population. If a patient in this cohort became a frequent visitor to the emergency department, obtaining cardiac catheterization may ultimately be the best option to clarify their medical status.

Clinical Syndrome: Gastrointestinal Disorders

Since before the time of Freud, there has been a known relationship between the gastrointestinal (GI) system and psychiatric disorders. Peptic ulcer disease, inflammatory bowel (including ulcerative colitis), and Crohn's disease were the classically described illnesses. Psychiatric comorbidity included anxiety, depression, and somatization. Often, this balance tended toward psychiatric, or so-called "functional," illnesses. As our understanding broadened, this was found to not always be correct, as when bacteria or anti-inflammatory drugs were found to be associated with peptic ulcer disease. Still, it is estimated that as many as 20% of peptic ulcer disease patients and up to 30% of those suffering from inflammatory bowel disease will be diagnosed with depression [27].

Perhaps, the biggest mental health factor associated with these disorders is the overall quality of life. Guthrie [28] demonstrated that physical function, role limitation, pain, and overall health perception were significantly worse in this comorbid cohort. However, this is a complex association. A patient suffering from depression could have worsened bowel symptoms, but the patient with severe bowel disease is likely to depress. Many of the medications used to treat either symptom cluster can have side effects on the other. Social stress can become profound. It becomes increasingly more difficult for patients to leave home, go to work, or meet friends, and a vicious cycle ensues.

A detailed history can sometimes tease apart the two clinical presentations. It is vital to note the time of symptoms onset. Depression is marked by depressed mood, decreased interest, poor concentration, and feelings of worthlessness, to name a few. The Rome criteria for irritable bowel disease focus on pain, features of the bowel symptoms, and time course aimed to eliminate some of the diagnostic uncertainty inherent in this disease. There can be an overlap of symptom clusters. These patients can be referred early to mental health, with subsequent untreated physical suffering. More often, the diagnosis and treatment focus on the physical, with mental anguish being treated symptomatically, if at all. This then becomes a dilemma for the busy emergency department, with a frequent visitor refusing to consider the possibility of a comorbid situation. Sometimes, great progress will be made with a patient by simply listening and letting them know you are trying to understand their situation.

Definitive pharmacologic interventions will rarely be started in the emergency department. A focus on the acute presentation is probably the best starting point, and short-acting benzodiazepines are certainly reasonable to consider if significant anxiety exists. Pain also needs to be addressed. Traditional tricyclic antidepressants have been shown to be effective over placebo [29]. The benefit of these medications is likely due to a combination of anticholinergic properties, as well as some analgesic effect. Duloxetine, a serotonin-norepinephrine reuptake inhibitor was marketed with a specific indication as an analgesic, though most of the SSRIs likely share some of this benefit. It is important to identify whether these medications are being started for their antidepressant or analgesic properties. In conjunction with the primary care provider, an emergency physician may have a window of opportunity, when a patient is in crisis, to initiate this type of medication.

Clinical Syndrome: Pain

Pain is an extremely common presenting complaint in the ED, with patients citing the inability to cope with pain as the most frequent reason for the ED visit [30]. It is imperative to be aware of the high rates of comorbidity of chronic pain with depression, anxiety, and post-traumatic stress disorder. Chronic pain and depression exacerbate one another; in fact, rates of major depressive disorder increase in proportion to greater pain severity [31]. Also, sometimes patients presenting with pain will even be labeled as having somatization or somatic symptom disorder. These are very difficult terms with multiple meanings ranging from any patient with physical complaints to a DSM-V psychiatric diagnosis for a patient with distressing somatic symptoms plus related abnormal distress and dysfunction. The label can be descriptive or pejorative. As always, a good history is vital, and diagnostic accuracy is very important.

Pain, however, can cause a range of psychosocial distress short of a major depression. These patients are inwardly focused and acutely aware of every bodily sensation, resulting in objectively minor complaints presenting as an impending catastrophe. This can quickly lead to isolation due to fears of leaving home, overuse of medications, frequent calls to the doctor, or visits to the ED, and burnout of friends and caregivers. Self-reported depression, feelings of worthlessness, and anhedonia (a pervasive inability to experience pleasure) are more likely to reflect a primary psychiatric disorder. A patient in severe pain may report feelings of being better off dead as a way to end the suffering, but not be interested in taking their own life. Anxiety complaints can be directly related to the pain, or fear of the pain, even if not currently present. Anger at the doctor's inability to find a resolution to their condition can quickly lead to an impasse, limiting proper evaluation and effective treatment.

Until proven otherwise, a complaint of pain should be taken at face value. Physicians tend to undermedicate pain with inadequate dosing and improper frequency. Many reasons are given for this, including overcrowding, fears of causing addiction, over medication causing complications, and poor understanding of basic pharmacokinetics. Also, psychiatric medications are often unfamiliar, comorbid psychopathology is frightening, and fears of making the mental health patient worse can be added obstacles. Opioids may not be the "gold standard" of years past for control of acute pain control, but they have the added benefit of being effective anxiolytics and are rarely contraindicated due to drug–drug interactions.

Treating pain in the ED creates a dilemma. Prior emphasis on improving patient analgesia likely has contributed to a rapidly growing epidemic of opioid use problems [32]. Ideally, pain management is tailored to specific cause and type of pain; however, the ED is rarely the optimal setting for addressing pain, particularly if it is chronic. Compared to other specialties, emergency medicine ranks as one of the highest for prescribing opioids [33]. However, prescriptions tend to be appropriate doses for very short periods of time. Patients with chronic noncancer pain who persistently use opioids have increased the risk of adverse effects, including side effects, the potential for misuse, and mortality. The American College of Emergency Physicians developed an Opioid Guideline Writing Panel guiding for management of opioids in the ED [34]. Utilizing a statewide prescription drug monitoring program when available can help reduce risk of doctor shopping, diversion of opioids, and opioid misuse [35]. Honoring pain medication contracts with other physicians is important and can reduce pressure to prescribe opioids for chronic pain. If opioids are prescribed, writing for the lowest reasonable dose and limited duration can mitigate some risk. Utilizing alternative medications such as nonsteroidal anti-inflammatory agents and muscle relaxants can have additive benefits. Psychiatric patients are often taking adjunctive medications such as tricyclic antidepressants, SSRIs, anticonvulsants, and benzodiazepines that can be adjusted to serve a dual therapeutic purpose.

Conclusion

Bias is an inherent part of the human psyche but is not inherently detrimental to patient care. Not being aware of bias, however, can be catastrophic. Medical and psychiatric illnesses often represent an overlapping and complex spectrum of symptoms and diagnoses. Both emergency physicians and psychiatrists must avoid early diagnostic closure and look at the whole patient. A duality of approach will almost always result in improved overall care.

References

1. Center for Behavioral Health Statistics and Quality. Key substance use and mental health indicators in the United States: Results from the 2015 National Survey on Drug Use and Health. HHS Publication No. SMA 16–4984, NSDUH Series H-51; 2016. Available at http://www.samhsa.gov/data/.
2. Kroenke K, Spitzer RL, Janet BW, Williams DSW. Physical symptoms in primary care: predictors of psychiatric disorders and functional impairment. Arch Fam Med. 1994;3:774–9.
3. Lipowski ZJ. The interface of psychiatry and medicine: towards integrated health care. Can J Psy. 1987;32(9):743–8.
4. Owens PL, Mutter R, Stocks C. Mental Health and Substance Abuse-Related Emergency Department Visits Among Adults, 2007. HCUP Statistical Brief #92. 2010. Rockville, MD; US Agency for Healthcare Research and Quality.
5. Curran GM, Sullivan G, Williams K, et al. Emergency department use of persons with comorbid psychiatric and substance abuse disorders. Ann Emerg Med. 2003;41(5):659–67.
6. Santucci KA, Sather J, Baker MD. Emergency medicine training programs' educational requirements in the management of psychiatric emergencies: current perspective. Pediatr Emerg Care. 2003;19(3):154–6.

7. Felker B, Yazel JJ, Short D. Mortality and medical comorbidity among psychiatric patients: a review. Psychiatr Serv. 1996;47(12):1356–63.
8. Mykletun A, Bjerkeset O, Overland S, et al. Levels of anxiety and depression as predictors of mortality: the HUNT study. Br J Psy. 2009;195(2):118–25.
9. Glassman AH, Bigger T, Gaffney M. Psychiatric characteristics associated with long-term mortality among 361 patients having an acute coronary syndrome and major depression. Arch Gen Psychiatry. 2009;66(9):1022–9.
10. Pan A, Sun Q, Okereke O, et al. Depression and risk of stroke morbidity and mortality: a meta-analysis and systematic review. JAMA. 2011;306(11):1241–9.
11. Wittstein IS. The broken heart syndrome. Cleve Clin J Med. 2007;74(suppl 1):S17–22.
12. May HT, Horne BD, et al. The association of depression at any time to the risk of death following coronary artery disease diagnosis. Eur Heart J Qual Care Clin Outcomes. 2017. https://academic.oup.com/ehjqcco/articleabstract/doi/10.1093/ehjqcco/qcx017/4036401.
13. Vandeleur CL, et al. Prevalence and correlates of DSM-5 major depressive and related disorders in the community. Psy Res. 250:50–8.
14. Claassen CA, Larkin GL. Occult suicidality in an emergency department population. Br J Psy. 2005;186:352–3.
15. The Joint Commission. Sentinel Event Alert 56: detecting and treating suicide ideation in all settings; 2016.
16. Schwab JJ, Clemmons RS, Bialow M, et al. The affective symptomatology of depression in medical inpatients. Psychosomatics. 1966;7:214–7.
17. American Psychiatric Association. Diagnostic and statistical manual of mental disorders. Fifth ed. Arlington, VA: American Psychiatric Publishing; 2013.
18. Ng TP, Niti M, Tan WC, et al. Depressive symptoms and chronic obstructive pulmonary disease: effect on mortality, hospital readmission, symptom burden, functional status, and quality of life. Arch Intern Med. 2007;167(1):6–7.
19. National Heart, Lung, and Blood Institute. Data fact sheet. Chronic obstructive pulmonary disease. Available at http://www.apsfa.org/docs/copd_fact.pdf. Accessed 6 June 2016.
20. Abrams TE, Sarrazin MV, VanderWeg MW. Acute exacerbations of chronic obstructive pulmonary disease and the effect of existing psychiatric comorbidity on subsequent mortality. Psychosomatics. 2011;52:441–9.
21. Usmani ZA, Carson KV, Heslop K, Esterman AJ, De Soyza A, Smith BJ. Psychological therapies for the treatment of anxiety disorders in chronic obstructive pulmonary disease. Cochrane Database Syst Rev. 2017;3:CD010673.
22. Shapiro PA. Psychiatric aspects of Heart disease (and cardiac aspects of psychiatric disease) in critical care. Crit Care Clin. 2017;33:619–34.
23. Fleet RP, Dupuis G, Marchand A, et al. Panic disorder in emergency department chest pain patients: prevalence, comorbidity, suicidal ideation, and physician recognition. Am J Med. 1996;101:371–801.
24. Frasure-Smith N, Lesperance F, Talajic M. Depression following MI: impact on 6 month survival. JAMA. 1993;270:1819–25.
25. Berkman LF, Blumenthal J, Burg M, et al. Enhancing recovery in coronary heart disease (ENRICHD). JAMA. 2003;289(23):3106–16.
26. Andrade C, Sandarsh S, Chethan KB, et al. Serotonin reuptake inhibitor antidepressants and abnormal bleeding: a review for clinicians and a reconsideration of mechanisms. J Clin Psychiatry. 2010;71(12):1565–75.
27. Craig TKJ. Abdominal pain. In: Brown GW, editor. Life events and illness. New York: Guilford; 1989. p. 233–59.
28. Guthrie E, Jackson J, Shaffer J, et al. Psychological disorder and severity of inflammatory bowel disease predict health related quality of life in ulcerative colitis and Crohn's disease. Am J Gastroenterol. 2002;97:1994–9.
29. Jackson JL, O'Malley PG, Tomkins G, et al. Treatment of functional GI disorders with antidepressant medications. Am J Med. 2000;108:65–72.
30. Poulin PA, Nelli J, Tremblay S, et al. Chronic pain in the emergency department: a pilot mixed-methods cross-sectional study examining patient characteristics and reasons for presentations. Pain Res Manag. 2016;2016:3092391.
31. Currie SR, Wang J. Chronic back pain and major depression in the general Canadian population. Pain. 2004;107(1–2):54–60.
32. Paulozzi LJ, Budnitz DS, Xi Y. Increasing deaths from opioid analgesics in the United States. Pharmacoepidemiol Drug Saf. 2006;15:618–27.
33. Volkow ND, McLellan TA, Cotto JH. Characteristics of opioid prescriptions in 2009. JAMA. 2011;305:1299–301.
34. Cantrill SV, Brown MD, Carlisle RJ, et al. American College of Emergency Physicians Opioid Guideline Writing Panel. Clinical policy: critical issues in the prescribing of opioids for adult patients in the emergency department. Ann Emerg Med. 2012;60(4):499–525.
35. Reifler LM, Droz D, Bailey JE, et al. Do prescription monitoring programs impact state trends in opioid abuse/misuse? Pain Med. 2012;13(3):434–42.

Medical Mimics of Psychiatric Illnesses

18

Samidha Tripathi, Rachel Littlefield, and Scott Sulik

Introduction

Acute psychosis can manifest in a variety of medical settings, from outpatient primary care clinics to emergency departments, urgent care, or even inpatient medical or surgical units. The presence of psychosis can create a diagnostic challenge for any physician, especially for patients who present with an apparent psychiatric symptom that might be masking an acute medical condition.

This chapter will discuss five life-threatening medical mimics of psychosis that may prove diagnostically challenging for physicians: catatonia, serotonin syndrome, neuroleptic malignant syndrome, psychiatric manifestations of seizure disorder, and anti-NMDA-receptor encephalitis.

S. Tripathi (✉)
Department of Psychiatry, University of Arkansas for Medical Sciences, Little Rock, AR, USA

R. Littlefield
Department of Emergency Medicine, University of Arkansas for Medical Sciences, Little Rock, AR, USA

S. Sulik
Department of Emergency Medicine, Ochsner Medical Center, Jefferson, LA, USA

Case Example

A 50-year-old male presented to the ER with acute mania. In the exam room, he was constantly moving in circles with a plastic spoon in hand and scraping the walls. He spoke rapidly and shuffled back and forth as he spoke. When greeted by his last name, Mr. Smith, he responded rather emphatically, "My name is Mr. Smith, Mr. Smith, Mr. Smith." His mood was elevated, and he had bizarre delusions about an alien invasion. Haloperidol was administered for agitation, but it did not yield much benefit. He consequently became tachycardic and hypertensive. Admission to medicine was sought, given an incidental finding of an acute kidney injury. A psychiatric consultant recommended lorazepam, and his excitement and autonomic instability resolved.

Catatonia

What Is It?

The concept of catatonia was formulated by Karl Ludwig Kahlbaum (1874). Although commonly thought to mean absence of movement, it is more precisely defined as a syndrome of motor dysregulation associated with disturbances in mood, cognition, affect, and thought [1]. As catatonic signs in other medical and psychiatric disorders

L. S. Zun et al. (eds.), *Behavioral Emergencies for Healthcare Providers*, https://doi.org/10.1007/978-3-030-52520-0_18

were discovered, the specificity of Kraepelin and Bleuler's perception of catatonia as a subtype of schizophrenia was challenged [2, 3].

As a result, catatonia is no longer linked under schizophrenia in the DSM-5, and can be invoked as a specifier in both major psychiatric and medical conditions. In addition, an "unspecified" category is also included until an underlying condition can be identified [4].

Deficits in the gamma-aminobutyric acid (or GABAergic) system in the dorsolateral prefrontal cortex, ventromedial prefrontal cortex, orbitofrontal cortex, and parietal lobe, in addition to dopamine hypoactivity and glutamate (NMDA) hyperactivity, are thought to play a role in the pathophysiology of catatonia. This results in a dysregulation in the motor loop or the cortico-subcortical circuits between the motor/premotor cortex and basal ganglia, leading to its variable features described below [5–8]. This concept helps clarify the benefits of lorazepam, ECT, amantadine, and memantine, and the deleterious effects of neuroleptics in the treatment of catatonic syndrome.

Surveys using standardized rating scales suggest that 7–15% of patients in an acute psychiatric hospital or psychiatric emergency room have signs consistent with catatonia. Unfortunately, catatonia is often underreported and underrecognized in a general hospital setting [9–11].

Are There Different Types?

Primary catatonia, or catatonia secondary to primary psychiatric or mood disorders, has a prevalence rate of 13–30% and appears commonly in bipolar disorder [12, 13]. Acute psychosis comprises 7–17% [13–15]. Medical or "organic" causes of catatonia make up 4–46% of cases, which are referred to as secondary catatonia (please see Table 18.1) [13–18]. Catatonic state has been recognized in limbic encephalitis, and the etiology for this is extensive [19–20]. Most notable is anti-NMDAR encephalitis, which is discussed in more detail later in this chapter.

Subtypes

There are four main subtypes of catatonia. Retarded catatonia, also known as Kahlbaum's syndrome, is the most widely recognized form of catatonia. It is marked by motoric immobility or psychomotor retardation, withdrawal features, rigidity, posturing, failure to respond to painful stimuli, mutism, and stupor in severe cases. Another variant is excited catatonia, which can mimic akathisia or mania. This is marked by excitement, increased motor activity, repetitious behavior, and frenzy [21–22]. Delirious mania, or Bell's mania, is closely related to catatonia and is characterized by rapid onset of delirium, mania, and psychosis that is not associated with prior psychiatric or systemic illness. Autonomic and catatonic signs are commonly present [23–24]. Proponents of excited delirium syndrome (please see chapter elsewhere in this book) have argued that this is the current manifestation of Bell's mania.

Lethal, pernicious, or malignant catatonia is a true medical emergency and is accompanied by increased morbidity and mortality. Hallmarks are fever, autonomic instability, and rigidity, which occur in conjunction with other catatonic signs [14, 25]. Neuroleptic malignant syndrome (NMS) and serotonin syndrome (SS) are considered forms of secondary malignant catatonia with high mortality and are discussed later in this chapter [26–30].

How Is It Recognized?

The core features of malignant catatonia include stupor, mutism, negativism, rigidity, posturing, catalepsy (a medical condition that is marked by seizure), waxy flexibility, withdrawal (refusal to eat or drink), repetitive movements or speech (stereotypy, mannerisms, and verbigeration), and echo-like behavior (echolalia and echopraxia) (Please see Table 18.2).

The Bush–Francis Catatonia Rating Scale (BFCRS) is a 23-item standardized rating scale that is widely used both clinically and in research

Table 18.1 Etiologies of catatonia by category

Category	Causes
Psychiatric	Mood disorders, acute psychosis and schizophrenia, conversion disorders, obsessive-compulsive disorders, postpartum/puerperal catatonia, post-traumatic stress disorder, pervasive developmental disorder (autistic spectrum)
Neurological	Brain stem, diencephalic and basal ganglia disorders, limbic and temporal lobe disorders, bilateral parietal infarcts, frontal lobe disorders, injuries, atrophy, tumors, generalized CNS disorders: Atrophy, Multiple Sclerosis; epilepsy, cortical venous thrombosis, subarachnoid hemorrhage, subdural hematoma, arteriovenous malformations, degenerative lesions: cerebellar and cerebromacular, paraneoplastic encephalopathy, hydrocephalus, tuberous sclerosis, systemic lupus erythematosus
Infectious	Acute and postencephalitic states, viral encephalitis: Herpes, Chicken Pox, tick-borne, rabies, acquired immunodeficiency syndrome, hydatid disease, postimmunization encephalopathy, subacute sclerosing panencephalitis, neurosyphilis, tuberculosis, progressive multifocal leukoencephalopathy
Metabolic and hereditary and endocrine	Tay-Sach's disease, Wilson's disease, Prader-Willie syndrome, hypercalcemia from parathyroid adenoma, homocystinuria, acute intermittent porphyria, hereditary coproporphyria, hepatic and renal failure, hyponatremia, membranous glomerulonephritis, hypo and hyperthyroidism, hyperparathyroidism, adrenal carcinoma
Nutritional deficiency	Pellagra, nicotinic acid deficiency, Wernicke's encephalopathy, vitamin B12 deficiency
Drug and Toxic agents	Drug intoxication and withdrawal syndromes: Alcohol, benzodiazepines, opiates, stimulants, hallucinogens Neuroleptic agents including atypical agents (clozapine, risperidone) Disulfiram Intoxication with: Aspirin, Lithium, NMDA antagonists, baclofen, steroids Anticonvulsants and gabapentin withdrawal Dopamine withdrawal (Levodopa) Antibiotics: ciprofloxacin Fluorinated hydrocarbons Coal gas CO poisoning
Miscellaneous disorders	Electrocution, burns, toxic epidermal necrolysis, thrombotic thrombocytopenic purpura, uremia, peripeural, autoimmune disorders

Adapted from Refs. [13, 15–18]

[31]. The first 14 items of this scale form the Bush–Francis Catatonia Screening Instrument (BFCSI). Item definitions of both scales are the same, and two or more signs identify catatonia.

Alternatively, the DSM-V requires three or more features from a similar list of 12 signs [4]. A series of changes have been made in the DSM-5 formulation of catatonia [32] and are discussed elsewhere in this book. Despite its broader definition, limitations of DSM-5 criteria include limited ability to recognize various subtypes and an inability to distinguish between benign and malignant forms of catatonia.

Immediate relief, or a positive response, characterized by at least 50% reduction in catatonic signs and symptoms measured by a standardized rating scale following administration of lorazepam 1–2 mg (also known as the "Lorazepam Challenge Test") is considered a verification of the diagnosis of catatonia [9–10].

Workup and Treatment

The differential diagnosis in catatonia is challenging, as the history and physical examination might be limited, due to mental status. Certain conditions may be comorbid with catatonia of any etiology. Elective mutism, stiff-person syndrome, akinetic mutism of Parkinson's disease,

Table 18.2 Features of catatonia

Symptoms	Description of pathology
Excitement	Hyperactivity, motor unrest which is nonpurposeful, cannot be attributed to akathisia or goal directed agitation
Mutism	Verbally unresponsive or minimally responsive, refusal to speak
Immobility/stupor	Decreased responsive to external stimuli, hypoactive behavior, immobile
Staring	Eyes fixed and open for long periods of time, decreased blinking, limited scanning of environment
Posturing	Purposely maintaining a posture for long periods of time
Catalepsy	Passive adoption of a posture
Grimacing	Maintenance of odd facial expressions
Echo phenomenon	Echolalia: senseless repetition of the words of other Echopraxia: mimicking the movements of other
Stereotypy	Repetitive, nongoal-directed motor activity (e.g., tapping finger), abnormality not inherent in act but in frequency
Mannerisms	Odd, purposeful movements (e.g., walking on tiptoes, etc.), abnormality inherent in the act itself
Verbigeration	Repetition of phrases or sentences (like a scratched record)
Rigidity	Maintenance of a rigid posture despite efforts to be moved
Negativism	Motiveless resistance to attempts to examine or commands, at times doing the exact opposite, e.g., gegenhalten, mitgehen
Waxy flexibility	Initial slight resistance to being moved before allowing self to be repositioned
Withdrawal	Refusal to eat, drink, or interact
Automatic obedience	Exaggerated cooperation with examiner's request or spontaneous continuation of movement requested
Ambitendency	Patient appears "stuck", indecisive, hesitant movement
Autonomic abnormalities	Temperature, blood pressure, pulse, respiratory rate, diaphoresis
Miscellaneous	Grasp reflex, perseveration (returning to same topic or movement), combativeness

Adapted from Refs. [4, 31]

locked-in-syndrome, noncatatonic stupor, encephalopathy, stroke, metabolic-induced stupor, severe obsessive-compulsive disorder, and malignant hyperthermia have remarkable similarity to catatonic syndromes [14, 33–34].

Once catatonia is recognized, a medical and toxicological workup should be performed to avoid the misattribution of psychosis to a psychiatric illness. In addition to routine studies, urine toxicology, creatine phosphokinase (CPK), workup for infectious disease, encephalitis, autoimmune screening, and neuroimaging should also be considered. Supportive measures such as frequent vital signs, intravenous hydration, enteral feeds, anticoagulant therapies, mobilization, and high level of nursing care can help reduce the risk of morbidity and mortality [34]. If the patient is in an outpatient setting, transfer to an emergency department or other emergent setting is appropriate.

Antipsychotics have been known to worsen symptoms and precipitate NMS, and antipsychotics are generally discouraged in patients presenting with catatonia [9, 35–36]. Benzodiazepines are considered first-line for management of primary and secondary catatonia [37–38]. Lorazepam 1–2 mg (with a lower dose for children and the elderly) is given every 3–8 hours, usually 30–60 minutes before meals. Dosages from 8 mg to 24 mg daily have been shown to be effective and well tolerated without sedation. If lorazepam is not available, diazepam and zolpidem have been reported as acceptable alternatives [39–43]. NMDA antagonists such as amantadine and memantine have also shown efficacy in the treatment of catatonic syndromes [44–49]. In treatment-refractory cases or cases of malignant catatonia, emergent treatment with ECT is indicated [38, 50].

Table 18.3 Complications of catatonia by organ system

Organ system	Complications
General	Dehydration and malnutrition due to poor oral intake, sepsis, disseminated intravascular coagulation
Dermatological	Skin breakdown and decubitus ulcers from immobility
Ophthalmological	Ocular surface irritation and pain, along with visual impairment as complication of prolonged staring and diminished blinking (xerophthalmia)
Musculoskeletal	Contractures due to catalepsy and posturing
Cardiovascular	Increased risk of deep vein thrombosis (DVT) and pulmonary embolism (PE) due to prolonged immobility, cardiac arrest
Respiratory	Respiratory failure, aspiration pneumonitis, laryngospasm
Gastrointestinal	Hypoglycemia, gastrointestinal bleeding, constipation, ileus
Renal	Acute renal failure and complications of rhabdomyolysis
Genitourinary	Urinary retention or incontinence, infections

Adapted from Refs. [13, 15, 51–58]

Disposition

Catatonia can lead to complications involving virtually every organ system (please see Table 18.3). If untreated, morbidity and mortality rates are extremely high, and admission for stabilization is therefore recommended [13, 15, 51–58]. The remission rate is considered to be high, approaching 70–80% [10, 59].

Serotonin Syndrome (SS)

What Is It?

Serotonin syndrome was formally described in 1982, is a condition that results from excess of serotonin in the central nervous system [29, 60]. Excessive serotonergic activity is most often medication-induced, either intentionally or unintentionally. Usually, SS involves combination treatments or interactions due to inhibition of cytochrome P450 enzymes, altering the hepatic breakdown of serotonergic agents [61].

There are countless central nervous system (CNS) serotonergic agents, including:

- Selective serotonin reuptake inhibitors (SSRIs)
- Serotonin-norepinephrine reuptake inhibitors (SNRIs)
- Monoamine oxidase inhibitors (MAOIs)
- Serotonin receptor (5-HT) agonists
- Antiparkinsonian agents
- Cough suppressants (dextromethorphan)
- Herbs (St. John's Wort)
- Narcotics (meperidine, tramadol, methadone)
- Triptans and ergotamine compounds
- Lithium
- Weight-loss agents (fenfluramine, sibutramine)
- Antiemetics
- Anticonvulsants
- Antibiotics (linezolid)
- Illicit substances like cocaine [62]

How Is It Recognized?

Clinical symptoms of SS exist on a spectrum and range from mild and self-limited to severe and potentially life-threatening. Symptoms can be arranged in four categories, as listed below [63–65].

1. Gastrointestinal (GI) symptoms: nausea, vomiting, diarrhea, incontinence, hyperactive bowel sounds
2. Autonomic instability: diaphoresis, shivering, sialorrhea, mydriasis, fever, tachycardia, tachypnea, and blood pressure lability
3. Neuromuscular symptoms: ataxia or incoordination, rigidity, myoclonus, ankle clonus, ocular clonus, and hyperreflexia, which is

usually most pronounced in the lower extremities
4. Mental status changes: range from mild disorientation, anxiety, and restlessness to confusion, agitation, and even coma.

Workup and Treatment

Diagnosis of serotonin syndrome is difficult, owing to the wide range and severity of symptoms. Several diagnostic criteria have been developed in order to assist clinicians. Sternbach described the first in 1991 [30]. Since that time, several studies have attempted to improve upon Sternbach's criteria, further characterizing serotonin syndrome on a scale of severity [62, 66–67]. The Hunter criteria, described in 2003, have been found to be simpler, more sensitive, and more specific than Sternbach's criteria [64]. According to these criteria, a patient can be diagnosed with SS if exposed to a serotonergic drug within the past 5 weeks and:

1. Spontaneous clonus or,
2. There is inducible clonus or ocular clonus with agitation or diaphoresis; or,
3. Presence of tremor and hyperreflexia; or,
4. Presence of hypertonicity, temperature greater than 38°C (100.4°F), and either ocular or inducible clonus.

Once identified, management of serotonin syndrome should begin with cessation of any inciting medications. Supportive therapy comprises the basis of treatment, with goals to address abnormal vital signs and control agitation and autonomic symptoms. Mild symptoms (tremor, hyperreflexia) typically resolve in 24 hours with observation and conservative management. More severe symptoms, including agitation and altered mental status, should be addressed with benzodiazepines, which can help reduce autonomic tone and hyperthermia. Severe hyperthermia should be managed with sedation, orotracheal intubation, and muscle paralysis, as significant elevations in temperature are largely attributed to increased muscle tone [29, 68].

Targeted pharmacotherapy with serotonin receptor antagonists remains a controversial option in serotonin syndrome management. Cyproheptadine (4–24 mg/day), a nonspecific antihistamine, has been effective at controlling symptoms in some cases, though improvement in patient outcomes has not been proven [69–70]. It is available in an oral preparation, which may be crushed and administered via nasogastric tube to intubated and sedated patients.

Neuroleptic Malignant Syndrome (NMS)

What Is It?

NMS was first named and described by Delay and Deniker in 1968 as a type of drug-induced extrapyramidal syndrome [115]. With an increasing understanding of its pathophysiology and recognized overlap with catatonia, it is now considered an iatrogenic form of malignant catatonia, mostly associated with use of neuroleptic agents [6, 71–74]. Dopamine depletion or blockade in the central nervous system appears to drive its characteristic manifestation [75–76].

How Is It Recognized?

Risk factors for development of NMS include the following:

1. Exposure to high-potency neuroleptics but atypical antipsychotics can also lead to NMS but with significantly less rigidity and elevation in CPK [77–80].
2. History of catatonia [81–83].
3. Abrupt cessation of dopaminergic agents [84].
4. Low levels of serum iron [85–87].
5. Basal ganglia disorders.
6. Nonneuroleptic agents with anti-dopaminergic activity like lithium, metoclopramide, phenelzine, clomipramine, tetrabenazine [88–92].

Signs and symptoms include autonomic instability (tachycardia, hypertension or hypotension, tachypnea, diaphoresis), thermodysregulation (hyperthermia ≥38°C), rigidity (usually "lead-pipe"), stupor, and altered mental status.

Workup and Treatment

NMS features can overlap at times with many other medical emergencies. Conditions in which hyperthermia and/or rigidity are prominent must be considered as a differential diagnosis for NMS and SS [93–99].

1. CNS infections and anatomic lesions affecting midbrain and brainstem: Presence of prodromal illness, localizing neurological signs, abnormal CSF, and neuroimaging.
2. Heatstroke: History of exposure to sun and high temperature, dry skin, muscle flaccidity.
3. Malignant hyperthermia: History of exposure to inhaled anesthetics or depolarizing muscle relaxants.
4. Central anticholinergic syndromes: History of exposure to anticholinergic agents, no rigidity, CPK levels normal, flushed dry skin and mucous membranes, mydriasis, and urinary retention.
5. Intoxication syndromes from cocaine, amphetamine (Ecstasy), and phencyclidine, along with withdrawal from alcohol, sedative hypnotics, and baclofen can also produce hyperthermia, autonomic instability, and altered mental status.
6. Considerable overlap between the NMS and SS, given fever and rigidity. Distinguishing findings in SS include tremor, ataxia, mydriasis, clonus (ocular, myoclonus), hyperreflexia, hyperactive bowel sounds, and diarrhea. Elevated CPK, leukocytosis, and myoglobinuria are uncommon in SS.

The workup should begin with a broad evaluation of electrolytes, urinalysis, creatine phosphokinase (CPK), an electrocardiogram, and initiation of IV hydration. Laboratory findings that may be characteristic for NMS include leukocytosis, elevated creatine phosphokinase (CPK) or myoglobinuria, and occasionally metabolic acidosis, but these are not specific [13, 27, 94].

Once NMS is identified, patients are generally admitted to the ICU, given the high lethality of this disease [100]. In addition to supportive measures, cessation of the offending agent is essential for recovery. Lorazepam is considered a first-line treatment, starting with 1–2 mg parenterally every 2–6 hours. If this fails, ECT has been known to be highly effective and improves recovery [38, 101–103]. Additionally, dopamine agonists, such as bromocriptine, amantadine, and levodopa, have shown to be effective by counteracting the neuroleptic dopaminergic inhibition. The recommended dose for bromocriptine is to start with 2.5 mg TID and increase to 2.5–7.5 mg per day, up to a maximum of 45 mg daily. Bromocriptine in high doses can exacerbate psychosis, lower blood pressure, and induce vomiting, leading to risk of aspiration pneumonitis. Amantadine is generally initiated at 200–400 mg/day in divided doses administered orally or through a nasogastric tube [104–107].

Dantrolene, a postsynaptic muscle relaxant that acts by inhibiting the release of calcium from the sarcoplasmic reticulum, helps control both muscle rigidity and hyperthermia. It is administered intravenously at a dose of 1–2.5 mg/kg body weight. If benefit is not apparent in 48 hours, an alternate treatment is warranted. Dantrolene is hepatotoxic in high doses and should be avoided in patients with liver disease [108–114].

Anti-NMDA Receptor Encephalitis

What Is It?

Encephalitis, or an inflammatory process involving the brain, is most commonly attributed to a viral infection. As many as 60% of cases have no identified source. Although no precise number exists, anti-N-methyl-D-aspartate receptor (NMDA-R) encephalitis, a recently characterized autoimmune cause, may be responsible for more cases of encephalitis than common viral agents, particularly in patients less than 30 years of age [115, 116].

First identified in 2005, anti-NMDA-R encephalitis was predominantly considered a paraneoplastic syndrome, found in previously healthy young females with an associated ovarian teratoma. Since the first report, however, the disease has since been observed in both males and females of varying ages without associated neoplasm. The disease process involves autoantibodies that bind to the NMDA receptor in the brain. Internalization of the complex ensues, leading to decreased expression of the receptor. Decreased NMDA receptor function has been attributed to some of the physical manifestations of the disease [117–119].

How Is It Recognized?

The clinical presentation of NMDA-R encephalitis is highly variable. Classically, patients experience a pattern involving two stages of illness, often preceded by a nonspecific viral syndrome that may last around 5 days, but no more than 2 weeks, prior to the start of behavioral symptoms. Viral prodrome symptoms typically include lethargy, headache, upper respiratory symptoms, nausea, diarrhea, myalgias, and fever. The first stage of behavioral symptoms consists of primarily psychiatric, including paranoia, hallucinations, and agitation. Isolated psychosis is rare, but, if present, may be falsely attributed to a primary psychiatric disorder. The disease then typically progresses to a second stage that includes catatonia, unresponsiveness, and autonomic instability. Seizures may occur and are more closely associated with anti-NMDA-R encephalitis than other causes. Hypoventilation is not uncommon and may require intubation and assisted ventilation [120–123].

Workup and Treatment

Initial evaluation is often limited by the patient's presentation, making definitive diagnosis difficult. Workup should include ruling out infectious or drug-induced causes of psychosis. Imaging studies, including CT and MRI, are of limited utility, as a majority will be normal. When present, significant MRI findings include T2 hyperintensity in the cerebral and cerebellar cortex, hippocampus, frontobasal, or insular regions. MRI findings are often transient in nature. Electroencephalography is often abnormal but usually reveals nonspecific, generalized slowing. Definitive diagnosis requires cerebrospinal fluid analysis with an immunoassay, as antibodies to the NMDA-R are present in most patients. A lymphocytic pleocytosis in the CSF is more common early in the disease course, but may normalize over time [118, 124–125].

Management of anti-NMDA-R encephalitis generally involves treatment with steroids, along with IVIG or plasma exchange. Resection of an associated tumor has been associated with improved outcome when combined with immune therapy. Second-line agents include rituximab and cyclophosphamide, and are typically reserved for patients with insufficient response, worsening of condition, or subsequent episodes. There is little evidence regarding the effective treatment of psychiatric symptoms. Both first-generation and second-generation antipsychotics have been utilized for agitation and aggression, but they pose a theoretical risk of worsening dystonia and movement disorders. Benzodiazepines, clonidine, and trazodone have been shown to improve abnormalities in sleep–wake cycle. Catatonia may be treated with scheduled benzodiazepines, while electroconvulsive therapy is reserved for resistant cases [125–127].

Epilepsy

What Is It?

Epilepsy is a chronic condition characterized by the recurrence of seizures that are typically unprovoked and unpredictable [128]. An epileptic seizure is due to an abnormal paroxysmal discharge of cerebral neurons, causing clinically detectable (via EEG) and observable events. Seizures may be partial (electrical activity abnormality in one area of the brain) or generalized (abnormal electrical activity occurring throughout the cortex) [129].

Some estimated 20–30% of patients with epilepsy also have psychiatric disorders, but these are often underrecognized or untreated [130, 131]. Depression is the most common psychiatric comorbidity associated with epilepsy [132]. Patients with depression are at higher risk of developing epilepsy than the general population, possibly due to abnormal CNS activity of multiple neurotransmitters, structural changes, and/or functional abnormalities [133]. Along with depression, suicide has a known increased risk with epilepsy. In fact, the average risk of suicide in epileptic patients is about 13% (vs. 1.4% for the general population) [131]. This is especially of concern with temporal lobe epilepsy, described below, where risk of suicide can be as high as 25 times greater than the general population [134]. Bipolar disorder, schizophrenia, ADHD, and personality disorders also have higher incidence in the epileptic population compared to the general population.

What Are the Types and Features?

There are several classifications of seizures, as well as types of psychoses thought to be secondary to seizure activity. A breakdown of the main seizure types is summarized in Table 18.4 [128, 129, 135].

Status epilepticus is described as a single seizure lasting at least 5 minutes, or two or more seizures without return to baseline consciousness between seizures. As the seizure passes 5 minutes of duration, the seizure threshold is lowered, neuronal damage occurs, and patients are less likely to be controlled with antiepileptic drugs. In nonconvulsive status epilepticus, no obvious seizure activity is present, but the patient is generally altered or comatose, and may have subtle motor symptoms such as twitching, blinking, and eye deviation [135].

It can be difficult to distinguish seizure behavior from acute psychosis. Typically, complex partial seizures (CPS) are associated with sudden onset and offset symptoms that typically last less than 3 minutes and have olfactory, gustatory, and tactile hallucinations that generally occur with automatisms. Alternatively, psychosis is gradual in onset, has longer length of symptoms (from 20 minutes up to weeks), and is more commonly associated with auditory hallucinations occurring without automatisms. Consciousness and recall are commonly altered in CPS; they are generally intact with psychosis [129]. Of patients with intractable CPS, 70% may have one or more concurrent psychiatric diagnoses—about 58% with depression, 32% with agoraphobia without panic or other anxiety disorder, and 13% with psychoses [134].

Ictal psychosis refers to psychosis that occurs in association with ictal discharges on EEG and

Table 18.4 Main categories of epileptic seizures

Type	Seizure activity
Generalized seizures	
Tonic clonic (grand mal)	Unconscious, rigid trunk and extremities, rhythmic jerking generally lasting 60–90 seconds; postictal period of confusion and fatigue may last several hours or longer
Absence (petit mal)	Staring spell with lapse in awareness, maintains posture
Myoclonic	Brief, sudden muscle contractions; unilateral or bilateral; occurring singly or repeatedly
Atonic	Sudden loss of muscle tone; localized or generalized
Partial seizures	
Simple	Consciousness not affected; sometimes considered "auras," progressing to generalized seizure
Complex	Focal, affect mentation; commonly "temporal lobe seizures"; can involve lip smacking, picking, repeating short phrases, hallucinations, déjà vu, fear, anxiety, paranoia, and depression
Intractable seizures	
Status epilepticus	

is described as psychosis caused by combination of cognitive, affective, and hallucinatory symptoms of partial epilepsy. Prolonged ictal psychosis is rare and may occur as a nonconvulsive status epilepticus with simple or complex partial or absence seizures [135].

Postictal psychosis (PIP) occurs in up to 7.8% of epileptics and is characterized by hallucinations, delusions, and/or gross behavior or affect abnormalities occurring up to 7 days after a seizure. Diagnostic criteria include episode of psychosis within 1 week after seizure; psychosis lasting greater than 15 hours but less than 3 months; delusions, hallucinations in clear consciousness, bizarre or disorganized behavior, formal thought disorder, or affective changes; and no evidence of AED toxicity, nonconvulsive status epilepticus, recent head trauma, alcohol or drug intoxication or withdrawal, or prior chronic psychotic disorder. Mood abnormalities predominate and include depressed affect, manic symptoms, irritable and aggressive behavior, and hallucinations. Voice commenting, thought insertion, and negative symptoms are not common in PIP. One unique characteristic of PIP is the lucid interval that commonly occurs 2.5–48 hours following return to baseline from last seizure and the onset of psychosis [135].

Interictal psychosis (or chronic inter-ictal psychosis (CIP)) is often caused by a long history of uncontrolled seizures that, in more than 5% of patients, can lead to a chronic psychotic state. It is characterized by insidious onset of paranoid delusions and hallucinations. Persecutory auditory hallucinations are common, and religiosity can occur. Thought disorder is uncommon. While positive symptoms such as delusions and hallucinations predominate, negative symptoms (such as isolation, decreased socialization, and affective blunting) also seem to have higher incidence in patients with temporal lobe epilepsy [135].

Workup and Treatment

Diagnosing seizures relies heavily on the history obtained. Abrupt onset, lack of recall, and a postictal phase are important features in determining seizure vs. nonseizure attack [135]. If seizures are suspected, first-line treatment with a benzodiazepine such as lorazepam is appropriate. Treatment of psychosis in epilepsy generally requires multidisciplinary treatment, including separate treatment of both epilepsy with AEDs and psychosis with antipsychotics [135]. Early recognition and initiation of therapy are imperative, as these can affect long-term quality of life and treatment compliance [131].

Conclusion

Medical mimics of psychiatric disorders form a fascinating mix of disorders spreading from behavioral-motoric syndrome to autoimmune disorders. Maintaining a broad differential outside of primary psychiatric diagnoses is essential to identify these potentially life-threatening illnesses. Physicians in all settings are encountering these cases and should be trained to identify and appropriately treat or refer these syndromes.

References

1. Kahlbaum KL. Catatonia. Johns Hopkins: Baltimore. 1974. Psychol Med. 1975;5(03):319.
2. Kraepelin E. Dementia praecox and paraphrenia. J Nerv Ment Dis. 1921;54(4):384.
3. Tillman C. Dementia Praecox or the Group of Schizophrenias. Eugen Bleuler; translated by Joseph Zinkin. New York: International Universities Press. 1950. Science. 1951;113(2935):368.
4. American Psychiatric Association. Diagnostic and Statistical Manual of Mental Disorders (DSM-5®): American Psychiatric Pub; 2013.
5. Northoff G. What catatonia can tell us about "top-down modulation": a neuropsychiatric hypothesis. Behav Brain Sci. 2002;25(05) Available at https://doi.org/10.1017/s0140525x02000109.
6. Northoff G. Catatonia and neuroleptic malignant syndrome: psychopathology and pathophysiology. J Neural Transm. 2002;109(12):1453–67.
7. Northoff G, Kotter R, Baumgart F, Danos P, Bauker H, Kaulisch T et al. Orbitofrontal Cortical Dysfunction in Akinetic Catatonia: A Functional Magnetic Resonance Imaging Study during Negative Emotional Stimulation. Schizophr Bull. 2004;30(2):405–27.
8. Fink M, Taylor MA. Catatonia: a clinician's guide to diagnosis and treatment: Cambridge University Press; 2003.

9. Rosebush PI, Hildebrand AM, Furlong BG, Mazurek MF. Catatonic syndrome in a general psychiatric inpatient population: frequency, clinical presentation, and response to lorazepam. J Clin Psychiatry. 1990;51(9):357–62.
10. Fink M, Taylor MA. The catatonia syndrome: forgotten but not gone. Arch Gen Psychiatry. 2009;66(11):1173–7.
11. Bräunig P, Krüger S, Shugar G. Prevalence and clinical significance of catatonic symptoms in mania. Compr Psychiatry. 1998;39(1):35–46.
12. Levenson JL. The American Psychiatric Publishing Textbook of Psychosomatic Medicine: Psychiatric Care of the Medically Ill: American Psychiatric Pub; 2011.
13. Taylor MA, Fink M. Catatonia in psychiatric classification: a home of its own. Am J Psychiatry. 2003;160(7):1233–41.
14. Caroff SN. Catatonia: from psychopathology to neurobiology: American Psychiatric Pub; 2004.
15. Stern TA. Massachusetts General Hospital Handbook of General Hospital Psychiatry: Elsevier Health Sciences; 2010.
16. Ahuja N. Organic catatonia: a review. Indian J Psychiatry. 2000;42(4):327–46.
17. Gelenberg AJ. The catatonic syndrome. Lancet. 1976;1(7973):1339–41.
18. Kruse JL, Lapid MI, Lennon VA, Klein CJ, Toole OO, Pittock SJ, et al. Psychiatric autoimmunity: N-methyl-D-aspartate receptor IgG and beyond. Psychosomatics. 2015;56(3):227–41.
19. Oldham M. Autoimmune encephalopathy for psychiatrists: when to suspect autoimmunity and what to do next. Psychosomatics. 2017;58(3):228–44.
20. Morrison JR. Catatonia. Retarded and excited types. Arch Gen Psychiatry. 1973;28(1):39–41.
21. Fink M, Taylor MA. The many varieties of catatonia. Eur Arch Psychiatry Clin Neurosci. 2001;251(S1):I8–13.
22. Fink M. Delirious mania. Bipolar Disord. 1999;1(1):54–60.
23. Bond TC. Recognition of acute delirious mania. Arch Gen Psychiatry. 1980;37(5):553.
24. Mann SC, Caroff SN, Bleier HR, Welz WK, Kling MA, Hayashida M. Lethal catatonia. Am J Psychiatry. 1986;143(11):1374–81.
25. Fricchione G, Mann SC, Caroff SN. Catatonia, lethal catatonia, and neuroleptic malignant syndrome. Psychiatr Ann. 2000;30(5):347–55.
26. Mann SC, Caroff SN, Ungvari GS, Cabrina Campbell E. Catatonia, malignant catatonia, and neuroleptic malignant syndrome. Curr Psychiatr Rev. 2013;9(2):111–9.
27. Strawn JR, Keck PE, Caroff SN. Neuroleptic malignant syndrome. Am J Psychiatry. 2007;164(6):870–6.
28. Boyer EW, Shannon M. The serotonin syndrome. N Engl J Med. 2005;352(11):1112–20.
29. Sternbach H. The serotonin syndrome. Am J Psychiatry. 1991;148(6):705–13.
30. Bush G, Fink M, Petrides G, Dowling F, Francis A. Catatonia. I. Rating scale and standardized examination. Acta Psychiatr Scand. 1996;93(2):129–36.
31. Tandon R, Heckers S, Bustillo J, Barch DM, Gaebel W, Gur RE, et al. Catatonia in DSM-5. Schizophr Res. 2013;150(1):26–30.
32. Stoudemire A. The differential diagnosis of catatonic states. Psychosomatics. 1982;23(3):245–52.
33. Clinebell K, Azzam PN, Gopalan P, Haskett R. Guidelines for preventing common medical complications of catatonia: case report and literature review. J Clin Psychiatry. 2014;75(6):644–51.
34. Gelenberg AJ. Catatonic reactions to high-potency neuroleptic drugs. Arch Gen Psychiatry. 1977;34(8):947.
35. Lee JWY. Neuroleptic-induced catatonia: clinical presentation, response to benzodiazepines, and relationship to neuroleptic malignant syndrome. J Clin Psychopharmacol. 2010;30(1):3–10.
36. Ungvari GS, Kau LS, Wai-Kwong T, Shing NF. The pharmacological treatment of catatonia: an overview. Eur Arch Psychiatry Clin Neurosci. 2001;251 Suppl 1:I31–4.
37. Bush G, Fink M, Petrides G, Dowling F, Francis A. Catatonia. II. Treatment with lorazepam and electroconvulsive therapy. Acta Psychiatr Scand. 1996;93(2):137–43.
38. Mastain B, Vaiva G, Guerouaou D, Pommery J, Thomas P. Favourable effect of zolpidem on catatonia. Rev Neurol. 1995;151(1):52–6.
39. Peglow S, Prem V, McDaniel W. Treatment of catatonia with zolpidem. J Neuropsychiatry Clin Neurosci. 2013;25(3):E13.
40. Thomas P, Rascle C, Mastain B, Maron M, Vaiva G. Test for catatonia with zolpidem. Lancet. 1997;349(9053):702.
41. Huang YC, Lin CC, Hung YY, Huang TL. Rapid relief of catatonia in mood disorder by lorazepam and diazepam. Biom J. 2013;36(1):35–9.
42. Huang TL. Lorazepam and diazepam rapidly relieve catatonic signs in patients with schizophrenia. Psychiatry Clin Neurosci. 2005;59(1):52–5.
43. Thomas C. Memantine and catatonic schizophrenia. Am J Psychiatry. 2005;162(3):626.
44. Carroll BT, Goforth HW, Thomas C, Ahuja N, McDaniel WW, Kraus MF, et al. Review of adjunctive glutamate antagonist therapy in the treatment of catatonic syndromes. J Neuropsychiatry Clin Neurosci. 2007;19(4):406–12.
45. Ellul P, Rotgé JY, Choucha W. Resistant catatonia in a high-functioning autism spectrum disorder patient successfully treated with amantadine. J Child Adolesc Psychopharmacol. 2015;25(9):726.
46. Hervey WM, Stewart JT, Catalano G. Treatment of catatonia with amantadine. Clin Neuropharmacol. 2012;35(2):86–7.
47. Obregon DF, Velasco RM, Wuerz TP, Catalano MC, Catalano G, Kahn D. Memantine and catatonia: a case report and literature review. J Psychiatr Pract. 2011;17(4):292–9.

48. Roy K, Warnick SJ, Balon R. Catatonia delirium: 3 cases treated with memantine. Psychosomatics. 2016;57(6):645–50.
49. Mann SC, Caroff SN, Bleier HR, Antelo RE, Un H. Electroconvulsive therapy of the lethal catatonia syndrome. Convuls Ther. 1990;6(3):239–47.
50. Carroll BT. Complications of catatonia. J Clin Psychiatry. 1996;57(2):95.
51. Lachner C, Sandson NB. Medical complications of catatonia: a case of catatonia-induced deep venous thrombosis. Psychosomatics. 2003;44(6):512–4.
52. Woo BKP. Basal ganglia calcification and pulmonary embolism in catatonia. J Neuropsychiatr. 2007;19(4):472–3.
53. Kaufmann RM, Schreinzer D, Strnad A, Mossaheb N, Kasper S, Frey R. Case report: intestinal atonia as an unusual symptom of malignant catatonia responsive to electroconvulsive therapy. Schizophr Res. 2006;84(1):178–9.
54. Swartz C, Galang RL. Adverse outcome with delay in identification of catatonia in elderly patients. Am J Geriatr Psychiatry. 2001;9(1):78–80.
55. Marik PE. Aspiration pneumonitis and aspiration pneumonia. N Engl J Med. 2001;344(9):665–71.
56. Bort RF. Catatonia, gastric hyperacidity, and fatal aspiration: a preventable syndrome. Am J Psychiatry. 1976;133(4):446–7.
57. Boyarsky BK, Fuller M, Early T. Malignant catatonia-induced respiratory failure with response to ECT. J ECT. 1999;15(3):232–6.
58. Lee JW, Schwartz DL, Hallmayer J. Catatonia in a psychiatric intensive care facility: incidence and response to benzodiazepines. Ann Clin Psychiatry. 2000;12(2):89–96.
59. Oates JA, Sjoerdsma A. Neurologic effects of tryptophan in patients receiving a monoamine oxidase inhibitor. Neurology. 1960;10(12):1076.
60. Mitchell PB. Drug interactions of clinical significance with selective serotonin reuptake inhibitors. Drug Saf. 1997;17(6):390–406.
61. Keck PE, Arnold LM. The serotonin syndrome. Psychiatr Ann. 2000;30(5):333–43.
62. Bodner RA, Lynch T, Lewis L, Kahn D. Serotonin syndrome. Neurology. 1995;45(2):219–23.
63. Dunkley EJC, Isbister GK, Sibbritt D, Dawson AH, Whyte IM. The hunter serotonin toxicity criteria: simple and accurate diagnostic decision rules for serotonin toxicity. QJM. 2003;96(9):635–42.
64. Cooper BE, Sejnowski CA. Serotonin syndrome. AACN Adv Crit Care. 2013;24(1):15–20.
65. Hegerl U, Bottlender R, Gallinat J, Kuss HJ, Ackenheil M, Möller HJ. The serotonin syndrome scale: first results on validity. Eur Arch Psychiatry Clin Neurosci. 1998;248(2):96–103.
66. Radomski JW, Dursun SM, Reveley MA, Kutcher SP. An exploratory approach to the serotonin syndrome: an update of clinical phenomenology and revised diagnostic criteria. Med Hypotheses. 2000;55(3):218–24.
67. Gillman PK. The serotonin syndrome and its treatment. J Psychopharmacol. 1999;13(1):100–9.
68. Graudins A, Stearman A, Chan B. Treatment of the serotonin syndrome with cyproheptadine. J Emerg Med. 1998;16(4):615–9.
69. McDaniel WW. Serotonin syndrome: early management with cyproheptadine. Ann Pharmacother. 2001;35(7–8):870–3.
70. Fricchione GL. Neuroleptic catatonia and its relationship to psychogenic catatonia. Biol Psychiatry. 1985;20(3):304–13.
71. Fink M. Neuroleptic malignant syndrome and catatonia: one entity or two? Biol Psychiatry. 1996;39(1):1–4.
72. Fink M, Taylor MA. Neuroleptic malignant syndrome is malignant catatonia, warranting treatments efficacious for catatonia. Prog Neuro-Psychopharmacol Biol Psychiatry. 2006;30(6):1182–3.
73. Caroff SN, Mann SC, Campbell EC. Neuroleptic malignant syndrome and the catatonic dilemma. Psychopharmacology. 2015;232(3):661–2.
74. Mann SC, Caroff SN, Lazarus A. Pathogenesis of neuroleptic malignant syndrome. Psychiatr Ann. 1991;21(3):175–80.
75. Mann SC, Caroff SN, Fricchione G, Cabrina Campbell E. Central dopamine hypoactivity and the pathogenesis of neuroleptic malignant syndrome. Psychiatr Ann. 2000;30(5):363–74.
76. Caroff SN. Neuroleptic malignant syndrome. Arch Gen Psychiatry. 1987;44(9):838.
77. Levenson JL. Neuroleptic malignant syndrome after the initiation of olanzapine. J Clin Psychopharmacol. 1999;19(5):477–8.
78. Strawn J. Neuroleptic malignant syndrome. Am J Psychiatry. 2007;164(6):870.
79. Tseng PT, Chang YC, Chang CH, Wang HY, Cheng YS, Wu CK, et al. Atypical neuroleptic malignant syndrome in patients treated with aripiprazole and clozapine: a case-series study and short review. Int J Psychiatry Med. 2015;49(1):35–43.
80. White DA, Robins AH. Catatonia: harbinger of the neuroleptic malignant syndrome. Br J Psychiatry. 1991;158(3):419–21.
81. Carroll BT, Lee JWY. Catatonia is a risk factor for neuroleptic malignant syndrome. J Clin Psychiatry. 2004;65(12):1722–3.
82. Paparrigopoulos T, Tzavellas E, Ferentinos P, Mourikis I, Liappas J. Catatonia as a risk factor for the development of neuroleptic malignant syndrome: report of a case following treatment with clozapine. World J Biol Psychiatry. 2009;10(1):70–3.
83. Frucht SJ. Movement disorder emergencies: diagnosis and treatment: Springer Science & Business Media; 2012.

84. Rosebush PI, Mazurek MF. Serum iron and neuroleptic malignant syndrome. Lancet. 1991;338(8760):149–51.
85. Carroll BT, Goforth HW. Serum iron in catatonia. Biol Psychiatry. 1995;38(11):776–7.
86. Lee JWY. Serum iron in catatonia and neuroleptic malignant syndrome. Biol Psychiatry. 1998;44(6):499–507.
87. Fava S, Galizia AC. Neuroleptic malignant syndrome and lithium carbonate. J Psychiatry Neurosci. 1995;20(4):305–6.
88. Gill J, Singh H, Nugent K. Acute lithium intoxication and neuroleptic malignant syndrome. Pharmacotherapy. 2003;23(6):811–5.
89. Abbar M, Carlander B, Castelnau D. Tricyclics and malignant syndrome. Eur Psychiatry. 1996;11(4):212–3.
90. Isbister GK, Buckley NA. Clomipramine and neuroleptic malignant syndrome: literature on adverse reactions to psychotropic drugs continues to confuse. BMJ. 2005;330(7494):790–1; author reply 791.
91. Heyland D, Sauvé M. Neuroleptic malignant syndrome without the use of neuroleptics. CMAJ. 1991;145(7):817–9.
92. Lazarus A. Differentiating neuroleptic-related heatstroke from neuroleptic malignant syndrome. Psychosomatics. 1989;30(4):454–6.
93. Caroff SN, Mann SC, Lazarus A, Sullivan K, MacFadden W. Neuroleptic malignant syndrome: diagnostic issues. Psychiatr Ann. 1991;21(3):130–47.
94. Turner MR, Gainsborough N. Neuroleptic malignant-like syndrome after abrupt withdrawal of baclofen. J Psychopharmacol. 2001;15(1):61–3.
95. Kaufman KR, Levitt MJ, Schiltz JF, Sunderram J. Neuroleptic malignant syndrome and serotonin syndrome in the critical care setting: case analysis. Ann Clin Psychiatry. 2006;18(3):201–4.
96. Lee JWY. Catatonic variants, hyperthermic extrapyramidal reactions, and subtypes of neuroleptic malignant syndrome. Ann Clin Psychiatry. 2007;19(1):9–16.
97. Perry PJ, Wilborn CA. Serotonin syndrome vs. neuroleptic malignant syndrome: a contrast of causes, diagnoses, and management. Ann Clin Psychiatry. 2012;24(2):155–62.
98. Paden MS, Franjic L, Halcomb SE. Hyperthermia caused by drug interactions and adverse reactions. Emerg Med Clin North Am. 2013;31(4):1035–44.
99. Shalev A, Hermesh H, Munitz H. Mortality from neuroleptic malignant syndrome. J Clin Psychiatry. 1989;50(1):18–25.
100. Jessee SS, Anderson GF. ECT in the neuroleptic malignant syndrome: case report. J Clin Psychiatry. 1983;44(5):186–8.
101. Trollor JN, Sachdev PS. Electroconvulsive treatment of neuroleptic malignant syndrome: a review and report of cases. Aust N Z J Psychiatry. 1999;33(5):650–9.
102. Davis JM, Caroff SN, Mann SC. Treatment of neuroleptic malignant syndrome. Psychiatr Ann. 2000;30(5):325–31.
103. Henderson VW, Wooten GF. Neuroleptic malignant syndrome: a pathogenetic role for dopamine receptor blockade? Neurology. 1981;31(2):132–7.
104. McCarron MM, Boettger ML, Peck JJ. A case of neuroleptic malignant syndrome successfully treated with amantadine. J Clin Psychiatry. 1982;43(9):381–2.
105. Rosebush PI, Mazurek MF. Bromocriptine and neuroleptic malignant syndrome. J Clin Psychiatry. 1991;52(1):41–2.
106. Nisijima K, Noguti M, Ishiguro T. Intravenous injection of levodopa is more effective than dantrolene as therapy for neuroleptic malignant syndrome. Biol Psychiatry. 1997;41(8):913–4.
107. Coons DJ, Hillman FJ, Marshall RW. Treatment of neuroleptic malignant syndrome with dantrolene sodium: a case report. Am J Psychiatry. 1982;139(7):944–5.
108. Martin ML, Lucid EJ, Walker RW. Neuroleptic malignant syndrome. Ann Emerg Med. 1985;14(4):354–8.
109. Sakkas P, Davis JM, Janicak PG, Wang ZY. Drug treatment of the neuroleptic malignant syndrome. Psychopharmacol Bull. 1991;27(3):381–4.
110. Rosenberg MR, Green M. Neuroleptic Malignant Syndrome. Review of response to therapy. Arch Intern Med. 1989;149(9):1927–31.
111. Stemp LI. Management of lethal catatonia with dantrolene sodium. Crit Care Med. 1993;21(9):1403.
112. Tsutsumi Y, Yamamoto K, Matsuura S, Hata S, Sakai M, Shirakura K. The treatment of neuroleptic malignant syndrome using dantrolene sodium. Psychiatry Clin Neurosci. 1998;52(4):433–8.
113. Vora NM, Holman RC, Mehal JM, Steiner CA, Blanton J, Sejvar J. Burden of encephalitis-associated hospitalizations in the United States, 1998–2010. Neurology. 2014;82(5):443–51.
114. Gable MS, Sheriff H, Dalmau J, Tilley DH, Glaser CA. The frequency of autoimmune N-methyl-D-aspartate receptor encephalitis surpasses that of individual viral etiologies in young individuals enrolled in the California Encephalitis Project. Clin Infect Dis. 2012;54(7):899–904.
115. Dalmau J, Tüzün E, Wu H-Y, Masjuan J, Rossi JE, Voloschin A, et al. Paraneoplastic anti-N-methyl-D-aspartate receptor encephalitis associated with ovarian teratoma. Ann Neurol. 2007;61(1):25–36.
116. Irani SR, Bera K, Waters P, Zuliani L, Maxwell S, Zandi MS, et al. N-methyl-D-aspartate antibody encephalitis: temporal progression of clinical and paraclinical observations in a predominantly non-paraneoplastic disorder of both sexes. Brain. 2010;133(Pt 6):1655–67.

117. Hughes EG, Peng X, Gleichman AJ, Lai M, Zhou L, Tsou R, et al. Cellular and synaptic mechanisms of anti-NMDA receptor encephalitis. J Neurosci. 2010;30(17):5866–75.
118. Kayser MS, Dalmau J. Anti-NMDA receptor encephalitis in psychiatry. Curr Psychiatr Rev. 2011;7(3):189–93.
119. Kayser MS, Titulaer MJ, Gresa-Arribas N, Dalmau J. Frequency and characteristics of isolated psychiatric episodes in anti–N-methyl-d-aspartate receptor encephalitis. JAMA Neurol. 2013;70(9):1133–9.
120. Granerod J, Ambrose HE, Davies NW, Clewley JP, Walsh AL, Morgan D, et al. Causes of encephalitis and differences in their clinical presentations in England: a multicentre, population-based prospective study. Lancet Infect Dis. 2010;10(12):835–44.
121. Mann AP, Grebenciucova E, Lukas RV. Anti-N-methyl-D-aspartate-receptor encephalitis: diagnosis, optimal management, and challenges. Ther Clin Risk Manag. 2014;10:517–25.
122. Titulaer MJ, McCracken L, Gabilondo I, Armangué T, Glaser C, Iizuka T, et al. Treatment and prognostic factors for long-term outcome in patients with anti-NMDA receptor encephalitis: an observational cohort study. Lancet Neurol. 2013;12(2):157–65.
123. Dalmau J, Lancaster E, Martinez-Hernandez E, Rosenfeld MR, Balice-Gordon R. Clinical experience and laboratory investigations in patients with anti-NMDAR encephalitis. Lancet Neurol. 2011;10(1):63–74.
124. Mann A, Machado NM, Liu N, Mazin A-H, Silver K, Afzal KI. A multidisciplinary approach to the treatment of anti-NMDA-receptor antibody encephalitis: a case and review of the literature. J Neuropsychiatry Clin Neurosci. 2012;24(2):247–54.
125. Chapman MR, Vause HE. Anti-NMDA receptor encephalitis: diagnosis, psychiatric presentation, and treatment. Am J Psychiatry. 2011;168(3):245–51.
126. Louis ED, Mayer SA, Rowland LP. Merritt's neurology: Lippincott Williams & Wilkins; 2015.
127. Stern TA, Fricchione GL, Rosenbaum JF. Massachusetts General Hospital Handbook of General Hospital Psychiatry: Elsevier Health Sciences; 2010.
128. Vuilleumier P, Jallon P. Epilepsy and psychiatric disorders: epidemiological data. Rev Neurol. 1998;154(4):305–17.
129. Psychiatric Disorders Associated With Epilepsy: Overview, Psychotic Disorders, Bipolar Affective Disorders. Cited 2017 Sep. 9. Available at http://emedicine.medscape.com/article/1186336-overview#a11.
130. Kanner AM. Depression and epilepsy: a new perspective on two closely related disorders. Epilepsy Curr. 2006;6(5):141–6.
131. Kanner AM. Depression in epilepsy: a neurobiologic perspective. Epilepsy Curr. 2005;5(1):21–7.
132. Harris EC, Barraclough B. Suicide as an outcome for mental disorders: a meta-analysis. Br J Psychiatry. 1997;170:205–28.
133. Tintinalli J, Stapczynski J, John Ma O, Cline DM, Meckler G. Tintinalli's emergency medicine: a comprehensive study guide. 8th ed: McGraw Hill Professional; 2016.
134. Tucker GJ. Seizure disorders presenting with psychiatric symptomatology. Psychiatr Clin North Am. 1998;21(3):625–35, vi.
135. Nadkarni S, Arnedo V, Devinsky O. Psychosis in epilepsy patients. Epilepsia. 2007;48 Suppl 9:17–9.

Acute Care of Eating Disorders

19

Suzanne Dooley-Hash

Introduction

Eating disorders (EDs) are serious mental illnesses that are often associated with potentially life-threatening psychiatric comorbidities and medical complications. Eating disorders have one of the highest mortality rate of any mental illness [1]. About one-half to two-thirds of all deaths seen in individuals with EDs are due to suicide or cardiac causes, both of which are likely to initially present to an emergency department or other acute-care settings. Given that the majority of individuals with EDs do not readily self-disclose their illness to health-care providers, it is imperative that all providers be able to recognize the signs and symptoms of EDs and maintain a high index of suspicion for associated complications. The purpose of this chapter is to (1) give a brief overview of the EDs, (2) discuss recognition of EDs and commonly associated complications, (3) describe the management of EDs and their complications in the acute setting, and (4) provide suggestions for appropriate disposition and referral decisions.

S. Dooley-Hash (✉)
Department of Emergency Medicine, University of Michigan, Ann Arbor, MI, USA
e-mail: sldh@umich.edu

Impact of Eating Disorders

Eating disorders are among the most prevalent psychiatric conditions in adolescents and young adults, and are third only to obesity and asthma as the most common chronic illnesses in these age groups [2]. Experts estimate that as many as 14% of adolescents have some form of clinically significant ED [2, 3]. Increasing numbers of adults have been found to struggle with an ED, as well. Rates as high as 7–21% of EDs are found in screening studies in the general population, primary care settings, and emergency departments [1, 2, 4–7].

Individuals with EDs have also been found to have overall increased utilization of all health-care services, including emergency departments [8–10]. At least one study has shown that the average number of emergency department visits is increased in ED patients who eventually died from their illness when compared to controls [11]. This finding raises concerns that those who present to the emergency department for care may have increased severity of disease and increased risk of mortality.

Individuals with EDs are also at significantly increased risk of death when compared to their peers. Anorexia nervosa has an estimated lifetime mortality rate of 5–10%, making it the among the deadliest mental illnesses [1, 12–15]. As many as an estimated one-third to one-half of ED-related

L. S. Zun et al. (eds.), *Behavioral Emergencies for Healthcare Providers*,
https://doi.org/10.1007/978-3-030-52520-0_19

deaths are attributable to suicide [13, 14]. The standardized mortality rate (SMR) for suicide in a patient with anorexia nervosa (AN) is 32.4 vs. 27.8 for a major depressive disorder, 18.2 for alcohol abuse, and 8.0 for schizophrenia [1]. Eating disorders other than AN have similar overall mortality rates for all EDs [15–17], with suicide rates also increased in those with bulimia nervosa (BN) and possibly binge eating disorder (BED) [18]. Individuals with EDs also have increased rates of psychiatric comorbidities compared to the general population, which contributes to increased health-care utilization and risk of serious complications or death. The emergency department and other acute-care settings represent critical points of entry into the health-care system for many people and may be the only available access for some. Any health-related visit may also serve as an ideal "teachable moment," during which an individual is more receptive to information and intervention. The same visit may be the only opportunity for any health-care provider to recognize the ED and intervene on behalf of the patient. Therefore, it is imperative that all health-care providers be aware of the signs and symptoms that are consistent with EDs and be prepared to treat them appropriately.

Prevalence and Types of Eating Disorders

Although AN is often the first eating disorder many may think of, it is the least common ED diagnosis. Traditional estimates for lifetime prevalence of AN have consistently been around 0.5–1%, but recent studies suggest prevalence as high as 2.2% [19, 20]. Recent changes in diagnostic criteria found in the Diagnostic and Statistical Manual of Mental Disorders (DSM-V) that loosen the requirements for a diagnosis of AN may increase the number of people diagnosed with it. AN is characterized by restriction of energy intake, resulting in significantly low body weight, an intense fear of gaining weight or becoming fat, and undue influence of body weight or shape on self-evaluation. AN can be either of a purely restrictive type or a binge/purge type [21]. Amenorrhea was removed from the diagnostic criteria in the DSM-V. Patients with AN often deny the seriousness of their illness despite very low body weights [22].

Bulimia nervosa (BN) also involves self-evaluation that is unduly influenced by body shape and weight. BN is, however, characterized by recurrent episodes of binge eating that are accompanied by a sense of lack of control over eating during the episode, as well as repetitive inappropriate compensatory behavior (purging) to prevent weight gain. Compensatory methods include self-induced vomiting; misuse of laxatives, diuretics, enemas, or other medications; fasting; and excessive exercise. These behaviors occur, on average, at least once per week for 3 months [21]. Bodyweight in individuals with BN is usually average or even above normal. Lifetime prevalence estimates for BN are generally around 1–3% but may be as high as 4.6% [19, 23], also perhaps related to the reduction of the frequency of episodes needed to meet diagnostic criteria for BN in the DSM-V.

Binge eating disorder (BED), which was formerly not considered a distinct disorder, was defined in DSM-V. It is the most common ED [24]. A BED is characterized by recurrent episodes of binge eating without any compensatory behaviors. Feelings of loss of control when eating, shame or guilt about eating, and eating in secret are some of the other characteristics of the disorder [21]. Binge eating disorder is unique among EDs, in that approximately 40% of cases occur in males. It has a total lifetime prevalence of 0.5–5.5% [24, 25]. Much less research has been done on the complications of BED, due to its recent definition and the lack of studies focused directly on BED. Many believe that the complications of a BED are simply those presumed to be caused by obesity, but studies have shown that BED may be a risk factor for metabolic complications independent of weight [25]. It should not be assumed that all BED patients are obese, as 30–40% are normal weight. Conversely, not all higher weight individuals have BED.

The final diagnostic categories for eating disorders include those that describe EDs that meet some, but not all, of the diagnostic criteria for the other EDs:

- Other specified feeding and eating disorder (OSFED)
- Unspecified feeding and eating disorder (UFED)

as well as disorders that are exceedingly rare and/or are primarily seen in children:

- Pica
- Rumination disorder
- Avoidant restrictive intake disorder [21]

It is important to note that individuals with these disorders can also be very ill and have many of the same risks and complications as those who meet full criteria for AN, BN, or BED.

Although EDs can occur in anyone, they most often have their onset during adolescence and young adulthood (older for BED), and are more common in females than males. Recent studies have seen much higher rates of EDs in males, and it is likely this gender gap is closing [26]. Eating disorders are found in nearly every developed country, and minorities have rates equivalent to those of Caucasian populations [27]. Eating disorders also affect people of all weights. Patients with abnormally low body weight are easier to identify but represent the minority of individuals with EDs, and those in individuals of normal or higher weight are often overlooked [22]. Family history, personality type, dieting, sports that emphasize weight or extreme fitness, adolescent females with Type I diabetes mellitus, and post-bariatric surgery patients are other high-risk groups [28, 29].

Time constraints in the emergency departments limit the utility of widespread screening for EDs. Instead, health-care providers must maintain a high index of suspicion for these potentially fatal illnesses. Targeted screening for EDs based on risk factors and presenting complaints can lead to early identification and vastly improved outcomes for these patients. While there are many screening tools for EDs available, the majority are too lengthy or complicated to administer in the emergency department. The SCOFF questionnaire (Table 19.1) is a brief screening tool that is easy to remember and manage, and that has been shown to have good sensitivity and specificity for identification of potential EDs [30].

Table 19.1 The SCOFF questionnaire [30]

Do you make yourself sick because you feel uncomfortably full?
Do you worry you have lost control over how much you eat?
Have you recently lost over 14 pounds[a] in a three-month period?
Do you believe yourself to be fat when others say you are too thin?
Would you say that food dominates your life?

[a]Changed from 1 stone in the original version of SCOFF from the United Kingdom. 1 stone = 14 pounds

Medical Complications of Eating Disorders

There are a multitude of medical complications associated with EDs described below. These complications can be directly related to the effects of starvation and malnutrition, as well as to the frequency and type of binge eating and purging behaviors used. These complications range in severity from mild to potentially life-threatening. Individuals with EDs are often quite reluctant to disclose their illness and may present for care with vague, nonspecific symptoms, rather than complaints that are more easily directly attributable to their ED. Identification and proper management of these patients require the health-care provider to maintain a high index of suspicion and to readily recognize signs and symptoms consistent with ED pathology.

Cardiovascular Complications

Cardiovascular (CV) complications can be seen in up to 80% [20] of individuals with EDs. Patients may present with complaints of chest pain, shortness of breath, edema, palpitations, lightheadedness, or syncope, or they may be asymptomatic. A thorough evaluation, including a complete blood count (CBC), comprehensive metabolic panel (CMP), magnesium (Mg), phosphorus (P), and an ECG, should be initiated for any concerns for CV disease. Arrhythmias, notably sinus bradycardia, and ECG changes are the most frequent abnormalities seen [20, 31]. Sinus bradycardia (HR < 60) is an adaptive physiologic response to starvation thought to be at least partially mediated by increased vagal tone to cardiac muscle [20, 32]. The degree of bradycardia correlates with the severity of the illness, as measured by BMI. Almost all significantly undernourished patients will be bradycardic [33]. A "normal" heart rate (60–90 bpm) is a cause for concern in these patients and should trigger a further evaluation for the etiology of this relative tachycardia (fever, dehydration, medications) [34].

Multiple other ECG changes can be seen in individuals with EDs. Prolonged QTc interval is mostly related to secondary causes such as electrolyte abnormalities, dehydration, and medications, and not due to the ED itself [20, 31, 35]. Given the association of prolonged QTc with malignant arrhythmias such as torsades de pointes, this finding should always prompt admission for monitoring and further evaluation. Administration of medications that could further prolong QTc (antiemetics, psychotropics, and cardiac medications) should be avoided [31]. Electrolyte abnormalities such as hypokalemia, hypocalcemia, and others may also contribute to the development of other arrhythmias and ECG changes.

Hypotension is also frequently seen in individuals with EDs and is likely multifactorial. Volume depletion from fluid restriction and purging, structural changes in the heart, and increased vagal tone can contribute to a significant decrease in blood pressure (BP). Cardiac muscle atrophy can result in decreased left ventricular wall and septal muscle mass, weakened myocardium, diminished strength of contraction, papillary muscle dysfunction, and possibly reduced cardiac output [20, 36]. Autonomic dysfunction can also lead to a decreased cardiovascular response to exercise and decreased heart rate variability, as well as a decreased peripheral vascular tone with resultant orthostasis [20, 36]. These changes are seen in low-weight patients but can also be seen in normal- or higher weight patients with significant malnutrition due to purging and other behaviors. Postural orthostatic tachycardia syndrome has also been described in individuals with AN [20]. Most of these changes are reversible with adequate nutrition and weight restoration, but fibrosis and scarring due to myocardial remodeling can occur with chronic severe illness and may contribute to permanent cardiac dysfunction [36].

A word of caution regarding treatment of these patients in the acute setting: Avoid aggressive IV fluid resuscitation in the ED patient who is hypotensive but asymptomatic and otherwise stable. It is important to recognize that a low BP such as 78/50 may be the baseline for an individual with a significantly low weight. Rapid infusion of fluids may quickly lead to volume overload and resultant congestive heart failure (CHF) in a patient whose heart has been weakened by starvation [19, 35]. Slow, continuous infusions of 50–75 cc/hour are recommended in patients with EDs—even those who experience tachycardia and are hypotensive but alert, mentating appropriately, and otherwise at baseline [34].

Cardiomyopathy in individuals with EDs may be related to complications of refeeding, electrolyte abnormalities, and myocardial atrophy [36]. Patients may present with mild symptoms or in extremis with respiratory distress due to weakened respiratory muscles, pulmonary edema, increased jugular venous distension, and other signs of florid heart failure. Syrup of ipecac, a cardiotoxic emetic agent, has been removed from US markets, reducing the incidence of this particular cause of cardiomyopathy. Treatment of cardiomyopathy in patients with EDs is the same as for other causes of CHF (diuresis, preload reduction, etc.), although the clinician must proceed carefully with diuresis in hypotensive patients and those who are likely to be total body hypovolemic. Vasopressors may be needed to accomplish preload reduction safely [34, 37].

Other cardiac complications seen in ED patients are of unclear clinical significance.

Mitral valve prolapse (MVP) has an increased incidence in ED patients. MVP has been reported in as many as 33–66% of individuals with AN and is thought to be related to the relatively large size of the mitral valve relative to the atrophied left ventricular wall that results from starvation [20, 34, 36]. MVP is associated with an increased risk of arrhythmias and, questionably, sudden death, but is sometimes a benign condition. Pericardial effusion is also seen in 22–35% of individuals with AN, but is typically small and does not cause significant compromise. Both of these findings resolve with weight restoration [20, 23].

Pulmonary Complications

Although less common than some other ED-related problems, pulmonary complications are seen and can be life-threatening. Self-induced vomiting can lead to aspiration pneumonitis, pneumothorax, pneumomediastinum, and subcutaneous emphysema [19]. Spontaneous pneumothorax has been seen in individuals with AN who may also develop early COPD, possibly related to decreased surfactant levels [34, 35]. Also, weakened respiratory muscles can lead to the development of respiratory insufficiency with hypoxia and hypercarbia. Appropriate laboratory studies (CBC, CMP, +/− blood cultures), chest X-ray, and ECG should be obtained for patients presenting with complaints of dyspnea, decreased exercise tolerance, cough, and chest pain. Treatment of respiratory failure and other pulmonary symptoms is the same as that of anyone with similar complaints.

Gastrointestinal Complications

Gastrointestinal (GI) complaints such as abdominal pain, bloating, and constipation are among the most common symptoms for which ED patients seek medical care [10, 25]. These symptoms may reflect relatively mild disease or may indicate a life-threatening condition. Indigestion or heartburn caused by repeated exposure of the esophagus to gastric acids with repeated self-induced vomiting may lead to gastroesophageal reflux (GERD), esophagitis, and esophageal spasm. Hematemesis can result from small lacerations of the esophageal mucosa, known as Mallory-Weiss tears, or may indicate more severe pathology such as esophageal rupture due to forceful vomiting (Boerhaave's syndrome) [38]. Complaint of severe chest pain with excessive yawning (due to diaphragmatic irritation) is consistent with Boerhaave's. Concerns for this syndrome necessitate a thorough evaluation of esophageal rupture: chest X-ray, direct visualization of the esophagus (endoscopy), and CT scan of the chest. Mediastinitis with sepsis due to esophageal rupture can develop rapidly, and carries a high mortality rate [39].

Prolonged starvation, chronic vomiting, and laxative abuse can all contribute to the significant slowing of the entire GI tract. Gastroparesis, or delayed gastric emptying, is common and results in nausea and vomiting, abdominal bloating, and discomfort, all increased with food intake [40]. Treatment is mostly supportive, using IV fluids, antiemetics, and promotility agents such as erythromycin, bethanechol, or metoclopramide. Abdominal X-rays may be necessary to differentiate gastroparesis from small bowel obstruction or other conditions. Although relatively rare, acute gastric dilatation has been reported in individuals with EDs as the result of massive binging or secondary to gastric outlet obstruction during refeeding. Gastric dilatation can lead to gastric perforation or rupture, which carries an 80% mortality rate [25, 41]. Constipation is almost universal in malnourished patients. It is often the result of slowed colonic motility, a consequence of chronic laxative abuse, electrolyte abnormalities, hypovolemia, and dehydration [25]. Long-term use of stimulant laxatives may directly damage colonic nerves and result in cathartic colon syndrome, the lack of colonic motility [41].

Less common GI complications reported in individuals with EDs include acute hepatitis, fulminant hepatic failure, pancreatitis, and superior mesenteric artery (SMA) syndrome [25, 32, 41]. Biliary colic and cholecystitis are seen in individuals who have had rapid weight loss or repeated cycles of weight gain and loss. In addition to a CMP, lipase should also be assessed in individuals with EDs who present with complaints of epigastric or right-upper-quadrant abdominal pain.

Metabolic and Electrolyte Abnormalities

Multiple electrolyte disturbances are found in patients with EDs. Abnormalities are more common in patients who purge and are largely related to the method(s) of purging. Restriction of fluid intake and starvation can also result in significant abnormalities. Electrolyte abnormalities affect nearly every organ system, and their consequences can be fatal. However, many individuals with EDs, particularly those with purely restrictive disorders, will have normal laboratory studies despite even severe malnourishment. Therefore, the lack of electrolyte abnormalities does not necessarily exclude severe malnourishment or other ED complications.

Hypokalemia is the most frequent electrolyte abnormality. Very low serum potassium (< 2.5 mEq/L), as well as elevated bicarbonate (<38 mEq/L) without another known cause, is almost exclusively seen in individuals who purge by vomiting and abuse laxatives/diuretics. In the absence of a clear cause, significant hypokalemia is found in <1% of healthy people with normal kidneys. These findings are suggestive of purging by vomiting and should prompt further investigation [42]. Treatment of hypokalemia is with oral and IV potassium supplementation. Moderate-to-severe hypokalemia increases the risk of potentially fatal cardiac arrhythmias and should be treated aggressively [19, 42]. Severe (<2.5 mEq/L) or moderate hypokalemia (2.5–3.0 mEq/L) in the setting of metabolic alkalosis should prompt admission for cardiac monitoring and treatment. Alkalosis must be corrected along with potassium to prevent ongoing renal losses of potassium due to increased aldosterone production in chronic dehydration.

Hyponatremia due to dehydration or excess free-water intake (or "water-loading") is another common electrolyte deficiency seen in EDs. Diuretics and selective serotonin reuptake inhibitors may exacerbate hyponatremia in these patients [19, 42]. Serum sodium levels below 120 mEq/L can result in seizures and death. Treatment includes IV normal saline (NS) with a goal of increasing the serum sodium by 4–6 mEq/L in the first 1–2 hours and no more than 8–10 mEq/L in the first 24 hours. Even slower rates may be appropriate in those with chronic hyponatremia [42]. Rapid increases in serum sodium should be avoided due to the risk of central pontine myelinolysis, and the use of hypertonic (3%) saline should be reserved for symptomatic (seizing or comatose) patients. Other electrolyte abnormalities, such as hypochloremia, hypomagnesium, and hypocalcemia, as well as micronutrient deficiencies, can also be seen in individuals with EDs. Hypomagnesium can cause muscle cramping, weakness, paresthesias, and arrhythmias. Low magnesium must be corrected to prevent further renal losses of potassium. Consider admission for significant electrolyte abnormalities, metabolic acidosis, or signs of chronic dehydration in any patient with inadequate resources, lack of follow-up, or those who are unlikely to correct the purging behaviors.

Metabolic alkalosis is the most common acid-base disturbance seen in individuals who purge, and serum bicarbonate of >35–38 mEq/L is highly suggestive of self-induced vomiting [33, 42]. Severe diarrhea secondary to laxative abuse may result in a non-ion gap metabolic acidosis acutely, but with chronic use, most patients develop hypokalemia and a mild metabolic alkalosis due to chronic dehydration with respiratory compensation. Renal dysfunction in individuals with EDs may also contribute to acid-base disturbances. Most renal abnormalities are pre-renal secondary to purging or decreased fluid intake; however, chronic AN patients are also at risk for renal salt wasting, intrinsic renal disease, and renal failure [34, 38].

Patients with very low body weights may also be hypothermic [35]. Low body temperature is a reflection of reduced basal metabolic rate resulting from chronic starvation. The inability to maintain body temperature usually indicates severe malnutrition. A core body temperature of <95 °F in the absence of other causes is an indication of severe compromise and warrants immediate hospitalization.

Endocrine Complications

Long-term complications of EDs including infertility, pregnancy complications, fetal abnormalities, amenorrhea or oligomenorrhea, osteoporosis, increased risk of fractures, overuse injuries, arrested growth, hypercortisolemia, and thyroid irregularities can occur and are beyond the scope of this text [34, 35, 42, 43]. Acute endocrine abnormalities such as significant hypo- or hyperglycemia in individuals with EDs can be life-threatening. Hypoglycemia is usually mild (≥70 mg/dL). When severe (<50 mg/dL), it is concerning for advanced hepatic dysfunction or depletion of glycogen stores and may result in death [35, 44, 45].

Young females with Type I diabetes mellitus (DM) are at increased risk for the development of an ED. Intentional manipulation of insulin in conjunction with other ED behaviors to achieve weight loss contributes to serious medical complications that can arise quickly. Poor glucose control leads to recurrent diabetic ketoacidosis (DKA), as well as a much higher incidence and younger onset of many long-term complications of diabetes [45]. These patients are also at risk of suicide by insulin overdose. Treatment of DKA includes IV fluids, electrolyte replacement, and insulin in an intensive-care setting, and is similar to that of other patients. The risks of cardiomyopathy and potential fluid overload are high and transfer to a facility with expertise in treating this dangerous combination should be considered [34, 45].

Neurologic Complications

Brain imaging has shown significant cerebral atrophy and ventricular enlargement similar to that seen in Alzheimer's disease in malnourished individuals with EDs. This atrophy may manifest in cognitive impairment such as decreased concentration and memory loss [35, 46]. Peripheral neuropathies are also seen and may be related to vitamin B or other micronutrient deficiencies [31]. These changes are usually reversible with weight restoration, but some patients may experience permanent cognitive deficits. Seizures have also been reported and may be related to electrolyte abnormalities, medications, or hypoglycemia [35].

Other Complications

Although not acutely life-threatening, some of the classic signs and symptoms of EDs may be helpful in identifying an occult ED. Parents may bring their child or adolescent in for concerns of weight loss or failure to grow. Older patients might complain of generalized fatigue or weakness, cold intolerance, or dizziness, none of which are diagnostic in and of themselves, but when taken into consideration with other clinical and diagnostic findings, should heighten suspicion for an ED.

Other commonly described findings include the development of lanugo hair (fine hair growth), hair loss, carotenoderma (yellowish skin discoloration due to high levels of carotene), brittle nails, dry skin, poor wound healing, and acrocyanosis due to peripheral vasoconstriction [34–36]. Russell's sign (callus on the dorsum of hand) is considered a classic sign of BN but is not a common finding [36]. Oral trauma, dental erosion, perimolysis (increased erosion on the lingular surface of maxillary teeth), cheilosis (cracking and erythema at the corners of the mouth), and parotid and other salivary gland enlargements can also be seen both during active illness and in the recovery period [19, 34–36]. Significant hematologic abnormalities are not common in individuals with EDs but may be present. Mild abnormalities such as iron-deficiency anemia are relatively common in low-weight patients due to inadequate dietary iron intake but may be masked by volume contraction. Starvation is one of the few causes of decreased sedimentation rate but is nonspecific. Bone-marrow hypoplasia and failure in severe malnutrition can result in reductions in any blood cell line or pancytopenia. Interestingly, individuals with severe AN do not show signs of immunosuppression and do not have increased rates of infection even in the setting of mild-to-moderate leukopenia [36]. Hematologic abnormalities are generally rapidly reversible with adequate nutrition [19].

Substances and Eating Disorders

Individuals with EDs are at increased risk for substance-use disorders (SUD), including misuse of prescribed medications, and may also be on psychotropic medications. These medications can have side effects that contribute to symptoms and are frequently used in suicide attempts [31, 46–48]. The availability of stimulant medications and the misuse/abuse of these medications on high school and college campuses have increased dramatically over the past two decades. The use of these medications, as well as illicit drugs such as amphetamines and cocaine for appetite suppression, is seen [47–49]. Overuse of stimulants in individuals with EDs puts them at greatly increased risk of cardiac sequelae, including heart failure. Treatment of stimulant toxicity is primarily supportive with cardiac monitoring, IVF, and benzodiazepines.

Abuse of other substances, including alcohol, is also increased in ED patients. Some studies have found that as many as 41% of patients with EDs will be affected by a SUD at some point in their illness [47, 48]. On the other hand, substance-abuse treatment centers report as many as one-third of their patients having comorbid EDs. The use of alcohol and other substances increases the risk of many complications of both disorders, including the risk of death by suicide and other causes. Providers should consider comorbid substance use when making treatment and disposition decisions for their patients with EDs [35].

Complications of Recovery

Complications seen during recovery from an ED range from benign and self-resolving to potentially fatal. While the most severely malnourished patients are usually initially stabilized in an inpatient setting, a significant number never seek treatment or are treated on an outpatient basis and may present to an acute-care facility due to complications of refeeding.

Sialadenosis, caused by hypertrophy of the parotid and other salivary glands due to chronic vomiting, can be seen during BN or three to 4 days after the cessation of vomiting. This is a benign, self-limiting condition, and reassurance is the only treatment necessary [34, 50].

Other problems in the recovery period are much more serious and can lead to fatal complications. Purging and diuretic use can lead to chronic dehydration, which stimulates renal aldosterone production. During the first two to three weeks after these patients stop purging, they are at risk of developing severe edema, along with worsening metabolic alkalosis and electrolyte abnormalities. This condition, Pseudo-Bartter's syndrome, is due to hyperaldosteronism caused by renal adaptations to chronic dehydration [34, 35, 51]. Slow fluid replacement (50–75 cc/hr. NS), along with potassium and magnesium supplementation, is the key to treatment. Rapid boluses of large volumes of IV fluid should be avoided [34, 35].

Refeeding syndrome may develop during the initial recovery period [19, 31, 34]. This syndrome is caused by rapid fluid and electrolyte shifts that occur with refeeding. During prolonged starvation, the body maintains homeostasis by shifting intracellular electrolytes to the extracellular space such that measured serum levels of electrolytes may appear relatively normal despite severe total body depletion. In early stages of refeeding, increased insulin released in response to the sudden presence of nutrition leads to increased cellular uptake of glucose, along with phosphorus and other electrolytes. Levels can drop rapidly, resulting in multiple symptoms primarily related to hypophosphatemia such as neurologic (confusion, seizures, coma), cardiac (arrhythmias, heart failure), hematologic (hemolysis), and muscular (weakness, rhabdomyolysis, diaphragm weakness leading to respiratory failure) complications [31, 34]. Regardless of weight, individuals are at risk of refeeding syndrome if they have had little or no nutritional intake for >5 days, a history of alcohol abuse, and the use of medications including insulin, chemotherapy, antacids, or diuretics [22, 34]. Emergency department treatment of patients with suspected refeeding syndrome includes slow administration of IV fluids (50–70 cc/hr. of NS) to avoid volume overload, aggressive replacement of electrolytes, and admission to a monitored bed or intensive-care unit. Cardiac monitoring and ongoing supplementation are indicated for any suspicion of refeeding syndrome.

Management of Eating Disorder Patients in the Acute Care Setting

It is imperative that all health-care providers maintain a supportive, nonjudgmental stance toward individuals with EDs. Equally important is the recognition that the vast majority of individuals with eating disorders are normal weight or higher. EDs can also occur in people of all races, genders, socioeconomic statuses, and ages. Providers must maintain a high index of suspicion for signs and symptoms concerning for an ED, regardless of the outward appearance of the individual. Whenever possible, involve family, friends, and significant others. It is also imperative that the EM physician recognizes and treats all potentially life-threatening abnormalities. With a few exceptions (see Table 19.2), management of acute symptoms in individuals with EDs is a quite similar treatment of any other patient.

Table 19.2 The academy for eating disorders criteria for acute medical or psychiatric stabilization [22]

Presence of one or more of the following:	*Or one or more of the following:*
≤ 75% median BMI for age, sex, and height	Acute food refusal
Hypoglycemia	Suicidal thoughts or behaviors
Electrolyte disturbance (hypokalemia, hyponatremia, hypophosphatemia, and/or metabolic acidosis or alkalosis)	Other significant psychiatric comorbidity that interferes with ED treatment (anxiety, depression, obsessive-compulsive disorder)
ECG abnormalities (e.g., prolonged QTc > 450, bradycardia, other arrhythmias)	*Other considerations regarding hospitalization:*
Hemodynamic instability Bradycardia Hypotension Hypothermia	Failure of outpatient treatment
Orthostasis	Uncontrollable bingeing and/or purging by any means
Acute medical complications of malnutrition (e.g., syncope, seizures, cardiac failure, pancreatitis, etc.)	Inadequate social support and/or follow-up medical or psychiatric care
Comorbid psychiatric or medical condition that prohibits or limits appropriate outpatient treatment (e.g., severe depression, suicidal ideation, obsessive-compulsive disorder, Type 1 diabetes mellitus)	
Uncertainty of the diagnosis of an ED	

Disposition

Generally accepted indications for hospital admission apply. Also, there are indications for admission specific to EDs. Many of the most egregious errors made by acute-care providers during the care of individuals with EDs are related to disposition. Table 19.2 contains guidelines for hospitalization (adult or adolescent) recently published by the Academy for Eating Disorders [22].

Older similar guidelines for children and adolescents are available from the Society for Adolescent Health [52] and for adults from the American Psychiatric Association and the UK's National Institute for Health and Care Excellence. It is strongly recommended that the acute-care provider consult one of these guidelines or, if available, a provider with expertise in the treatment of EDs when determining the disposition of these patients. A commonly made error is the discharge of a patient who is deemed "stable," based on normal vital signs and normal or only slightly abnormal laboratory studies without due consideration of weight and/or complicating factors such as comorbid medical or psychiatric conditions, lack of access to follow-up care, or severity of current ED behaviors. Given the high risk of complications and increased mortality seen in individuals with EDs, it is better to err on the side of caution by admitting or transferring to an appropriate facility, rather than discharging a potentially very ill individual.

The majority of patients with EDs recover fully; however, the prognosis is much improved by early diagnosis and effective early treatment. The risk of developing a chronic, treatment-resistant ED increases with every year that the patient goes untreated or inadequately treated [2, 53]. Successful, definitive treatment is most often quite lengthy (3–5 years) and will obviously not be accomplished in the acute-care setting. It is imperative, however, that any health-care provider in an acute-care setting who has identified a patient suspected to suffer from an ED refer this patient to appropriate specialty care. For individuals who do not require hospitalization, ensure adequate follow-up care with the patient's primary care provider (PCP) and ED specialist if available, and provide ED-related resources to the patient and family members. Ideally, the provider who has concerns for an occult ED will relate these concerns to the individual's PCP. Know the resources in your local area. If you are unsure, or there aren't any, consult reputable online sources of information on EDs and treatment specialists, including the Academy for Eating Disorders (www.aedweb.org), the Binge Eating Disorder Association (bedaonline.com), and the National Eating Disorders Association (www.neda.com).

Conclusions

Eating disorders are serious mental illnesses that have multiple psychiatric and medical comorbidities, as well as one of the highest mortality rates of any psychiatric condition. Contrary to popular opinion, they are not rare (more than 10% of the general population will develop a clinically significant ED at some point in their life) and can be seen in individuals of any race, size, gender, level of education, and socioeconomic status [22]. Effective interventions do exist, and most patients recover fully with good treatment. Emergency department and other health-care visits represent an opportunity for early recognition and intervention in patients who are often otherwise reluctant to disclose their illness. It is important that providers be able to identify and manage the signs and symptoms of eating disorders, especially in high-risk populations. If you suspect an eating disorder in one of your patients, say something! A visit to the emergency department is a frightening experience for many individuals with EDs. It may also represent an excellent "teachable moment" and an opportunity to provide life-saving intervention and referral. Saying nothing may be interpreted by the individual as tacit approval of the illness or "evidence" that there is nothing seriously wrong, and a key opportunity for early identification and referral will have been missed.

References

1. Harris E, Barraclough B. Excess mortality of mental disorder. Br J Psy. 1998;173:11–53.
2. Chamay-Weber C, Narring F, Michaud P. Partial eating disorders among adolescents: a review. J Ado Health. 2005;37(3):417–27.
3. Fairburn C, Cooper Z, Doll H, Norman P, O'Connor M. The natural course of bulimia nervosa and binge eating disorder in young women. Arch Gen Psych. 2000;57:659–65.
4. Hautala L, Junnila J, Alin J, Gronroos M, Maunula AM, Karukivi M, et al. Uncovering hidden eating disorders using the SCOFF questionnaire: cross-sectional survey of adolescents and comparison with nurse assessments. Int J Nurs Stud. 2009;46:1439–47.
5. Johnston O, Fornai G, Cabrini S, Kendrick T. Feasibility and acceptability of screening for eating disorders in primary care. Fam Pract. 2007;24:511–7.
6. Mond J, Myers T, Crosby R, Hay P, Rodgers B, Morgane J, et al. Screening for eating disorders in primary care: EDE-Q versus SCOFF. Behav Res Ther. 2008;46:612–22.
7. Dooley-Hash S, Banker J, Walton M, Ginsburg Y, Cunningham R. The prevalence and correlates of eating disorders among emergency department patients aged 14–20 years. Int J Eat Disord. 2012;45(7):883–90.
8. Ogg E, Millar H, Pusztai E, Thom A. General practice consultation patterns preceding diagnosis of eating disorders. Int J Eat Disord. 1997;22:89–93.
9. Striegel-Moore R, Dohm F, Kraemer H, Schreiber G, Crawford P, Daniels S. Health services use in women with a history of bulimia nervosa or binge eating disorder. Int J Eat Disord. 2005;37:11–8.
10. Dooley-Hash S, Lipson S, Walton M, Cunningham R. Increased emergency department use by adolescents and young adults with eating disorders. Int J Eat Disord. 2013;46(4):308–15.

11. Crow S, Praus B, Thuras P. Mortality from eating disorders: a 5-to-10-year record linkage study. Int J Eat Disord. 1999;26(1):97–101.
12. Birmingham C, Su J, Hlynsky J, Goldner E, Gao M. The mortality rate from anorexia nervosa. Int J Eat Disord. 2005;38:143–6.
13. Fichter M, Quadflieg N, Hedlund S. Twelve-year course and outcome predictors of anorexia nervosa. Int J Eat Disord. 2006;39:87–100.
14. Hoek H. Incidence, prevalence and mortality of anorexia nervosa and other eating disorders. Curr Opin Psy. 2006;19(4):389–94.
15. Arcelus J, Mitchell AJ, Wales J, Nielsen S. Mortality rates in patients with anorexia nervosa and other eating disorders: a meta-analysis of 36 studies. Arch Psy. 2011;68:724.
16. Keel P, Dorer D, Eddy K, Franko D, Charatan D, Herzog D. Predictors of mortality in eating disorders. Arch Gen Psych. 2003;60:179–83.
17. Pompili M, Girardi P, Tatarelli G, Ruberto A, Tatarelli R. Suicide and attempted suicide in eating disorders, obesity and weight-image concern. Eat Behav. 2006;7:384–94.
18. Crow S, Peterson C, Swanson S, Raymond N, Specker S, Eckert E, et al. Increased mortality in bulimia nervosa and other eating disorders. Am J Psy. 2009;166:1342–6.
19. Agras W, editor. The oxford handbook of eating disorders. First ed. New York: Oxford University Press; 2010.
20. Spaulding-Barclay M, Stern J, Mehler P. Cardiac changes in anorexia nervosa. Card in Young. 2016;26(4):623–8.
21. Amercian Psychiatric Association. Diagnostic and statistical manual of mental disorders. Fifth ed. Arlington: American Psychiatric Publishing; 2013.
22. The Academy for Eating Disorders. AED report 2016. In: Eating disorders: a guide to medical care. Third ed. Deerfield; 2016.
23. Keel P, Heatherton T, Dorer D, Joiner T, Zalta A. Point prevalence of bulimia nervosa in 1982, 1992, and 2002. Psychol Med. 2006;36:119–27.
24. Hudson J, Hiripi E, Pope HG, Kessler R. The prevalence and correlates of eating disorders in the National Comorbidity Survey Replication. Biol Psy. 2007;61:348–58.
25. Mitchell J. Medical comorbidity and medical complications associated with binge eating disorder. Int J of Eat Dis. 2016;49(3):319–23.
26. Domine F, Berchtold A, Akre C, Michaud P, Suris J. Disordered eating behaviors: what about boys? J Ado Health. 2009;44:111–7.
27. Shaw H, Ramirez L, Trost A, Randall P, Stice E. Body image and eating disturbances across ethnic groups: more similarities than differences. Psychol Addict Behav. 2004;18(1):12–8.
28. Young-Hyman D, Davis C. Disordered eating behavior in individuals with diabetes: importance of context, evaluation and classification. Diab Care. 2010;33(3):683–9.
29. Segal A, Kussunoki D, Larino M. Post-surgical refusal to eat: anorexia nervosa, bulimia nervosa or a new eating disorder? A case series. Obes Surg. 2004;14:353–60.
30. Hill L, Reid F, Morgan J, Lacey J. SCOFF, the development of an eating disorder screening questionnaire. Int J Eat Disord. 2010;43:344–51.
31. Katzman D. Medical complications in adolescents with anorexia nervosa: a review of the literature. Int J Eat Disord. 2005;37(Supplement):S52–9.
32. Nudel D, Gootman N, Nussbaum M, Shenker I. Altered exercise performance and abnormal sympathetic responses to exercise in patients with anorexia nervosa. J Pediatr. 1984;105(1):34–7.
33. Panagiotopoulos C, McCrindle B, Hick K, Katzman D. Electrocardiographic findings in patients with eating disorders. Pediatrics. 2000; 105(5):1100–5.
34. Mehler P, Anderson A. Eating disorders: a guide to medical care and complications. Second ed. Baltimore: The Johns Hopkins University Press; 2010.
35. Mehler P, Brown C. Anorexia nervosa: medical complications. Int J Eat Disord. 2015;3:11.
36. Sachs K, Mehler P. Medical complications of bulimia nervosa and their treatments. Eat Weight Disord. 2016;21(1):13–18.9.
37. Silber T. Ipecac syrup abuse, morbidity, and mortality: Isn't it time to repeal its over-the-counter status? J Ado Health. 2005;37(3):256–60.
38. Pomeroy C, Mitchell J. Medical complications of anorexia nervosa and bulimia nervosa. In: Eating disorders and obesity: a comprehensive handbook. Second ed. New York: Guilford Press; 2002. p. 278–85.
39. Chen K, Chen J, Kuo S, Huang P, Hsu H, Lee J, et al. Descending necrotizing mediastinitis: a 10-year surgical experience in a single institution. J Thor Cardiov Surg. 2008;136(1):191–8.
40. Zipfel S, Sammet I, Rapps N, Herzog W, Herpertz S, Martens U. Gastrointestinal disturbances in eating disorders: clinical and neurobiological causes. Auton Neurosci. 2006;129(1–2):99–106.
41. Mitchell J, Crow S. Medical complications of anorexia nervosa and bulimia nervosa. Curr Opin Psy. 2006;19(4):438–43.
42. Mehler P, Walsh K. Electrolyte and acid-base abnormalities associated with purging behaviors. Int J Eat Disord. 2016;49(3):311–8.
43. Misra M, Golden N, Katzman D. State of the art systematic review of bone disease in anorexia nervosa. Int J Eat Disord. 2016;49(3):276–92.
44. Mattingly D, Bhanji S. Hypoglycaemia and anorexia nervosa. J R Soc Med. 1995;88(4):191–5.
45. Goebel-Fabbri A. Disturbed eating behaviors and eating disorders in type 1 diabetes: clinical significance and treatment recommendations. Curr Diab Rep. 2009;9:133–9.
46. Lask B, Gordon I, Christie D, Frampton I, Chowdhury U, Watkins B. Functional neuroimag-

ing in early onset anorexia nervosa. Int J Eat Disord. 2005;37:S49.
47. Holderness C, Brooks-Gunn J, Warren M. Co-morbidity of eating disorders and substance abuse review of the literature. Int J Eat Disord. 1994;16(1):1–34.
48. Krug I, Treasure J, Anderluh M, Bellodi L, Cellini E, di Bernardo M. Present and lifetime comorbidity of tobacco, alcohol and drug use in eating disorders: a European multicenter study. Drug Alcohol Depend. 2008;97:169–79.
49. Bogle K, Smith B. Illicit methylphenidate use: a review of prevalence, availability, pharmacology, and consequences. Curr Drug Abuse Rev. 2009;2(2):157–76.
50. Forney K, Buchman-Schmitt J, Keel P, Frank G. The medical complications associated with purging. Int J Eat Disord. 2016;49(3):249–59.
51. Mitchell J, Pomeroy C, Seppala M. Pseudo-Bartter's syndrome, diuretic abuse and eating disorders. Int J Eat Disord. 1988;7:225–37.
52. Golden N, Katzman D, Kreipe R, Stevens S, Sawyer S, Rees J, et al. Eating disorders in adolescents: position paper of the society for adolescent medicine. J Ado Health. 2003;33:496–53.
53. Steinhausen H. The outcome of anorexia nervosa in the 20th century. Am J Psy. 2002;159:1284–93.

Part V

Treatment of the Psychiatric Patient

When to Admit the Psychiatric Patient

20

Carmen R. Serpa

Introduction

The emergency department (ED) is an intense, stressful work environment that plays a unique and critical role in the modern-day health-care system. The ability to evaluate and initiate treatment for unplanned medical emergencies 24 hours a day, 7 days a week, sets the ED apart from other medical facilities. The unplanned nature of patient attendance and challenges involving access to health care have led to emergency departments becoming a primary source of treatment for those with mental illnesses. A shortage of psychiatrists and inpatient psychiatric facilities often leave ED staff members ill-equipped to manage increasingly frequent behavioral emergencies.

As emergency providers are faced with performing a rapid evaluation of symptoms, identifying patients at high risk for self-harm or injury to others is critical. Providing initial psychiatric treatment and creating a safe disposition to an appropriate level of care help to ensure high-risk cases are managed effectively.

The purpose of this chapter is to provide an overview of what aspects to consider when determining whether to admit an individual to a psychiatric unit. We will also discuss in detail how to conduct a comprehensive risk assessment when evaluating various populations with psychiatric pathologies. (Please also see Chap. 8, "Discharge of the Emergency Patient with Risk Factors for Suicide: Psychiatric and Legal Perspectives.")

Case Example

Ms. M. is a thirty-six-year-old woman with a history of bipolar disorder brought to the emergency department by the police after being involved in an altercation at home with her brother. Her brother tried to stop her from cutting her wrist in a suicide attempt following a break-up with her boyfriend. It appears that her brother found out that Ms. M. had been Googling ways of "how to die quickly." Upon arrival at the ED, during her triage, Ms. M. reported to the nurse that she wanted to die but later denied it to the psychiatrist and social worker who had consulted with the patient while in the ED. The patient was discharged. The next evening, Ms. M. texted a friend "I just want to end it all." She had been drinking, and her friend didn't take her text seriously and advised her to go to sleep. The next morning, her friend decided to check on her and found Ms. M.

C. R. Serpa (✉)
Macomb County Community Mental Health Services, Clinton Twp, MI, USA

Common Ground, Pontiac, MI, USA

L. S. Zun et al. (eds.), *Behavioral Emergencies for Healthcare Providers*,
https://doi.org/10.1007/978-3-030-52520-0_20

hanging off a tree branch in her back yard. On the day of her funeral, Ms. M.'s mother was crying and shared with relatives that 2 weeks prior, Ms. M. had been talking about wanting "to disappear."

Risk Assessment

It is important to be skillful and precise when determining the risk individuals pose to themselves or others. Given the nature of what is discussed during the assessment, establishing a good rapport, and demonstrating empathy to the patient are two important aspects to keep in mind. Documentation showing that the clinician a) performed a reasonable assessment of risk and b) provided a rationale for implementing a reasonable management plan will be likely to meet the standard of care [1]. The assessment should also focus on factors that elevate the patient's risk of intentional or unintentional danger [2]. This implies that aside from exploring any suicidal and homicidal ideations, imminent vulnerability to danger also includes evidence of intoxication, debilitating drug use, unexpected life crisis, expressions of hopelessness, irritable mood, global insomnia, impulsivity, chronic debilitating physical conditions, thought disorganization, disheveled appearance, and agitation [1, 2].

Criteria for Psychiatric Hospitalization

Involuntary commitment, also known as civil commitment, is the legal process of hospitalizing a person against his or her stated wishes. The criteria for involuntary admission to a psychiatric unit are met when a patient is deemed to be at danger to themselves or others, or is unable to provide for himself or herself because of mental illness [2]. In the United States, forcing someone to enter a facility to undergo treatment is considered a significant curtailment of his or her rights. Two major legal principles have been used by lawmakers to protect individuals who are involuntarily admitted. The first is to protect the citizenry from harm, via "police powers." The second is to protect the individual from harming themselves, via parens patriae. Parens patriae is Latin for "parent of the nation" and has its greatest application via the treatment of children, mentally ill persons, and other individuals who are legally incompetent to manage their affairs [3]. When the state invokes its police powers, it usually results in someone being arrested for breaking the law. In psychiatry, this power is, therefore, invoked if someone's actions threaten the safety or welfare of others [4]. Parens patriae powers are also used to help those who can't help themselves, as its key principle is to protect the individual. Individuals have a right to the least restrictive treatment. However, when their actions are believed to represent an imminent danger to themselves or others as the result of a psychiatric etiology, admission to a psychiatric facility is granted. Physicians should be aware of the laws that govern involuntary hospitalization in their state, as the criteria may vary. These can easily be found by an internet search for involuntary commitment laws or by directly speaking with legal representatives [5].

Suicidality

Suicide has become a major public health issue worldwide and accounts for an estimated 2% of all emergency room visits [6]. There were approximately 34,000 suicides in the United States in 2007, accounting for roughly 100 suicides per day. Per the American Foundation for Suicide Prevention, in 2016, the numbers increased to 123 suicides per day. In 2016, firearms were the most common method of death by suicide, accounting for a little more than half (51.01%) of all suicide deaths [7]. Suicide ranks tenth among causes of death nationwide and is the third leading cause of death in youths between the ages of 15–24 years [6, 7].

An estimated 8–25 suicide attempts occur for every suicide among children and adolescents. This ratio is much lower among individuals aged 65 and older, with approximately four attempts for every completed suicide [6]. A study in the 1970s reported that 82% of patients who committed suicide visited a physician within 6 months of their death; retrospectively, 51% of these patients had evidence of depression, but only 38% of those who committed suicide were diagnosed with depression [8].

Competent clinical care for suicidal patients requires that medical staff recognize and determine the patient's suicidal risk by conducting a thorough interview to identify current suicidal desire, ideations, plans, means, intent, past attempts, and protective factors. Once the level of risk is determined, a collaborative intervention plan appropriate for the situation should be developed and documented [9]. (Please see Chap. 8, "Discharge of the Emergency Patient with Risk Factors for Suicide: Psychiatric and Legal Perspectives") Patients in acute crisis with a moderate-to-high suicide risk should be admitted. In such cases, voluntary hospitalization is preferable when possible to provide a more collaborative, patient-centered care plan [10]. Otherwise, involuntary commitment is necessary.

The use of standardized rating scales in the emergency department as part of the assessment process has provided evidence that their use can help to improve the identification of additional patients with recent suicide attempts. A study by Gregory Brown et al. identified that 18% of the patients who were classified as making a recent attempt by using a standardized assessment such as the Columbia Suicide Severity Rating Scale were not identified as such by the clinical assessment upon review of the medical records [11]. The same study concluded that the sensitivity and accuracy of identifying suicidal behavior and non-suicidal self-injury behavior using standardized scales resulted in a valuable asset to a comprehensive clinical assessment.

Homicidality

Homicidal ideation, intent, attempts, and plans can be difficult to assess. As with suicide, no clinician can confidently predict what is going to happen. As in the assessment of suicide, rating scales may be helpful in making a thorough assessment of homicidal risk. The Danger Assessment (DA) is a twenty-question assessment tool designed to assess the likelihood of lethality or near-lethality occurring in a case of intimate partner violence. It can accurately identify the vast majority of abused women who are at increased risk of femicide or attempted femicide [12].

A logical assessment of the prevailing risk of violence can help develop and justify a reasonable treatment plan for these patients. Studies have shown that the only factor clearly associated with future violent behavior is a history of violence [13]. A comprehensive violence assessment should also include exploring historical and clinical factors. Table 20.1 depicts various factors to consider that can assist the clinician in carrying out a structured assessment [1].

The Modified Overt Aggression Scale (MOAS) is a four-part behavior rating scale designed to measure four types of aggressive behaviors as witnessed in the past week. See

Table 20.1 Historical and clinical factors associated with violence risk [1]

Historical factors	Clinical factors
Past violence (affective, predatory)	Homicidal/violent thoughts
Frequency of recurrence of violent acts	Substance abuse
Use of weapons during the act	Impulsivity
Age (esp. late teens, early twenties)	Poor insight into mental illness or to past violent acts
Male gender	Psychosis (command-type hallucinations)
Low IQ	Delusions (persecutory, history of acting on the delusions)
Major mental illness	Depression
Criminal record/ juvenile delinquency	Acutely manic
Combat training	Organic brain dysfunction (TBI, frontal lobe syndrome, intermittent explosive ds)
Animal cruelty/ antisocial traits	Acute symptoms of PTSD
Childhood abuse	

Table 20.2 Modified overt aggression scale calculation score [15]

Behavior score	Score	Weights	Total sum
Verbally aggressive		x1	
Destruction of property		x2	
Self-injurious acts		x3	
Physically aggressive		x4	
Total score			

Table 20.2 [14]. Aggression is divided into four categories: verbal, physical against objects, physical against self, and physical against others. Each category is rated from 0 to 4, depending on the level of severity. Total scores on the MOAS range from 0 to 40, with a higher score indicating more aggressive behavior. The scores of the scale have shown good reliability in helping to predict future aggressive behaviors [15].

Another helpful tool is the Brøset Violence Checklist (BVC) developed by Linaker and Bush-Iversen. The BVC is an easy-to-use instrument that can help predict the risk of violence and is based on the presence or absence of six characteristics: confusion, irritability, boisterousness, verbally threatening, physically threatening, and attacks on objects [15]. Research performed on the BVC has shown that it has a moderate sensitivity and high specificity with an adequate inter-rater reliability in its ability to predict violence within the next 24-hour period [16].

While tools such as DAT, MOAS, and BVC are a useful resource, clinicians must be aware that the use of rating scales does not replace the need for clinical judgment about a patient's current risk of violence. A thorough assessment of the patient's homicidal risk must include a detailed interview in efforts to identify current homicidal or suicidal desires, ideations, plans, means, intent, history of violence, and protective factors. The disclosure of intent to the authorities or parties involved does not represent a violation of HIPAA laws. A clinician's duty to protect overrides the confidentiality of the therapist–patient relationship. The professional may discharge this duty in several ways, including notifying police, warning the intended victim, or taking other reasonable steps to protect the threatened individual [9].

The Elderly

Psychiatric emergencies are common among the elderly and carry significant morbidity and mortality rates. The most common psychiatric emergencies among the elderly population are delirium, depression with suicidality, substance abuse, and dementia accompanied by aggression [17]. Early identification of delirium and appropriate management of the underlying medical precipitants will reduce its severity and lead to improved outcomes for the patient [18]. Delirium is missed anywhere from 12.5% to 75% of the time in the emergency room [19]. An appropriate assessment of cognitive function was the clinical element most often neglected both in 69.1% patients admitted to psychiatric units and in 38.2% of those admitted to medical units [9]. It has been found that key assessments to rule out organicity are less likely to be performed in patients with mental status changes who are admitted to psychiatric units than in those admitted to medical units [20]. The Confusion Assessment Method (CAM) is a standarized and validated algorithm that is helpful in the assessment of delirium and to help non-psychiatrically trained clinicans to identify delirium in a quick and accurate way. The CAM focuses on rating confusion by understanding acute onset vs fluctuating and inattention; and either, disorganized thinking or level of altered consciousness [21]. It should be considered as part of a comprehensive evaluaiton of these patients.

Elderly patients are more likely to experience feelings of worthlessness and guilt [16]. When compared to other segments of the population with depression, elderly patients have the highest rate of suicide [19]. The rate of deaths by suicide is the highest in this age group, with an estimated 14.3 per 100,000 [17]. The reasons for increased lethality include the use of more violent means, decreased physical resilience, and increased isolation [22].

The presence of depressive symptoms should prompt emergency staff to introduce questions about death, thoughts of suicide, intent to harm self, and access to means [23]. However, an appropriate ED assessment of depression in the elderly should also include strong consideration for medical illness as an etiology of the patient's signs and symptoms. There are many depression scales in existence that are specific to the elderly, including the Geriatric Depression Scale (GDS) and the Center for Epidemiological Studies Depression (CES-D) Scale. Many will consider that spending 15 minutes performing this exercise might be impractical, given the busy pace of the ED. However, when in doubt of the diagnosis, this could be 15 minutes well spent and help in the decision of when to admit.

Up to 50% of elderly patients with dementia may develop depression. Depression with psychotic features is the most common variant of depression among this segment of the population. Around 23% of the elderly will experience psychotic symptoms that may be associated with aggressive or disruptive behavior [19]. Dementia is the most common cause of psychosis in the elderly. Approximately 50% of Alzheimer's dementia patients experience delusions or hallucinations within the first 3 years of clinical onset [19]. Primary psychiatric disorders make up a significant but less common cause of psychosis in the elderly. The assessment of psychosis in the ED for elderly patients should include a thorough medical screening with special attention to a neurologic evaluation, including consideration of head trauma, malignancy, infection, and seizures.

Furthermore, psychotic symptoms may also be present in substance intoxication and withdrawal. Physicians should have a lower threshold for laboratory testing in elderly patients. Approximately 14% of elderly patients in the emergency department and more than 20% of those psychiatrically hospitalized meet the criteria for alcohol abuse or dependence [24]. The UDIT-C (Adult Use Disorder Identification Test) questionnaire and the Michigan Alcoholism Screening Test-Geriatric Version (MAST-G) are the most commonly used tools to facilitate detection of alcohol use [25]. A history of detoxifications, seizures, delirium tremens, or unstable medical comorbidities may warrant inpatient detoxification. In addition, many of the commonly used medications among the elderly, such as corticosteroids, anti-inflammatories, antihistamines, or antidepressants, may precipitate psychosis.

Children and Adolescents

There has been an increase in the number of children and adolescents seeking psychiatric care in the ED. Approximately 10% of children in the USA have been diagnosed with mental illness. It is estimated that roughly 13 million of the children in the USA are in need of mental health or substance-abuse services [26]. It has been found that emergency room staff commonly struggle with how to handle these cases. According to the Institute of Medicine, ED evaluation of such cases tends to be inadequate. Child and adolescents who use the ED repeatedly represent 18.6% of youth psychiatric emergencies [27]. When determining the need for admission to a psychiatric unit, the criteria used for children and adolescents are similar to the criteria used for adults. However, assessing factors such as parental/guardian involvement, home environment, and the ability of the caretakers to provide a safe environment are paramount.

Individuals with Personality Disorders

Assessing the risk of harm in individuals with a personality disorder is complicated. A period of observation is advisable, and it is recommended that the ED staff is extremely diligent when documenting observations and behaviors. Research suggests that having borderline personality disorder increases the odds that a person may be misdiagnosed with bipolar disorder [28]. This will be helpful in highlighting discrepancies between claims voiced by the patient and overall imminent risk. When evaluating patients with a personality disorder, it is important to consider the following warning signs [29]:

- History of recent suicide attempt that was unreported or only accidentally survived
- Occurrence of a violent episode immediately prior to presentation in the ED
- Severe life stressors or interpersonal conflicts
- Suicidal and or homicidal intent with a well-thought-out plan
- Carried out actions to implement the plan

- Intense rage against an identified person
- Intense guilt, self-hatred, or shame
- Extreme psychomotor agitation or anxiety
- Episode of physically or verbally threatening behaviors while in the ED

Patients with Substance-Use Disorder

When assessing risk in individuals with an ongoing substance use, the mental health provider should take into consideration how impairing use of the substance(s) may affect the individual's physical and psychological well-being. A period of observation is also helpful in these cases. In many instances, erratic behaviors and/or suicidal ideations will resolve once the patient is able to regain sobriety or as the effects of the drugs wear off. It is important to determine that a patient is medically and cognitively able to participate in the psychiatric interview, as intoxication often confounds the patient's behavioral reactions [30]. Extensive questioning about how the patient sees his/her use affecting their life and obtaining collateral information from relatives or other close contacts are critical factors in determining the level of lethality. In many cases, those who have lost control have already endangered themselves by getting involved in previous accidents while under the influence. A history of multiple unintended overdoses, visits to the emergency department, or aggression while intoxicated may indicate an increased level of risk. Patients who fail to comprehend the extent of their uncontrolled use and continue engaging in the behavior should be considered for inpatient commitment.

Conclusion

Predicting risk and determining who needs to be admitted to inpatient services is not easy, nor is there a magical formula that can be applied to guarantee safe outcomes. Mental health and emergency providers must justify, through comprehensive documentation, that the medical decisions were reasonable and professional. The increased pace of the ED environment should never become an excuse to derail us from a thorough consideration of all clinical data and resources. Facts should be documented in an objective tone and comprehensive manner, especially when considering disposition. As providers, we should maintain objectivity and avoid letting countertransference come between us and the impartiality of our clinical judgment.

References

1. Knoll JL. The psychiatric ER survival guide blog. New York: James Knoll; 2017. Cited 2017 Sept 15. Available at https://storage.googleapis.com/quantumunitsed.com/materials/3032_Psychiatric%20ER%20Survival%20Guide.pdf.
2. Ravindranath D, Newman M. Managing a psychiatric emergency: what every psychiatrist needs to know to be prepared. Psychiatr Times. 2010;27(7):17.
3. Mentalillnesspolicy.org. New York. Involuntary treatment and involuntary commitment laws: Basis in law and history; 2017. Cited 2017 Oct 15. Available at https://mentalillnesspolicy.org/ivc/involuntary-commitment-concepts.html.
4. Feuerstein S, Fortunati F, Morgan CA, Coric V, Temporini H, Southwick S. Civil commitment: a power granted to physicians by society. Psychiatry. 2005;2(8):53.
5. Johnson JM, Stern TA. Involuntary hospitalization of primary care patients. The Primary Care Companion for CNS Dis. 2014;16(3)
6. Gray C. Assessment of the suicidal patient in the emergency department. In: Zun L, Chepenik LG, Mallory MN, editors. Behavioral emergencies for the emergency physician. First ed. New York: Cambridge University Press; 2013. p. 60–6.
7. afsp.org/about-suicide/suicide-statistics/. New York: American Foundation for Suicide Prevention. 2018. Cited 2018 Apr 30. Available at https://afsp.org/about-suicide/suicide-statistics/.
8. Ronquillo L, Minassian A, Vilke GM, Wilson MP. Literature-based recommendations for suicide assessment in the emergency department: a review. J Emerg Med. 2012;43(5):836.
9. Assessing client dangerousness to self and others: Stratified risk management approaches. Berkeley: University of California; 2013. Updated 2013 Sept 18. Cited 2017 Dec 17. Available at https://socialwelfare.berkeley.edu/sites/default/files/users/gregmerrill/Assessing%20client%20dangerousness%20to%20self%20and%20others%2C%20stratified%20risk%20management%20approaches%2C%20Fall%202013.pdf.

10. Betz ME, Boudreaux ED. Managing suicidal patients in the emergency department. Ann Emerg Med. 2016;67(2):276.
11. Brown GK, Currier GW, Jager-Hyman S, Stanley B. Detection and classification of suicidal and non-suicidal self-injurious behavior in emergency department. J Clin Psy. 2015;76:10.
12. Campbell JC, Webster DW, Glass N. The danger assessment. J Interpers Violence. 2009;24(4):653.
13. Thienhaus OJ, Piasecki M. Assessment of psychiatric patients' risk of violence toward others. Psychiatr Serv. 1998;49(9):1129.
14. Kay SR, Wolkenfeld F, Murrill LM. Profiles of aggression among psychiatric patients: I. nature and prevalence. J Nerv Ment Dis. 1988;176(9):539.
15. Woods P, Almik R. The Brøset violence checklist. Acta Psychiatr Scand Suppl. 2002:103–5.
16. Yudofsky SC, Silver JM, Jackson W, Endicott J, Williams D. The overt aggression scale for the objective rating of verbal and physical aggression. Am J Psy. 1986;143(1):35.
17. Piechniczek-Buczek J. Psychiatric emergencies in the elderly population. Emerg Med Clin North Am. 2006;24(2):467.
18. American College of Emergency Medicine Practice Committee of the American College of Emergency Physicians. Care of the psychiatric patient in the emergency department—A review of the literature. 2014 Oct. Cited 2017 Sept 15. Available at https://www.acep.org/uploadedFiles/ACEP/Clinical_and_Practice_Management/Resources/Mental_Health_and_Substance_Abuse/Psychiatric%20Patient%20Care%20in%20the%20ED%202014.pdf.
19. Ward MA, Ahn J. Geriatric psychiatric emergencies. In: Zun L, Chepenik LG, Mallory MN, editors. Behavioral emergencies for the emergency physician. First ed. New York: Cambridge University Press; 2013. p. 219–23.
20. Reeves RR, Parker JD, Burke SR. Unrecognized physical illness prompting psychiatric admission. Ann Clin Psyc. 2010;22(3):180–3.
21. Inouye SK, van Dyck CH, Alessi CA, Balkin S, Siegal AP, Horwitz RI. Clarifying confusion: the confusion assessment method—a new method for detection of delirium. Ann Intern Med. 1990;113(12):941.
22. Centers for Disease Control. Prevention understanding suicide fact sheet; 2009. Cited 2017 Aug 30. Available at http://www.cdc.gov/violenceprevention/pdf/Suicide_FactSheet-a.pdf.
23. Waern M, Beskow J, Runeson B, Skoog I. Suicidal feelings in the last year of life in elderly people who commit suicide. Lancet. 1999;354(9182):917.
24. O'Connell H, Chin A, Cunningham C, Lawlor B. Alcohol use disorders in elderly people—redefining an age old problem in old age. Br Med J. 2003;327(7416):664.
25. Blow FC, Brower KJ, Shulenberg JE, Demo-Dananberg LM, Young JP, Beresford TP. The Michigan alcoholism screening test-geriatric version (MAST-G): a new elderly-specific screening instrument. Alcohol Clin Exp Res. 1992;16:372.
26. Dolan MA, Fein JA. Pediatric and adolescent mental health emergencies in the emergency medical services system. Pediatrics. 2011;127(5):e1356.
27. Boyer L, Henry J, Samuelian J, Belzeaux R, Auquier P, Lancon C, et al. Mental disorders among children and adolescents admitted to a french psychiatric emergency service. Emer Med International. 2013;2013:1.
28. Ruggero CJ, Zimmerman M, Chelminski I, Young D. Borderline personality disorder and the misdiagnosis of bipolar disorder. J Psychiatr Res 2009. 2010;44(6):405.
29. Beedle D. Personality disorder in the acute setting department. In: Zun L, Chepenik LG, Mallory MN, editors. Behavioral emergencies for the emergency physician. First ed. New York: Cambridge University Press; 2013. p. 109.
30. Lukens TW, Wolf SJ, Edlow JA, Shahabuddin S, Allen MH, Currier GW, et al. Clinical policy: critical issues in the diagnosis and management of the adult psychiatric patient in the emergency department. Ann Emerg Med. 2006;47(1):79.

De-escalation in the Emergency Department

21

Janet S. Richmond

Introduction

Agitation is a state of hyperarousal that can occur on a continuum ranging from anxiety to outright violence. Patients in emergency departments who present in an agitated state require immediate relief from their mounting tension [1–6]. Involuntary medication and restraint have been traditionally considered standard treatments for agitation. However, both are time-consuming and require many resources and much planning. Involuntary medication and restraint are considered coercive treatments and put the patient into a submissive position. When restraints are used, the main message is that physical force is the only method to resolve conflict, which is something that the agitated patient already believes to be true. These methods also reinforce that the patient cannot control his own behavior and that others are responsible for doing so. These methods can be dehumanizing, humiliating, and traumatizing [5, 7] or may have the unintended consequence of increasing agitation and thus lengthening the hospital stay [8, 9].

For the patient who is agitated but still in control, verbal de-escalation is an effective, easily learned, and quickly implemented intervention that can often obviate the need for restraint or forced medication. While the need for these latter interventions is necessary for patients who have moved beyond the point of reason and containment, verbal de-escalation can still be utilized at some point in the management of even the most agitated patients. When verbal de-escalation is used, staff morale is enhanced because "managing a behavioral emergency competently can be very rewarding" [7].

This chapter discusses techniques based on this author's experience and an expert consensus of The American Association for Emergency Psychiatry (AAEP) [1].

Case Example

A twenty-two-year-old man was brought to the emergency department (ED) after police received several calls by his neighbors complaining that he had been up for several nights screaming, slamming doors, and appeared "out of it." He had just moved into the rooming house and was not known to the community.

The patient was agitated, attempted to leave the ED, and repeatedly yelled about needing to get to "Randy." This was interspersed with

J. S. Richmond (✉)
Department of Psychiatry, VA Boston Healthcare System, Boston, MA, USA

McLean Hospital, Belmont, MA, USA

Tufts University School of Medicine, Boston, MA, USA

L. S. Zun et al. (eds.), *Behavioral Emergencies for Healthcare Providers*,
https://doi.org/10.1007/978-3-030-52520-0_21

statements that he was a psychiatrist and needed to speak with the director of the hospital to be deemed "sane." Staff began the process of getting physical restraints and drawing up IM haloperidol and lorazepam. The clinician, however, on a hunch, sat in front of the patient, made eye contact, and asked, "Who's Randy?"

The patient stopped all his movement, stared at the clinician, and began to cry. Randy was his dog who had just died. This had prompted him to move from his home in another state and rent his current room. He had been off his medication for several weeks, had not been sleeping, and had decompensated into a psychotic state. The clinician and he talked about his deep loss. Then he requested to resume his usual medication. The clinician was able to reach the man's clinicians in the other state and arrange hospitalization.

Signs of Escalating Agitation

Signs and symptoms of agitation include excessive, repetitive, and purposeless motor or verbal activity [1]. Examples are pacing, fidgeting, clenching fists or teeth, a prolonged stare, picking at clothing or skin, threatening to or throwing objects, or responding to internal stimuli (usually auditory or visual hallucinations). Psychotic patients often look around the room, trying to "track" or locate the source of their voices. The goal is to keep agitation from escalating.

Increased pacing, irritability, impatience, frustration, verbal outbursts, slamming or banging objects, an exaggerated startle response, increased sweating or hyperventilation, labile affect, paranoia, defiance; demanding or threatening behaviors are signs that the agitation is escalating. The clinician needs to monitor even small changes in behavior and respond quickly to avoid further escalation [1, 5, 7].

Safety: The Environment, Physical Space, and Staffing

Verbal de-escalation also involves nonverbal and environmental components. [4, 5]. If the clinician or other staff do not feel safe, then no treatment can occur. Since existing emergency departments have different physical layouts, each facility must deal with their specific space issues. The ideal location would be a quiet area away from the more active ED but with accessibility to emergency restraints, adequate space, and additional staffing should the patient escalate to violent behavior. Since furniture and equipment may be a distraction or used as a weapon by the patient, these objects should be kept to a minimum. Video cameras can be helpful so that patients can be monitored from the nursing station. However, patients who are truly at risk for harmful activity to themselves or others require continuous in-person observation. Before placement into a room, a "health and safety" search is recommended to look for items that could be used as weapons. Patients may be instructed to change into a hospital gown to ensure that there are no concealed weapons and to allow for a complete physical examination [2, 5]. These patients are also less likely to leave before evaluation is complete.

Staffing

When working with an agitated patient, staff must always be prepared for the worst-case scenario, which generally involves physical restraint. Thus, working with an agitated patient is a team effort, and there must be an adequate number of people to fill each role on the team. Ideally, the de-escalation team should consist of four to six team members made up of nurses, clinicians, technicians, and police and security officers, if available [1]. A mechanism such as a centrally located panic button or overhead intercom should exist to call upon additional help as needed. Staff members and police should be at the bedside of any patient who is or has the potential to be moderately or severely agitated.

General Approaches to Verbal De-escalation

The goals of verbal de-escalation are to contain the patient's emotional turmoil, define the problem, and elicit the patient's "request" [1, 10]. Asking the patient what outcome he or she would like from his

ED visit builds rapport and a therapeutic alliance. There is evidence that the better the relationship, the less likelihood of further escalation [11, 12]. In building this relationship, caution should be given to presuming a working alliance prematurely or trying to establish one when one is already present. Younger clinicians can especially err in this area, not recognizing that an adequate alliance has been made. The clinician should be aware that some patients are defensive because they have had past traumatic experiences such as difficult medical treatments or procedures, or problematic interactions with physicians. A trauma-informed approach is recommended. In other words, the clinician should be aware that any patient could have a traumatic past that can arouse feelings of vulnerability and loss of control. Patients with a history of sexual or physical abuse may be hypervigilant around being disrobed or touched. If the patient refuses to speak or disrobe, ask the patient to write or draw what is on their mind. Finally, some patients perceive the need to seek help as shameful and humiliating. This may cause some patients to become anxious or defensive, which then can escalate to agitation. If the clinician is not sensitive to this possibility, power struggles can occur when both patient and provider feel disempowered and feel (or fear being) humiliated [13].

Verbal de-escalation requires staff attitudes to change from power and control to engagement and cooperation, without sacrificing one's authority and the safety of the patient and those involved in his care [4]. De-escalation is a team effort, and any member of the staff can intervene. As in cardiac arrest, one staff person (preferably someone skilled and comfortable with de-escalation and who knows the patient) should be in charge of the de-escalation. If that person is not comfortable, then another staff member should take over. Hospital security and experienced nursing staff can be extremely helpful, as they often have years of experience in the management of agitated patients and are skillful at defusing tense situations. Unlike a traditional code, the person leading it does not have to be the physician. The ability to connect with the patient is key.

Like any other emergency, agitation must be addressed directly and swiftly, even when the etiology is unclear. The objective of any encounter with an agitated patient is to help him or her become cooperative, stay in control, and prevent further escalation [4]. This means that the clinician needs to stabilize the patient's level of agitation before attempting to further evaluate the patient. Obtaining vital signs, doing a physical examination, performing diagnostic studies, or attempting to explore the nature of the patient's distress may all result in escalation of the patient's agitation and even violence unless the patient is stabilized first. An initial attempt at de-escalation and measures to ensure the safety of all involved, including the patient, should take precedence.

The Clinician's Demeanor: Body Language, Speech, and Attitude

The clinician must demonstrate by body language that he will not harm the patient, that he or she wants to listen and would like everyone to be safe. Normal, friendly eye contact should be used, but excessive eye contact can be interpreted as an aggressive act. Even normal eye contact may be difficult for the paranoid patient who cannot tolerate that level of intimacy. If the patient is pacing, one recommendation is to walk with the patient, but at a slower pace. Stooping so as to make oneself appear smaller is also a consideration [1, 6].

Both the patient and clinician should have equal access to the exit—neither should feel trapped. The clinician should not crowd the patient and should stand or sit at least a leg's length from the patient so that the clinician will not be injured by kicking. If a patient tells you to get out of the room, do so [1, 5, 14]. This is not the time to set limits or assert one's authority. Understanding the meaning of the patient's order can come later. Speaking to a patient from the doorway is also a safety measure.

If the clinician becomes anxious while in the examination room, one option is to leave the room quickly and call for help [1, 5, 15]. Taking a break is often useful. If the patient is starting to get under the clinician's skin, state, "Okay, let's take a few minutes … Things seem to be getting too hot in here … Let's both calm down, and I'll be back in ten minutes." It is essential to then be back as stated in 10 minutes. Sometimes, this process needs to be repeated several times until the patient and clinician can have a reasonable conversation.

Hands should be visible and not clenched. Concealed hands, either behind one's back or in one's pockets, can raise the patient's suspicion that the clinician may have a concealed weapon [1, 6]. Closed body language, such as arm folding or turning away, can communicate lack of interest. The message, verbal and otherwise, is that "I want to help. I'm here to listen. Let's talk about this."

Slow, repetitive, soft speech is best with the escalating patient to help him regain control [1]. Agitated patients can be provocative and may challenge the authority, competence, or credentials of the clinician. Some patients deflect their own vulnerability by detecting the clinician's vulnerability and focusing on that. In these instances, the clinician should understand his own tendencies to retaliate, argue, or otherwise become defensive [1, 4, 5, 7, 16]. Such behaviors on the part of the clinician only serve to worsen the situation and create iatrogenic escalation.

If the clinician can remind himself that the patient's behavior is not willful, but part of his psychopathology, this can help diminish some of the frustration. For example, the delirious, psychotic, intoxicated, or intellectually disabled patient is impaired in his or her ability to cooperate. Others with dysfunctional personality traits are demonstrating ingrained, automatic behavior that are the only strategies these patients know that will get their needs met [1]. Patients do not come to the ED purposely to frustrate or get into arguments with the providers, but it may seem that way in a busy ED with a boisterous and agitated patient. Finally, flexibility, spontaneity, and authenticity are very useful character traits for working with the agitated patient.

Eliciting the Patient's "Request"

Determine what the patient wants to have happen and allow the patient the opportunity to state it, even if the request cannot be granted. Be patient and provide the patient with ample time to speak, Statements like "I really need to know what you expected when you came here" are as essential as is the caveat "Even if I can't provide it, I would like to know, so we can work on it." For an escalating patient, offering food, water, a blanket, or allowing the patient to make a telephone call might well decrease the degree of agitation. If an agitated patient comes to the ED demanding medication, it may be best to give him or her the desired medication if appropriate, even if the way it was requested was not appropriate [14, 15]. Given the need for quick symptom reduction, honoring the patient's request may prove useful, as the patient likely knows what works best. By not attending to the request, the patient may feel dismissed, misunderstood, or unheard. At the very least, a discussion about the medication should ensue. Sometimes, the answer to the request is "Yes, but not yet." Consider the following interchange:

Patient: "I want to get the f____ out of here!"

Staff: "Great. That's my job, to start the process of your getting out. (the "yes"). The bottom line is that people will need to see that it's safe for you to go. (the "not yet"). Maybe I can help with that. Perhaps some medication might help with that."

Finally, as with the case example above, attend to any real-life problems that need to be dealt with as urgently as the psychiatric condition because these may be part of the reason for the agitation.

Cultural, Ethnic, Age, and Gender Issues

Attention to the patient's gender, age, ethnicity, and cultural background is important. For example, direct eye contact and handshaking in some cultures are unacceptable. Some cultures require a same-sexed clinician to examine the patient. However, if this is not possible, the patient needs to know. "I regret that I cannot do as you ask. I understand that it would be more comfortable/acceptable for you to be examined by a female clinician, but I am the only clinician covering the emergency room this evening. I will certainly ask [a female staff person] to be in the room when I perform my examination." If the patient's cultural needs are unfamiliar to the clinician, asking the patient to educate him can also build an alliance by empowering the patient to teach the clinician about a subject in which he is an expert. Another consideration is whether the patient needs or wants an interpreter. Ideally, interpreters should be professionals.

Recommended Communication Techniques

Table 21.1 provides a summary of de-escalation techniques. Table 21.2 provides strategies when approaching the agitated patient, based on Fishkind's "10 domains of de-escalation" (see Table 21.3) [1, 14, 15].

Table 21.1 Summary of de-escalation strategies

Observation
Sympathy
Empathy, honesty, and prudent self-disclosure
Dilute the intensity of the interaction; bring in another staff member
Appeal to the patient's rationale
Bargaining
Offer choices
Limit-setting/informing patient about consequences
Giving instructions

Table 21.2 Avoiding interview mistakes

Arguing with the patient
Being judgmental
Being or being perceived as punitive or threatening
Failing to recognize when a therapeutic alliance has been achieved
Making assumptions/empathic failures
Being overly empathic
Inadvertently provoking the patient
Inadvertently humiliating the patient
Trying to dissuade a fixed belief or delusion
Failing to take a trauma-informed approach

Table 21.3 10 domains of de-escalation

Respect personal space
Monitor one's own emotional reactions
Do not be provocative
Establish verbal contact; identify wants and feelings
Use simple, concise language
Listen closely to what the patient is saying
Agree or agree to disagree
Set clear limits in a non-punitive manner
Offer choices and optimism
Debrief the patient and staff

Adapted from: Fishkind [15]

Observation Observing the patient is a good way to determine the level of agitation and determine if extra staff are needed.

Sympathy If the physician can sympathize with the patient and his situation, the patient will sense this. For example, one can readily sympathize with someone who is frightened or who has waited a long time to be seen. However, some patients misinterpret signs of sympathy with being pitied, so one must observe the patient's behavior and affect closely.

Empathy, Honesty, and Prudent Self-Disclosure Some measured self-disclosure may be helpful: "I can't concentrate on your needs if I'm worried about my own safety." Or ask the patient quite upfront, "Do I need to worry about my safety in here?" Or say, "I'm not feeling comfortable in here. Are you having the same feeling?" A general rule is that this type of self-disclosure can have a salutary effect on the patient, without violating boundaries or undermining the physician's role [1, 7].

Dilute the Intensity of the Interaction Bring in another staff member. Ideally, this would be someone who has established some rapport with the patient or who is neutral. Nursing staff are particularly helpful in these situations, as are peer specialists. Appealing to the patient's rational side [4, 7] partners the patient with the clinician in attempting to keep the peace. For example, statements such as "You know, there are some very ill and distressed people here who need things to be quiet" can distract the patient from his own agitation.

Bargaining Consider using bargaining to get the patient to take a medication that may reduce his level of agitation. "I'll give you a sandwich, but I would like you to also take this pill, which will make you feel better" [1, 5]. If the patient is experiencing pain, addressing their discomfort may result in a more cooperative patient.

Offer Choices For example, stating, "You can take the medication by mouth, or we can give you an injection ['shot']—which would you prefer?" This gives the patient control over one part of the decision, even though the overall decision is not his to make [1, 5, 14, 15].

Limit-Setting Less experienced clinicians may be at greater risk of being assaulted because they may be more hesitant to set limits and therefore are more likely to allow threatening behavior to escalate [7]. Limit-setting needs to be stated in a neutral, non-emotional manner and not when the clinician is feeling perturbed. If the clinician finds himself becoming annoyed with the patient, it is easy to inadvertently lapse into irrational thinking and maladaptive behaviors that can escalate the situation because the patient feels judged, humiliated, or provoked. Take a break and calm down either by speaking to another colleague or distracting yourself with another task until calmer. When calm, the clinician needs to apologize for his behavior. A heartfelt apology is an indicator of the clinician's ability to self-reflect, admit his errors, and role-model proper behavior for the patient [13]. The clinician needs to be keenly attuned to his own biases, temperament, and countertransference.

If the patient appears able to listen, initiate a discussion: "When you do/say that, I feel irritated, and if that happens, I can't be attentive to your needs" [1, 4, 14, 15].

Giving Instructions Use clear, specific statements such as "I want you to put down the chair" or state that violence will not be tolerated [1]. "You need to demonstrate to me that you can stay in control so that I can be of help to you." The patient may be able to turn his attention away long enough to distract himself from his own distress. However, telling a patient to "calm down" may not be useful [3] because the patient doesn't know how to calm down. He needs instruction and help doing so. "What do you do to help yourself calm down? How can I help you calm down?"

Confrontation This technique can quickly lead to further escalation and needs to be used very judiciously. If properly timed, however, confrontation can be very useful. An example might be an observation followed by exploration: "You appear to want to pick a fight. Please help me understand why you want to do this."

State Consequences of the Behavior [1, 3, 6, 15] Consequences of disruptive behavior must be stated in a matter-of-fact manner, giving the patient the facts without inadvertently humiliating or coming across as punitive. For example, stating clearly and calmly to the patient that "We need the blood drawn; you can either do this willingly, or we will have to restrain you to do this." Caution is that such statements should not be said until ample staff and equipment are available to act on the consequence should the patient not be able to engage. Threatening to call security is generally not helpful, interferes with any trust the patient may be developing, and can lead to more agitation [2]. If police are needed, then call them without announcement.

Agree with the Patient as Much as You Can; Don't Argue with a Delusion If a patient challenges the physician because he believes he has waited too long to be seen ("How would you feel if you had to wait this long?"), the physician can agree that "Waiting is difficult" or "No, I don't like to wait either." If the patient insults the clinician— "I don't want to see a rotten doctor!"—the response might be, "How do you know? You just met me. Can you give me a chance?"

If a delusional patient challenges you by stating, "You don't believe me, do you?" then the response could be "I have never personally had that experience, but I can agree that I wouldn't like that either." Or, "I can see how angry that would make anyone, but I don't agree that retaliation is the solution."

Avoiding Interview Mistakes

Failing to recognize when an adequate alliance is present, making assumptions, verbalizing observations prematurely, making too empathic a statement to paranoid patients, and failing to be sensitive to the possibility of a past traumatic experience are errors easily made. If made, do apologize. Arguing with the patient, appearing punitive, threatening, or judgmental can provoke a patient into (further) agitation [1, 4, 14, 15]. In addition, empathic failures can lead to iatrogenic escalation.

An example of an empathic failure is assuming you know how the patient feels. For example, "You must feel scared" might provoke the following response: "No! I'm furious! You're not listening to me!"

Another example of an empathic failure is failing to address the patient's request once it is elicited. "You've told me very clearly that you want to go home tonight, but that's not going to be possible, because things have reached such a crisis point that I believe you need to come into the hospital." (Once again, as a safety precaution, this should be conveyed when there are enough staff with the clinician to respond if the patient becomes more agitated or attempts to leave the ED).

As noted earlier, if not addressed, the patient may feel dismissed, misunderstood, or humiliated, and these feelings can lead to agitation.

Trying to Dissuade a Fixed Belief or Delusion can escalate a patient [1, 5, 7]. If he states that he is being followed by aliens, the clinician may gently challenge this to determine the degree of the delusion. However, it is of no use to suggest that it is impossible. The clinician can ask, "How do you know that your neighbor is bugging your apartment?" The more elaborate the explanation, the more delusional. If the patient states, "Well, I think he has some microphones, but I can't know for sure," then the delusion is less fixed.

Special Patient Situations

The anxious patient can become irritable and even hostile and aggressive when anxious enough. Reassurance and frequent checks by staff are helpful if there is a long wait to be seen. Leaving the examination room door open so that the patient does not feel isolated and alone can be helpful, even when intuitively and for confidentiality's sake it would seem that a closed door would be more appropriate.

The delirious patient is typically disoriented, usually paranoid, and may be experiencing hallucinations, including visual and tactile. There are multiple causes for delirium, some of which are life-threatening, and these need to be promptly investigated and treated by the provider. Most medical causes of delirium fall into four general categories: (1) toxicologic (including withdrawal); (2) metabolic (e.g., endocrine, fluid, and electrolytes); (3) infection; or (4) intracranial pathology. Reassurance, cold compresses, blankets, food, or water may help the agitated patient calm down. Repeated low-toned reminders as to where the patient is, why they are in the ED, and the roles of staff are key. If possible, one staff person can be assigned to the patient to repeatedly explain, orient, and speak calmly to the patient. This may also be necessary for safety concerns. Family members can also serve this function.

The Paranoid Patient By acknowledging the patient's difficulty with trust, the interviewer may be able to establish enough rapport so that the patient can participate in the evaluation [2, 5, 7]. For example: "I can understand your reluctance to believe that I want to help; could we sit down and talk? Perhaps I'll be able to demonstrate to you through my attitude and speech that what I say is trustworthy."

The Disorganized/Psychotic Patient The psychotic patient's thinking can become quite loose and tangential. When interviewing acutely psychotic patients, the clinician should assess symptoms without attempting to use logic or to convince the patient that his perceptions are wrong [1, 4, 5]. Short, simple statements and instructions should be utilized.

The acutely traumatized patient fears being (re) traumatized or humiliated, and can become defensive quite quickly. He or she may appear frightened, even paranoid, and defend himself or herself through anger and other distancing behaviors. Make no sudden movements so as not to startle them, explain what you are going to do and why you are doing it. For example, explain each step of the rape kit protocol. This may need to be stated repeatedly. State that you want to help the patient feel safe and in control. However, overly empathic statements can be misperceived as being seductive. Since a history of trauma is frequently unknown, it is best for the clinician to approach all patients in a trauma-informed manner.

The personality disordered patient often assumes that he or she won't get needs met in the ED and is often dissatisfied with care. He or she may try to wear the clinician down, hoping that he will "give in" to his demands. These patients are anxious, easily misinterpret interactions, project their feelings onto others, and blame others for their distress. They may have labile moods and move from restlessness to agitation to argumentativeness quickly. Dealing with them can be challenging and irritating [16]. Monitoring one's own minute-by-minute emotional reactions is key, and prudent self-disclosure is effective. Techniques include setting limits, appealing to the patient's rational side, and maintaining an attitude of genuine curiosity and honesty. Give consequences and instructions. Be empathic, but not overly so, because such statements can be perceived as pitying or infantilizing. Borghesani et al. [17] recommend motivational interviewing techniques and "problem solving therapy" to help contain the personality-disordered patient's agitation.

Approaching the Patient about Psychiatric Medication

Offering medication can help the patient feel cared for. Like food or water, giving medication can be soothing. Zeller offers a stepwise method of introducing the topic of medication [1, 4, 15].

Ask the patient "What has worked for you in the past?" If the patient refuses medication, an educational role is best: "It is important for you to calm down, and medication can help do that." If the patient still refuses, an authoritative (not authoritarian) technique is implemented: "It is my opinion that medication is necessary," and then give a choice—"Would you prefer drug X or drug Y?"—and explain some of the benefits and side effects if the patient is unfamiliar with them.

Another approach is to provide the patient with some "incentive," such as telling them you are going to give them a sandwich and some medication, or that you are going to give them a sandwich if they take a medication to help them feel better. Oral medication may be an easier alternative for medication administration (please see Chap. 23, "Agitation in the Emergency Department"). For example, olanzapine has both antipsychotic and sedative properties, and comes in the ODT formulation. This can easily be administered to most mildly agitated patients in the ED and can be combined with verbal de-escalation techniques to prevent these patients from escalating to a more severely agitated state.

Finally, stating, "This is an emergency, and I am going to give you [medication X]." Then, continue to offer choices: "Would you prefer a shot or a pill?" Fishkind [15] recommends using vernacular instead of clinical terms; hence, the word "shot" for "injection." In these situations, be prepared to have both oral and injectable forms of the medication on hand and ample number of staff to implement the plan if forceful administration is required due to safety concerns—and after all other attempts to de-escalate the patient have failed [1].

Debriefing

An often-neglected part of de-escalation is debriefing of both staff and patient [4]. The patient needs to be empowered to state what would be helpful in the future, should such an occurrence repeat. A patient might say, "If I'm upset, please don't give me haloperidal; give me risperidone." A flag can then be placed on the patient's chart for future reference.

Conclusion

Agitation is a common presentation in the emergency department. This chapter has addressed techniques of verbal de-escalation that the emergency clinician can quickly learn and implement as an alternative to seclusion and restraint. Ultimately, verbal de-escalation improves staff morale and patient adherence, because it utilizes a noncoercive, patient-centered approach. Verbal de-escalation takes no more than 5–10 minutes and enhances the doctor–patient relationship, while seclusion and restraint require more staff and ultimately take more time and resources to implement. The offering of medication can be considered part of verbal de-escalation, and methods of introducing the subject of taking medication can be done in increments as outlined in this chapter.

References

1. Richmond JS, Berlin JS, Fishkind AB, Holloman GH Jr, Zeller SL, Wilson MP, et al. Verbal de-escalation of the agitated patient: consensus statement of the american association for emergency psychiatry project BETA de-escalation workgroup. West J Emerg Med. 2012;13(1):17–25.
2. Rossi J, Swan MC, Isaacs ED. The violent or agitated patient. Emerg Med Clinics North America. 2010;28(1):235–56.
3. Lofchy J, Fage B. Practical tips for managing the agitated patient: avoiding violence in the clinical setting. Psychiatric Times. 2017. Available at http://www.psychiatrictimes.com/special-reports/practical-tips-managing-agitated-patient-avoiding-violence-clinical-setting.
4. Berlin JS. Collaborative de-escalation. In: Zeller SL, Wilson MP, editors. The diagnosis and management of agitation. Cambridge: Cambridge University Press; 2017. p. 144–55.
5. Novitsky MA. Non-pharmacological management of violence in psychiatric emergencies. Primary Psy. 2009;16:49–53.
6. Frueh BC, Knapp RG, Cusack KJ, Grubaugh AL, Sauvageot JA, Cousins VC, et al. Special section on seclusion and restraint: patients' reports of traumatic or harmful experiences within the psychiatric setting. Psychiatr Serv. 2005;56(9):1123–33.
7. Kleespies P, Richmond JS. Evaluating behavior emergencies: the clinical interview. In: Kleespies P, editor. Behavioral emergencies: an evidence-based resource for evaluating and managing risk of suicide, violence, and victimization. Washington, DC: American Psychological Association; 2009. p. 33–55.
8. Weiss AP, Chang G, Rauch SL, Smallwood JA, Schechter M, Kosowsky J, et al. Patient- and practice-related determinants of emergency department length of stay for patients with psychiatric illness. Ann Emerg Med. 2012;60(2):162–71. e5
9. Wilson MP, Pepper D, Currier GW, Holloman GH Jr, Feifel D. The psychopharmacology of agitation: consensus statement of the american association for emergency psychiatry project beta psychopharmacology workgroup. West J Emerg Med. 2012;13(1):26–34.
10. Lazare A, Eisenthal S, Wasserman L. The customer approach to patienthood: attending to patient requests in a walk-in clinic. Arch Gen Psychiatry. 1975;32(5):553–8.
11. Beauford JE, McNiel DE, Binder RL. Utility of the initial therapeutic alliance in evaluating psychiatric patients' risk of violence. Am J Psychiatry. 1997;154(9):1272–6.
12. Polaschek DL, Ross EC. Do early therapeutic alliance, motivation, and stages of change predict therapy change for high-risk, psychopathic violent prisoners? Crim Behav Ment Health. 2010;20(2):100–11.
13. Lazare A. Shame and humiliation in the medical encounter. Arch Intern Med. 1987;147(9):1653–8.
14. Fishkind A. Agitation II: de-escalation of the aggressive patient and avoiding coercion. In: Glick RL, Berlin JS, Fishkind A, Zeller SL, editors. Emergency psychiatry: principles and practice. Philadelphia: Wolters Kluwer Health/Lippincott Williams & Wilkins; 2008. p. 125–36.
15. Fiskind A. Calming agitation with words, not drugs: 10 commandments for safety. Curr Psychol. 2002;1(4):32–40. Available at http://www.currentpsychiatry.com/pdf/0104/0104_Fishkind.pdf. Accessed 29 Sept 2017.
16. Groves JE. Taking care of the hateful patient. New England J Med. 1978;29:883–7.
17. Borghesani PR, Romm S, Pasic J. Psychiatric causes of agitation: exacerbation of personality disorders. In: Zeller SL, Nordstrom KD, Wilson MP, editors. The diagnosis and management of agitation. Cambridge: Cambridge University Press; 2017. p. 104–25.

22 Peer Mentors in the Emergency Department

Samuel Mullinax and Michael P. Wilson

Introduction

> Near the end of that bleak November, I sat drinking in my kitchen. With a certain satisfaction, I reflected there was enough gin concealed about the house to carry me through that night and the next day. My wife was at work. I wondered whether I dared hide a full bottle of gin near the head of our bed. I would need it before daylight.
>
> My musing was interrupted by the telephone. The cheery voice of an old school friend asked if he might come over. He was sober. It was years since I could remember his coming to New York in that condition. I was amazed. Rumor had it that he had been committed for alcoholic insanity. I wondered how he had escaped. Of course, he would have dinner, and then I could drink openly with him. Unmindful of his welfare, I thought only of recapturing the spirit of other days. There was that time we had chartered an airplane to complete a jag! His coming was an oasis in this dreary desert of futility. The very thing—an oasis! Drinkers are like that.
>
> The door opened and he stood there, fresh-skinned and glowing. There was something about his eyes. He was inexplicably different. What had happened?
>
> I pushed a drink across the table. He refused it. Disappointed but curious, I wondered what had got into the fellow. He wasn't himself [1].

These paragraphs begin an account of what would arguably prove the most impactful peer-mentoring intervention of the twentieth century: Alcoholics Anonymous (AA). Bill Wilson, the narrator of the story above, is recounting a meeting he had with his friend Ebby Thacher. Wilson had endured numerous unsuccessful hospitalizations for alcoholism and had nearly given up hope that his condition could ever be treated when Thacher visited with the news that he had managed to remain abstinent from alcohol for a sustained period of time:

> He had come to pass his experience along to me—if I cared to have it. I was shocked but interested. Certainly, I was interested. I had to be, for I was hopeless [1].

The following month, Wilson was hospitalized for alcohol dependence for the last time; he attributed his willingness to seek a final round of treatment, as well as his motivation to maintain lifelong sobriety, to the conversation he had at his kitchen table:

> While I lay in the hospital the thought came that there were thousands of hopeless alcoholics who might be glad to have what had been so freely given me. Perhaps I could help some of them. They, in turn, might work with others [1].

S. Mullinax (✉) · M. P. Wilson
Department of Emergency Medicine, University of Arkansas for Medical Sciences, Little Rock, AR, USA
e-mail: mpwilso1@outlook.com

L. S. Zun et al. (eds.), *Behavioral Emergencies for Healthcare Providers*, https://doi.org/10.1007/978-3-030-52520-0_22

Alcoholics Anonymous would later go on to become a worldwide organization, with a membership estimated at over two million as of 2016 [2].

Much like Alcoholics Anonymous, evidence for the efficacy of other peer support interventions is mixed [3–5]. However, the premise of peer support is simple, yet appealing: Patients suffering from emergent psychiatric symptoms may be less inclined to engage in substance abuse or violence if they are given the opportunity to talk with a peer mentor who has experience with overcoming similar issues.

Definition of Peer Support

Peer mentoring (or peer support) is defined by Bouchard et al. as "a relationship in which persons voluntarily and spontaneously interact to give and receive help, addressing individual issues or shared concerns" [6]. Peer mentors may be effective because they serve as role models who display behaviors that their peers wish to emulate [7, 8]. Such an individual might be perceived as more approachable and less intimidating than other healthcare professionals, both because they do not exist within a traditional institutional hierarchy and because it is easier for them to empathize with the patient. While they may be seen as less authoritarian, peer mentors might still be regarded by patients as credible, compelling, and inspirational role models, due to their reliance upon their own firsthand empirical experience when making suggestions [9]. Furthermore, as Bill Wilson intuited, peer mentors (known as "sponsors" in AA) may simultaneously reinforce their own recovery from psychiatric illness through the provision of such support and increased identification with their role as a caregiver [6, 10].

Many studies have provided evidence suggesting that maintaining social connectedness is important for suicide prevention [11–15]. The interpersonal theory of suicide suggests that psychological constructs such as thwarted belongingness and perceived burdensomeness make an individual more likely to attempt suicide [16]. Given that the majority of suicides occur within 30 days after discharge from the hospital or emergency department [17, 18], peer mentors may provide a sense of social connectedness and self-acceptance during this critical period, thereby preventing suicide by modifying the interpersonal constructs of thwarted belongingness and perceived burdensomeness.

While Alcoholics Anonymous is perhaps the most recognizable peer mentoring organization, as a mutual support group, it represents only one specific type of peer support. At least three different models of peer support have been described in the literature: mutual support groups, auxiliary peer support services, and peer mental health service providers (please see Table 22.1).

The limited evidence available regarding the use of peer mentors in acute settings suggests that peer support services and peer mental health service providers are more likely than mutual support groups such as Alcoholics Anonymous to be integrated into acute settings such as emergency departments (EDs).

As defined in a recent systematic review, peer support service providers are peer mentors who provide supplemental assistance that complements the standard psychiatric care provided by medical staff [19]. An example of this model has been implemented in the ED at Maine Medical

Table 22.1 Models of peer support [19]

Mutual support groups	Peers who have varying degrees of lived experience dealing with a mental illness but who typically lack medical training mentor one another with recovery, usually outside of a medical setting
Peer support services	Peer mentors who have substantial lived experience dealing with mental illness patients and typically lack medical training provide additional therapeutic support to patients already receiving treatment in a medical setting
Peer mental health service providers	Peer mentors who have substantial lived experience dealing with mental illness patients and have also received medical training provide direct treatment to patients in a medical setting

Center by Amistad Peer Support and Recovery. According to their website:

> Peer Supporters will make sure that you get a meal or drink if that would be helpful. They make sure that you understand what is happening. They can share their experience with you, or just sit with you. They will help you pass the time, play cards with you, or offer you reading or writing material. They can share resources with you, or skills that they have found useful once you are out of the emergency room [20].

Similarly, Anchor Recovery Community Center in Rhode Island dispatches trained peer recovery coaches to local EDs as part of a program called AnchorED. Recovery coaches assist opioid overdose patients with discharge planning, harm reduction, and follow-up treatment [21].

Hypothetically, allowing patients to feel heard and receive emotional support from a nonmedical individual with lived experience, both in the ED and after discharge, could reduce ED resource utilization both at the intervention visit and in the future. However, there are no studies of this in the ED literature.

Peer mental health service providers are paid ED staff who have previous experience as consumers of psychiatric services. They deliver the standard ED psychiatric care traditionally provided by ED staff, as most medical staff presumably have less lived experience with mental illness [19].

Evidence for Peer Support

In a 2003 survey conducted by Allen et al., patients who had previously experienced behavioral emergencies expressed a preference for increased use of peer support services throughout the course of their psychiatric treatment [22]. Despite the enthusiasm from patients, peer support has had sometimes disappointing results in randomized trials. Much of the existing research on peer support is unfortunately limited by unstandardized interventions, variable settings, and a lack of large, randomized, controlled trials [23]. The literature has also largely focused on outpatient support groups or peer-delivered information, which is primarily unidirectional [19].

In other populations, such as those in pediatric emergency departments, however, the provision of emotional support by specially trained nonmedical personnel has had more success. Use of peer support in pediatric emergency departments has been shown to result in less distress, reduce anxiety, and promote coping [24, 25].

While further studies are needed to support the use of peer mentors in the treatment of behavioral emergencies, particularly in emergency department settings, at least one large, randomized, controlled trial found that a peer-led intervention decreased psychiatric symptoms and increased hopefulness, as well as quality of life among a population of severely mentally ill outpatients [26]. Another randomized, controlled trial showed a reduction in psychiatric hospitalizations for patients assigned a peer mentor [27]. Systematic reviews by Davidson et al. [28] and Chinman et al. [29] suggest that peer mentors may be equally as effective as conventional providers, but that more rigorous methodologies will be required in future studies to tease out the active ingredients of the intervention.

Mental health peer mentor training and certification programs already have wide popular support; such programs either currently exist or are under development in 43 states. While further study of its efficacy is needed, peer mentoring represents a promising and cost-effective intervention for behavioral emergencies that could benefit both patients and their peer mentors. Although increasingly popular in the outpatient setting, there are as of yet no randomized trials to support the use of peer mentors instead of traditional emergency department staff. Intuitively, however, peer supporters may have more insight into the nature of mental illness. In addition, if peer support was shown to significantly reduce symptoms of suicidal ideation, agitation, or substance abuse among psychiatric consumers in the ED, it might be a cheaper way of improving patient-centered care while freeing up more expensive staff and resources for those with acute medical illnesses or more severe psychiatric symptoms. Such conversations might also be followed by caring contacts such as phone calls, text messages, or postcards from their peer mentor. Another unanswered question is whether allowing those with emergent psychiatric conditions to speak with peer mentors in the ED might have the unintended consequence of actually increasing ED utilization by patients hoping to see their new friend.

Conclusion

Peer mentoring is a promising intervention for psychiatric emergencies because it has the potential to conserve behavioral healthcare resources while satisfying the stated desire of patients to speak with someone like themselves. Theoretically, recovery communities may represent an attractive alternative to overburdened local mental health services. In such a model, patients with emergent symptoms could utilize professional medical treatment while their peers freely support one another in daily maintenance to prevent such episodes from occurring. In an emergent setting, peer support may theoretically provide information and reassurance for patients who are in a busy, chaotic emergency department. Thus, use of peer mentors intuitively seems as though it would have obvious benefits for patients. However, this concept needs further study with more rigorous methodology in order to fully assess potential benefits.

References

1. Anonymous. Alcoholics anonymous: the story of how many thousands of men and women have recovered from alcoholism. Alcoholics anonymous world services. 2001.
2. Estimated worldwide A.A. individual and group membership. Alcoholics Anonymous, General Service Office. Available at http://www.aa.org/assets/en_US/smf-132_en.pdf.
3. Ferri M, Amato L, Davoli M. Alcoholics anonymous and other 12-step programmes for alcohol dependence. Cochrane Libr. 2006;
4. Kaskutas LA. Alcoholics anonymous effectiveness: faith meets science. J Addict Dis. 2009;28(2):145–57.
5. Humphreys K, Blodgett JC, Wagner TH. Estimating the efficacy of alcoholics anonymous without self-selection bias: an instrumental variables re-analysis of randomized clinical trials. Alcohol Clin Exp Res. 2014;38(11):2688–94.
6. Bouchard L, Montreuil M, Gros C. Peer support among inpatients in an adult mental health setting. Issues Ment Health Nurs. 2010;31(9):589–98.
7. Bandura A. Social learning theory Englewood cliffs. New Jersey: Prentice-Hall; 1977.
8. Kelly JA. Popular opinion leaders and HIV prevention peer education: resolving discrepant findings, and implications for the development of effective community programmes. AIDS Care. 2004;16(2):139–50.
9. Davidson L, Bellamy C, Guy K, Miller R. Peer support among persons with severe mental illnesses: a review of evidence and experience. World Psy. 2012;11(2):123–8.
10. Sarbin TR, Allen VL, Lindzey G, Aronson E. Handbook of social psychology. 1968.
11. Duberstein PR, Conwell Y, Conner KR, Eberly S, Evinger J, Caine ED. Poor social integration and suicide: fact or artifact? A case-control study. Psychol Med. 2004;34(7):1331–7.
12. Darke S, Williamson A, Ross J, Teesson M. Attempted suicide among heroin users: 12-month outcomes from the Australian treatment outcome study (ATOS). Drug Alcohol Depend. 2005;78(2):177–86.
13. Conner KR, Britton PC, Sworts LM, Joiner TE. Suicide attempts among individuals with opiate dependence: the critical role of belonging. Addict Behav. 2007;32(7):1395–404.
14. You S, Van Orden KA, Conner KR. Social connections and suicidal thoughts and behavior. Psychol Addict Behav. 2011;25(1):180.
15. Ling WS, Yaacob SN. Peer relationship satisfaction, self-efficacy, and adolescents' suicidal ideation in Selangor, Malaysia. J Manag Res. 2015;7(2):286.
16. Van Orden KA, Witte TK, Cukrowicz KC, Braithwaite SR, Selby EA, Joiner TE Jr. The interpersonal theory of suicide. Psychol Rev. 2010;117(2):575.
17. Geddes JR, Juszczak E, O'Brien F, Kendrick S. Suicide in the 12 months after discharge from psychiatric inpatient care, Scotland 1968–92. J Epidemiol Community Health. 1997;51(4):430–4.
18. Appleby L, Shaw J, Amos T, McDonnell R, Harris C, McCann K, et al. Suicide within 12 months of contact with mental health services: national clinical survey. BMJ. 1999;318(7193):1235–9.
19. Lloyd-Evans B, Mayo-Wilson E, Harrison B, Istead H, Brown E, Pilling S, et al. A systematic review and meta-analysis of randomised controlled trials of peer support for people with severe mental illness. BMC Psy. 2014;14(1):39.
20. Peer Support at the Maine Med Emergency Room: Amistad Peer Support and Recovery. Available at http://amistadinc.com/emergency-room-at-maine-medical-center/.

21. Anchor ED: The Providence Center. Available at https://providencecenter.org/services/crisis-emergency-care/anchored.
22. Allen MH, Carpenter D, Sheets JL, Miccio S, Ross R. What do consumers say they want and need during a psychiatric emergency? J of Psy Practice. 2003;9(1):39–58.
23. Cabassa LJ, Camacho D, Vélez-Grau CM, Stefancic A. Peer-based health interventions for people with serious mental illness: a systematic literature review. J Psychiatr Res. 2017;84:80–9.
24. Li HCW, Lopez V, Lee TLI. Psychoeducational preparation of children for surgery: the importance of parental involvement. Patient Educ Couns. 2007;65(1):34–41.
25. Perry JN, Hooper VD, Masiongale J. Reduction of preoperative anxiety in pediatric surgery patients using age-appropriate teaching interventions. J Perianesth Nurs. 2012;27(2):69–81.
26. Cook JA, Copeland ME, Jonikas JA, Hamilton MM, Razzano LA, Grey DD, et al. Results of a randomized controlled trial of mental illness self-management using wellness recovery action planning. Schizophr Bull. 2011;38(4):881–91.
27. Sledge WH, Lawless M, Sells D, Wieland M, O'Connell MJ, Davidson L. Effectiveness of peer support in reducing readmissions of persons with multiple psychiatric hospitalizations. Psychiatr Serv. 2011;62(5):541–4.
28. Davidson L, Chinman M, Sells D, Rowe M. Peer support among adults with serious mental illness: a report from the field. Schizophr Bull. 2006;32(3):443–50.
29. Chinman M, George P, Dougherty RH, Daniels AS, Ghose SS, Swift A, et al. Peer support services for individuals with serious mental illnesses: assessing the evidence. Psychiatr Serv. 2014;65(4):429–41.

Agitation in the Emergency Department

23

Lauren R. Klein and Marc L. Martel

Introduction

The management of acute agitation is a complex medical issue. In acute settings, clinicians are frequently required to care for patients with acute undifferentiated agitation. The health care team must be able to ensure the safety of the patient, and be positioned to consider the safety of caregivers, as well as other patients and visitors. In these circumstances, the etiology of the patient's agitation must be rapidly determined, as several life-threatening causes need to be considered in the differential diagnosis.

Agitation is defined by one or more of the following: motor restlessness, heightened responsivity to stimuli, irritability, inappropriate or purposeless verbal or motor activity, decreased sleep, and fluctuation of symptoms over time [1]. Although most commonly associated with psychiatric disorders (such as bipolar disorder or schizophrenia) or alcohol and illicit substance abuse, agitation can also be associated with other diagnoses, such as major depression, generalized anxiety disorder, panic disorder, personality disorders, and Parkinson's and Alzheimer's diseases. Agitation has also been linked to life-threatening medical etiologies such as hypoglycemia, toxins, head injury, infection, encephalopathy, and endocrine and metabolic abnormalities.

The degree of agitation manifesting in an individual patient can be highly variable [2]. Considered a life-threatening condition, excited delirium is a term commonly used to describe an extreme of this spectrum. Excited delirium is characterized by confusion, anxiety, disorientation, psychomotor agitation, violent behavior, and hyperthermia. This severe form of agitation is believed to cause significant metabolic acidosis and is closely linked to sudden unexpected death [3–6]. This syndrome highlights the importance of early and aggressive treatment of agitation by frontline practitioners. Emergency physicians, in particular, need to have a clear algorithm for management of these patients.

Agitation, regardless of the etiology, is a behavioral emergency. It requires immediate attention in order to treat the patient's symptoms, prevent injury, and facilitate a medical and psychiatric evaluation [7, 8]. This should be approached in a respectful, nonpunitive manner to safely evaluate a patient or as part of a coordinated treatment plan.

L. R. Klein (✉) · M. L. Martel
Department of Emergency Medicine, Hennepin County Medical Center, Minneapolis, MN, USA
e-mail: lauren.klein@hcmed.org

L. S. Zun et al. (eds.), *Behavioral Emergencies for Healthcare Providers*,
https://doi.org/10.1007/978-3-030-52520-0_23

A General Approach

Emergency providers can use their clinical gestalt, as well as assistance from agitation assessment instruments such as the Behavioral Activity Rating Scale (BARS) [2] or Altered Mental Status Scale (AMSS) [9] to characterize the severity of the agitation. To anticipate violent behaviors, they may also consider using prediction tools such as the Brøset Violence Checklist, the Classification of Violence Risk tool, or the McNeil-Binder Violence Screening Checklist [10, 11].

Treatment of agitation in many scenarios can be accomplished using well-executed verbal de-escalation techniques. Experts suggest that this may include a variety of behaviors such as respecting the patient's personal space, avoiding provocative language, identifying patient needs, and offering choices to the patient [12]. (See Chap. 21, "Verbal De-escalation in the Emergency Department," for more information on this topic.)

In certain cases, verbal de-escalation techniques alone may be sufficient. However, in some instances, particularly in moderate to severe agitation, or when verbal de-escalation techniques are not successful, pharmacologic treatment may be indicated if patient and provider safety is compromised. Of note, the phrase "chemical restraint" should be avoided when referring to this pharmacological treatment of acute agitation. The terminology chemical restraint implies that the medication is being "used as a restriction to manage the patient's freedom of movement" [13]. In contrast, the pharmacologic options discussed below are part of a thoughtful treatment plan to safely evaluate a medical patient.

Medications

Antipsychotics

Typical (conventional or first-generation) and second-generation antipsychotics are frequently used in the management of agitation. The specific mechanism of action is not known, but these drugs have varying effects on dopamine, serotonin, and other neurotransmitter function [14].

First-generation antipsychotics are generally classified into low-, medium-, and high-potency classes. The reference to "potency" is related to the degree of affinity for the dopamine receptors and relative dosing of the drugs, rather than efficacy. Low-potency antipsychotics are generally more sedating and often cause orthostatic hypotension, dizziness, and anticholinergic symptoms. High-potency antipsychotics are considered less sedating but are more often associated with extrapyramidal side effects. These effects most commonly manifest as tremors, rigidity, acute dystonia, and akathisia. Medium-potency antipsychotics have mixed effects between high- and low-potency medications.

The atypical antipsychotics are a newer generation of drugs, developed primarily to treat schizophrenia. The medications tend to more selectively block central dopaminergic receptors or inhibit serotonin reuptake. Whereas first-generation antipsychotics generally impact the positive effects of schizophrenia, second-generation antipsychotics are effective in the management of negative symptoms, as well. It is believed that this improved receptor specificity is responsible for less sedation, fewer extrapyramidal effects, and less effect on QT prolongation [15].

It is important to note that both classes of antipsychotic medications have been associated with significant adverse events. As a result, the US Food and Drug Administration (FDA) has placed several warnings, including the more serious "black box" warning, on both classes of drugs. The two that apply to acute management of agitation are discussed below; further details on the specific medications are listed in Table 23.1.

The FDA has issued a black box warning "that both conventional and atypical antipsychotics are associated with an increased risk of mortality in elderly patients treated for dementia-related psychosis" [16]. A meta-analysis conducted by the FDA in 2005 found a 1.6–1.7 times increase in the risk of death in patients treated with second-generation antipsychotics versus placebo when used for dementia-related behavioral disorders [17]. In 2008, this black box warning was added to the first-generation antipsychotics, as well. The causes of death varied, but cardiovascular and infectious etiologies were the most common [16].

The other black box warning on several antipsychotics warns against QT prolongation and torsade de pointes [18, 19]. Thioridazine is the conventional antipsychotic agent that is most associated with QTc prolongation; intravenous haloperidol also carries an increased risk. Of the second-generation antipsychotics, ziprasidone appears most likely to prolong the QTc interval [19]. Prolongation of the QTc interval raises concern for abnormal cardiac conduction and possi-

Table 23.1 Common antipsychotics used in the treatment of acute agitation

Drug (brand name)	FDA-approved indications	Warnings and select side effects
First-generation antipsychotics		
Chlorpromazine (Thorazine)	Psychotic disorders, schizophrenia, nausea/vomiting	QTc prolongation, EPS (specifically akathisia, dystonia)
Thioridazine (Mellaril)	Schizophrenia	*QTc prolongation*, hypotension, retinopathies, EPS
Perphenazine (Trilafon)	Schizophrenia, nausea/vomiting	EPS (specifically tardive dyskinesia)
Trifluoperazine (Stelazine)	Schizophrenia, nonpsychotic anxiety	EPS (severe), somnolence, xerostomia
Fluphenazine (Prolixin)	Psychotic disorders	EPS, somnolence, weight gain
Loxapine (Loxitane)	Schizophrenia, agitation due to schizophrenia/bipolar disorder	Bronchospasm, EPS, somnolence, taste alterations
Thiothixene (Navane)	Dementia related psychosis/agitation	EPS, somnolence, weight gain
Haloperidol (Haldol)	Schizophrenia, behavioral disorders, Tourette disorders	QTc prolongation, TdP, EPS (frequent), hypotension, weight gain
Droperidol (Inapsine)	Postoperative nausea/vomiting	*QTc prolongation*, TdP, EPS, sedation, hypotension
Second-generation antipsychotics		
Clozapine (Clozaril)	Treatment-resistant schizophrenia, reduction of suicidal behaviors in schizophrenia	*Agranulocytosis, seizures, myocarditis, hypotension*, sedation, dizziness, hyperthermia
Olanzapine (Zyprexa)	Schizophrenia, bipolar disorder, acute agitation in schizophrenia/bipolar mania	*Postinjection delirium/sedation syndrome*, CVAE, hypotension, hyperglycemia, weight gain, sedation
Quetiapine (Seroquel)	Schizophrenia, bipolar disorder, major depressive disorder	*Suicidal thoughts*, cataracts, hyperglycemia, sedation, hypotension
Risperidone (Risperdal)	Schizophrenia, bipolar disorder	EPS, hyperglycemia, hypotension, weight gain, hyperprolactinemia
Ziprasidone (Geodon)	Schizophrenia, bipolar mania, acute agitation in schizophrenia	QTc prolongation, sedation, rash, hypotension, hyperglycemia, EPS
Aripiprazole (Abilify)	Schizophrenia, bipolar disorder, acute agitation in schizophrenia or bipolar	*Suicidal thoughts*, CVAE, EPS, hyperglycemia, seizure, hypotension

Notes: *EPS* extrapyramidal side effects, *CVAE* cardiovascular side efects, *TdP* Torsades de pointes

bly the risk for fatal arrhythmias like torsade de pointes (TdP) [19]. If electrocardiographic data are available prior to administration, the QTc interval should be assessed and considered by the treating clinician. Cardiac monitoring may not be possible prior to initiating control of a patient's agitated state. If aggressive behavior is exhibited, the unlikely potential for medication-induced cardiac arrhythmias must be weighed against the real risk of violence. Other adverse effects of antipsychotic use in the treatment of acute agitation are discussed below.

Seizures

Although there is little literature on the effects of antipsychotics on lowering the seizure threshold when used in single-dose therapy for acute agitation, both the first- and second-generation antipsychotics can lower the seizure threshold when used chronically (range of 0.1–1.5% incidence rate in patients with therapeutic doses) and can significantly increase the risk of seizure in overdose. Chlorpromazine and clozapine are associated with the highest known risk [20].

Anticholinergic Effects

Certain antipsychotics have particularly high anticholinergic receptor affinity, such as olanzapine, clozapine, and quetiapine. As such, with these medications, sedation (an anticholinergic side effect) may be more notable. Along these lines and when considering this side effect, there are limited data that suggest any added benefit from the use of diphenhydramine in combination with haloperidol and lorazepam (the "B-52") [7].

Other anticholinergic effects are common and variable, and include dry mouth, blurred vision, constipation, urinary retention, and adynamic ileus. Dysarthria, mydriasis, and delirium can be seen as a result of the central effects of these medications [21]. Anticholinergic-related cardiovascular effects are also often clinically evident. Orthostatic hypotension and tachycardia may be compounded by the medications' adrenergic effects, but this hypotension is typically responsive to intravenous fluids.

Movement Disorders

Acute antipsychotic-induced movement disorders include akathisia and acute dystonia. Both are likely caused by alterations in the dopaminergic pathways of the basal ganglia, specifically the D2 receptors of the nigrostriatum [22]. These reactions are unfortunately common, with one study reporting more than 60% of chronic use associated with at least one form of antipsychotic-induced movement disorder [23].

Akathisia is an uncomfortable sense of motor restlessness manifested by an intense desire to move, usually the legs. This side effect can occur with acute or chronic use, and is worsened if misdiagnosed or inappropriately treated as progressive agitation. Propranolol (30–60 mg po), anticholinergics including benzatropine (1–2 mg IM or po) or diphenhydramine (25–50 mg IM/IV/po), and benzodiazepines (lorazepam 1–2 mg IM/IV) are generally effective treatment strategies. Patients may benefit from ongoing treatment to prevent recurrence [24].

Acute dystonia is typically an idiosyncratic reaction to antipsychotic medications. Dystonic reactions are characterized by intermittent spasmodic or sustained involuntary contractions of the face, neck, trunk, or extremities. More serious forms of dystonia manifest clinically as oculogyric crisis and laryngospasm. Anticholinergics including benzatropine (1–2 mg IM or po) or diphenhydramine (25–50 mg IM/IV/po) are indicated to treat dystonia and can be combined if symptoms are resistant to either independently. Benzodiazepines may be added, if necessary. Patients should be also continued on this treatment regimen for 3–5 days to prevent recurrence.

Neuroleptic Malignant Syndrome

Neuroleptic malignant syndrome (NMS) is a rare, idiosyncratic reaction to the antipsychotics [25]. The high-potency agents are more frequently associated with the syndrome, but both first-generation and second-generation have been implicated. NMS is life-threatening disorder characterized by fever, muscular rigidity, autonomic instability (tachycardia, blood pressure instability, and diaphoresis), and altered mental status. A medical emergency, mortality in NMS has been reported as high as 20%. Mortality has been related to respiratory fail-

Table 23.2 Common benzodiazepines available for use in control of acute agitation

Name	Route of administration	Dosing (mg)	Duration (half-life in hours)	Relative dosing potency (mg)
Alprazolam	Oral	0.5–1 mg	9–20	0.5–1
Chlordiazepoxide	Parenteral and oral	10–25 mg	24–48	10–25
Clonazepam	Oral	1–2 mg	30–40	0.25–0.5
Clorazepate	Oral	15–30 mg	48	7.5–15
Diazepam	Parenteral, oral, rectal	5–10 mg	35	5–10
Lorazepam	Parenteral and oral	1–2 mg	10–20	1–2
Midazolam	Parenteral and oral	5–10 mg	1.8–6.4	Intravenous: 1.3–2.7 Oral: 3.3–7
Oxazepam	Oral	20–30 mg	4–15	15–30
Triazolam	Oral	0.25–0.5 mg	1.5–5	0.25–0.5

ure, cardiovascular collapse, acute renal failure, arrhythmias, and disseminated intravascular coagulation. Management is predominantly supportive in an intensive-care setting and includes discontinuation of antipsychotics, hydration, temperature regulation (cooling), and possibly dantrolene or bromocriptine to reduce rigidity [25, 26].

Benzodiazepines

Benzodiazepines are commonly used in the acute management of agitation and may be particularly useful when treating agitation due to sympathomimetic use or withdrawal syndromes. They may be administered independently or combined with an antipsychotic for agitation control [8, 27–29]. There are several approved medications available for use in the United States. Table 23.2 outlines several of the available agents.

The main distinguishing features among the benzodiazepine class of medications are route of administration and duration of action. In the management of acute agitation, the shorter-acting parenteral medications are preferred. Both midazolam (short-acting) and lorazepam (intermediate-acting) are used extensively in the United States. In one study of severely agitated patients, the onset of action of intramuscular midazolam was found to be 13 minutes shorter than lorazepam [30].

Benzodiazepines, particularly the oral formulations, have a wide therapeutic window. Aside from the intended sedation, which can be excessive, adverse effects include respiratory suppression, hypoventilation, apnea, hypotension, amnesia, dizziness, and ataxia. Midazolam carries a black box warning issued by the FDA related to the risk of respiratory suppression [31]. The recommendations encourage the use of midazolam solely in settings where continuous respiratory and cardiac monitoring, airway management equipment, resuscitative drugs, and providers skilled in airway are available.

Similarly, the combination of benzodiazepines with olanzapine has been reported to possibly potentiate the sedating effects of both medications and result in excessive sedation. The package inserts states, "Careful evaluation of clinical status for excessive sedation and cardiorespiratory depression is recommended" [32]. The clinical effect has been refuted in recent studies [28, 33, 34].

Ketamine

Ketamine is a dissociative anesthetic with clinical indications for anesthesia induction and anesthesia maintenance. The rapid sedative effects are particularly useful in the ED management of acute agitation, and ketamine is already commonly used in the ED for procedural sedation [35, 36]. Reports of ketamine use in the ED have been limited to several small cohorts [37], although nationally, emergency medical services appear to be adding ketamine to their formularies with success [38–42].

In addition to rapid sedation, ketamine's short duration of action, parenteral route of administration, and preservation of protective airway reflexes in particular are attractive properties in the management of patients with acute agitation. When given intramuscularly, sedation occurs within 3–4 minutes and lasts for up to 30 minutes [43]. The sedative effects of ketamine are profound, and in conjunction with its onset of action, agitation control can occur quickly and allows rapid stabilization of potentially dangerous situations [38, 40, 43].

After ketamine administration, antipsychotics should typically be used to extend sedation because of ketamine's short, clinical duration of action. It is unlikely that the treatment of severe agitation with ketamine alone will result in an adequate clinical response. Providers should select an appropriate additional sedative with a longer duration of action, such as intramuscular haloperidol or olanzapine, to avoid a rapid "down-up" effect of sedation. Providers should also be aware of numerous side effects of ketamine, including nausea, vomiting, hypersalivation, laryngospasm, and apnea. Therefore, close monitoring (end-tidal CO_2, pulse oximetry) post-ketamine administration is indicated. Emergence reactions, which are episodes of agitation, nightmares, or hallucinations following ketamine administration that are felt not to be a recurrence of previous agitation, may also occur [35]. These reactions require prompt attention and treatment, including the administration of benzodiazepines; midazolam 2–5 mg IV is preferred due to its rapid onset of action.

Similarly, early reports of the use of subanesthetic doses of ketamine in patients with schizophrenia were thought to worsen positive symptoms of the disease. Given this, schizophrenia was thought to be a contraindication to the use of ketamine [44, 45]. Several reports have refuted these initial concerns, and currently, it is felt to be safe. From the most conservative perspective, this may be considered a relative contraindication [46–50].

Routes of Administration

As outlined above, several treatment modalities exist for the management of acute agitation. Many of the medications are available in both oral and parenteral (intramuscular or intravenous) formulations. A systematic review of published articles on pharmacologic treatments for agitation by Zeller and Rhoades in 2010 suggested that oral, intramuscular, and intravenous administration modalities may all be effective, but noted that the onset of action varied according to the route of administration [51].

The American College of Emergency Physicians (ACEP) recommends oral medications in "agitated but cooperative patients" [52], as do other expert guidelines [7]. One published study remarked that non-parenteral methods also provide the potential benefit of an improved physician–patient relationship if injections can be avoided, and patient preference is considered when possible [53]. Options for oral medications include 5–10 mg of olanzapine oral disintegrating tablets (ODTs) or 1–4 mg tablets of lorazepam, to be used only in a subset of cooperative patients.

Though there are certain benefits to oral administration of agitation treatments, the nature of the patient's presentation frequently precludes oral administration [51], as patient cooperation is necessary to successfully and safely administer the medication in this manner. Oral formulations may also encourage "cheeking" behaviors (or not swallowing medications). Patient cooperation (or lack thereof) may also preclude the use of inhaled delivery systems (such as inhaled loxapine, which was recently shown to significantly reduce agitation in consenting patients who were able to follow study protocol) [54]. Intravenous routes of administration also depend on patient cooperation and the ability to obtain intravenous access. As such, intramuscular injections are often used, as they can be rapidly administered regardless of the patient's behavior [55]. These methods do carry the risk of placing providers at an increased risk of bloodborne pathogen exposure through needle-stick injuries.

Length of Stay

Safe medical and acute psychiatric evaluation is required after management of acute agitation. In patients who are being admitted for an acute medical issue, ED lengths of stay are less critical.

However, a significant issue in the management of acute agitation is the time after sedation is administered until the patient may be transferred to definitive care either for psychiatric consultation or inpatient mental health services. The duration of action and depth of sedation must be sufficient to safely allow evaluation and transport, but not excessively long or deep to delay these components of care. Emergency department evaluations may also be complicated by close observation, end-tidal CO_2, pulse oximetry, and cardiac monitoring.

As implied by the delay in onset of action for the oral formulations, lengths of stay may be affected by route of administration, as well as medication choice, dosing, and patient response. Although comparing agents based on half-lives may imply superiority with respect to times in the ED, no clinical trials to date have specifically addressed this issue. Short-acting agents may encourage more rapid recovery, or second-generation antipsychotics may provide less sedation.

Comparative Efficacy

Given the ongoing importance of this subject in clinical practice, a number of studies have emerged investigating comparative efficacy of different agents in treating acute agitation in the emergency department. Table 23.3 outlines the currently published randomized control trials on the subject [27–30, 56–59].

Table 23.3 Emergency department studies on agitation including patients with both psychiatric and nonpsychiatric diagnoses

Study	Arms	Outcome(s)	Results/conclusions
Battaglia (1997) [29]	Haloperidol (5 mg), lorazepam (2 mg), haloperidol+lorazepam (5 mg + 2 mg)	Agitated behavior scale (sedation scale)	Symptom reduction was achieved in each treatment group, but occurred most rapidly for the combination group
Richards (1998) [56]	Lorazepam (2–4 mg), droperidol (2.5–5 mg)	Sedation scores, repeat doses	Droperidol led to significantly lower sedation scores than lorazepam, and lorazepam required more repeat doses
Nobay (2004) [30]	Midazolam (5 mg), haloperidol (5 mg), lorazepam (2 mg)	Time to adequate sedation	Midazolam had a significantly shorter time to adequate sedation compared to haloperidol and lorazepam, but had a shorter time until arousal
Martel (2005) [57]	Droperidol (5 mg), midazolam (5 mg), ziprasidone (20 mg)	Change in altered mental status score (sedation scale)	Adequate sedation (AMS score < 1) was achieved at 15 minutes in patients receiving midazolam and at 30 minutes for patients receiving droperidol or ziprasidone. Droperidol or ziprasidone required rescue medications less frequently than midazolam
Knott (2006) [58]	Midazolam (5 mg), droperidol (5 mg)	Time to sedation, proportion sedated at 5–10 minutes	There were no differences in time to sedation; more patients were adequately sedated at 5 minutes in the midazolam group, but no differences at 10 minutes
Isbister (2010) [59]	Droperidol (10 mg), midazolam (10 mg), droperidol+midazolam (5 mg + 5 mg)	Duration of acute behavioral disturbance	There were no differences in the duration of the acute behavioral disturbance; more rescue sedation was required for midazolam
Chan (2013) [27]	Midazolam+placebo, midazolam+olanzapine, midazolam+droperidol	Time to adequate sedation	Droperidol or olanzapine + midazolam decreases the time to adequate sedation versus midazolam alone
Taylor (2017) [28]	Midazolam+droperidol (5 mg + 5 mg), droperidol (10 mg), olanzapine (10 mg)	Proportion of patients sedated at 10 minutes	The midazolam+droperidol group had the highest proportion of sedated patients at 10 minutes

Special Populations

Elderly Patients

For elderly patients who appear to be medically compromised, pharmacological treatments for agitation should be used cautiously and judiciously. Verbal de-escalation should be emphasized [12]. Elderly patients may also be more likely to have an organic or medical underlying etiology of their agitation, so the focus should be on identifying and treating these potentially reversible causes [60].

If medications are deemed clinically necessary, small doses of a single class of medication are recommended. There are several other unique considerations in the elderly, including particular attention to avoiding medications known to prolong the QTc interval (as they may already be on other QTc-prolonging medications at baseline), and avoiding antipsychotics if concomitant dementia is known or suspected (per the FDA black box warning). This presents a challenging situation in agitated elderly patients with dementia. The risk of serious complications is more associated with long-term use [17, 60, 61]. As such, reasonable options in this population include haloperidol (concentrate or tablets 0.5–1 mg every 6 hours), risperidone (0.25–0.5 mg solution or dissolving tablet every 6 hours), or, if necessary, lorazepam (1 mg IM or 1 mg solution). Antipsychotics with strong anticholinergic properties and benzodiazepines should be avoided if possible, as they may exacerbate any associated delirium.

Pregnant Women

There are no outcome studies for treating the agitated pregnant patient [62, 63]. The fetal risk of using several doses of psychotropic medication to treat agitated pregnant women remains unknown. In the absence of safety data, clinicians should use the minimal amount of medication necessary to safely reduce agitation and aggression in these patients. All efforts should be made to avoid physical restraints, especially in the second or third trimesters, as restraints may pose significant risks to the pregnant patient [63].

Children and Adolescents

There is a paucity of data regarding the treatment of adolescents and children who are severely agitated, though this subject is gaining popularity in recent years [64–66]. As children and adolescents are more vulnerable to side effects from first-generation antipsychotics, second-generation antipsychotics or lorazepam are considered preferable alternatives. Dosing of lorazepam is 0.5–2 mg orally or IM every hour as needed to achieve sedation. Some authors have also recommended antihistamines such as diphenhydramine or hydroxyzine for children and adolescents with less severe symptoms [67].

Conclusion and Recommendations

The real-world management of patients with acute agitation is exceedingly complex. As described, a variety of options for type and route of medical therapy exist. A simple algorithm is suggested in Fig. 23.1. In addition to the options outlined in Fig. 23.1, combination therapies are also possible, based on findings from various recent prospective trials; these combinations include haloperidol plus lorazepam, droperidol plus midazolam, and olanzapine plus midazolam [27–29].

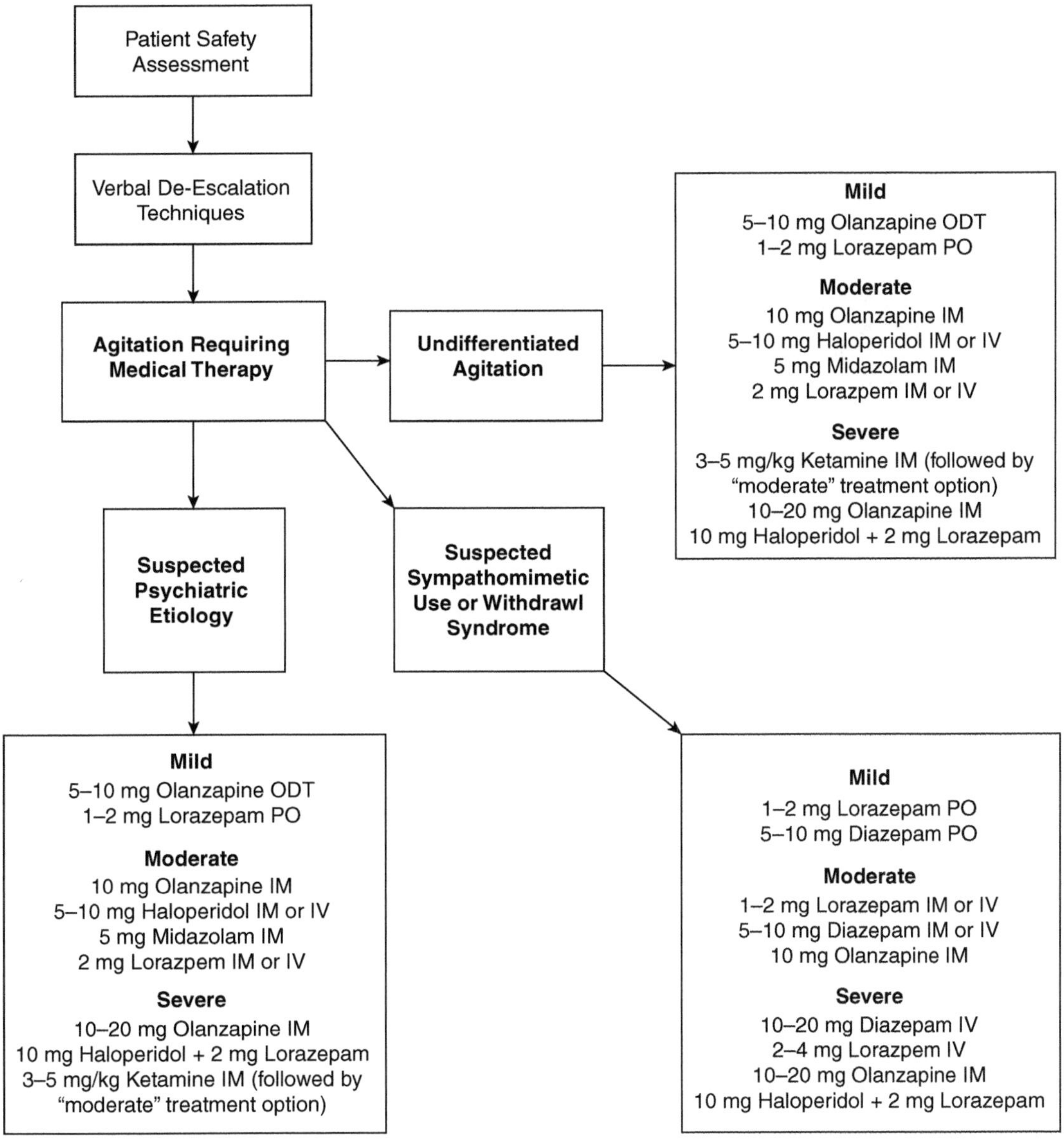

Fig. 23.1 Suggested Algorithm for Assessing Patients with Acute Agitation

References

1. Lindenmayer JP. The pathophysiology of agitation. J Clin Psy. 2000;61(Suppl 14):5–10.
2. Swift RH, Harrigan EP, Cappelleri JC, Kramer D, Chandler LP. Validation of the behavioural activity rating scale (BARS): a novel measure of activity in agitated patients. J Psychiatr Res. 2002;36:87–95.
3. Ho JD, Dawes DM, Nelson RS, Lundin EJ, Ryan FJ, Overton KG, et al. Acidosis and catecholamine evaluation following simulated law enforcement "use of force" encounters. Acad Emerg Med. 2010;17:e60–8.
4. Stratton SJ, Rogers C, Brickett K, Gruzinski G. Factors associated with sudden death of individuals requiring restraint for excited delirium. Am J Emerg Med. 2001;19:187–91.
5. Vilke GM, DeBard ML, Chan TC, Ho JD, Dawes DM, Hall C, et al. Excited Delirium Syndrome (ExDS): defining based on a review of the literature. J Emerg Med. 2012;43:897–905.
6. Pollanen MS, Chiasson DA, Cairns JT, Young JG. Unexpected death related to restraint for excited delirium: a retrospective study of deaths in police custody and in the community. CMAJ. 1998;158:1603–7.

7. Wilson MP, Pepper D, Currier GW, Holloman GH Jr, Feifel D. The psychopharmacology of agitation: consensus statement of the american association for emergency psychiatry project beta psychopharmacology workgroup. West J Emerg Med. 2012;13:26–34.
8. Battaglia J. Pharmacological management of acute agitation. Drugs. 2005;65:1207–22.
9. Miner JR, McCoy C, Biros M. A standardized intoxication scale vs. breath ethanol level as a predictor of observation time in the emergency department. Acad Emerg Med. 2003;10(5):520.
10. Abderhalden C, Needham I, Miserez B, Almvik R, Dassen T, Haug H-J, et al. Predicting inpatient violence in acute psychiatric wards using the Brøset-violence-checklist: a multicentre prospective cohort study. J Psychiatr Ment Health Nurs. 2004;11:422–7.
11. Whittington R, Hockenhull JC, McGuire J, Leitner M, Barr W, Cherry MG, et al. A systematic review of risk assessment strategies for populations at high risk of engaging in violent behaviour. Update 2002–8. Health Technol Assess. 2013;17:i–xiv, 1–128.
12. Richmond JS, Berlin JS, Fishkind AB, Holloman GH Jr, Zeller SL, Wilson MP, et al. Verbal de-escalation of the agitated patient: consensus statement of the American association for emergency psychiatry project BETA de-escalation workgroup. West J Emerg Med. 2012;13:17–25.
13. CMS.gov. Final Rule. Available at https://www.cms.gov/Regulations-and-Guidance/Legislation/CFCsAndCoPs/downloads/finalpatientrightsrule.pdf.
14. Laruelle M, Frankle WG, Narendran R, Kegeles LS, Abi-Dargham A. Mechanism of action of antipsychotic drugs: from dopamine D(2) receptor antagonism to glutamate NMDA facilitation. Clin Ther. 2005;27(Suppl A):S16–24.
15. Seeman P. Atypical antipsychotics: mechanism of action. Can J Psy. 2002;47:27–38.
16. Information for Healthcare Professionals: Conventional Antipsychotics, in U.S. Food and Drug Administration. Cited Sep. 2017. Available at https://www.fda.gov/Drugs/DrugSafety/ucm124830.htm.
17. Schneider LS, Dagerman KS, Insel P. Risk of death with atypical antipsychotic drug treatment for dementia: meta-analysis of randomized placebo-controlled trials. JAMA. 2005;294:1934–43.
18. Haddad PM, Anderson IM. Antipsychotic-related QTc prolongation, torsade de pointes and sudden death. Drugs. 2002;62:1649–71.
19. Beach SR, Celano CM, Noseworthy PA, Januzzi JL, Huffman JC. QTc prolongation, torsades de pointes, and psychotropic medications. Psychosomatics. 2013;54:1–13.
20. Pisani F, Oteri G, Costa C, Di Raimondo G, Di Perri R. Effects of psychotropic drugs on seizure threshold. Drug Saf. 2002;25:91–110.
21. Ozbilen M, Adams CE, Marley J. Anticholinergic effects of oral antipsychotic drugs of typicals versus atypicals over medium- and long-term: systematic review and meta-analysis. Curr Med Chem. 2012;19:5214–8.
22. Marsden CD, Jenner P. The pathophysiology of extrapyramidal side-effects of neuroleptic drugs. Psychol Med. 1980;10:55–72.
23. Janno S, Holi M, Tuisku K, Wahlbeck K. Prevalence of neuroleptic-induced movement disorders in chronic schizophrenia inpatients. Am J Psy. 2004;161:160–3.
24. Vinson DR, Drotts DL. Diphenhydramine for the prevention of akathisia induced by prochlorperazine: a randomized, controlled trial. Ann Emerg Med. 2001;37:125–31.
25. Strawn JR, Keck PE Jr, Caroff SN. Neuroleptic malignant syndrome. Am J Psy. 2007;164:870–6.
26. Levenson JL. Neuroleptic malignant syndrome. Am J Psy. 1985;142:1137–45.
27. Chan EW, Taylor DM, Knott JC, Phillips GA, Castle DJ, Kong DCM. Intravenous droperidol or olanzapine as an adjunct to midazolam for the acutely agitated patient: a multicenter, randomized, double-blind, placebo-controlled clinical trial. Ann Emerg Med. 2013;61:72–81.
28. Taylor DM, Yap CYL, Knott JC, Taylor SE, Phillips GA, Karro J, et al. Midazolam-droperidol, droperidol, or olanzapine for acute agitation: a randomized clinical trial. Ann Emerg Med. 2017;69:318–326.e1.
29. Battaglia J, Moss S, Rush J, Kang J, Mendoza R, Leedom L, et al. Haloperidol, lorazepam, or both for psychotic agitation? A multicenter, prospective, double-blind, emergency department study. Am J Emerg Med. 1997;15:335–40.
30. Nobay F, Simon BC, Levitt MA, Dresden GM. A prospective, double-blind, randomized trial of midazolam versus haloperidol versus lorazepam in the chemical restraint of violent and severely agitated patients. Acad Emerg Med. 2004;11:744–9.
31. Midazolam injection: Package Insert. Available at http://www.medsafe.govt.nz/profs/datasheet/m/MidazolaminjPfizer.pdf.
32. FDA. Olanzapine Package Insert. Available at https://www.accessdata.fda.gov/drugsatfda_docs/label/2009/020592s051,021086s030,021253s036lbl.pdf.
33. Wilson MP, MacDonald K, Vilke GM, Feifel D. Potential complications of combining intramuscular olanzapine with benzodiazepines in emergency department patients. J Emerg Med. 2012;43:889–96.
34. Wilson MP, MacDonald K, Vilke GM, Feifel D. A comparison of the safety of olanzapine and haloperidol in combination with benzodiazepines in emergency department patients with acute agitation. J Emerg Med. 2012;43:790–7.
35. Green SM, Roback MG, Kennedy RM, Krauss B. Clinical practice guideline for emergency department ketamine dissociative sedation: 2011 update. Ann Emerg Med. 2011;57:449–61.
36. Godwin SA, Burton JH, Gerardo CJ, Hatten BW, Mace SE, Silvers SM, et al. Clinical policy: procedural sedation and analgesia in the emergency department. Ann Emerg Med. 2014;63:247–58.e18.
37. Hopper AB, Vilke GM, Castillo EM, Campillo A, Davie T, Wilson MP. Ketamine use for acute agitation in the emergency department. J Emerg Med. 2015;48:712–9.

38. Ho JD, Smith SW, Nystrom PC, Dawes DM, Orozco BS, Cole JB, et al. Successful management of excited delirium syndrome with prehospital ketamine: two case examples. Prehosp Emerg Care. 2013;17:274–9.
39. Olives TD, Nystrom PC, Cole JB, Dodd KW, Ho JD. Intubation of profoundly agitated patients treated with prehospital ketamine. Prehosp Disaster Med. 2016;31:593–602.
40. Scaggs TR, Glass DM, Hutchcraft MG, Weir WB. Prehospital ketamine is a safe and effective treatment for excited delirium in a community hospital based EMS system. Prehosp Disaster Med. 2016;31:563–9.
41. Scheppke KA, Braghiroli J, Shalaby M, Chait R. Prehospital use of i.m. ketamine for sedation of violent and agitated patients. West J Emerg Med. 2014;15:736–41.
42. Le Cong M, Gynther B, Hunter E, Schuller P. Ketamine sedation for patients with acute agitation and psychiatric illness requiring aeromedical retrieval. Emerg Med J. 2012;29:335–7.
43. Cole JB, Moore JC, Nystrom PC, Orozco BS, Stellpflug SJ, Kornas RL, et al. A prospective study of ketamine versus haloperidol for severe prehospital agitation. Clin Toxicol. 2016;54:556–62.
44. Lahti AC, Koffel B, LaPorte D, Tamminga CA. Subanesthetic doses of ketamine stimulate psychosis in schizophrenia. Neuropsychopharmacology. 1995;13:9–19.
45. Lahti AC, Weiler MA, Tamara Michaelidis BA, Parwani A, Tamminga CA. Effects of ketamine in normal and schizophrenic volunteers. Neuropsychopharmacology. 2001;25:455–67.
46. Reames E, Rosenblatt R. Ketamine anesthesia of a catatonic schizophrenic patient. Anesthesiology. 1979;51:577–8.
47. Kranaster L, Hoyer C, Janke C, Sartorius A. Preliminary evaluation of clinical outcome and safety of ketamine as an anesthetic for electroconvulsive therapy in schizophrenia. World J Biol Psy. 2014;15:242–50.
48. Ishihara H, Kudo H, Murakawa T, Kudo A, Takahashi S, Matsuki A. Uneventful total intravenous anaesthesia with ketamine for schizophrenic surgical patients. Eur J Anaesthesiol. 1997;14:47–51.
49. Carpenter WT Jr. The schizophrenia ketamine challenge study debate. Biol Psy. 1999;46:1081–91.
50. Pomarol-Clotet E, Honey GD, Murray GK, Corlett PR, Absalom AR, Lee M, et al. Psychological effects of ketamine in healthy volunteers: phenomenological study. Br J Psy. 2006;189:173–9.
51. Zeller SL, Rhoades RW. Systematic reviews of assessment measures and pharmacologic treatments for agitation. Clin Ther. 2010;32:403–25.
52. American College of Emergency Physicians Clinical Policies Subcommittee (Writing Committee) on the Adult Psychiatric Patient, Nazarian DJ, Broder JS, MEW T, Wilson MP, Zun LS, et al. Clinical policy: critical issues in the diagnosis and management of the adult psychiatric patient in the emergency department. Ann Emerg Med. 2017;69:480–98.
53. Allen MH, Carpenter D, Sheets JL, Miccio S, Ross R. What do consumers say they want and need during a psychiatric emergency? J Psychiatr Pract. 2003;9:39–58.
54. Lesem MD, Tran-Johnson TK, Riesenberg RA, Feifel D, Allen MH, Fishman R, et al. Rapid acute treatment of agitation in individuals with schizophrenia: multicentre, randomised, placebo-controlled study of inhaled loxapine. Br J Psy. 2011;198:51–8.
55. Zimbroff DL. Pharmacological control of acute agitation: focus on intramuscular preparations. CNS Drugs. 2008;22:199–212.
56. Richards JR, Derlet RW, Duncan DR. Chemical restraint for the agitated patient in the emergency department: lorazepam versus droperidol. J Emerg Med. 1998;16:567–73.
57. Martel M, Sterzinger A, Miner J, Clinton J, Biros M. Management of acute undifferentiated agitation in the emergency department: a randomized double-blind trial of droperidol, ziprasidone, and midazolam. Acad Emerg Med. 2005;12:1167–72.
58. Knott JC, Taylor DM, Castle DJ. Randomized clinical trial comparing intravenous midazolam and droperidol for sedation of the acutely agitated patient in the emergency department. Ann Emerg Med. 2006;47:61–7.
59. Isbister GK, Calver LA, Page CB, Stokes B, Bryant JL, Downes MA. Randomized controlled trial of intramuscular droperidol versus midazolam for violence and acute behavioral disturbance: the DORM study. Ann Emerg Med. 2010;56:392–401.e1.
60. Aftab A, Shah AA. Behavioral emergencies: special considerations in the geriatric psychiatric patient. Psychiatr Clin North Am. 2017;40:449–62.
61. Gareri P, De Fazio P, Manfredi VGL, De Sarro G. Use and safety of antipsychotics in behavioral disorders in elderly people with dementia. J Clin Psychopharmacol. 2014;34:109–23.
62. Aftab A, Shah AA. Behavioral emergencies: special considerations in the pregnant patient. Psychiatr Clin North Am. 2017;40:435–48.
63. Ladavac AS, Dubin WR, Ning A, Stuckeman PA. Emergency management of agitation in pregnancy. Gen Hosp Psy. 2007;29:39–41.
64. Hilt RJ, Woodward TA. Agitation treatment for pediatric emergency patients. J Am Acad Child Adolesc Psy. 2008;47:132–8.
65. Sonnier L, Barzman D. Pharmacologic management of acutely agitated pediatric patients. Paediatr Drugs. 2011;13:1–10.
66. Cole JB, Klein LR, Strobel AM, Blanchard SR, Nahum R, Martel ML. The use, safety, and efficacy of olanzapine in a level I pediatric trauma center emergency department over a 10-year period. Pediatr Emerg Care. 2017; https://doi.org/10.1097/PEC.0000000000001231.
67. Heyneman EK. The aggressive child. Child Adolesc Psychiatr Clin N Am. 2003;12:667–77, vi–vii.

24 Restraint and Seclusion in the Emergency Department

Garrett K. Blumberg and Lynn P. Roppolo

Introduction

Restraints and seclusion once seemed to be the only option in our arsenal of defense against the agitated and combative patient. We now know that these aggressive measures must be used as a last resort due to the many concerning consequences associated with their use, including physical injury, psychological stress, and the medicolegal concerns associated with their application. These techniques should be utilized only when other safer measures have failed, and only in a final attempt to prevent injury to patients and others. In the event that physical restraints or seclusion are implemented, several general principles should be considered to optimize the outcome of patients and to mitigate any adverse consequences. This chapter will review the use of restraints and seclusion for patients with behavioral emergencies and will provide recommendations according to the best available evidence and practice guidelines.

G. K. Blumberg (✉)
Department of Emergency Medicine, University of Texas Southwestern Medical Center, Dallas, TX, USA

L. P. Roppolo
Department of Emergency Medicine, Parkland Health and Hospital System, Dallas, TX, USA
e-mail: Lynn.roppolo@utsw.edu

Definitions

Restraints: Any manual method, physical or mechanical device, material, or equipment that immobilizes or reduces the ability of a patient to move his or her arms, legs, body, or head freely [1]. When referring to restraints in this chapter, physical restraints are implied, as the term "chemical restraint" has been used to describe medications that are administered only to restrict movement. As medication is typically intended as therapy, the term "chemical restraint" is not recommended. Instead, providers should prescribe appropriate medications indicated in specific clinical conditions such as agitation, anxiolysis, or psychosis. The goal of medication in these situations is to calm the patient so that they can be more appropriately assessed and treated by clinicians.

Seclusion: The involuntary confinement of a patient alone in a room or area from which the patient is physically prevented from leaving. Seclusion may only be used for the management of violent or self-destructive behavior [1].

Case Example

A 39-year-old man with a history of unspecified psychiatric illness was brought to the emergency department via emergency medical services

L. S. Zun et al. (eds.), *Behavioral Emergencies for Healthcare Providers*, https://doi.org/10.1007/978-3-030-52520-0_24

(EMS) for agitated behavior. The patient became violent in the ambulance bay and was restrained by several hospital security guards. He was placed prone, with his arms behind him. The following medications were administered intramuscularly (IM) by nursing staff, as ordered by the attending emergency physician: 5 mg haloperidol, 50 mg diphenhydramine, and 2 mg lorazepam. During the restraint process, the patient became apneic and pulseless. He was moved across the hallway to the resuscitation room in the emergency department (ED) and immediately intubated. He was initially in a nonperfusing bradycardia, which deteriorated into ventricular fibrillation, and then asystole. Epinephrine, atropine, and bicarbonate were given, and return of spontaneous circulation was observed shortly after. An arterial blood gas was obtained and showed severe metabolic and respiratory acidosis. His hemodynamic status stabilized, and the acidosis reversed within 12 hours. Life support was subsequently withdrawn 2 days later, due to a persistent vegetative state. Urine toxicology was positive for cocaine; serum levels were not available.

Restraints

Although the case presented above sounds drastic, this is an unfortunate real-life example of the inappropriate use of physical restraint and pharmacotherapy in the ED. Despite the prevalent use of restraints and seclusion in the acute-care setting, there are no controlled studies evaluating their efficacy [2]. Many of the studies performed suffer from selection bias, lack of blinding, and weak data collection methods [3]. The goal of applying restraints is to keep a patient from moving in order to administer necessary treatments and to prevent harm if other measures to calm the patient, such as de-escalation and pharmacotherapy, have failed. Physical restraints should never be used to punish [4]. The Joint Commission's standards on physical restraint (and seclusion) are summarized in Table 24.1 [5].

Physical restraint of an agitated patient is not without complications. One prospective study reported a low rate of complications, with the most common being getting out of the restraints, vomiting, injury to self or others, and spitting [6]. A more recent study from the United Kingdom reported a more substantial amount of physical injuries to staff and patients during the restraint process [7]. Resisting against restraints should be considered a medical emergency [8]. Rhabdomyolysis can occur from severe agitation and become even more pronounced from prolonged resisting against restraints, which may lead to acute kidney damage or life-threatening hyperkalemia. Some patients may develop a profound acidosis as the result of lactic acid accumulation, co-ingestion stimulant medications such as cocaine, and restrictive movements during the restraint process, which may impede the appropriate respiratory compensation [6]. Cardiac arrest was reported in several unmedicated patients who had resisted against restraints. Although the cause of death was unknown, sympathetic overflow, severe lactic acidosis, or electrolyte disorders such as hyperkalemia may have been contributory [8]. In order to prevent such complications, medications for agitation must be given in a timely manner. Medications are often administered to agitated patients as isolated therapy or in combination with physical restraints in an effort to reduce escalation to violent behavior,

Table 24.1 Joint Commission Standards on Physical Restraint and Seclusion

The hospital uses restraint or seclusion only to protect the immediate physical safety of the patient, staff, or others.
The hospital does not use restraint or seclusion as a means of coercion, discipline, convenience, or staff retaliation.
The hospital uses restraint or seclusion only when less restrictive interventions are ineffective.
The hospital uses the least restrictive form of restraint or seclusion that protects the physical safety of the patient, staff, or others.
The hospital discontinues restraint or seclusion at the earliest possible time, regardless of the scheduled expiration of the order.

Adapted from: Joint Commission Standards on Restraint and Seclusion/Non-violent Crisis Intervention Training Program. Available at: https://www.crisisprevention.com/CPI/media/Media/Resources/alignments/Joint-Commission-Restraint-Seclusion-Alignment-2011.pdf [5]

but patients must be closely monitored with continuous pulse oximetry, cardiac monitoring, and waveform capnometry to avert complications associated with these medications.

A graded approach should be utilized in the implementation of physical restraints, as described in Fig. 24.1. Verbal de-escalation should be included in the initial approach to an agitated patient, although this may be used in combination with pharmacologic measures. Physical restraint, if the patient is not at an immediate risk of harming self or others, is a measure of last resort, which will be discussed later [3, 9]. Moreover, the least restrictive intervention should be used and only as long as necessary [1, 10]. Therefore, physical restraints are indicated if the patient is actively violent [10]. If the restrained patient is then able to be engaged and communicate, additional efforts should be made in verbal de-escalation during the restraining processes and thereafter. Medications should be given to calm patients in restraints. Which medications are given will depend on the patient's level of agitation, the amount of anxiety, and the degree of psychosis. If possible, patient cooperation with medication administration should be solicited and may influence the route that these medications are given; pills or oral dissolving tablets are ideal if the patient is alert and cooperative, while IM injections are often needed if the patient is severely agitated or exhibiting violent behaviors.

There are two general types of physical restraints used for agitated patients in the hospital setting. The first is manually restraining a patient who is an imminent threat to self or others, which is discussed in more detail below. The second are limb restraints that are applied to the extremities to limit movement. Soft wrist restraints are commonly used in the hospital setting and are made of comfortable foam material and secured with hook-and-loop fasteners. This form of physical restraint is typically used for mildly agitated or confused patients to prevent them from getting out of bed or pulling on essential tubes and catheters. Four-point limb restraints are required for severely agitated and combative patients. These restraints are typically wrapped around all four distal extremities at the wrist and ankles to prevent movement. In some institutions, these four-point restraints are composed of a much stronger material such as leather. However, other institutions have stopped using leather restraints due to concerns for adverse events and instead use locked limb-holders made of less abrasive material. Despite these differences in limb restraints, some generalities in their application exist. Providers must be familiar with proper restraint application prior to first-time use, including appropriate sizing based on the patient's weight and height. When applying restraints to the upper extremities or lower extremities, ensure two fingerbreadths of space to prevent neurovascular compromise and injury. Secure restraints to the bedsprings or frame of the bed. Never apply restraints to the side rails of a bed or mattress. Doing so would allow excessive movement that would place the providers and patient at risk. Lastly, avoid tying knots; most knots can be released easily and quickly or alternatively, may be difficult to remove.

To re-emphasize, the underlying goal of physical restraints is to prevent harm to self and others and should only be applied if all other methods have failed. Restraints should also be considered if there is a life-threatening injury that results in agitated behavior or prevents healthcare providers from delivering life-saving interventions. Some examples include hypoxia, hypoglycemia, overdose with stimulants, and traumatic injuries. Patients should be closely monitored for complications of restraint use and reassessed for the continued need for them, as patients may become cooperative as their condition is treated and may no longer need them.

Method of Application

Assuming the decision has been made that a patient requires restraints, certain prerequisites must be met. First and foremost, provider safety is the number one priority. Call for help and do not attempt to restrain the patient alone. Studies have indicated that safe application of restraints requires at least five to six individuals: one person to take control of the head (ensuring to avoid covering the

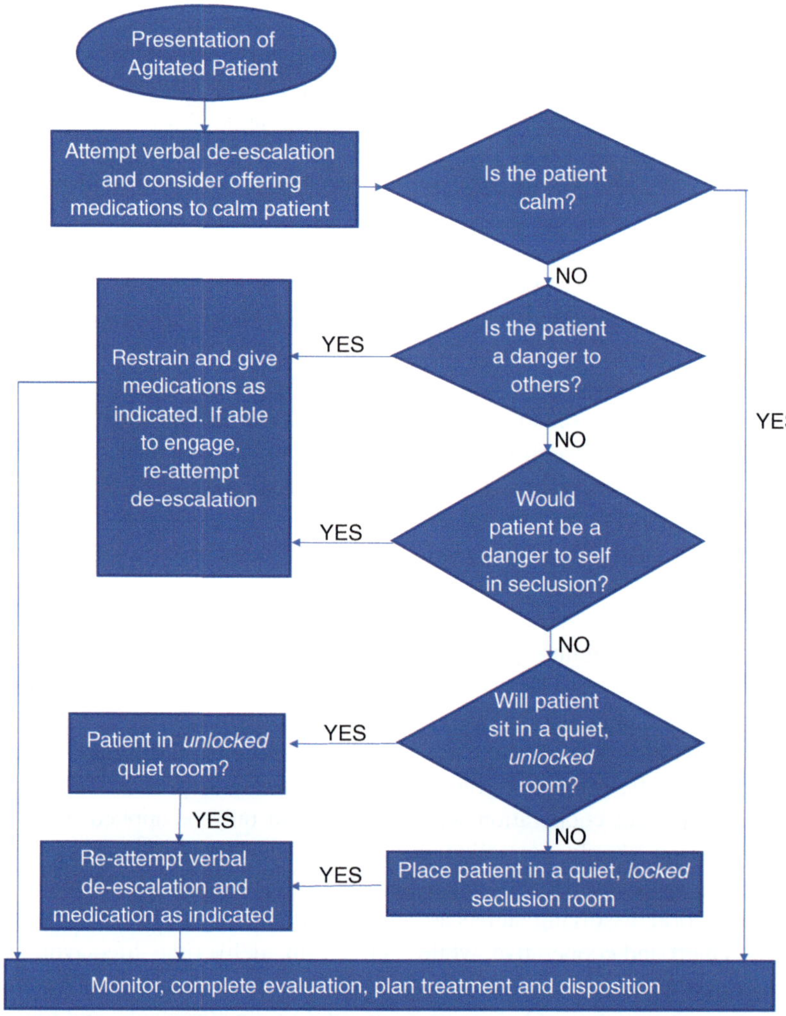

Fig. 24.1 Flowchart for use of restraints and seclusion on agitated patients

mouth and nose), one person for each extremity, and one person as the leader [11]. Prior to restraint application, the leader should attempt verbal de-escalation and tell the patient that if their behavior persists, they will need to be put into restraints. It is essential to verbalize the reason for placing the patient in restraints. Explain to the patient what you are doing, why you are doing it, and what the patient needs to do to prevent it from happening [11–13], and give the patient time to comprehend. This serves to give the patient options, a form of empowerment, and also provides them the opportunity (if able) to de-escalate.

If the patient does not show signs of de-escalation, action must be taken in a confident and swift manner. The leader provides a signal, at which time each team member holds their respective body part (arm, leg, head). If no bed is available, the patient is brought to the floor. Nearly all patients should be restrained in the supine position. Placing a patient in the "hog-tie" position usually involves applying pressure with unsafe holds onto the back, neck, or head. Many deaths have been associated with this position [14]. Although one study found that this position is not associated with hypoxia, the prone position should be avoided because patients who require medication (most restrained patients) cannot protect their airway [15]. Specific populations such as the elderly, acutely ill, or anyone at risk for aspiration may require being rolled onto their side. Once the patient is in restraints, release any harmful holds, such as pressure on the patient's face, neck, or chest.

If the agitated patient attempts to spit at providers, apply a spit mask to the patient's face. Never insert anything into the patient's mouth. Manufacturers have created spit masks for this purpose. It is very important to note the difference between each state's regulations regarding spit masks, since some states forbid application of such masks to agitated patients. Providers should, therefore, become familiar with the laws of their state. Regardless, providers should take the necessary precautions to protect themselves from body fluid exposure.

After the patient has been physically restrained, all attempts must be made to assess airway, breathing, and circulation (ABCs). To assess the patient's airway, ensure that they are able to speak. To assess breathing, look to ensure adequate chest rise and release any restraints that may compromise the patient's respiration. Patients should be placed on a continuous cardiopulmonary monitor, if possible. If medications are given for sedation, or if the patient becomes obtunded, place the patient on continuous waveform capnography to ensure adequate ventilation. The patient must be monitored closely and reassessed at 15-minute intervals. After the patient has met the goals for release from restraints, the provider should debrief the patient. Additionally, staff should undergo debriefing to help participants involved in the care of the patient cope and conceptualize what took place. This is also a good time to discuss what staff thought went well or could be done better next time.

Finally, given that there are several adverse consequences associated with the application of restraints, the American College of Emergency Physicians (ACEP) has outlined several principles regarding their application (see Table 24.2).

Table 24.2 ACEP endorses the following principles regarding patient restraints [16]

Restraints should be instituted only after verbal de-escalation has been attempted.
Restraint of patients should be individualized and employed in a manner that makes all reasonable attempts to maintain the patients' privacy and dignity.
The method of restraint should be the least restrictive necessary for the protection of the patient and others.
Staff should be properly trained in the appropriate use and application of restraints and in the monitoring of patients in restraint and seclusion.
Protocols to ensure patient safety should be developed to address observation and treatment during the period of restraint and periodic assessment as to the need and means of continuing or discontinuing restraint.
The use of restraints should be carefully documented, including the reasons for and means of restraint, alternatives to restraint, and the periodic assessment of the restrained patient.
ACEP opposes any requirement by hospital representatives or medical staff that emergency physicians provide inpatient restraint or seclusion orders. Patient restraint or seclusion requires comprehensive patient assessment, and the emergency physician's principal legal and ethical responsibility is to patients who present to be seen and treated in the emergency department.
The use of restraints should conform to applicable laws, rules, regulations, and accreditation standards [16].

Seclusion

Seclusion is defined as the involuntary confinement of a patient in a room or area from which the patient is physically prevented from leaving. Seclusion may only be used to prevent harm to the patient or others, or destruction of the physical environment, or if the patient is not redirectable [1]. Indications are outlined in Table 24.3. The treatment involves removing the patient from contact with staff, other patients, and external stimuli. The goal of this process is to give the patient space, free of harmful objects and external stimuli, to de-escalate alone or with the help of a healthcare provider. Like patients who require physical restraints, patients who are placed into seclusion must be closely monitored. Some patients may view seclusion as a form of punishment.

Table 24.3 Seclusion indications

Prevent imminent harm to the patient, other persons when other means of control are ineffective
Prevent significant damage to the physical environment
Unable to redirect

Like physical restraints, seclusion should be short-term and used only to protect and ensure the safety of both the patient and staff. Additionally, seclusion should take place in a room designed specifically for that purpose [17]. Providers should be mindful of using seclusion in patients with a known history of claustrophobia or in whom seclusion was used as a form of abuse. For example, seclusion should be avoided if a patient has been forcibly locked in a closet in the past, as the present seclusion may be a trigger and result in psychological trauma. As with restraints, there are no randomized or controlled trials exist supporting this practice [18].

Method of Application

The patient is placed in a room designed specifically for seclusion. This room must be devoid of physical objects that the patient may be able to use to harm him or herself. When placed in seclusion, at least one staff member must be within sight and sound of the patient [17, 19]. Goals for the patient to be out of seclusion must be communicated to the patient throughout the seclusion process. Maintaining close communication between staff and patient throughout the encounter is of the utmost importance. Redirection alone has been shown to decrease the negative experience of seclusion. For example, showing interest and talking with the patient has been shown to reduce stress and may promote a sense of calm [12, 13].

For patients who may be severely agitated and not redirectable, it is still very important to explain what is happening and provide frequent redirection [20]. While in seclusion, patients must have free access to a restroom, water, and food. In the United States, a physician must assess a patient placed in seclusion within 1 hour of the intervention [21].

Once the patient is a candidate for release from seclusion, debriefing should occur. In debriefing the patient, recap what happened and what may have led to seclusion, especially since seclusion is a form of failed prevention. This is often helpful for patients to prevent future use of seclusion and to minimize or reverse any negative effects [22]. Additionally, staff members can comment on what went well or poorly during the intervention.

Documentation and Medicolegal Issues

Regulations by the Department of Health and Human Services (DHHS) and the Center for Medicare and Medicaid Services (CMS) state that restraint or seclusion may only be imposed to ensure the immediate physical safety of the patient, staff members, or others, and that these measures must be discontinued at the earliest possible time [1]. Healthcare personnel have the responsibility to determine if a patient lacks the capacity to refuse treatment. If a patient requires restraints, proper documentation is a necessity and the need to keep the patient safe is of highest priority. Restraining a patient who has the capacity to refuse treatment puts providers at risk for battery and false imprisonment [23]. If the patient has the capacity, the patient must give expressed consent before proceeding with treatment. Alternatively, if deemed to not have the capacity, documentation of the factors that led to treatment without consent is imperative. If unable to determine capacity, then it is more appropriate to treat the patient than put them at risk by not treating. Moreover, it is easier to defend against battery and false imprisonment than it is to defend against negligence in the court of law for patients who are clearly a danger to themselves or others. The law tends to support health care provider's decisions in times of emergency regarding actions to preserve the patient's life or health. However, documentation is key and must include the three following components: (1) an emergency exists, (2) the reason consent could not be obtained, and (3) treatment provided was in the best interest of the patient. For example, "The patient is a threat to himself and others. He is unable to answer questions and provide insight into his illness. Medication and restraints were required to provide life-saving treatment and prevent harm to himself and others." Documentation of the behaviors and decisions of the patient that led to the assessment of the patient's lack of capacity is very important. If the patient's family or friends are present, it is essential to explain to them the need for action, and one should document their support [23]. Assessing capacity is discussed more thoroughly in Chap. 43.

When restraint or seclusion is used for the management of violent or self-destructive behavior that jeopardizes the immediate physical safety of the patient, a staff member, or others, the patient must be seen face-to-face within 1 hour after the initiation of the intervention. The patient may be assessed by a physician, other licensed independent practitioner (LIP), registered nurse, or physician assistant who has been trained in the CMS restraint-and-seclusion training requirements [24]. If the face-to-face evaluation is conducted by a trained registered nurse or physician assistant, that individual must consult the attending physician or other LIP who is responsible for the patient's care as soon as possible. Simultaneous restraint-and-seclusion use is permitted only if the patient is continually monitored face to face by an assigned, trained staff member or by trained staff using both video and audio equipment [1]. Patients requiring restraint or seclusion should be assessed every 15 minutes thereafter. See Table 24.4 for assessments that should be made by healthcare providers for patients in restraints or seclusion.

Table 24.4 Assessments on patients in restraints or seclusion

Signs of any injury associated with applying restraint or seclusion
Nutrition and hydration
Circulation and range of motion in the extremities
Vital signs
Level of distress and agitation
Skin integrity
Mental status
Cognitive functioning
Hygiene and elimination

Conclusion

Using restraints and seclusion is considered a last-ditch effort in treating the agitated patient. As illustrated in the initial case example, physical restraints and seclusion carry high risks for patients and providers. All attempts must be made to avoid these techniques. Early implementation of verbal de-escalation and medication administration is essential. Applying restraints or seclusion is a high-risk procedure that must be performed with care. Ensure not to restrain patients in the prone position, and release dangerous holds on the back, neck, chest, or face immediately. Once restrained or in seclusion, these patients require frequent monitoring and release as soon as possible. Lastly, proper documentation is important to minimize any medicolegal issues that may come up from appropriately restraining a patient against their will.

References

1. Department of Health and Human Services, Centers for Medicare and Medicaid Services [Internet]. CMS manual system: Pub. 100-07 states operations: Provider certification. Transmittal 37 2008. Updated October 2008. [cited 17 Sept 2018]. Available from https://www.cms.gov/Regulations-and-Guidance/Guidance/Transmittals/downloads/R37SOMA.pdf.
2. Nelstrop L, Chandler-Oatts J, Bingley W, Bleetman T, Corr F, Cronin-Davis J, et al. A systematic review of the safety and effectiveness of restraint and seclusion as interventions for the short-term management of violence in adult psychiatric inpatient settings and emergency departments. Worldview Evid Based Nurs. 2006;3(1):8–18.
3. Weiland T, Ivory S, Hutton J. Managing acute behavioral disturbances in the emergency department using the environment, policies and practices: a systematic review. West J Emerg Med. 2017;19(4):647–61.
4. Hodge A, Marshall A. Violence and aggression in the emergency department: a critical care perspective. Aust Crit Care. 2007;20(2):61–7.
5. Joint Commission Standards on Restraint and Seclusion/Non-violent Crisis Intervention Training Program [Internet]. Joint Commission on Accreditation of Healthcare Organizations. Reprinted 2010. [cited 17 Sept 2018]. Available from: https://www.crisisprevention.com/CPI/media/Media/Resources/alignments/Joint-Commission-Restraint-Seclusion-Alignment-2011.pdf.

6. Zun LS. A prospective study of the complication rate of use of patient restraint in the emergency department. J Emerg Med. 2003;24(2):119–24.
7. Renwick L, Lavelle M, Brennan G, Stewart D, James K, Richardson M, et al. Physical injury and workplace assault in UK mental health trusts: an analysis of formal reports. Int J Ment Health Nurs. 2016;25(4):355–66.
8. Hick J, Smith S, Lynch M. Metabolic acidosis in restraint-associated cardiac arrest: a case series. Acad Emerg Med. 1999;6(3):239–43.
9. Annas G. The last resort: the use of physical restraints in medical emergencies. N Engl J Med. 1999;341(18):1408–12.
10. Knox D, Holloman G. Use and avoidance of seclusion and restraints: consensus statement of the American Association for Emergency Psychiatry Project BETA Seclusion and Restraint Workgroup. West J Emerg Med. 2012;13(1):35–40.
11. Rintoul Y, Wynaden D, McGowan S. Managing aggression in the emergency department: promoting an interdisciplinary approach. Int Emerg Nurs. 2009;17(2):122–7.
12. Chan C, Chung C. A retrospective study of seclusion in an emergency department. Hong Kong J Emer Med. 2005;12(1):6–13.
13. Strike C, Rufo C, Spence J, Links P, Bergmans Y, Ball J, et al. Unintended impact of psychiatric safe rooms in emergency departments: the experiences of suicidal males with substance use disorders. Brief Treat Crisis Interv. 2008;8(3):264–73.
14. O'Halloran R, Janice F. Asphyxial death during prone restraint revisited: a report of 21 cases. Am J Forensic Med Pathol. 2000;21(1):39–52.
15. Chan TVG, Neuman T, Clausen J. Restraint position and positional asphyxia. Ann Emerg Med. 1997;20(5):578–86.
16. ACEP Board of Directors. Use of patient restraints. American College of Emergency Physicians. Updated April 2014. [cited 17 Sept 2018]. Available from: https://www.acep.org/patient-care/policy-statements/use-of-patient-restraints/#sm.0000sq4z6f33af00rfs2rqnp2rw3s.
17. Pereira S, Fleischhacker W, Allen M. Management of behavioural emergencies. J Psychiatr Intens Care. 2006;2(2):71–83.
18. Sailas E, Fenton M. Seclusion and restraint for people with serious mental illnesses. Cochrane Database Syst Rev [Internet]. 2000; [cited 2018 September 17]. Available from: https://www.cochrane.org/CD001163/SCHIZ_seclusion-and-restraint-for-people-with-serious-mental-illnesses.
19. Staten P. Restraint, seclusion standards raise questions. Nurs Manag. 2001;32(7, Part 1 of 2):17.
20. Mann-Poll P, Smit A, De Vries W, Boumans C, Hutschemaekers G. Factors contributing to mental health professionals' decision to use seclusion. Psychiatr Serv. 2011;62(5):498–503.
21. Rocca P, Villari V, Bogetto F. Managing the aggressive and violent patient in the psychiatric emergency. Prog Neuro-Psychopharmacol Biol Psychiatry. 2006;30(4):586–98.
22. O'Hagan M, Divis M, Long J. Best practice in the reduction and elimination of seclusion and restraint: Seclusion: Time for change. Te Pou o Te Whakaaro Nui: the National Centre of Mental Health Research, Information and Workforce Development. 2008; [cited 17 Sept 2018]. Available from: https://www.mentalhealth.org.nz/assets/ResourceFinder/FINAL-SECLUSION-REDUCTION-BEST-PRACTICE-Research-Report.pdf.
23. Thomas J, Moore G. Medical-legal issues in the agitated patient: cases and caveats. West J Emerg Med. 2013;14(5):559–65.
24. Centers for Medicare and Medicaid Services. In: Giacomo-Geffers E, Herrlin D, editors. The CMS restraint training requirements handbook. Brentwood: HCPro a division of BLR; 2016. [cited 17 Sept 2018]. Available from: https://hcmarketplace.com/aitdownloadablefiles/download/aitfile/aitfile_id/1880.pdf.

25 Boarding of Psychiatric Patients in the Emergency Department

Kimberly Nordstrom

Introduction

Since the peak of state-run mental health hospitals in 1955, which reached 344 beds per 100,000 population, there has been a steady decline. In 2014, the number was 11.7, with 5.4 beds filled with forensic patients [1]. As these public hospitals have declined in beds, patients have moved into the community. At first, this deinstitutionalization was thought to be preferable, but this change brought with it a rise in the mentally ill found in jails, prisons, or warehoused in emergency departments (ED) awaiting psychiatric hospitalization.

While immediate admission to a psychiatric facility is often the goal, it is not always an option. In many states, the number of people requiring admission far exceeds the number of available inpatient psychiatric beds. Patients who have been assessed, stabilized, and deemed appropriate for inpatient care by emergency physicians and psychiatrists must remain in the ED for hours to days, awaiting an appropriate inpatient bed. Termed "boarding," this queuing of inpatients in the ED is all too common. This phenomenon has become so widespread that the American Psychiatric Association has created a position statement [2] and resource document on the issue [3].

This chapter will serve to discuss longer-term treatment options for patient boarders. Acute treatment, which usually focuses on agitation stabilization, is detailed throughout the rest of the book and will only be briefly addressed in this chapter. Intermediate, or longer-term, care approaches the disease process in a more comprehensive way.

Definition of "Boarding"

Hospitals and accrediting agencies tend to define the word differently, based on time after the admission order is placed. Some hospitals consider boarding to begin at the time of the admission order, while others create an arbitrary clock to signify an extended stay. The Joint Commission settled on 4 hours as the standard, citing field and literature reviews for this determination [4]. The actual amount of time necessary for a patient to be called a boarder is somewhat controversial but in various facilities may start an administrative clock that changes clinical behaviors. Some EDs have created patient-care areas specific for boarders, as funding sources, including the Centers for Medicare and Medicaid Services, tend to require specific behaviors and documentation to accept charges for extended-stay care.

K. Nordstrom (✉)
Department of Psychiatry, University of Colorado Anschutz, Aurora, CO, USA

L. S. Zun et al. (eds.), *Behavioral Emergencies for Healthcare Providers*,
https://doi.org/10.1007/978-3-030-52520-0_25

Treatment Team Members

As in other areas of specialty care, it is often helpful to augment the treatment team for specific functions. When it comes to treating the long-stay or boarding psychiatric patient, adding a psychiatrist or clinician with specialty training in psychiatry can be very helpful. Another highly important team member is the social worker.

For facilities with a large psychiatric presence, the consult-liaison or inpatient psychiatrist can sometimes be called to take a direct role in patient care. Staff psychiatrists may provide useful phone consultation, even if unable to initiate direct care for the patient. Many hospitals do not have the luxury of calling on psychiatry staff and are forced to be more creative. With the advent of telepsychiatry, even rural hospitals may be afforded the opportunity to have a psychiatrist consultant. For the established patient, contacting the patient's outpatient psychiatrist or primary care physician may aid in understanding medication issues for the patient and help define treatment goals for the stay.

Social workers are invaluable to the treatment team. Roles may be dependent on the setting but could include obtaining collateral information from outside treaters and family, short-term therapy and family meetings, and disposition planning. Each of these will be described below in more detail.

Treatment Goals

The transition from acute to long-stay, as noted previously, may be an arbitrary point on the clock, but this point changes the care paradigm. The goals change from triage, identification of illness (especially ruling out delirium and other medical causes of psychiatric symptoms), treatment of agitation, and disposition, to a new focus on the underlying disorder.

The focus turns to stabilization of the psychiatric illness. Treatment is largely determined by past history:

- Is this disorder new-onset for the patient or long-standing?
- Is there a history of noncompliance with medication?
- Is there a history of responding negatively or favorably to specific medications?
- Are there psychosocial pieces that need to be considered?

New-Onset Disease

Psychosis

Psychosis in a patient with no history of mental illness should be evaluated medically. This point cannot be overstated. The differential diagnosis is long, and some medical causes of psychosis are associated with high mortality [5–9]. After a thorough workup, including information from collateral sources, treatment can begin.

For the initial treatment of the psychotic, unagitated patient, consideration should be given to patient preference. A psychotic patient is presumed to have decision-making capacity unless, on exam, the patient is found not to have the capacity for treatment decisions. This is an important concept, as psychotic patients should be afforded autonomy and allowed to participate in treatment decisions. There are various treatment strategies for psychosis, and the decision is based on several factors, such as patient preference, cost, and access to care. In the ED, an antipsychotic may be initiated, but follow-up care is typically necessary, as some psychotic disorders may be chronic in nature, such as schizophrenia or persistent substance-induced psychosis.

The other major consideration is side-effect profile. The first-generation antipsychotics have a greater rate of extrapyramidal effects, whereas second-generation antipsychotics have a higher propensity toward metabolic effects. Within the second-generation class, some medications are linked more to weight gain, diabetes, and cholesterol elevation with long-term use than others, though all of the medications in the class have risk. Similarly, some first-generation (chlorpromazine) and second-generation (quetiapine, olanzapine) antipsychotics have a higher propensity for sedation, which, unless once-a-night dosing is sufficient, tends to be considered a negative experience by patients. Also, patients tend to prefer one medication over polypharmacy. This may come into play if considering a high-potency first-generation antipsychotic, such as haloperidol.

The decision of initial medication may also be determined by the level of cooperation and the level of agitation of the patient. There are now antipsychotics available for a variety of routes of administration, including tablet/capsules, rapid-dissolving tablets, inhalation, intramuscular (IM) injection, and intravenous (IV) injection. A cooperative patient who is in distress may agree to oral medications, but as cooperation decreases, consideration must be given to both possible diversion ("cheeking") and safety of the patient and team while administering the medication. When diversion is suspected, a rapidly dissolving tablet, such as rapidly dissolving olanzapine or risperidone, might prove most useful. There is also increasing evidence to support the use of inhaled loxapine, as it can be quickly determined if the patient does not take a sufficient breath. When a patient is highly agitated, a tablet or inhaler may not be feasible, and an IM or IV formulation may be preferred, though restraints are often necessary at this point.

Bipolar Mania

Before considering treatment for new-onset mania, all other causes should be ruled out. For treatment, second-generation antipsychotics or mood stabilizers may be considered. Most of the second-generation antipsychotics have been approved for treatment in acute mania as monotherapy or as an adjunct with lithium or divalproate. Initiating a mood stabilizer, such as valproic acid/divalproate, carbamazepine, or lithium, may take a little more thought because of titration needs but may be more cost-effective. Valproic acid can be oral-loaded in the ED at 20–30 mg/kg/day in a healthy person with normal liver function [10]. Carbamazepine needs titration and has multiple drug–drug interactions, making it less attractive in the ED setting. Lithium, while also requiring titration, can be initiated in the ED. The advantages of the mood stabilizers are that there is extensive history with these medications and the therapeutic target dosing is known. The rule of 8s is a helpful mnemonic for target therapeutic levels for maintenance treatment: 0.8 for lithium; 8 for carbamazepine; and 80 for valproic acid. The major disadvantage of the mood stabilizers, especially lithium, is that they can be fatal in overdose. In the case of lithium, the therapeutic window is narrow, with toxicity beginning at blood levels just outside of this window. A meta-analysis of all of the second-generation antipsychotics used in the treatment of acute mania, except for asenapine, as well as lithium, carbamazepine, oxcarbazepine, divalproex, and haloperidol found that patients had an increased chance of response and remission (except for oxcarbazepine) than placebo, but also had a higher risk of discontinuation due to adverse events [11].

Depression

The long-stay patient suffering from depression may be admitted to the hospital for one of two reasons. The first reason is that the person is at high risk for suicide; the second has to do with the inability to care for self. Treatment for new-onset depression would be the same as long-standing depression, except that long-standing depression may be refractory.

The primary antidepressant selection determinants are cost, side effect profiles, and compliance likelihood. Most of the selective serotonin reuptake inhibitors (SSRIs) are now generic and readily available. If the patient has never had an adequate trial (defined by most as at least 6–8 weeks) on an SSRI, this is a good choice. Since there are serotonin receptors in the GI system, any SSRI can cause nausea. SSRIs are known to have a myriad of side effects that lead many to premature treatment discontinuation [12]. They can be initially activating, even increasing anxiety. For the anxious patient, initiating an SSRI at one-half the normal starting dose (with a plan for this to continue for 1–2 weeks) may mitigate this activation. On the spectrum of activation, fluoxetine tends to be the most activating, with paroxetine the least activating. Side effects are largely the same for serotonin and norepinephrine reuptake inhibitors (SNRIs).

The acute treatment of bipolar depression also requires caution. At best, typical antidepressants have been found to lack efficacy [13]. Of more concern is their potential role in manic relapse [14]. In the meta-analysis mentioned above, lamotrigine, aripiprazole, olanzapine, and quetiapine were included to determine efficacy as monotherapy. Only quetiapine—and, to a lesser degree, olanzapine—showed efficacy as monotherapy for acute bipolar depression [11].

Treatment of Patient with Chronic Mental Illness

This is where collateral information is highly helpful. As noted earlier, specific questions need to be answered that will aid in guiding treatment. Is there a history of noncompliance? If the answer is yes, clinicians tend to become judgmental, rather than ask the following question: "Why?" Noncompliance may be caused by a number of reasons: lack of insight into the disease, side effects, allergy, cost, or difficulty filling medications (transport), to name a few. When helping a patient choose a medication, past difficulties should be discussed.

In many cases, the treatment may simply be restarting the medication. For most patients, restarting and/or retitrating home medications, while covering for breakthrough symptoms, should be considered. Familiarity with side-effect profiles of psychotropics, as well as titration nuances of clozapine and lithium, are important. For example, retitrating lithium while also using an atypical antipsychotic and benzodiazepine is an effective bridge between acute stabilization and intermediate care. Akathisia and orthostatic hypotension are anticipated with some antipsychotics, particularly when restarting the home dose. Both can be managed easily in the ED. The use of fall precautions and urinals might be helpful for orthostasis. If the patient has been off medication for a long period, consider retitrating the medication, rather than restarting the previous dose.

Nonpharmacological Treatment

For the psychotic or manic patient, managing agitation levels while treating the source is key. A simple step can include destimulating the environment. This is accomplished through dimming lights, decreasing the number of hospital staff who interact with the patient, and moving the patient to an observation area that may be quieter than the main ED. Meeting basic needs such as providing food and a blanket can also go a long way. Verbal de-escalation can be a key ingredient to engagement with the patient [15]. This is largely covered elsewhere (see Chap. 23).

For the depressed patient, quick therapies have been found to be helpful in the emergency environment. Some of these therapies include supportive therapy, solution-focused therapy, motivational interviewing, and family meetings. Most social workers are adept at these therapies. In its simplest form, supportive therapy is listening and encouraging the patient. This can be very helpful in calming the patient who is overwhelmed. Solution-focused therapy basically helps the patient to problem-solve. This is particularly helpful for the depressed or anxious patient. The idea is not to problem solve but rather to create an environment and gently question the patient in order to help the patient become more goal directed.

In the ED, short-term therapy largely focuses on safety planning. A tool has been created for emergency physicians to use for patients when there is concern for suicide risk and may be a good place to start [16]. Safety planning begins with a safety risk assessment. An important piece in the assessment is determining modifiable risk factors for suicide. If modifiable risk factors are elucidated, they can become the focus of the therapy. An example of this is a recent argument with family. The individual therapy can focus on the patient's perspective as to the causes and outcomes. This can possibly evolve into a family session where the issues can be examined, with the end result of having a safety plan in place that the patient and family can support. Safety risk assessments are covered fully elsewhere.

Reevaluation

For the long-stay patient, reevaluation of the psychiatric condition is often overlooked. Many times, when a patient is placed on admission status, this is left unchallenged. If the patient is receiving active treatment while awaiting inpatient care, the severity of the condition may lessen, allowing for a diversion from inpatient hospitalization. In many communities, there are lower levels of short-term residential placement; acute treatment units and crisis stabilization units should be considered. For the depressed suicidal patient, psychosocial stressors may have lessened to the point that a patient can be safely discharged back into the community, especially if family is involved.

Reevaluation is also helpful in cases of drug-induced psychosis. Typically, patients will clear within 24–48 hours and be able to be discharged or transferred to a substance treatment facility.

Disposition

If the patient continues to require an inpatient level of care, a comprehensive handoff should occur, especially if treatment for the psychiatric disorder has been provided. This allows the next team to utilize the head start in treatment, rather than start over in care. Any problematic side effects or possible allergies should be part of this communication.

In some cases, as noted above, treatment of patients while boarding can end in discharge to a lower level of care. If the patient is discharged back to the community, a referral to a primary care physician, psychiatrist, or mental health clinic is helpful but not sufficient. If medication is initiated, an actual follow-up appointment, within 1–2 weeks, should be secured for the patient, with patient education around needing to return if symptoms worsen or suicidal thoughts return.

After starting an antidepressant in the ED, an increase in suicidal behavior is a concern. The depressed patient is classically thought to be more likely to attempt suicide after the initiation of treatment, when energy and motivation are stronger. A 27-year longitudinal, observational study has refuted this belief [17]. Despite noting that antidepressants were more likely to be used in participants with greater symptom severity or symptom worsening, an overall reduction in the risk of suicidal behavior after antidepressant initiation was observed [17]. Nonetheless, quick follow-up is necessary after the initiation of a psychiatric medication at discharge.

Conclusion

With inpatient psychiatric beds less available in the community, EDs have had to shoulder the burden of holding patients awaiting these beds, sometimes for days or weeks. New thoughts on the boarding of patients have created a paradigm shift from housing to treating the primary psychiatric disorder. This can best be done through a team approach, with psychiatric consultation and social work team members. Treatment can begin in the form of medication and short-term therapies. Reevaluation should occur at least daily to determine if the patient continues to require the highest level of care. Care alternatives should be understood by team members and used, if able to do so safely.

References

1. Beyond beds: the vital role of a Full Continuum of Psychiatric Care. National Association of State Mental Health Program Directors. 2017 Oct. Available at http://www.treatmentadvocacycenter.org/storage/documents/beyond-beds.pdf. Accessed on 25 Mar 2020.
2. APA official actions: position statement on emergency boarding of patients with acute mental illness. 2016 July. Available at: https://www.psychiatry.org/File%20Library/About-APA/

Organization-Documents-Policies/Policies/Position-2016-Emergency-Department-Boarding-of-Patients-with-Acute-Mental-Illness.pdf, Accessed on 25 Mar 2020.
3. Nordstrom K, Berlin JS, Nash SS, Shah SB, et al. Boarding of mentally ill patients in emergency departments: American Psychiatric Association Resource Document. West J Emerg Med. 2019;20(5):690–5.
4. Manual A, Longer AMN, Seal UG. The patient flow standard and the 4-hour recommendation. Jt Comm Perspect. 2013;33(6):1–4.
5. Corbett B, Nordstrom K, Vilke G, Wilson MP. Psychiatric emergencies for clinicians: Emergency department diagnosis and management of steroid psychosis. J Emerg Med. 2016;51(5):557–60.
6. Lasoff D, Vilke G, Nordstrom K, Wilson MP. Psychiatric emergencies for clinicians: Detection and management of Anti-N-Methyl-D-Aspartate receptor encephalitis. J Emerg Med. 2016;51(5):561–3.
7. Nordstrom K, Vilke GM, Wilson MP. Psychiatric emergencies for clinicians: The ED management of serotonin syndrome. J Emerg Med. 2016;50(1):89–91.
8. Sharp CS, Wilson MP, Nordstrom K. Psychiatric emergencies for clinicians: The ED management of thyroid storm. J Emerg Med. 2016;51(2):155–8.
9. Wilson MP, Vilke GM, Hayden SR, Nordstrom K. Psychiatric emergencies for clinicians: the ED management of neuroleptic malignant syndrome. J Emerg Med. 2016;51(1):66–9.
10. Hirschfeld RM, Baker JD, Wozniak P, et al. The safety and early efficacy of oral-loaded divalproex versus standard-titration divalproex, lithium, olanzapine, and placebo in the treatment of acute mania associated with bipolar disorder. J Clin Psychiatry. 2003;64(7):841–6.
11. Tamayo JM, Zarate CA, Vieta E, et al. Level of response and safety of pharmacological monotherapy in the treatment of acute bipolar I disorder phases: a systematic review and meta-analysis. Int J Neuropsychopharmacol. 2010;13(6):813–32.
12. Warden D, Madhukar H, Trivedi MD, et al. Early adverse events and attrition in SSRI treatment: a suicide assessment methodology study. J Clin Psychopharmacol. 2010;30(3):259–66.
13. Sachs GS, Nierenberg AA, Calabrese JR, et al. Effectiveness of adjunctive antidepressant treatment for bipolar depression. N Engl J Med. 2007;356(17):1711–22.
14. Lewis J, Winokur G. The induction of mania: a natural history study with controls. Arch Gen Psychiatry. 1982;39(3):303–6.
15. Richmond JS, Berlin JS, Fishkind AB, et al. Verbal de-escalation of the agitated patient: consensus statement of the American Association for Emergency Psychiatry Project BETA De-Escalation Workgroup. West J Emerg Med. 2012;13(1):17–25.
16. Wilson MP, Moutier C, Wolf L, Nordstrom K, et al. Emergency department recommendations for suicide prevention in adults: the ICAR2E mnemonic and a systematic review of the literature. Am J Emerg Med. 2019;37:2246; [Epub ahead of print]. https://doi.org/10.1016/j.ajem.2019.06.031.
17. Leon AC, Solomon DA, Li C, et al. Antidepressants and risks of suicide and suicide attempts: a 27-year observational study. J Clin Psychiatry. 2011;72(5):580–6.

Rapidly Acting Treatment in the ED for Psychiatric Patients

26

Michael P. Wilson and Ross Heller

Introduction

Psychiatric patients in the emergency department (ED) present unique and difficult challenges for the emergency medicine physician. Ostensibly, the primary role of the ED physician with regard to the psychiatric patient is to "medically clear" the patient prior to psychiatric evaluation. By "clear," standard practice is to reasonably ensure that the patient has no medical cause for their psychiatric symptoms. Yet, the evaluation and treatment of the psychiatric patient are often not done in a linear fashion. The initial management of any psychiatric patient is to assure their safety and health, as well as the safety of others in the ED. A calm, quiet patient with a history of depression who presents to the ED with complaints of their typical depression and feeling of hopelessness may be fairly uncomplicated to evaluate. However, patients who are acutely agitated, hostile, aggressive, psychotic, altered in sensorium, or aggressively homicidal or suicidal present an entirely different challenge. Given the danger to the physician, the staff, and the patient, it is often necessary to rapidly treat a patient's psychiatric symptoms with medications even before a full workup is completed. This chapter will review current therapies, as well as newer and investigational treatment options that are useful in the treatment of acute psychiatric symptoms.

M. P. Wilson (✉)
Department of Emergency Medicine, University of Arkansas for Medical Sciences, Little Rock, AR, USA

Department of Emergency Medicine, Saint Louis University School of Medicine, St. Louis, MO, USA
e-mail: mpwilso1@outlook.com

R. Heller
Department of Emergency Medicine, Saint Louis University School of Medicine, St. Louis, MO, USA

Treatment of the Acute Psychotic, Aggressive, and Violent Patient

DSM-5 describes a brief psychotic episode as having one or more of the following: delusions, hallucinations, disorganized speech, or grossly disorganized behavior. These patients may also have a rapidly changing mood, disorientation, and impaired attention, and can have emotional volatility, outlandish behavior, and rampant screaming. A careful mental status examination is required to distinguish this from delirium, dementia, organic brain syndrome, or another medical condition.

Immediate Medical Assessment and Intervention

While it is incumbent on the ED physician to ensure that a patient exhibiting psychiatric symptoms is medically assessed, often the patient must

L. S. Zun et al. (eds.), *Behavioral Emergencies for Healthcare Providers*,
https://doi.org/10.1007/978-3-030-52520-0_26

be treated acutely with medications to prevent aggressive and agitated symptoms from progressing and to allow for an effective medical examination process. This may require a flexible and simultaneous combination of pertinent medical assessment and stabilization, along with the use of restraints. Particular attention to abnormal vital signs, including blood pressure, pulse, respiratory rate, pulse oximetry, temperature, and the bedside glucose measurement are important for any patient with an altered sensorium. Appropriate interventions are made as abnormalities are identified.

Restraint

During early stabilization and evaluation, and prior to an understanding of the underlying cause of the altered sensorium, restraint of the patient may be necessary. (Please see Chap. 24.) All ED staff involved in the use of restraints must be familiar with the use of restraints and their proper and appropriate application [1, 2]. Studies have found that the application of restraints in and of themselves can increase agitation. Techniques for de-escalation should also be applied when time permits to avoid the use of restraints, as there are well-recognized risks involving restraints including serious injury and death to the patient [3]. The use of restraints must be minimal in duration and appropriate in the application, but may be necessary so that the staff can safely administer medications to extremely agitated patients. Early initiation of medications for agitation can assist in reducing seclusion and physical restraint use and improve the safety of patients and staff [4].

Psychopharmacological Treatments

Rapid treatment to stop acute psychotic symptoms should be initiated whenever the patient is out of control or escalating in such a manner as to put them or staff at risk of injury (please see also Chap. 23). Traditionally, the acute psychotic state was treated with first-generation antipsychotics [4–8]. These agents have been used for many decades, have a well-known therapeutic range, and may have known risks. In the past decade, a group of drugs known as second-generation antipsychotics have shown increasing use in the management of the psychotic patient. There has been extensive evaluation in the management of the acutely psychotic patient's symptoms in the emergency department setting utilizing these agents [9–22]. The key for the emergency physician is to be knowledgeable about the risks and benefits, as well as know which drugs to use in specific subsets of patients.

First-Generation Antipsychotics (FGAs)

This class of antipsychotics has been shown to provide rapid, predictable, and effective sedation in the management of patients who are acutely psychotic [6, 23]. The most often used antipsychotics in this class have been haloperidol (Haldol) and droperidol (Inapsine) [23]. Intramuscular (IM) Haldol in typical doses of 5–10 mg is traditionally used to treat thought disorders, hallucinations, and delusional activity but is contraindicated as a single agent [24]. Haloperidol can be given both orally and IM in the emergency department setting at 2–5 mg doses, utilizing multiple doses of haloperidol intramuscularly over a 3-hour period [7]. The dose range over the 3 hours was a low of 13 mg IM up to a high of 33 mg IM. Approximately 35% of the patients suffered the major side effect of acute dystonia and extra-pyramidal symptoms (EPS), which are known to be dose-dependent, thus limiting the use of high-dose haloperidol.

EPS side effects and the association of haloperidol with the neuroleptic malignant syndrome (NMS) has prompted a search for other treatments. Although an early study showed a decrease in side effects with the combination of haloperidol and lorazepam, meta-analyses have shown no benefit [7, 24].

Droperidol is another first-generation antipsychotic that has been long used to treat acutely psychotic patients [4]. However, in 2001, this drug received a black-box warning from the

FDA, given in the association of QT interval prolongation and sudden death [25]. As a result, the use of droperidol for antipsychotic treatment in the emergency department setting drastically declined. However, some studies have disputed the clinical significance of QT interval prolongation, stating a lack of a convincing causal relationship between droperidol and life-threatening cardiac events [8].

Benzodiazepines and Combination Therapy

Benzodiazepines—such as lorazepam (Ativan) at 1–2 mg IM or orally, or clonazepam (Klonopin) at 1–2 mg IM—may be given as single agents [26, 27]. Although there is only low-quality evidence, benzodiazepines may be a reasonable alternative or adjunct to antipsychotics in order to avoid antipsychotic toxicity. It has been found that given by itself, lorazepam may be as effective as haloperidol in sedation but has fewer extrapyramidal side effects. Although there are fewer EPS side effects, the use of lorazepam can lead to serious complications, including excessive sedation, confusion, disinhibition, ataxia, and respiratory depression, and patients should, therefore, be monitored continuously [27].

Second-Generation Antipsychotics (SGAs)

The advent of the second-generation antipsychotics was promising, with the suggestion that patients would be treated for their symptoms with much less concern for the EPS and other side effects than FGAs. The SGAs (see Table 26.1) most commonly used in the ED include risperi-

Table 26.1 Medications useful for the "lysis" of acute psychiatric symptoms in the ED

Drug	Indication	Dosage	Primary side effects	Secondary side effects	Warnings
Haloperidol[a] (Haldol)	Acute psychosis and agitation	2–5 mg IM may repeat	EPS, other movement disorders	NMS	Prolongs QT
Droperidol[a]	Acute psychosis/agitation	2.5–5 mg IM	Sedation	EPS	Not safe in patients with prolonged QT or arrhythmias
Ziprasidone (Geodon)[b]	Acute psychosis/agitation	10–20 mg IM up to 40 mg	Sedation, EPS, orthostatic hypotension	NMS	Can cause increased QT—do not use in patients with known QT prolongation
Olanzapine (Zyprexa)[b]	Acute psychosis/agitation	10 mg IM or oral tablet	Sedation, EPS, orthostatic hypotension	NMS	Do not use with other CNS depressants; caution in patients with dementia
Quetiapine (Seroquel)[b]	Acute psychosis/agitation but primarily shown in bipolar/schizophrenia and ICU delirium	25–50 mg PO starting dose BID	Sedation, EPS, orthostatic hypotension	NMS	Can cause increased QT—do not use in patients with known QT prolongation; caution in patients with dementia
Risperidone (Risperdal)[b]	Acute psychosis/agitation but primarily shown in bipolar/schizophrenia	1–2 mg PO or ODT	Sedation, EPS, orthostatic hypotension	NMS	Caution if using in dementia patients
Lorazepam (Ativan)	Rapid tranquilization of the agitated patient	1–2 mg IM or PO; may repeat	Sedation and respiratory depression	CNS depression	Can cause respiratory arrest; must monitor

[a]FGA
[b]SGA

done, quetiapine, olanzapine, and ziprasidone, which effectively control a broad range of symptoms associated with psychosis, including agitation and aggression with a much-reduced side-effect profile [4]. These agents are believed to work through the D2 (dopamine) receptors, as well as inhibiting serotonin reuptake. These differing receptors may contribute to the more favorable side-effect profile, although SGAs are still associated, albeit to a lesser extent, with the development of neuroleptic malignant syndrome [28]. Although the combination of SGAs and benzodiazepines is not as well studied as the combination of FGAs and benzodiazepines, some studies have claimed that this combination is safe in acute use, although have recommended against the use of injectable SGAs in alcohol intoxication [29–32].

Rapid Treatment of Acute Depression and Suicidal Ideation

The acute management of the depressed or suicidal patient requires a comprehensive approach. Disposition of these patients can be difficult, lengthy, and fraught with potential hazards [33]. While impractical to admit all patients with suicidal ideation or attempts, the use of a high-risk screen is not a panacea. Such techniques as a no-harm contract are of little benefit and are not recommended in the ED [34, 35]. However, joint safety planning is recommended and may reduce the risk of a future suicide attempt. Collaboration with a mental health clinician is necessary to develop a treatment plan, especially if the patient is to be discharged from the ED. The prescribing of antidepressant medications is typically not performed in the ED and is not yet considered standard care. Most of these medications do not have a clinical effect for at least 2 weeks after initiation of treatment. In addition, some antidepressants have been associated with an initial increased risk for suicidal behavior, particularly the SSRI class.

An agent that would alleviate thoughts of self-harm while providing for a "cooling-off period" for patients while they achieve therapeutic benefit from antidepressant therapy would be quite useful in an ED setting. Ketamine, a well-known agent used as an anesthetic and for pain management, has been recently studied for this purpose. Its use in treating acute depression with relief of symptoms such as depression, anxiety, and hopelessness is relatively new, and the use of ketamine is not yet considered standard care [36]. However, some early studies of ketamine have shown promise for stopping the suicidal thoughts in patients for up to 7–10 days [37, 38]. If proven effective, ketamine therapy may allow discharge and follow-up with some patients, without the need for emergency psychiatric hospitalization.

In conclusion, acute psychiatric conditions that present to the ED often require a multifaceted approach. Underlying medical conditions must be evaluated, treated, or excluded. To assist in the process, rapid treatment of psychotic symptoms is useful. Understanding the available medication armamentarium for rapid control of the acutely agitated, psychotic, or depressed patient is mandatory for the safety evaluation, treatment, and disposition. These medications not only stabilize the patient but may also prevent immediate harm to self or others. In addition, these medications may facilitate further psychiatric intervention when needed and may potentially reduce the patient's symptoms enough to allow for safe discharge from the ED. The future of mental health care, especially in an era of dwindling resources, will require additional research to identify safe treatment alternatives for the appropriate disposition of patients.

References

1. Zun LS, Downey LA. Level of agitation of psychiatric patients presenting to an emergency department. Prim Care Companion J Clin Psychiatry. 2008;10(2):108–13.
2. Knox DK, Holloman GH. Use and avoidance of seclusion and restraint: consensus statement of the American Association for Emergency Psychiatry Project BETA seclusion and restraint workgroup. West J Emerg Med. 2012;13(1):35–40.
3. Richmond JS, Berlin JS, Fishkind AB, Holloman GH Jr, Zeller SL, Wilson MP, et al. Verbal de-escalation of the agitated patient: consensus statement of the

American Association for Emergency Psychiatry Project BETA De-escalation Workgroup. West J Emerg Med. 2012;13(1):17–25.
4. Wilson MP, Pepper D, Currier GW, Holloman GH Jr, Feifel D. The psychopharmacology of agitation: consensus statement of the American Association for Emergency Psychiatry Project BETA Psychopharmacology Workgroup. West J Emerg Med. 2012;13(1):26–34.
5. Hirayasu Y, Korn ML. Management of patients with acute psychosis. Medical Education Collaborative. 2018 March 20. Available at https://www.medscape.org/viewarticle/420241.
6. Anderson WH, Kuehnle JC. Rapid treatment of acute psychosis. Am J Psychiatry. 1976;133(9):1076–8.
7. Battaglia J, Moss S, Rush J, Kang J, Mendoza R, Leedom L, et al. Haloperidol, lorazepam, or both for psychotic agitation? A multicenter, prospective, double-blind, emergency department study. Am J Emerg Med. 1997;15:335–40.
8. Kao LW, et al. Droperidol, QT prolongation and sudden death: what is the evidence? Ann Emerg Med. 2003;41:546–58.
9. Brook S, Lucey JV, Gunn KP. Intramuscular ziprasidone compared with intramuscular haloperidol in the treatment of acute psychosis. Ziprasidone I.M. Study Group. J Clin Psychiatry. 2000;61(12):933–41.
10. Mendelowitz AJ. The utility of intramuscular ziprasidone in the management of acute psychotic agitation. Ann Clin Psychiatry. 2004;16(3):145–54.
11. Zimbroff DL. Management of acute psychosis: from emergency to stabilization. CNS Spectr. 2003;8(11 Suppl. 2):10–5.
12. Zimbroff DL, Allen MH, Battaglia J, Citrome L, Fishkind A, Francis A, et al. Best clinical practice with ziprasidone IM: update after 2 years of experience. CNS Spectr. 2005;10(9):1–10.
13. Karagianis JL, Dawe IC, Thakur A, Begin S, Raskin J, Roychowdhury SM. Rapid tranquilization with olanzapine in acute psychosis: a case series. J Clin Psychiatry. 2001;62(Suppl. 2):12–6.
14. Mohr P, Pecenak J, Svestka J, Swingler D, Treuer T. Treatment of acute agitation in psychotic disorders. Neuro Endocrinol Lett. 2005;26(4):327–35.
15. Bartko G. New formulations of olanzapine in the treatment of acute agitation. Neuropsychopharmacol Hung. 2006;8(4):171–8.
16. Battaglia J. Pharmacological management of acute agitation. Drugs. 2005;65(9):1207–22.
17. Lim HK, Kim JJ, Pae CU, Lee CU, Lee C, Paik IH. Comparison of risperidone orodispersible tablet and intramuscular haloperidol in the treatment of acute psychotic agitation: a randomized open, prospective study. Neuropsychobiology. 2010;62(2):81–6.
18. McAllister-Williams RH, Ferrier IN. Rapid tranquilization: time for a reappraisal of options for parenteral therapy. Br J Psychiatry. 2002;180:485–9.
19. Hsu WY, Huang SS, Lee BS, Chiu NY. Comparison of intramuscular olanzapine, orally disintegrating olanzapine tablets, oral risperidone solution and intramuscular haloperidol in the management of acute agitation in an acute care psychiatric ward. J Clin Psychopharmacol. 2010;30(3):230–4.
20. Currier GW, Simpson GM. Risperidone liquid concentrate and oral lorazepam versus intramuscular haloperidol and intramuscular lorazepam for treatment of psychotic agitation. J Clin Psychiatry. 2001;62(3):153–7.
21. Currier GW, Chou JC, Feifel D, Bossie CA, Turkoz I, Mahmoud RA, et al. Acute treatment of psychotic agitation: a randomized comparison of oral treatment with risperidone and lorazepam versus intramuscular treatment with haloperidol and lorazepam. J Clin Psychiatry. 2004;65(3):386–94.
22. Veser FH, Veser BD, McMullan JT, Zealberg J, Currier GW. Risperidone versus haloperidol, in combination with lorazepam, in the treatment of acute agitation and psychosis: a pilot, randomized, double-blind, placebo-controlled trial. J Psychiatr Pract. 2006;12(2):103–8.
23. Campillo A, Castillo E, Vilke GM, Hopper A, Ryan V, Wilson MP. First-generation antipsychotics are often prescribed in the emergency department but are often not administered with adjunctive medications. J Emerg Med. 2015;49(6):901–6.
24. Ostinelli EG, Brooke-Powney MJ, Li X, Adams CE. Haloperidol for psychosis-induced aggression or agitation (rapid tranquillisation). Cochrane Database Syst Rev. 2017;7:CD009377.
25. Gan TJ. "Black box" warning on droperidol: report of the FDA Convened Expert Panel. Anesth Analg. 2004;98(6):1809.
26. Gillies D, Sampson S, Beck A, Rathbone J. Benzodiazepines for psychosis-induced aggression or agitation. Cochrane Database Syst Rev. 2013;9:CD003079.
27. Zaman H, Sampson SJ, Beck ALS, Sharma T, Clay FJ, Spyridi S, et al. Benzodiazepines for psychosis-induced aggression or agitation. Cochrane Database Syst Rev. 2017;12:CD003079.
28. Wilson MP, Vilke GM, Hayden SR, Nordstrom K. Psychiatric emergencies for clinicians: Emergency Department Management of Neuroleptic Malignant Syndrome. J Emerg Med. 2016;51(1):66–9.
29. Wilson MP, MacDonald K, Vilke GM, Feifel D. Potential complications of combining intramuscular olanzapine with benzodiazepines in emergency department patients. J Emerg Med. 2012;43(5):889–96.
30. Wilson MP, Chen N, Vilke GM, Castillo EM, MacDonald KS, Minassian A. Olanzapine in ED patients: differential effects on oxygenation in patients with alcohol intoxication. Am J Emerg Med. 2012;30(7):1196–201.
31. Wilson MP, MacDonald K, Vilke GM, Ronquillo L, Feifel D. Intramuscular ziprasidone: influence of alcohol and benzodiazepines on vital signs in the emergency setting. J Emerg Med. 2013;45(6):901–8.
32. Wilson MP, Minassian A, Bahramzi M, Campillo A, Vilke GM. Despite expert recommendations,

second-generation antipsychotics are not often prescribed in the emergency department. J Emerg Med. 2014;46(6):808–13.
33. Wilson MP, Brennan JJ, Modesti L, Deen J, Anderson L, Vilke GM, et al. Lengths of stay for involuntarily held psychiatric patients in the ED are affected by both patient characteristics and medication use. Am J Emerg Med. 2015;33(4):527–30.
34. Ronquillo L, Minassian A, Vilke GM, Wilson MP. Literature-based recommendations for suicide assessment in the emergency department: a review. J Emerg Med. 2012;43(5):836–42.
35. Wilson MP, Nordstrom K, Zeller SL. Practical management of the suicidal patient in the emergency department. Emerg Med Rep. 2014;35(1):1–12.
36. DiazGranados N, Ibrahim LA, Brutsche NE, Ameli R, Henter ID, Luckenbaugh DA, Machado-Vieira R, et al. Rapid resolution of suicidal ideation after a single infusion of an NMDA antagonist in patients with treatment-resistant major depressive disorder. J Clin Psychiatry. 2010;71(12):1605–11.
37. Price R, Nock MK, Charney DS, Mathew SJ. Effects of intravenous ketamine on explicit and implicit measures of suicidality. Biol Psychiatry. 2009;66(5):522–6.
38. Larkin GL, Beautrais AL. A preliminary naturalistic study of low-dose ketamine for depression and suicide ideation in the emergency department. Int J Neuropsychopharmacol. 2017;20(7):611.

Prehospital Behavioral Emergencies

27

Thom Dunn

Introduction

Prehospital providers, specifically those working in the emergency medical services (EMS), play a unique role in the healthcare system. Unlike their counterparts working in hospitals and clinics, EMS providers typically encounter their patients in the patient's environment. These providers are equipped to cope with the widest possible range of patient types and presentations, including the capacity to care for all ages of patients, from geriatrics to neonates. Similarly, patient presentations can be quite varied, including all acute and subacute medical conditions, those intoxicated on drugs or alcohol, polytrauma, and those with neurological or psychiatric conditions. While not only contending with a wide range of patient types and presentations, EMS providers also expertly handle these patients expediently and without the benefit of specialty resources such as radiography, laboratory studies, or expert consultation.

The manner in which emergency medical services are provided varies in the United States [1]. Some municipalities have emergency medical technicians (EMTs) who are trained in basic life support and whose practice does not include medications. These first responders, often firefighters, will reach the patient and provide basic life support (BLS) until paramedics arrive. Paramedics provide advanced life support (ALS) and have access to a limited formulary of medications, typically advanced cardiovascular life-support medicines, antiemetic drugs, sedating agents, and narcotic analgesics. Some regions may have only EMTs who transport the patient, while some larger municipalities may have paramedic first responders, as well as ALS transport capabilities. EMS is delivered not only by ambulances, but also by helicopter, bicycles, motorcycles, and by providers who ski to their patient.

Paramedics and EMTs frequently come into contact with those suffering from mental illness. Larkin and others found that nearly 33% of psychiatric patients in the emergency department are brought in by ambulance, compared to only 14% of other patient types [2]. Due to fewer and fewer inpatient psychiatric beds, EMS is also frequently called upon to perform interfacility transports to move behavioral health patients from one facility to another [3]. This chapter outlines the important roles paramedics and EMTs play in a broader system of care for patients having a behavioral health emergency.

T. Dunn (✉)
Behavioral Health Service, Denver Health, Denver, CO, USA

School of Psychological Sciences, University of Northern Colorado, Greeley, CO, USA
e-mail: thom.dunn@dhha.org

L. S. Zun et al. (eds.), *Behavioral Emergencies for Healthcare Providers*,
https://doi.org/10.1007/978-3-030-52520-0_27

Case Example 1

A 16-year-old girl working at an ice cream parlor experiences an episode of syncope; 911 is called. An ALS ambulance and BLS fire engine are sent to the scene. The patient spontaneously recovers consciousness and there is no evidence of a post-ictal state. The attending paramedic appreciates no trauma after syncope and the physical examination is significant only for skin abrasions on the dorsum of the patient's right hand. Vital signs are measured to be a blood pressure of 90/68, a heart rate of 112, and a respiratory rate of 22. The electrocardiogram reveals sinus tachycardia with ST depression, inverted T waves, the presence of a U wave, and a corrected QT value of 520. The paramedic recognizes that these findings are consistent with hypokalemia and elects to transport the patient to a nearby hospital. While en route, the paramedic asks whether the patient is vomiting to manage her diet, and the girl confides she is. The patient is later found to have a serum potassium level of 2.5 mmol/l (normal 3.6–5.2 mmol/l) from repeated vomiting. She responds well to oral potassium. Her parents, previously believing her purging was a "phase," make arrangements for her to be admitted to an eating disorder center.

It can be difficult to determine when a person's behavior becomes pathological, particularly in milder forms of many psychiatric conditions [4]. The involvement of community resources, such as EMS, can be an indicator of pathology. In the case above, a teenage girl who faints and then recovers quickly may be falsely considered a low-acuity event. However, a thorough evaluation by a skilled prehospital provider who is knowledgeable about a wide range of patient types is in the position both to detect a potentially significant medical problem and to elicit a history to derive its psychiatric etiology. In this case, transport of the patient to the hospital by ambulance can serve as an indicator to parents in denial that there is a serious problem.

While there are opportunities for EMS providers to intervene in more subtle presentations of psychiatric illness, such as one that has triggered a medical emergency, it is more likely that EMS is activated for more frank presentations of decompensated mental illness. Erratic behavior is often first observed by friends, family, or bystanders who call 911. Traditionally, erratic behavior in the field setting has often been addressed by law enforcement [5]. Such an approach, however, can have poor outcomes, as studies have found that persons with mental illness have higher rates of violence by resisting police contact [6], as well as a greater likelihood of requiring use of force by law enforcement [7].

Additionally, agitation is a common presentation of a number of life-threatening conditions, including hypoxia, alcohol withdrawal, intoxication, infection, neurological insult, and metabolic derangement. Coupled with the growing awareness about the deleterious health effects of erratic behavior, particularly excited delirium, agitation is increasingly being viewed as an acute medical emergency [8–11]. This is an important distinction, as it may help prevent injuries and deaths of agitated individuals who are taken into police custody [12]. Therefore, it is essential not only that EMS providers respond alongside law enforcement to reports of an agitated individual but also that the paramedic or EMT leads the interaction with the patient. This creates the dynamic of coping with erratic behavior, including agitation, as a symptom of underlying pathology, rather than a law enforcement problem of managing a troublesome person [13].

Case Example 2

A city's 911 call center receives the report of a man acting strangely. He is reported to be walking down the center of a busy street. He is not wearing clothes and is breaking windows. While most callers are asking for the police to respond, dispatchers also assign a BLS fire engine crew, along with an ALS ambulance. Several police officers, paramedics in an ambulance, and four firefighters arrive to find a man in his thirties frantically moving around cars in a parking lot. He makes nonverbal vocalizations and does not engage with any of the first responders around him. He is clearly diaphoretic, tachypneic, and agitated.

Certainly, there are concerns about risks of violence toward prehospital providers [14]. Paramedics and EMTs report high rates of being verbally abused, spat upon, and physically assaulted [15]. One mechanism to cope with such violence is to require responding units to "stage," or wait nearby before responding to the patient once law enforcement has declared the scene safe [16]. This approach may cause unnecessary delays and may defeat the purpose of having EMS respond alongside law enforcement. Thoughtfully coordinating an approach to the patient between EMS and law enforcement can safely mitigate many of the risks of violence against prehospital providers and reduce law enforcement contact with individuals who are not suspected of having committed a crime. This coordination should entail an assessment of whether the individual being contacted is having an acute medical problem (including a psychiatric decompensation) or whether the behavior is criminal in nature.

If it is believed that the person is having a medical emergency, then the paramedic or EMT should lead the encounter between patient and the responders, including police. This shifts law enforcement officers into a support position, where their role is to protect the safety of the EMS providers. However, if the individual is thought to be acting erratically or is agitated, and a medical problem is not suspected, then law enforcement leads the encounter. EMS is then available to provide postarrest medical evaluation. Obviously, in instances where the EMT or paramedic feels like their safety may be in jeopardy, EMS should defer to law enforcement. There may also be instances when it is impractical to coordinate a response between EMS and law enforcement. In these instances, law enforcement should lead the interaction, as the safety for all those involved is of utmost importance. As agitation may have an organic etiology, even if police officers lead the interaction, many of these individuals still require assessment by EMS. If indicated, the person being detained by law enforcement should be transported to an emergency department for further evaluation and treatment.

Table 27.1 outlines indications and contraindications for when prehospital providers should lead the interaction during a field contact with an agitated person or when an individual is otherwise acting erratically. It is important to note that in these situations, individuals with agitation may have diminished medical decision-making capacity. Since patients who are unable to make informed medical-decisions are unable to refuse care in the field, EMS providers should evaluate decision-making capacity for those who do not wish to be transported. Those found to lack the capacity to refuse care can be treated and transported under implied consent [17].

Table 27.1 Indications and contraindications of EMS provider leading the field intervention of an individual who is acting erratically or is agitated

Indications	Contraindications
Prominent feature of patient presentation is altered mental status.	Any suggestion that the person is armed or may have access to weapons.
There are physical indicators of an acute medical compromise, such as tachypnea, diaphoresis, or ataxia.	Law enforcement backup is delayed or unavailable.
Information from bystanders or family members that the patient suffers from mental illness, is on the autism spectrum, has dementia, or is intellectually disabled.	The individual is suspected to have committed a crime or otherwise will be placed into police custody at the end of the interaction.
Patient known to the EMS providers or law enforcement and is not known to be violent.	Patient is known to EMS providers or law enforcement and known to be violent.
The individual is a child.	The patient has barricaded themselves.
The patient is being evaluated in a healthcare facility.	Insufficient number of providers to safely manage the patient.

Case Example 2, Continued

The attending paramedic and senior police officer briefly confer. Other than being naked in public, the individual is not believed to have committed a serious crime. Unless the patient is later found to have warrants for his arrest, it is unlikely that he will be arrested. The consensus is that the individual is having a medical emergency and that EMS will lead contact with the patient and intervene in his behavior.

Figure 27.1 provides a framework for the EMS provider to contact, assess, and treat the agitated patient. Part of this framework is recognition that there are some patient presentations that may be life-threatening and that safely restraining the patient early in the prehospital course may be indicated. Central to this framework is Table 27.2, which shows the "ERASER" mnemonic, an approach to verbal de-escalation techniques based on the Project BETA De-escalation Workgroup [18]. Obviously, this approach works best when EMS agencies are trained using the framework and mnemonic, when they have protocols that support their use, and when law enforcement and prehospital providers train together. It should also

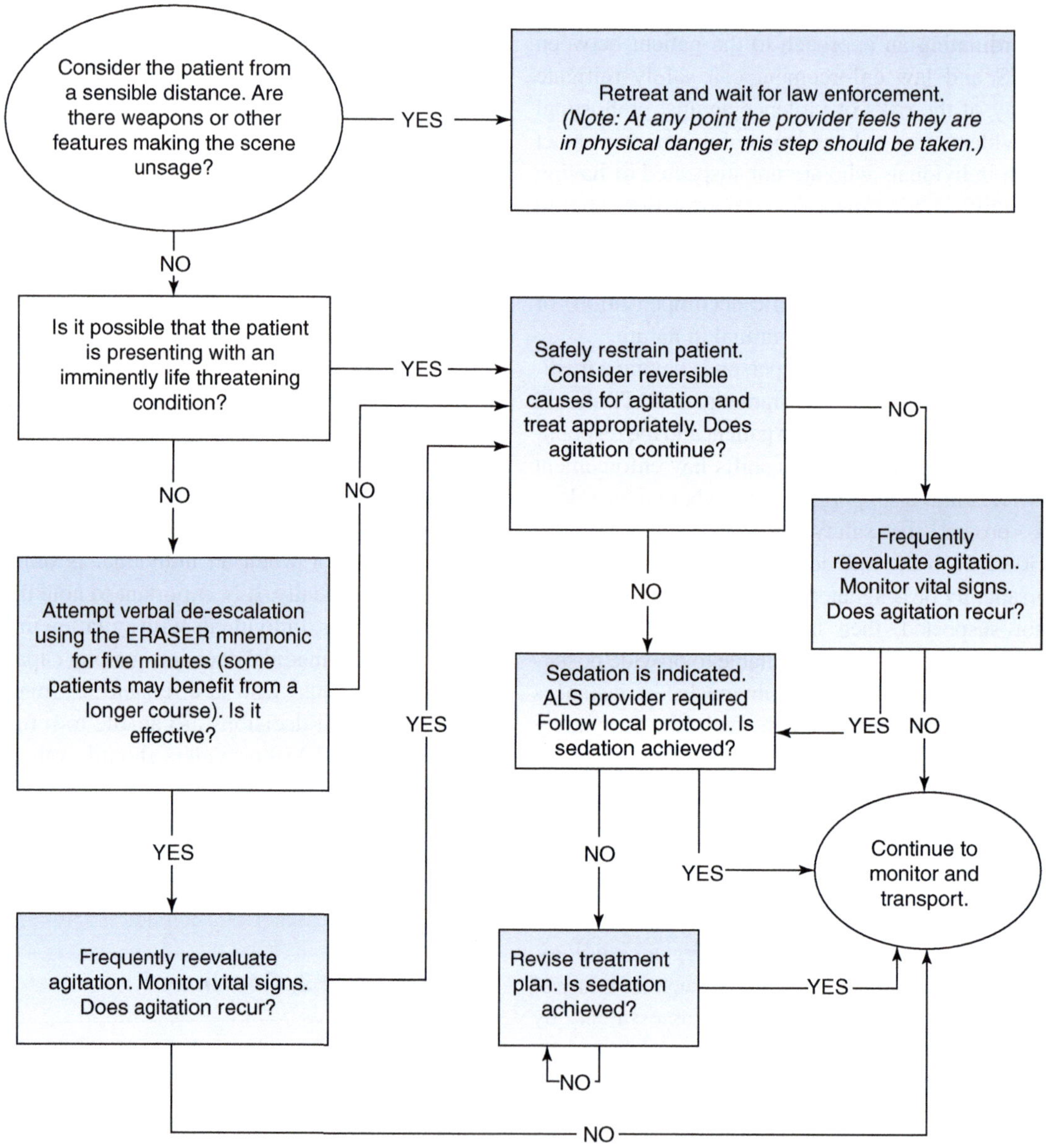

Fig. 27.1 Flowchart of managing agitation in the field. (Adapted from Dunn and Dempsey [5]. Reprinted with permission)

Table 27.2 ERASER mnemonic for verbal de-escalation, based on the project BETA De-escalation Workgroup [18]

Step	Action
E: EYEBALL the patient	Evaluate the patient from a safe distance. Are there weapons or other features that make the scene unsafe? Retreat and wait for law enforcement. Are there signs that the patient will not respond to verbal de-escalation or may be suffering from an imminent life-threatening condition? It may be prudent to safely and rapidly restrain the patient for further evaluation and treatment.
R: RESPECT patient's space	Patients may escalate when there is intrusion into the personal space. The provider should maintain a respectful distance while being aware of escape routes should the patient become violent.
A: A single provider does the talking and builds rapport	With multiple providers on a scene, a single individual should be charged with talking with the patient. The provider charged with this task must not become "emotionally involved" in the patient (such as becoming angry or frightened of the patient).
S: SENSIBLE listening	Often, agitated patients want to be heard. The provider making contact with the patient needs to calmly listen to the patient without being drawn into a prolonged conversation or reacting to demands. This step is likely when iatrogenic escalation may occur. Another provider may need to step in and continue if this happens.
E: ESTABLISH expectations and set boundaries	Boundaries should be set with the patient about behavior that will not be tolerated, consequences of actions, and what the patient is likely to expect, such as, "You may not threaten people," "We need to make sure you are alright, so we are going to take some vital signs and ask you some questions," or "Unfortunately, we are worried you cannot make informed medical-decisions because you are intoxicated, so we are going to take you to the hospital so you can be treated for your injuries."
R: REASONABLE choices are given to the patient	By retaining some degree of control, many patients will comply with direction if given reasonable choices. For example, a provider could say, "Would you like to walk over to the ambulance and sit on the bed inside, or do you prefer we bring the bed over here for you to sit on?"

The ERASER mnemonic first appeared in Dunn and Dempsey [5]. The table is reprinted with permission

be employed only after it is believed that risk of intervening with the patient through de-escalation is much less than the benefits that may be achieved. Unfortunately, there is no standardized method of assessing agitation in field settings, although the Behavioral Agitation Rating Scale (BARS) shows promise, as it has only seven items and is not cumbersome to use [19]. (Please see Chap. 23, for more information on agitation assessment.)

Case Example 2, Continued

The lead paramedic believes that her patient is unarmed, as he is not holding a weapon, nor is he wearing clothes that might conceal one. Other features to the scene that might make it unsafe (such as intoxicated bystanders, the patient being close to the edge of a bridge, or the possibility that the patient could lunge for a weapon) are also not noted. The paramedic is quite concerned that the patient is having an acute medical condition and needs immediate care. Knowing that prolonged restraint of such patients can lead to cardiovascular collapse, the paramedic opts to aggressively sedate the patient after attempts to de-escalate do not appear to be working. His agitation is clearly dangerous, and without a careful approach, it is possible that someone will be assaulted. The paramedic coordiantes her plan with the police officers. Once roles are assigned and the medication is ready, the firefighters and police officers safely take the patient to the ground. The paramedic administers 5 mg/kg of ketamine (400 mg) intramuscularly. Less than 2 minutes later, the patient's agitation has resolved.

Key to the safe management of the patient is a coordinated approach to physical restraint that is systematic and designed to keep both the patient and first responders safe. Some hospital-based providers might find quickly moving to restraint as missing an opportunity to offer sedating medicines by mouth, as this approach is common [20, 21]. In the field, however, securing the patient takes a greater priority. This permits the patient to be quickly evaluated for reversible causes of agitation, keeps the patient safe by not permitting them to engage in harmful behavior like running or acting violently, and keeps EMS providers safe. Recall that unlike hospital settings, EMTs or paramedics are typically one-on-one with their patients and without the ancillary personnel found in a hospital, such as additional providers and security.

Case Example 2, Continued

The patient is placed in the ambulance and evaluated. He is atraumatic. He is found to be tachycardic at 140, his blood pressure is elevated at 190/90, and his breathing is tachypneic at 38. Hypoglycemia is ruled out with a finger-stick blood-glucose check. Hypoxia is ruled out with pulse oximetry. The paramedic does not appreciate some signs of a cerebral vascular accident, such as hemiparesis or facial droop. She also does not appreciate oral trauma or incontinence that may suggest a generalized tonic–clonic seizure. Intravenous access is secured in the patient's antecubital fossa, and his oxygen saturation, end-tidal carbon dioxide level, and electrocardiogram are monitored as he is transported to the hospital.

Pharmacological management of behavioral emergencies in the field can be challenging.

Some systems do not have paramedics, and without these ALS providers, administration of medication is not possible. In some EMS systems, ALS providers may not have calming medications in their formulary. Still, in other systems, medicine-managed agitation is at the discretion of a base physician providing medical control, who may not permit the paramedic to administer certain medications. Best practice for pharmacological management of agitation in the field is when the paramedic is able to choose an agent from a number of different drug classes in order to properly treat the patient without first contacting a base physician. Early management of agitation is critical in the field. In this example, the paramedic elects to use ketamine, as some advocate its utility in quickly managing agitated patients when there is no IV access without hemodynamic and respiratory side effects [22]. However, Cole and others warn that while ketamine is superior to haloperidol for managing prehospital agitation, it does have other complications, such as hypersalivation, emergence reactions, and higher rates of requiring intubation [23].

Typically, the sedating agents in the paramedic formulary are limited to first-generation antipsychotics, most often haloperidol. Benzodiazepines are also common, such as midazolam or diazepam, as these medicines can also be used for presentations other than agitation. Noticeably absent is lorazepam, commonly used to treat in-hospital agitation. Given that this agent is intolerant of wide variations in temperature, it is impractical for use in many EMS systems. Finally, even in more progressive systems where ALS providers have broad discretion when medicating an agitated patient, it should be noted that the treating paramedic has other challenges. For example, the paramedic is often solely responsible for retrieving the medication (typically a scheduled drug that is kept in a double-locked cabinet), drawing it into a syringe, and administering it while also monitoring the patient.

Case Example 2, Continued

The patient is safely transported to a community hospital and has no hypersalivation or other complications from receiving ketamine. He is recognized by hospital staff. "Oh, it's ML. He's off his meds again," says a nurse. ML is known to suffer from schizoaffective disorder and often uses stimulants. He is admitted, and once he sobers from methamphetamine intoxication, he is found to be psychiatrically decompensated and requires admission to a psychiatric unit. A bed is found on a unit in a nearby city. ML is placed on an involuntary psychiatric hold and his parents are notified.

One of the effects of the decreasing capacity of inpatient psychiatric care [24] is that patients having a behavioral emergency often do not reach definitive care once they are transported to the hospital. It is not unusual that patients with an emergent psychiatric condition (agitation, mania, psychosis, acute suicidality, etc.) must be transported a second time to definitive care. This again requires EMS providers to care for a patient with a behavioral emergency during transport. In rural systems, it may be the municipal ambulance pulled from its 911 response duties to complete the patient transfer. In suburban and urban areas, a private ambulance company may be responsible for interfacility transfers. In both systems, contacts with psychiatric patients are often seen as unglamorous and beneath providers, who are trained to act quickly and skillfully to save lives [25]. Transporting behavioral emergencies from one facility to another is often left to the least trained and most junior of EMS providers [25].

Case Example 2, Continued

A private ambulance company is contacted, an ambulance staffed by EMTs and dedicated to the interfacility transfer of patients is dispatched to pick up ML and transport him to the psychiatric unit. "Oh, great," says one of the EMTs. "Psych transfer. Dispatch hates us." The EMTs find ML sleeping in his bed. A nurse hands one of the EMS providers a packet of paperwork and says, "He is in room 16." The EMTs grumble that their patient cannot simply walk to the ambulance and they go about moving him to their stretcher for transport. As he is placed into the ambulance, the senior EMT says to his partner, "You are attending on this patient, I've been here long enough that I don't have to ride with psych patients any longer." The senior EMT closes the doors and climbs into the driver's seat.

There are challenges to managing a patient with a behavioral emergency when being transported from one hospital to another. EMS providers who would normally be quite aware of their safety and surroundings may have a sense of complacency during a transfer. There are also complicated decisions that have to be made by an EMT who may not have the training or experience to make them. Should the patient be permitted to walk to and from the ambulance? Once in the ambulance, should the patient be restrained, or are seat belts sufficient? Where should the patient sit? During transport, if the patient announces that he changed his mind and no longer wants care, can he simply be released on the street? What if the patient starts getting agitated? Should sedation be offered? Can the ambulance return to the sending facility?

It is imperative that clinicians who are involved in the transfer of a psychiatric patient provide guidance to the transport team regarding the patient's capacity to refuse care after leaving the hospital, whether restraints should be used, and advice for managing agitation. If there is a concern for agitation or elopement, an ALS transport team should be requested, as a BLS ambulance without a paramedic provider is poorly equipped to deal with agitation during transport. Similarly, protocols to simply restrain *all patients* during transport are often too broad, and such direction may be clinically contraindicated. Table 27.3 shows how one EMS system makes transport decisions based on patient presentation and history. This protocol is followed when deciding what crew configuration should be used when transferring a psychiatric patient. This saves ALS resources for the 911 system when not indicated for the transfer, as well as assigning specialized resources for higher acuity psychiatric patient transfers.

EMS agencies also have a responsibility for training their crews to safely transport patients having a behavioral emergency. As there are regular reports of patients dying by suicide during interfacility transfer by leaping from a moving ambulance [26], safe management of these patients is crucial. While there are several different places for people to sit in the back of an ambulance, patients suffering from a behavioral emergency should always be placed on the stretcher of the ambulance, as this is where the

Table 27.3 Eagle County Paramedic Services (Vail, CO) risk stratification for interfacility transport of the psychiatric patient

Risk	Presentation and crew configuration
Very high risk: *Patient has a history of violence*	Any patient who has been violent or threatening toward staff. Any patient thought to be at high risk for harming themselves or the transfer crew. Strongly consider a paramedic attendant, sedation, and early restraint.
Very high risk: *Patient has a history of elopement*	Exiting a moving ambulance is often fatal. Strongly consider a paramedic attendant, sedation, and early restraint.
High risk: *Patient who is, or has been, restrained during their hospital course*	If the patient required physical restraint or sedation during their course, these are red flags. Consider paramedic attendant and prepare for restraint.
High risk: *Patient who is manic or actively psychotic*	Verbal de-escalation techniques may not be successful if transport lasts more than an hour. Consider paramedic attendant and prepare for restraint.
At risk: *History of actual suicide attempt*	This is a step above ideation or gesturing; the patient who made a true attempt to end their life is at risk. Consider paramedic as part of crew configuration.
At risk: *History of needing to be redirected; anyone staff wants out of the hospital*	This is a patient who hasn't followed the rules and had to be "redirected." This patient is showing a tendency to misbehave. Consider paramedic as part of crew configuration.
Low risk: *None of the above*	The patient is either not on a hold or likely on an involuntary hold for only suicidal ideation or gesture. They have not displayed any of the higher risk features above. Consider BLS crew configuration.

Note: From the field medical protocols of Eagle County Paramedic services. These protocols were developed by the author and clinical manager of this EMS agency, Will Dunn.

patient's center of gravity is at its lowest. This permits the attending provider to sit beside the patient and remain vigilant for escalating agitation. The patient's hands should always be in view (never under a blanket, for example). The provider should explain that seat belts are to be worn for the entire transfer and at no point is the patient permitted to touch the buckles. The buckles should be reversed so their release button is facedown and against the patient. A patient attempting to take off the seat belts may need restraint or sedation. Once the ambulance has reached its destination, thought should be given to carefully consider whether the patient should be permitted to walk. Patients who may be an elopement risk or have otherwise become agitated likely need to be brought in on the stretcher.

Case Example 2, Continued

ML is safely admitted to an inpatient psychiatric unit and responds well to pharmacotherapy consisting of risperidone and valproic acid. The patient agrees to a long-acting injectable antipsychotic medication, as he has a tendency to stop taking his medication. Being off medication often leads to a psychosis developing and paranoia that medicine is poison. ML's parents agree to come and pick him up, but do not believe that he will stay at their house for long. He has a tendency to prefer being homeless and stays along the bank of a river in town. There is concern that the patient will not follow-up with office visits to assure that the patient's valproic acid blood level is in the therapeutic range. It is also not clear whether the patient will come into the office for a repeat injection of Risperdal Consta in 14 days. The social worker responsible for discharge arranges for a community paramedic referral.

Recently, there has been a proliferation of programs that are designed to train paramedics to perform duties more akin to primary care than emergency care [27]. These providers, known as "community paramedics," working in "mobile integrated health care" have an expanded scope of practice and protocols that permit them to visit patients in their homes and address wellness, postdischarge care, and additional surveillance of the chronically ill [28]. However, use of community paramedics with psychiatric populations is not common [29]. This is unfortunate, as community paramedics are ideal providers to interact with those living with severe mental illness. Community paramedics:

- Can meet those living with mental illness in the patient's environment
- Are capable of performing important postdischarge follow-up tasks, such as drawing blood for therapeutic blood monitoring, evaluating for side effects of medicine, and assessing for worsening of psychiatric symptoms
- Integrate well with other field providers, such as law enforcement
- Can be paired with a mental health provider and make treatment decisions (reducing transport to emergency departments) and, in some cases, arrange admission directly to a psychiatric facility [30]

Community paramedics who are integrated with local mental health centers or other behavioral health providers have the potential to intervene earlier in the course of those experiencing psychiatric decompensation. Early and effective interventions by community paramedics could have a dramatic decrease in the number of persons who have a behavioral emergency in a community. Realizing this benefit can have far-reaching effects: The patient can be kept out of the hospital and emergency departments will have fewer psychiatric patients to place. As a result, fewer community resources, like law enforcement and EMS, will have to be spent on these emergencies. The burden on inpatient psychiatric beds can be reduced. It may be that the best response to a behavioral emergency is finding ways to prevent it from happening in the first place.

Understanding the role of EMS providers in behavioral emergencies is critical. As complicated as such emergencies are in the hospital, intervening with these patients in the field can be exceptionally difficult. It behooves both emergency psychiatry providers and EMS systems to partner in training, protocol development, and collaboration for safe patient treatment and transport. Even if EMS is not directly involved in the initial contact of a patient in the field (e.g., the patient is brought in by police), many patients may ultimately require ambulance transport to definitive care. Finally, as community paramedic programs are developed, these providers are ideal for collaborating with mental health systems in patient follow-up. Patient care can be improved with increased involvement between psychiatry and the emergency medical services.

References

1. Wang HE, Mann NC, Jacobson KE, Mears G, Smyrski K, et al. National characteristics of emergency medical services responses in the United States. Prehosp Emerg Care. 2013;17(1):8–14.
2. Larkin GL, Claassen CA, Pelletier AJ, Camargo CA. National study of ambulance transports to United States emergency departments: importance of mental health problems. Prehosp Disaster Med. 2006;21(2):82–90.
3. Cheney P, Haddock T, Sanchez L, Ernst A, Weiss S. Safety and compliance with an emergency medical service direct psychiatric center transport protocol. Am J Emerg Med. 2008;26(7):750–6.
4. American Psychiatric Association. Diagnostic and statistical manual of mental disorders. 5th ed. Washington, D.C.: APA; 2013.
5. Dunn T, Dempsey C. Agitation in field settings: emergency medical services providers and law enforcement. In: Zeller SL, Nordstrom KD, Wilson MP, editors. The diagnosis and management of agitation. Cambridge: Cambridge University Press; 2017. p. 156–72.
6. Mulvey P, White M. The potential for violence in arrests of persons with mental illness. Policing. 2014;37(2):404–19.
7. Morabito MS, Socia K, Wik A, Fisher WH. The nature and extent of police use of force in encounters with people with behavioral health disorders. Int J Law Psychiatry. 2017;50:31–7.
8. Svenson JE, Abernathy MK. Ketamine for prehospital use: new look at an old drug. Am J Emerg Med. 2007;25(8):977–80.
9. Burnett AM, Peterson BK, Stellpflug SJ, Engebretsen KM, Glasrud KJ, Marks J, et al. The association between ketamine given for prehospital chemical restraint with intubation and hospital admission. Am J Emerg Med. 2015;33(1):76–9.
10. Otahbachi M, Cevik C, Bagdure S, Nugent K. Excited delirium, restraints, and unexpected death: a review of pathogenesis. Am J Forensic Med Pathol. 2010;31(2):107–12.
11. Vilke GM, DeBard ML, Chan TC, Ho JD, Dawes DM, Hall C, et al. Excited delirium syndrome (ExDS): defining based on a review of the literature. J Emerg Med. 2012;43(5):897–905.

12. Karch SB. The problem of police-related cardiac arrest. J Forensic Legal Med. 2016;41:36–41.
13. Ford-Jones PC, Chaufan C. A critical analysis of debates around mental health calls in the prehospital setting. Inquiry. 2017;54:1–5.
14. Koritsas S, Boyle M, Coles J. Factors associated with workplace violence in paramedics. Prehosp Disaster Med. 2009;24(05):417–21.
15. Dunn TM, Johnston J, Dunn WW, Doty C. Violence against emergency medical service providers: reports from over 2,500 EMTs and paramedics. San Francisco: Association for Psychological Science; 2014.
16. Gratton M, Garza A, Salomone JA, McElroy J, Shearer J. Ambulance staging for potentially dangerous scenes: another hidden component of response time. Prehosp Emerg Care. 2010;14(3):340–4.
17. McCullough LB, McGuire AL, Whitney SN. Consent: informed, simple, implied and presumed. Am J Bioeth. 2007;7(12):49–50; discussion W3–4.
18. Richmond JS, Berlin JS, Fishkind AB, Holloman GH Jr, Zeller SL, Wilson MP, et al. Verbal de-escalation of the agitated patient: consensus statement of the American Association for Emergency Psychiatry Project BETA De-escalation Workgroup. West J Emerg Med. 2012;13(1):17–25.
19. Swift R, Harrigan E, Cappelleri J, Kramer D, Chandler L. Validation of the behavioural activity rating scale (BARS): a novel measure of activity in agitated patients. J Psychiatr Res. 2002;36(2):87–95.
20. Knox DK, Holloman GH. Use and avoidance of seclusion and restraint: consensus statement of the American Association for Emergency Psychiatry Project BETA Seclusion and Restraint Workgroup. West J Emerg Med. 2012;13(1):35–40.
21. Wilson MP, Pepper D, Currier GW, Holloman GH Jr, Feifel D. The psychopharmacology of agitation: consensus statement of the American Association for Emergency Psychiatry Project BETA Psychopharmacology Workgroup. West J Emerg Med. 2012;13(1):26–34.
22. Scheppke KA, Braghiroli J, Shalaby M, Chait R. Prehospital use of IM ketamine for sedation of violent and agitated patients. West J Emerg Med. 2014;15(7):736–41.
23. Cole JB, Moore JC, Nystrom PC, Orozco BS, Stellpflug SJ, Kornas RL, Fryza BJ, Steinberg LW, O'Brien-Lambert A, Bache-Wiig P, Engebretsen KM. A prospective study of ketamine versus haloperidol for severe prehospital agitation. Clin Toxicol (Phila). 2016;54(7):556–62.
24. Salinsky E, Loftis C. Shrinking inpatient psychiatric capacity: cause for celebration or concern? Issue Brief George Wash Univ Natl Health Policy Forum. 2007;(823):1–21.
25. Prener C, Lincoln AK. Emergency medical services and "psych calls": examining the work of urban EMS providers. Am J Orthopsychiatry. 2015;85(6):612–9.
26. Dunn TM. Handle with care: the challenges of transporting suicidal patients. JEMS. 2008;33(10):86–92.
27. Ball L. Setting the scene for the paramedic in primary care: a review of the literature. Emerg Med J. 2005;22(12):896–900.
28. Bigham BL, Kennedy SM, Drennan I, Morrison LJ. Expanding paramedic scope of practice in the community: a systematic review of the literature. Prehosp Emerg Care. 2013;17(3):361–72.
29. Choi BY, Blumberg C, Williams K. Mobile integrated health care and community paramedicine: an emerging emergency medical services concept. Ann Emerg Med. 2016;67(3):361–6.
30. Stanaway N. Community paramedic program cuts mental health patient call volume. 2016. Available at https://www.ems1.com/community-paramedicine/articles/93357048-Community-paramedic-program-cuts-mental-health-patient-call-volume/. Accessed on 26 May 2016.

Part VI

Special Populations

Mental Health Issues in Adolescents

28

Vint Blackburn and John S. Rozel

Introduction

Psychiatric emergencies in the pediatric and adolescent population are often as intimidating for the caregivers as for the patient. Many practitioners are less accustomed to working with adolescents; their perceived unpredictability and intense emotional responses can often make clinicians second-guess themselves. Challenges in differentiating normal teenage behavior from bona fide pathology, for instance, can lead to any number of misperceptions. Like most emergency settings, normal behavior is seldom a reason for a referral, although it does occur and needs to be considered. Compounding all of this is the fact that we have not just the child to deal with but their family, as well, who can often be just as overwrought as the patient. A calm, educated demeanor and effective communication skills often are as important—if not more so—than diagnostic acumen or familiarity with pharmacology.

V. Blackburn (✉)
Department of Psychiatry, University of Pittsburgh Medical Center, Pittsburgh, PA, USA
e-mail: blackburnvr@upmc.edu

J. S. Rozel
Department of Psychiatry, UPMC Western Psychiatric Hospital, Pittsburgh, PA, USA

Case Example 1

A 16-year-old male comes into the emergency room, terrified that he is losing his mind, convinced that he has developed a severe mental illness such as schizophrenia. He reports that he is hearing and seeing things, his thoughts are racing, and the world simply seems "unreal … evil and wrong." Initial considerations may include primary psychotic disorders or a psychotic mood disorder. Further questioning, along with reassurance, reveals that the patient has been smoking marijuana.

Psychiatric emergencies, while sometimes requiring pharmacological or medical intervention, are best first approached and treated with understanding and reassurance. In the case above, once the treating clinician fully understands the situation, they can reassure the patient that he is likely suffering the effects of a substance that will soon wear off. Also, reminding the patient he is safe and not being judged aids the patient in de-escalating himself.

Child and adolescent behavioral emergencies can be a major operational challenge for emergency departments. They are increasingly frequent, often occur in people with limited insurance or other resources, have limited referral resources, and often extend boarding times [1–3]. And while child emergency psychiatry is a growing field, the science remains young,

L. S. Zun et al. (eds.), *Behavioral Emergencies for Healthcare Providers*,
https://doi.org/10.1007/978-3-030-52520-0_28

compared to pediatric emergency medicine and adult emergency psychiatry [4–7]. For a generation, the field has lacked anything like a manual or textbook; thankfully, that has recently changed with two valuable books [8, 9]. Finally, it is increasingly well established that like adults, children and adolescents neither need nor benefit from excessive laboratory or imaging, except as specifically indicated by a history and screening physical [10–12].

Thus, the provider is left with limited technical resources but a firm reminder that, regardless of etiology, the first goal of the assessment is a compassionate, objective evaluation where the clinician will have to rely on their humanity, knowledge, and curiosity.

Evaluation Settings

It should be noted that there are several settings in which these psychiatric emergencies are seen. Arguably, direct evaluation by a child and adolescent emergency psychiatrist in a specialized setting is optimal; such programs are uncommon but do exist [11]. Telepsychiatric evaluation has also been shown to be helpful for child and adolescent psychiatric emergencies and may be an option in some settings as well [12, 13].

Often, however, children and adolescents may present to ersatz settings: adult psychiatric emergency services, adult medical emergency departments, or pediatric emergency departments. Evaluation of children and adolescents with psychiatric emergencies in these settings may be clinically appropriate depending on several factors, including the expertise of available clinicians, available consultation, and the dynamic variable of ease of access to more specialized assessment settings. An adolescent with benign anxiety may not need to be transferred to a dedicated child emergency psychiatric program even if it is across the street; however, a team may wish to expend considerable resources to get a complex, high-risk patient across the state for evaluation. It will all depend on the known and knowable facts of the case, the resources of the emergency department, and the judgment of the clinician.

The Family System

Unlike working with an adult patient, the adolescent generally comes with a group of other concerned individuals. Usually parents, family members, or a legal guardian, these people may be as uncertain of facts and dysregulated in emotions as the patient. Often, the patient will be returning to this household at the end of the evaluation or the admission; engaging the family is vital.

Early intervention has long been recognized as a critical tool for working with higher risk children and adolescents [13, 14]. Many of the stressors and etiologies of our adolescent's pathologies can be either exacerbated or mitigated by how their family interacts with them at home [15, 16]. Family interventions can be especially important and useful in the context of emergency care [17].

At the same time, the family can also be an impediment or even the cause of a psychiatric emergency. Sexual or physical abuse, neglect, parental pathology, or even intrafamilial conflict can play a major role in driving psychiatric emergency presentations. Collateral information is essential in any adolescent psychiatric emergency assessment; direct observation of parent–child interactions can be invaluable.

Who to Interview First

Ideally, in every assessment, adolescents should be interviewed on their own at some point. This allows for more detailed or personal assessment of routine aspects of assessment and also improved quality of assessment on sensitive topics (e.g., substance use, abuse, and sexuality). Younger children may become too anxious on separation from their parent or caregiver to provide useful information; a judgment call must be made. Adolescents need to be given an opportunity to speak alone, without fear of immediate repercussions or judgments from family members.

The same opportunity should be offered to the parents or family members. Often, the caregivers will be uncomfortable expressing their concerns—or sensitive aspects of the family history—in front of the patient. Conflicting information and views from the patient and the family often are noted and should be reflected upon thoughtfully and without judgment. The truth often lies somewhere in between the offered narratives. Most parents or family members who have brought a child to the emergency department or a clinic are interested in the child's well-being, even if they don't know how to achieve it. There is no quicker way to undermine a clinical assessment than to make the family feel marginalized or judged when it comes to the care of their child.

Self-Injury, Suicidal Ideation, Contingent Suicide, or Homicidal Threats

Suicidal threat or gesture and a family's discovery of self-injury are often reasons for presentation to the psychiatric emergency service. Clinicians should remember that many nonprofessionals may not understand that nonsuicidal self-injury (NSSI) and suicidality are often two distinct clinical issues and require different clinical interventions. As with adults, adolescents should be asked directly about suicidal thoughts and similar issues [18]. This is a question best asked of the patient privately but with the caveat that a caregiver may need to be informed if there are acute safety concerns.

Nonsuicidal Self-Injury

While it is true that individuals who intentionally self-injure are at higher risk for suicidality, it must be understood that NSSI is not the same as suicidal ideation or intent [19]. An important question to ask any patient who shows up in the emergency department for assessment of self-injury is "Were you trying to end your life?" With NSSI, the answer will usually be "I was just trying to feel something," or similarly, "I felt like I needed some relief." NSSI can be viewed as a coping skill and often reflects a paucity of other, more effective coping strategies. NSSI often begins in adolescence. The most common areas for cutting include the arms, thighs, shoulders, and abdomen. Exploration of NSSI should be a common element of the exam of adolescents in the psychiatric emergency service. Adolescents may use long sleeves (even during warm weather) or bracelets and bangles to cover the wrist. NSSI is an important warning sign for pathology and should be referred to therapy and psychiatry for follow-up treatment; however, NSSI does not itself warrant an inpatient hospitalization. NSSI should prompt careful exploration of suicidality and related risk factors.

Suicidal Threats or Gestures

Suicidal threats or gestures can be one of the most frightening psychiatric emergencies faced by clinicians (and parents). Inpatient referral or further specialized evaluation should be considered for any patient who has made an act or attempt or expresses specific intent to kill themselves. Often, however, the reason an adolescent is present is for evaluation of ideation or a passive death wish, either reported directly by the patient or expressed to a parent, friend, or other interested party.

Passive Death Wish

The patient themselves may have some uncertainty about whether they are considering suicide or are merely expressing a passive death wish. Clarifying questions with the patient or parent can be essential. Passive death wish is far less likely to result in immediate lethality and is generally an expression of significant depression. Nonetheless, the presence of passive death wish in a child can be extremely distressing to other professionals, as well as the parents. Outpatient therapy referral is often appropriate for patients with passive death wish. Safety planning—important in all psychiatric emergency care—is essential in a person with any degree of suicidality, including passive death wish.

Suicidal Ideation

Suicidal ideation involves the thought or desire to kill themselves. It can be with or without method, such as "I want to kill myself. I haven't thought about how yet." It can be with a clear method, such as jumping off a high building or bridge. The next question that we tend to follow up with is "Do you intend to do this?" Any active suicidality, with or without intent or method, should lead to further and careful assessment.

Contingent Suicidal or Homicidal Threats

Often in the psychiatric emergency room, we are presented with young patients who have made contingent threats to kill themselves to parents along the lines of "If you don't let me go out with my friends, I will kill myself." This is a simplistic example, but any time a threat of suicidality accompanies a request, it is contingent and is often the sign of significant affect intolerance and emotion dysregulation. Great care needs to be taken with these patients, as it is easy to reinforce this behavior—something that has often already taken place in the patient's life.

Parents of these patients often report that they feel that they are being held hostage by the behaviors. Patients of this sort often have low short-term risk but do require appropriate clinical intervention. This intervention may not be what the patient or family wants or expects; interventions grounded in dialectical behavior therapy (DBT) may be preferred both in the emergency setting and for a longer term outpatient care [20, 21].

Reacting calmly and appropriately to these patients and their threats is important. Overreacting or emoting can reinforce the unwanted behavior. However, ignoring it completely can also escalate the behavior. This is another case in which an assessment by a skilled clinician can be very helpful before making a disposition decision. Validating the feelings of a patient making contingent threats—while not validating or reinforcing the behaviors—is an excellent way to establish rapport and de-escalate these individuals, and it is a primary tenant of DBT [21].

Post Visit Safety

If a patient is going to go home, safety in the home must be discussed. If the patient engages in NSSI, removal of sharp objects should be considered and may include somebody going through the patient's room to look for possible implements and removing objects such as knives from the kitchen or other areas. Also, locking up all medications, including nonprescription medications, and making sure that the patient is provided only their daily doses and watched as they take them is good practice.

Discussing a safety plan, such as who the patient will reach out to (parent, relative, adult friend, teacher), effective coping skills, and preferred interventions or responses by the parents, and providing a crisis phone number are also important. Safety plans should be developmentally appropriate and reflect the input of the patient and family members.

Discussing firearm access should be considered during any evaluation of suicidal or aggressive children and adolescents. Counseling safer storage is an important part of any safety plan (see the related chapter on firearm safety). Adolescents with significant mental health issues, including suicidality, are as likely to have access to firearms in the home as those without mental health issues [22, 23]. Children and adolescents will often report that they know where and how to access firearms, even when the parents believe otherwise [24, 25]. Parents are often open to appropriate education about firearm safety [26].

Homicidal Threats

Homicidal threats, especially in school settings, can be a common and concerning issue [27]. While threats are common and may be immature pranks or impulsive exclamations, careful evaluation is always essential; prior threats or leakage (indirect statements about intent to harm made to nontargets) are common in school violence and violence in general [28, 29]. Careful evaluation by an appropriate clinician should be routine in all such situations. Critical risk factors to consider in any threat of violence include prior acts of violence, explicit threats, hostile attributional style, access to/carrying of weapons, substance use, impulsivity, and reasons for acting or not acting on the aggressive urges.

If at any time the clinician feels uncomfortable or concerned about the safety of the patient, it is reasonable to ask for a psychiatric consultation. Also, regardless of the clinical decisions made, thorough documentation, including safety plans, protective factors, and risk factors, is always good practice.

The "Freak Out"

Often, patients will be brought to the emergency department because they are experiencing an intense emotional crisis. The reasons for a child or adolescent meltdown vary widely and may require a variety of approaches for stabilization and evaluation [30]. Evaluating and managing pediatric agitation is a complex process but may be quite common in acute settings and pediatric hospitals; well-considered guidelines and tools for clinicians may be useful [31]. For pharmacologic management of acute agitation, see related chapter.

Case Example 2

A 9-year-old boy was brought to the emergency room after he threw a pencil at a peer in school while they were getting ready to go to a surprise assembly. His mother described him as a very intelligent and sensitive child, who was well above average when it came to his speech and reading and writing skills, but who had struggled with peers most of his life. In the emergency department, he was curled up under a chair and would bark like a dog at anyone who approached him. This is not the first time that he had suffered from such an extreme emotional reaction. He had always been subject to "tantrums." Grandparents, who accompanied the child and his mother to the emergency department, said, "He just needs a lot more discipline. He gets away with too much as it is." On further examination and discussion, most obtained by history, a strong suspicion for high-functioning autism became apparent. This recent meltdown was triggered by a change in his normal schedule at school. On further questioning, it was clear that he did very poorly with any variation from a schedule and that many of his emotional meltdowns would be triggered by surprises or unexpected occurrences.

Table 28.1 General guidance on the patient who is "freaking out"

1. Assess the safety of the patient and those around them before anything else.
2. Do not overreact if immediate safety is not an issue.
3. Get as much collateral as you can, especially regarding the trigger of this incident.
4. Reassure the patient, if possible (do not argue with psychosis).
5. Use PRNs judiciously, but as needed, with the goal of relieving the stress on the patient but not subduing them.

While it is beyond the scope of this chapter to teach the diagnostic criteria for autism spectrum disorder, the example above does reflect one important fact: Most emotional meltdowns are triggered by something, and the triggers can vary for each—and even for each episode (Table 28.1).

Remember to ask the question "Do I need to physically or medically intervene at this moment?" If the answer is no, allowing the behavior to burn out or dissipate is not an unreasonable approach. Use of PRN medications for child and adolescent agitation can be precarious, with limited research to guide selection and dosage.

Differential for the Meltdown

The differential for the emotional breakdown can be quite broad, including psychosis, anxiety or fear, oppositionality, trauma, or substance use. Agitation as an adverse effect of a medication, psychiatric or somatic, can also be an option—including paradoxical agitation from medications usually considered sedating (e.g., antihistamines or benzodiazepines) or akathisia due to antipsychotic medications. Intervention, as always, should be tailored to etiology and concern.

Psychosis is most likely going to respond to a combination of medication and maintaining a calm environment. If the crisis is so acute that they are not able to keep themselves safe or are risking others, admission may be warranted. Psychosis with agitation or new-onset psychosis may also warrant an inpatient psychiatric admission. In young patients with a known history of psychosis and treatment, nonadherence with prescribed medications can be surprisingly common and easily missed in the assessment.

Anxiety or fear, whether due to an anxiety disorder, severe obsessive–compulsive disorder, or an intellectual disability, often responds well to reassurance, a clear explanation of what is going on and what will happen next, maintaining a safe space, a nonthreatening approach, and, if necessary, medication. Arguably, this type of approach is prudent in most psychiatric evaluations but can be critical in working with severely anxious children and adolescents. Response to these treatments will further determine disposition.

Oppositional defiant adolescents and children can often be extremely difficult to work with, especially if one approaches them authoritatively. They often feel unheard or that their lives are unfair. These are patients who are going to need more extensive therapy and should be referred for treatment. In the short term, confrontation, arguments, and unnecessary power struggles can be exceedingly unhelpful [32]. Patients with an acute risk of danger to themselves or others may warrant brief inpatient treatment.

Posttraumatic stress can be a very difficult situation to handle in the emergency department, but significant reassurance and selective use of medication are often good approaches. Childhood trauma and its associated symptoms can have a broad spectrum of presenting features, including oppositional resistance (freezing), agitation or aggression (activation or recapitulation), or avoidance and withdrawal [33]. Early childhood or repeated traumas can be especially challenging to evaluate and understand. Referral to specialized, trauma-focused treatment is often optimal, and brief inpatient stabilization may be helpful. Reporting to child protective services may be legally required, depending on the context and facts of the case.

Substance use is a common reason for emergency department visits. They may result from recreational drug use or adverse reactions to therapeutically prescribed medications. Emergency presentations are broad and varied. As emphasized throughout much of this chapter, collateral is extremely helpful. Intoxication may warrant a brief medical admission; ongoing substance use in and of itself is seldom appropriate for inpatient psychiatric admission but may warrant linkage to definitive substance-use treatment providers. Medically complicated withdrawal from alcohol, benzodiazepines, or opioids is rare in this age group but may require admission for detoxification when present.

Review of prescription drug monitoring databases is often appropriate; note that the stimulants commonly used for ADHD are controlled substances and should be trackable through such databases.

Keep in mind that addiction is a pernicious problem, often with onset in adolescence, and may not be spontaneously disclosed by or easily recognized in an adolescent. Involuntary rehabilitation and inpatient hospitalizations for substance-use disorders are controversial and without meaningful evidence to support their use. However, brief motivational interviewing has been shown to be quite effective in the emergency room setting [34]. These are often patients who are primed for change. Take advantage of this when you can.

Legal Considerations for Emergency Psychiatric Care of Minors

By its very definition, the term "minor" connotes that a person has diminished legal rights by their age [35]. Legal minority often impacts a person's rights relating to some healthcare issues regarding a person's legal ability to maintain confidentiality and to consent to medical treatment. Most relevant are the domains of mental health and substance use; additional categories include reproductive health (including prenatal care) and general medical issues. For each of these domains, providers need to navigate complex and sometimes conflicting standards from state and federal sources. Legal consultation is often advisable; well-written hospital policies and guidelines prepared in advance to guide clinicians through such scenarios are ideal. Some important legal questions to consider are listed in Table 28.2.

Again, as the theme often is in child psychiatric emergencies, effective communication with the child and the parent can forestall many risks. This certainly extends to clear communication, when possible, about the relative risks and benefits of various interventions such as admission, discharge, and medications. Providers should be mindful of black box warnings on medications, as well as labeling-related age limits. Off-label prescribing is common—arguably essential—in child and adolescent psychiatry but should not be done without informing the patient and parent, as appropriate.

Many states, especially heavily populated ones, may have resources (including manuals, fact sheets, or training) to provide answers to these questions from interested nonprofit organizations such as juvenile law centers or the state chapter of the American Civil Liberties Union. A cursory exploration with a search engine for keywords such as "minors' healthcare legal rights" and your state may be fruitful.

Table 28.2 Important legal questions for your jurisdiction

What is the age at which a patient can consent to medical or reproductive healthcare treatment? Are there exceptions for pregnancy-related issues, including abortion?
What is the age at which a patient can consent to psychiatric treatment?
Are their different standards for inpatient or outpatient treatment? Are there different standards for medication treatment versus psychotherapy only?
What are the legal standards for resolving conflicts about treatment decisions between minors and parents? Between parents who disagree?
What is the age at which a patient can consent to substance-use disorder treatment?
What are the standards for the reporting of child abuse?
What is the legal age of consent for sexual activity?
What is the standard for records retention for minors?

As with adults, minors involved in the criminal justice system may present for emergency care. Clinically, juvenile offenders have elevated rates of an array of psychiatric morbidity and high rates of psychosocial complexity, and may be managed (as with behavioral emergencies) in settings intended for adult offenders [36]. Legal rights of minors involved in the criminal justice system can be especially complex to understand. Legal consultation is often advisable, and boarding these patients in the emergency department pending clear advice may be necessary. While boarding is never desirable, it may provide intermediate options for careful decision-making: Law enforcement may push for quick decisions before all the facts or legal rules are understood, and a "soft admission" may become a "disposition nightmare" for the inpatient team because of the clinical complexity of these cases.

Finally, providers should note that medical malpractice liability for psychiatric treatment of minors may be unusually complex and enduring. An adult who believes that they were the victim of malpractice must sue within a specified number of years, as dictated by the relevant jurisdiction's statute of limitations. In many states, the statute of limitations does not begin to toll until the person reaches the age of 18, potentially extending the window of liability exposure (and having a correlating impact on malpractice insurance policy considerations such as tail coverage).

Conclusion

Child psychiatric emergencies can be especially challenging due to some factors, both clinical and systematic. While these presentations can be stressful for all involved, careful attention to the fundamentals of good behavioral emergency management—good communication, gathering collateral, and reflecting before responding or acting—can continue to provide the resources needed to navigate many of these presentations. Dedicated child and adolescent emergency psychiatric services may be unavailable. Consultation with a child psychiatrist experienced in emergency evaluation should be sought whenever appropriate by clinicians and should be fought for as a priority resource by administrators and leaders. No matter what the decision may be, careful documentation of the assessment, decision-making, safety plans, and protective and risk factors is always prudent.

References

1. Carubia B, Becker A, Levine BH. Child psychiatric emergencies: updates on trends, clinical care, and practice challenges. Curr Psychiatry Rep. 2016;18(4):41.
2. Chakravarthy B, Yang A, Ogbu U, Kim C, Iqbal A, Haight J, et al. Determinants of pediatric psychiatry length of stay in 2 urban emergency departments. Pediatr Emerg Care. 2017;33(9):613.
3. Mercado MC, Holland K, Leemis RW, Stone DM, Wang J. Trends in emergency department visits for nonfatal self-inflicted injuries among youth aged 10 to 24 years in the United States, 2001–2015. JAMA. 2017;318(19):1931–3.
4. Nunn K. Emergency paediatric psychiatry: an emerging sub-specialty. J Paediatr Child Health. 2017;53(7):628–9.
5. Goldstein AB, Horwitz SM. Child and adolescent psychiatric emergencies: the need for a clear research agenda. Pediatr Emerg Care. 2006;22(4):282.
6. Rozel JS. Child and adolescent emergency psychiatry: a review of recent developments. Curr Emerg Hosp Med Rep. 2015;3(4):202–8.
7. Newton AS, Hartling L, Soleimani A, Kirkland S, Dyson MP, Cappelli M. A systematic review of management strategies for children's mental health care in the emergency department: update on evidence and recommendations for clinical practice and research. Emerg Med J. 2017;34:376; emermed-2016-205939.
8. Haddad F, Gerson RS, American Psychiatric Association, editors. Helping kids in crisis: managing psychiatric emergencies in children and adolescents. 1st ed. Washington, D.C.: American Psychiatric Publishing, a division of American Psychiatric Association; 2015. p. 213.
9. Prager LM, Donovan AL. Suicide by security blanket, and other stories from the child psychiatric emergency service: what happens to children with acute mental illness. Santa Barbara: Praeger; 2012. p. 115. (Praeger series on contemporary health and living.)
10. Santillanes G, Donofrio JJ, Lam CN, Claudius I. Is medical clearance necessary for pediatric psychiatric patients? J Emerg Med. 2014;46(6):800–7.
11. Donofrio JJ, Santillanes G, McCammack BD, Lam CN, Menchine MD, Kaji AH, et al. Clinical utility of screening laboratory tests in pediatric psychiatric patients presenting to the emergency department for medical clearance. Ann Emerg Med. 2014;63(6):666–675.e3.
12. Donofrio JJ, Horeczko T, Kaji A, Santillanes G, Claudius I. Most routine laboratory testing of pediatric psychiatric patients in the emergency department is not medically necessary. Health Aff (Millwood). 2015;34(5):812–8.
13. Bronfenbrenner U. Is early intervention effective? Day Care Early Educ. 1974;2(2):14–8.
14. McGorry PD. Early intervention in psychosis: obvious, effective, overdue. J Nerv Ment Dis. 2015;203(5):310–8.
15. Claxton M, Onwumere J, Fornells-Ambrojo M. Do family interventions improve outcomes in early psychosis? A systematic review and meta-analysis. Front Psychol. 2017;8:371.
16. James KM, Woody ML, Feurer C, Kudinova AY, Gibb BE. Disrupted physiological reactivity among children with a history of suicidal ideation: moderation by parental expressed emotion-criticism. Biol Psychol. 2017;130:22–9.
17. Wharff EA, Ginnis KB, Ross AM, White EM, White MT, Forbes PW. Family-based crisis intervention with suicidal adolescents: a randomized clinical trial. Pediatr Emerg Care. 2017;35:170.
18. Dazzi T, Gribble R, Wessely S, Fear NT. Does asking about suicide and related behaviours induce suicidal ideation? What is the evidence? Psychol Med. 2014;44(16):3361–3.
19. Olfson M, Wall M, Wang S, Crystal S, Gerhard T, Blanco C. Suicide following deliberate self-harm. Am J Psychiatry. 2017;174(8):765–74.
20. Lynch TR, Trost WT, Salsman N, Linehan MM. Dialectical behavior therapy for borderline personality disorder. Annu Rev Clin Psychol. 2007;3(1):181–205.
21. Sneed JR, Balestri M, Belfi BJ. The use of dialectical behavior therapy strategies in the psychiatric emergency room. Psychotherapy. 2003;40(4):265–77.
22. Simonetti JA, Mackelprang JL, Rowhani-Rahbar A, Zatzick D, Rivara FP. Psychiatric comorbidity, suicidality, and in-home firearm access among a nationally representative sample of adolescents. JAMA Psychiatry. 2015;72(2):152–9.
23. Simonetti JA, Theis MK, Rowhani-Rahbar A, Ludman EJ, Grossman DC. Firearm storage practices in households of adolescents with and without mental illness. J Adolesc Health. 2017;61:583. Available at http://www.sciencedirect.com/science/article/pii/S1054139X17302239. Accessed 15 Sept 2017.
24. Azrael D, Miller M, Hemenway D. Are household firearms stored safely? It depends on whom you ask. Pediatrics. 2000;106(3):e31.

25. Baxley F, Miller M. Parental misperceptions about children and firearms. Arch Pediatr Adolesc Med. 2006;160(5):542–7.
26. Garbutt JM, Bobenhouse N, Dodd S, Sterkel R, Strunk RC. What are parents willing to discuss with their pediatrician about firearm safety? A parental survey. J Pediatr. 2016;179:166. Available at http://linkinghub.elsevier.com/retrieve/pii/S0022347616306862. Accessed 19 Sept 2016.
27. Glick RL, Hirshbein LD, Patel N. Emergency psychiatry: how should emergency psychiatrists respond to school violence? Psychiatr Serv. 2004;55(3):223–4.
28. Vossekuil B, Fein RA, Reddy M, Borum R, Modzeleski W. The final report and findings of the safe school initiative: implications for the prevention of school attacks in the United States. Washington, D.C.: U.S. Department of Education, Office of Elementary and Secondary Education, Safe and Drug-Free Schools Program and U.S. Secret Service, National Threat Assessment Center; 2002.
29. Meloy JR, O'Toole ME. The concept of leakage in threat assessment. Behav Sci Law. 2011;29(4):513–27.
30. Rozel JS, Stowell KR, Thorkelson GD. Diagnosis and management of agitation in children and adolescents. In: Zeller S, Nordstrom K, Wilson M, editors. Diagnosis and management of agitation in children and adolescents. New York: Cambridge University Press; 2017. p. 253–70.
31. Malas N, Spital L, Fischer J, Kawai Y, Cruz D, Keefer P. National survey on pediatric acute agitation and behavioral escalation in academic inpatient pediatric care settings. Psychosomatics. 2017;58:299. Available at http://www.sciencedirect.com/science/article/pii/S0033318217300233. Accessed 28 May 2017.
32. Greene RW, Ablon JS. Treating explosive kids: the collaborative problem-solving approach. New York: Guilford Press; 2006.
33. Perry BD, Pollard RA, Blakley TL, Baker WL, Vigilante D. Childhood trauma, the neurobiology of adaptation, and "use-dependent" development of the brain: how "states" become "traits". Infant Ment Health J. 1995;16(4):271–91.
34. Newton AS, Dong K, Mabood N, Ata N, Ali S, Gokiert R, et al. Brief emergency department interventions for youth who use alcohol and other drugs: a systematic review. Pediatr Emerg Care. 2013;29(5):673–84.
35. Garner BE, editor. Black's law dictionary. 9th ed. St. Paul: West; 2009.
36. Whitley K, Rozel JS. Mental health care of detained youth and solitary confinement and restraint within juvenile detention facilities. Child Adolesc Psychiatr Clin N Am. 2016;25(1):71–80.

Mental Health Considerations After Sexual Assault

29

Lauren R. Klein and Jeffrey D. Ho

Introduction

The Centers for Disease Control and Prevention estimates that one in five women in the United States will be sexually assaulted at some point during their lifetime, creating a greater burden on the health care system than any other type of crime [1, 2]. However, understanding the scope of the sexual assault problem in the United States may be limited due to inherent underreporting. Approximately 60–70% of sexual assaults are not disclosed to the police, according to the Department of Justice [3–5], and only half of those who report to the police receive any medical treatment.

When the sexual assault victim arrives at the emergency department (ED), a unique set of circumstances arise. The provider needs to understand that this patient population is indeed a group of victims that requires a careful balance of advocacy, flexibility, and neutrality on the part of the examiner. In a typical provider–patient relationship, patients generally present by their own volition. Even in circumstances when a patient is unresponsive, the provider approaches care from the standpoint of implied consent, meaning that the provider proceeds with care decisions under the assumption that the incapacitated patient would want aggressive interventions made on their behalf. In the case of the sexual assault victim, that is not necessarily the case, and there may be victims who present with ambivalence (or even resistance) toward issues related to their care and the documentation of evidence in their case. It is therefore important to remember that the examiner must approach these cases advocating for the interests of the victim, while remaining neutral with regard to gathering evidence and documenting the details and allowing flexibility for the victim to maintain decision authority over their care, even if their decisions change long after the assault. For instance, an alleged victim may be identified by a family member and brought in for evaluation but is reluctant to report this to law enforcement. This requires that the examiner respect the victim's wishes and not report this, while maintaining the evidence in an acceptable way that it is not tainted should the victim wish to report this several weeks later.

Few other types of emergency presentations involve such an in-depth consideration of the potential for physical injury, potential infectious disease, serious legal consequences, and devastating mental health sequelae, making this a particularly challenging scenario for emergency providers. The focus of this chapter will be those mental health issues, including considerations for the initial victim's assessment, as well as considerations regarding the long-term care of this complex population.

L. R. Klein (✉) · J. D. Ho
Department of Emergency Medicine, Hennepin County Medical Center, Minneapolis, MN, USA
e-mail: lauren.klein@hcmed.org

L. S. Zun et al. (eds.), *Behavioral Emergencies for Healthcare Providers*,
https://doi.org/10.1007/978-3-030-52520-0_29

The Initial ED Presentation

There is no "classic" initial presentation for the sexual assault victim; this is true when it comes to their physical manifestations as well as their mental health issues [6–8]. The initial presentation is also likely to be unpredictable, regardless of whether they present hours, days, or weeks after their assault. For these reasons, there are very limited data available characterizing what providers may come to expect regarding their victim's initial mental health assessment, and the literature that does exist is largely expert consensus or based on surveying victims and the providers who care for them.

The victim's post-assault behavior can be highly variable and can be influenced by both personal attributes and external factors. Therefore, a wide variety of emotional reactions can be expected by emergency providers [6, 7]. This may include feelings of guilt, shame, anxiety, depression, hypervigilance, or denial, to name just a few. Other important contributing factors may include pre-existing social support networks, the relationship of the victim to the assailant, previous assault/life experiences, spiritual beliefs, and the severity of the assault [9]. There are also extremes of a sexual assault presentation, which may include acute agitation requiring immediate medical attention. Also complicating the presentation is the fact that it can be common for sexual assault victims to present with some form of intoxication. Any type of trauma, whether it is sexual assault or otherwise, can cause significant psychomotor agitation, and providers should consider the use of chemical sedation if the victim's or provider's immediate physical safety is at risk [10].

In addition to variability in the victim's responses, the history and account of the assault provided by the victim can change drastically during this initial evaluation. Experts recognize that trauma can lead to "extremes of (memory) retention and forgetfulness" [11], where traumatic memories can be recalled with great precision or may not be consolidated at all. This is referred to in the psychological literature as memory fragmentation and has been noted for decades, as it pertains to many different traumatic presentations [11–13]. This traumatic amnesia can last for minutes or years, and may not return without cognitive therapy or, in unfortunate circumstances, a recurrence of the scenario or environment surrounding the initial traumatic event. Traumatic dissociation is another important process, similar to memory fragmentation, where memories are recalled in pieces, but the unified narrative cannot be recollected in its entirety [11]. This dissociative memory may be what most emergency providers are familiar with, regarding seeing victims attempting to account for their assaults in the acute setting.

The scant primary literature on this subject, though largely in the psychiatric and law enforcement literature, is still quite informative for emergency providers. One study performed by psychiatrists interviewed 46 assault victims (30 of which were sexual assault victims) and noted marked variability in victim memory processing, as well as a high prevalence of traumatic memory recollection in the form of initial dissociated elements of the assault [11]. They noted that over time a narrative often developed, but concluded that, "[I]t is the very nature of traumatic memory to be dissociated, stored as sensory fragments without a coherent semantic component." Another study from the law enforcement literature came to similar conclusions; investigators used questionnaires among recent sexual assault victims and found that among their participants, there were high rates of traumatic dissociation, memory fragmentation, and incoherence of the account. A notable finding in this study was that dissociation/fragmentation scores were negatively associated with the likelihood to proceed with their legal case [14].

Presentation Variability, Memory Dissociation, and Emergency Providers

The manner in which the victim presents can have a strong impact on the provider's perception of the victim, and the provider's perception of the victim can have a strong impact on their treatment of the victim. This initial exposure to the medical system and the relationship established by providers can play an enormous role in the sexual assault victim's subsequent mental health and psychological well-being; this concept is illustrated by the notion of secondary victimization, which we will now discuss.

Secondary victimization is defined as the "attitudes, beliefs, and behaviors of social system personnel that victims experience as victim blaming and insensitive" [15]. It has also been referred to as "secondary rape" or "secondary assault." One expert explains that secondary victimization is a process that "exacerbates (the victim's) trauma, and makes them feel like what they are experiencing is a second rape" [15]. Secondary victimization has been described regarding all aspects of the sexual assault victim's interaction with the system, including interactions with their medical providers, social services providers, and mental health providers as well as law enforcement.

Early work on the subject of secondary victimization studied the opinions of mental health professionals, and the results identified that there was a negative impact on the victims from contact with social system personnel [16]. Overall, 86% of participants agreed that the behavior of professionals further traumatizes the assault victim; 84% of those surveyed felt the interaction led to victims feeling guilty, and 89% believed it led to victim's distrust. Regarding system-specific interactions, 81% thought that reporting to the criminal justice system was psychologically detrimental, and 58% felt that mental health professionals contributed to further traumatization. These findings only begin to highlight the scope of this problem [16].

A more recent work examined the perspective of the sexual assault victims themselves. In one study, investigators found that among 112 victims, nearly one-third of participants felt contact with the medical system was hurtful from a mental health standpoint [17]. Subjects who identified a contact with the medical system as hurtful highlighted that a lack of communication regarding important medical needs was a source of their dissatisfaction. Those victims who felt the medical system was hurtful were less likely to have received information about emergency contraception or emergency sexually transmitted disease treatment [17].

Another study interviewed victims specifically regarding their emergency department care as they were waiting for discharge paperwork after their initial post-assault assessment [18]. This study found that secondary victimization behaviors were extremely common; over 90% of women experienced at least one secondary victimization behavior, and this included doctors questioning their behavior/choices (33%), questioning their relationship with the perpetrator (52%), questioning their resistance to the assault (100%), and questioning what clothing they wore (33%). These behaviors made the victims feel depressed (88%), anxious (91%), guilty (74%), violated (94%), and distrusting of others (74%). Interestingly, this study also went on to ask the medical team (doctors and nurses) their perception of these same behaviors and found notable discrepancies between their responses and the responses of the victims. The inter-rater agreement among victims and medical personnel was only 58% (which the authors point out is just slightly better than chance), where the medical providers were consistently under-reporting victimization behaviors, as well as demonstrating a lack of appreciation of the victim's acute mental health concerns (e.g., depression, anxiousness, and guilt) [18].

The findings of this study and the others described suggest that emergency providers should consider their interactions with the sexual assault victim with great care. While the trauma itself is probably still the most important contributor to the future mental health of the sexual assault victim, the initial experience with the medical system can have profound effects on an already vulnerable individual. This interaction may be one of the only modifiable factors regarding the victim's long-term prognosis that the emergency providers can meaningfully influence. Figure 29.1 provides some specific recommendations for the interview with the sexual assault victim.

- **Consider:**
  - Using language that allows for a comfortable dialogue with the patient
  - Using open-ended questions
  - Expressing appreciation that the patient came to the ED
  - Carefully articulating the medical needs of the encounter, such as emergency contraception and sexually transmitted disease testing
  - Encouraging the use of ancillary support staff, such as social workers or sexual assault nurse examiners
- **Attempt to Avoid:**
  - Language that can be interpreted as blaming
  - Questioning the patient's behavior during the assault (ie., substance use, resistance during the assault)
  - Questioning the patient's relationship with the perpetrator
  - Questioning the patient's account of events (with respect to memory fragmentation)
  - Criticizing when the patient presented to the ED (if they do not present immediately after the assault)

Fig. 29.1 Recommendations for emergency providers during the patient interview

Long-Term Mental Health Considerations

Long-term mental health consequences for victims of sexual assault have been described in the literature for decades. Dating back to the 1970s, Burgess et al. described a rape trauma syndrome as "a syndrome of behavioral, somatic, and psychological reactions (to) a life-threatening situation" [19]. In a series of 146 women, they described a constellation of symptoms that develop over time, including nightmares, phobias, fear, and anxiety, as well as physical/somatic manifestations such as muscle tension and gynecological symptoms.

Many other studies have since cited this association between sexual assault and the long-term development of multiple mental health sequelae, including depression, anxiety, post-traumatic stress disorder (PTSD), sleep disorders, eating disorders, personality disorders, chronic pain disorders, and suicide [20]. We will now provide an overview of some of these important mental health processes.

Depression and Anxiety

Depression and anxiety can manifest soon after the assault occurs, but has been investigated most comprehensively as a long-term consequence of sexual assault. A recent meta-analysis evaluated 30 years of research on this topic and looked specifically at the development of anxiety disorders and depression among sexual assault victims. They reported that the odds ratio for developing depression post-assault was 3.1 (95% confidence interval, 2.4–3.9), and developing anxiety disorders was 2.7 (95% confidence interval, 2.1–3.3). They also investigated to see if the severity of the assault played a role; they found that rape specifically was more likely to be associated with a lifetime diagnosis of depression (odds ratio = 6.3; 95% confidence interval, 1.9–20.1). This severity–response relationship has been identified in other work, as well, suggesting that the details and circumstances of the assault may be important for the victim's risk for developing these mental health sequelae [21].

Despite much evidence describing the relationship between sexual assault and the development of anxiety and depression, the mechanism of this association is not fully understood. Many, however, have proposed a possible role of a genetic predisposition. One of the early publications describing this concept was a longitudinal study investigating a functional polymorphism in a serotonin transporter gene. Individuals with the short allele of this gene were more likely to develop clinical depression in response to a stressful life event [22]. Though many studies replicated these findings in subsequent work, a recent meta-analysis did not find any association, highlighting some of the complexities in this line of research [23].

Considerations for the emergency department provider regarding treatments and therapies for depression and anxiety in the sexual assault victim will be similar to other encounters where patients report such symptoms. One of the most useful interventions the emergency provider can provide for this population is timely and appropriate recognition of the diagnosis and proper referral for outpatient programs (if appropriate) or emergent escalation of care if these symptoms are severe. Emergency providers may be interested in referring the victim to resources that are specifically designed for sexual abuse victims, such as the National Sexual Assault Telephone Hotline offered by the Rape, Abuse & Incest National Network (RAINN) [24].

Post-Traumatic Stress Disorder

Post-traumatic stress disorder (PTSD) occurs very commonly among sexual assault victims, and the prevalence of symptoms may be as high as 80% according to national-level data [1, 25]. One prospective study following 94 women found the prevalence of PTSD symptoms among their cohort to be even as high as 94% in the weeks after the assault [26]. The previously discussed meta-analysis also noted a lifetime odds ratio for the development of PTSD of 2.3 (95% confidence interval, 1.6–3.4) [20].

A variety of characteristics regarding the victim and the assault may all be correlated with the development and the severity of PTSD [27, 28]. Features such as the degree of the violence during the assault, number of lifetime sexual assaults, childhood sexual abuse history, and the victim–offender relationship have all been shown to be associated with long-term PTSD symptoms. There are other features associated with PTSD development—such as delay in the disclosure, self-blaming behaviors, social support, and coping mechanisms—that are considered to be modifiable factors. These modifiable factors are particularly important for emergency providers to take note of, as this may be an opportunity for the encounter with emergency services to have a positive impact on future mental health prognosis [27, 28].

Another area in which emergency providers could potentially make a positive impact on the victims is in the detection of this mental health condition. Symptoms of PTSD in the sexual assault victim may include nightmares, anxiety, avoidance, and feelings of detachment, among many others [25]. Challenging its diagnoses is the fact that each victim will present with a different constellation of these symptoms, making it potentially difficult for the emergency provider to identify, especially if the encounter is not necessarily focused on mental health. However, given such a high prevalence among assault victims, it is reasonable for emergency providers to have a very low threshold to screen if there is a known history of sexual assault. A number of validated screening tools exist, several of which are brief and can be easily adopted for use in the emergency department setting [29].

Currently, there is a multi-center study underway to gather victim DNA samples while interviewing the victims over time to determine if there is a genetic component that predisposes some victims toward developing PTSD. This represents a developing network contributing to a novel way of possibly identifying those at risk. Similar to how cancer registry network development improved survival outcomes for cancer patients by allowing for sharing of information between numerous centers, prospectively identifying those at risk and sharing this information is an emerging concept that may help to provide better PTSD outcomes through early identification of risk and targeted intervention.

Suicide Ideation and Suicide Attempt

Two of the most serious potential mental health consequences of sexual assault are suicide and suicide attempts [30–33]. Because of their devastating nature, suicide among sexual assault victims has been the subject of much research. The statistics on suicide are quite staggering; one study estimated that sexual assault victims are four times more likely to experience suicidal ideation and 13 times more likely to have attempted suicide [33]. Another group found a lifetime increased odds of suicide attempts of 4.1 (95% confidence interval 2.9–5.8) [20].

The National Comorbidity Survey is a large-scale representative survey conducted to examine mental health issues and has provided much insight regarding the prevalence of various mental health conditions in the United States. Ullman and colleagues [31] performed a subgroup analysis, specifically looking at 627 women who stated they had experienced sexual assault (either in childhood or in adulthood). Their findings constitute much of what we know about the demographic and psychosocial factors associated with suicidal ideation and suicide attempts in this population. In their cohort, 35% of women who had experienced a sexual assault had at some point had suicidal thoughts, and 17% had attempted suicide in their lifetime. Several variables were found to be associated with suicidal ideation; the authors identified demographic associations such as younger age, being unemployed, being unmarried, and experiencing a number of traumatic events over the course of one's lifetime. Other associated psychosocial variables included less social support, but the most significant relationship was noted for concomitant PTSD, concomitant depression, and alcohol dependence symptoms. The authors comment that these findings were similar for both suicidal ideations, as well as a history of a suicide attempt [31].

To this point, we have focused mostly on mental health considerations for female sexual assault victims; the topic of suicide, however, demonstrates some important gender discrepancies. Though there are fewer male victims of sexual assault, they may be more likely to contemplate and attempt suicide. One cross-sectional study by Martin and colleagues looked specifically at gender differences in this relationship between sexual abuse and suicidality [34]. They found in their study that 55% of the male sexual assault victims attempted suicide, compared to 29% of females. Interestingly, they also found that among males, suicidal ideation (including plans, threats, and history of self-injury) did not necessarily correlate with depression or other psychosocial factors. However, suicidal ideation among female sexual assault victims was found to be "fully mediated by depression, hopelessness, and family dysfunction." This highlights some potentially important considerations when considering the suicidal ideation among male versus female victims in the emergency setting.

Sexual Assault Nurse Examiners

Sexual assault nurse examiner (SANE) programs specialized training programs for nurse examiners who have completed a focused education in forensic nursing related to the examination of sexual assault victims and suspects. This pathway provides eligibility for SANE-A (adult and adolescent) and SANE-P (pediatric) certification through the International Association of Forensic Nursing. SANE programs are increasing in popularity around the country and worldwide; currently, there are nearly 800 programs in the United States and almost 900 internationally.

Achievement of a SANE certification requires education in many areas related to the care and counseling of sexual assault victims, including crisis intervention, referral for follow-up counseling, and support services. They also receive specialized training on mental health issues, including victim responses and advocacy. As such, SANE providers can be an invaluable resource for the mental health needs of the sexual assault victim and should be utilized by emergency providers when appropriate.

Conclusion

The evaluation of the sexual assault victim in the emergency department can be a complex process, given the spectrum of physical, emotional, legal, and mental health considerations. There are many competing factors that may be present when dealing with a sexual assault victim that can complicate their evaluation and create in them an immediate fragile state of mental health. These factors can include the presence of intoxicating substances, concomitant physical illness or trauma, shame or embarrassment, fear of a known assailant or fear of the unknown, and apprehension related to the exposure that may occur if the assault is reported to authorities. Sexual assault victims are also at high risk for developing delayed mental health issues related to post-traumatic stress, depression, and even suicidality. Present-day research is focusing on identifying victims most at risk for this, with the hope of possible early intervention. Current best practices in managing these victims will include the use of specially trained forensic nurse examiner teams when feasible.

References

1. National intimate partner and sexual violence survey: 2010 summary. Available at https://www.cdc.gov/violenceprevention/pdf/nisvs_report2010-a.pdf.
2. National Institute of Justice. National criminal justice reference. Available at https://www.ncjrs.gov/pdffiles/victcost.pdf.
3. Planty M, Langton L, Krebs C, Berzofsky M, Smiley-McDonald H. Female victims of sexual violence, 1994–2010. Special Report (No NCJ 240655). Washington, D.C.: Bureau of Justice Statistics US Department of Justice. Available at http://responsesystemspanel.whs.mil/public/docs/meetings/20130627/04_Bkgrnd_Prep_Materials/Binder_1/Tab_11_US_DoJ_Special_RPT.pdf.
4. Statistics about sexual violence. National Sexual Violence Resource. Available at https://www.nsvrc.org/sites/default/files/publications_nsvrc_factsheet_media-packet_statistics-about-sexual-violence_0.pdf.
5. Rape and sexual assault: reporting to police and medical attention. Available at https://www.bjs.gov/content/pub/pdf/rsarp00.pdf.
6. Frazier PA. The role of attributions and perceived control in recovery from rape. J Pers Interpers Loss. 2000;5(2–3):203–25.
7. Koss MP, Goodman LA, Browne A, Fitzgerald LF, Keita GP, Russo NF. Responses to sexual harassment. In: No safe haven: male violence against women at home, at work, and in the community. Washington, D.C.: American Psychological Association; 1994. p. 133–48.
8. Wyatt GE, Notgrass CM, Newcomb M. Internal and external mediators of women's rape experiences. Psychol Women Q. 1990;14(2):153–76.
9. Littleton H, Breitkopf CR. Coping with the experience of rape. Psychol Women Q. 2006;30(1):106–16.
10. Wilson MP, Pepper D, Currier GW, Holloman GH Jr, Feifel D. The psychopharmacology of agitation: consensus statement of the American Association for Emergency Psychiatry Project Beta Psychopharmacology Workgroup. West J Emerg Med. 2012;13(1):26–34.
11. van der Kolk BA, Fisler R. Dissociation and the fragmentary nature of traumatic memories: overview and exploratory study. J Trauma Stress. 1995;8(4):505–25.
12. Bedard-Gilligan M, Zoellner LA. Dissociation and memory fragmentation in post-traumatic stress disorder: an evaluation of the dissociative encoding hypothesis. Memory. 2012;20(3):277–99.
13. O'Kearney R, Perrott K. Trauma narratives in post-traumatic stress disorder: a review. J Trauma Stress. 2006;19(1):81–93.
14. Hardy A, Young K, Holmes EA. Does trauma memory play a role in the experience of reporting sexual assault during police interviews? An exploratory study. Memory. 2009;17(8):783–8.
15. Campbell R. Research for the real world seminar: the neurobiology of sexual assault. December 2012.
16. Campbell R, Raja S. Secondary victimization of rape victims: insights from mental health professionals who treat survivors of violence. Violence Vict. 1999;14(3):261–75.
17. Campbell R, Wasco SM, Ahrens CE, Sefl T, Barnes HE. Preventing the "second rape:" rape survivors' experiences with community service providers. J Interpers Violence. 2001;16:1239–59.
18. Campbell R. What really happened? A validation study of rape survivors' help-seeking experiences with the legal and medical systems. Violence Vict. 2005;20(1):55–68.
19. Burgess AW, Holmstrom LL. Rape trauma syndrome. Am J Psychiatry. 1974;131(9):981–6.
20. Chen LP, Murad MH, Paras ML, et al. Sexual abuse and lifetime diagnosis of psychiatric disorders: systematic review and meta-analysis. Mayo Clin Proc. 2010;85(7):618–29.
21. Pegram SE, Abbey A. Associations between sexual assault severity and psychological and physical health outcomes: similarities and differences among African American and Caucasian survivors. J Interpers Violence. 2016;34:4020. https://doi.org/10.1177/0886260516673626.
22. Caspi A, Sugden K, Moffitt TE, et al. Influence of life stress on depression: moderation by a polymorphism in the 5-HTT gene. Science. 2003;301(5631):386–9.
23. Risch N, Herrell R, Lehner T, et al. Interaction between the serotonin transporter gene (5-HTTLPR), stressful life events, and risk of depression: a meta-analysis. JAMA. 2009;301(23):2462–71.
24. Finn J, Garner MD, Wilson J. Volunteer and user evaluation of the National Sexual Assault Online Hotline. Eval Program Plann. 2011;34(3):266–72.
25. Chivers-Wilson KA. Sexual assault and posttraumatic stress disorder: a review of the biological, psychologi-

cal and sociological factors and treatments. Mcgill J Med. 2006;9(2):111–8.
26. Rothbaum BO, Foa EB, Riggs DS, Murdock T, Walsh W. A prospective examination of post-traumatic stress disorder in rape victims. J Trauma Stress. 1992;5(3):455–75.
27. Peter-Hagene LC, Ullman SE. Sexual assault-characteristics effects on PTSD and psychosocial mediators: a cluster-analysis approach to sexual assault types. Psychol Trauma. 2015;7(2):162–70.
28. Ullman SE, Filipas HH, Townsend SM, Starzynski LL. Psychosocial correlates of PTSD symptom severity in sexual assault survivors. J Trauma Stress. 2007;20(5):821–31.
29. PTSD Screening Instruments. US Department of Veterans Affairs. Available at https://www.ptsd.va.gov/PTSD/professional/assessment/screens/index.asp. Accessed Aug 2017.
30. Davidson JR, Hughes DC, George LK, Blazer DG. The association of sexual assault and attempted suicide within the community. Arch Gen Psychiatry. 1996;53(6):550–5.
31. Ullman SE, Brecklin LR. Sexual assault history and suicidal behavior in a national sample of women. Suicide Life Threat Behav. 2002;32(2):117–30.
32. Ullman SE, Najdowski CJ. Correlates of serious suicidal ideation and attempts in female adult sexual assault survivors. Suicide Life Threat Behav. 2009;39(1):47–57.
33. Kilpatrick D. The mental health impact of rape. Charleston: Medical University of South Carolina; 2000.
34. Martin G, Bergen HA, Richardson AS, Roeger L, Allison S. Sexual abuse and suicidality: gender differences in a large community sample of adolescents. Child Abuse Negl. 2004;28(5):491–503.

30 Mental Health Issues in Veterans

Janet S. Richmond

Introduction

This chapter focuses on the unique issues of military veterans and how these factors can impact their medical encounters. Military culture and specific medical conditions unique to veterans are described as are special considerations regarding the behavioral challenges to the doctor–patient relationship that can occur in the emergency setting.

Medical Illnesses in Veterans

Veterans have a higher unadjusted prevalence of health conditions than the general population [1]. Veterans with post-traumatic stress disorder (PTSD) have a higher prevalence of diabetes and gastroesophageal reflux disease (GERD), hypertension, metabolic syndrome, and hyperglycemia than nonveterans. They are more likely to be diagnosed with cancer, hearing loss, and post-traumatic stress disorder (PTSD) than civilians [2, 3]. Veterans are considered "less healthy" than the general population and have an increased proportion of "poor" health habits such as smoking and substance abuse than the general population. Veterans report feeling older than their peers, and there is speculation that PTSD may be associated with premature aging [4] and premature death. It is not unusual to see a patient with the following comorbidities: diabetes mellitus, hypertension, chronic renal failure, chronic obstructive pulmonary disease (COPD), alcoholism, depression, and chronic pain from military injuries. Table 30.1 shows medical conditions common to veterans in each era.

Veterans also have a higher incidence of socioeconomic issues, including homelessness. However, since 2010, the rate of homelessness among veterans has declined, and projections are that it will continue to decline [5].

Veterans have specific ("signature") medical conditions as a result of combat such as hearing loss, Da Costa's Syndrome ("soldier's heart"), Gulf-War syndrome, traumatic brain syndrome, and toxic states (Agent Orange). One signature injury of the Iraq and Afghanistan wars is traumatic brain injury (TBI), which has a myriad of signs and symptoms that can make communication difficult in the doctor–patient relationship: personality changes; cognitive impairments in memory, attention, and concentration; and poor judgment.

J. S. Richmond (✉)
VA Boston Healthcare System, Boston, MA, USA

McLean Hospital, Belmont, MA, USA

Tufts University School of Medicine, Boston, MA, USA

L. S. Zun et al. (eds.), *Behavioral Emergencies for Healthcare Providers*,
https://doi.org/10.1007/978-3-030-52520-0_30

Table 30.1 Signature illnesses by era

Civil war
Da Costa's syndrome ("Soldier's heart")
World war II
Cold injury
Chemical warfare agent experiments
Exposure to nuclear weapons (including testing or clean-up)
Korea
Agent Orange exposure
Cold injury (frostbite)
Chemical warfare agent experiments
Exposure to nuclear weapons (including testing or clean-up)
Vietnam
Agent Orange/pesticide exposure (*soft tissue sarcoma, non-Hodgkin's lymphoma, Hodgkin's disease, chloracne, porphyria* cutanea tarda, *respiratory cancers, multiple myeloma, prostate cancer, acute peripheral neuropathy,* and *spina bifida* in offspring)
Hepatitis C
Malaria
Embedded shrapnel
Traumatic war neurosis
Substance abuse
Bacterial and *fungal infections ("jungle rot")*
Gulf wars
Chemical or biological agents (e.g., mustard/nerve gas, oil-well fires, radiation)
Depleted uranium (DU)
Spinal cord injuries
Animal bites
Burns
Exposures to smoke
Embedded fragments
Infectious diseases (i.e., leishmaniasis)
Reproductive health issues
Cold war
Radiation-related disorders, including *leukemia, various cancers,* and *cataracts*
Operation Iraqi Freedom/Operation Enduring Freedom/ Operation New Dawn (OIF/OEF/OND):
Combined penetrating, blunt trauma, and burn injuries (blast injuries)
Embedded fragments (shrapnel)
Leishmaniasis
PTS (post-traumatic stress)
Multidrug-resistant Acinetobacter
Reproductive health issues
Traumatic amputation
Traumatic brain or spinal cord injury
Vision loss

Adapted from the US Department of Veterans Affairs Military Health History Pocket Card. Available at https://www.va.gov/oaa/pocketcard/m-index.asp

Amputation and limb salvage are now another issue that veterans face. In recent conflicts, soldiers who in past wars would have died on the battlefield, are living, often from attempts at limb salvage or amputation [6].

Post-Traumatic Stress Disorder

Not all veterans have PTSD. Being in combat or having multiple deployments are stressors, but soldiers are warriors who are trained to tolerate much. The usual horrific encounters that would qualify as traumatic events in civilian life are sometimes just part of routine combat. Yet, there are events that happen that are outside the bounds of the usual combatant's experience. Therefore, PTSD in military personnel may look quite different from what we usually think of as PTSD. There is literature on "combat stress reaction," where symptoms can be delayed in onset, often years after military service [7–10]. These characteristics are reminiscent of traumatic war neurosis first described by Kardiner [11] and Grinker and Spiegel [12], which eventually led to the modern diagnosis of PTSD in 1987 [13, 14].

For others, subclinical symptoms of PTSD can go on for decades. Symptoms may include sleep disturbances, decreased concentration, anger, hypervigilance, avoidance, psychic numbing, irritability, depression, and substance abuse. These subclinical features can become full-blown and usually develop after life-cycle events such as the birth of a child, retirement, or physical illness [8, 9].

An example of war-related PTSD was reported in 1918 by Rivers, who described as follows:

> a case … "of a young officer who was flung down by the explosion of a shell so that his face struck the distended abdomen of a German [soldier] several days dead, the impact of his fall rupturing the swollen corpse. Before he lost consciousness, the patient had clearly realized his situation and knew that the substance which filled his mouth and produced the most horrible sensations of taste and smell were derived from the decomposed entrails of an enemy. When he came to himself he vomited profusely and was much shaken, but "carried on" for several days, vomiting frequently, and haunted by persistent images of taste and smell" [15].

When that veteran comes to see the doctor often years after his military experience, he may complain of unrelenting nausea, vomiting, anorexia, diarrhea, or constipation. Thus, the military history is vital to the clinician. However, for a myriad of reasons, veterans frequently do not volunteer this history, and taking a military history is often overlooked in the medical encounter. Multiple workups with no clear remedy and a sense of intense urgency and frustration often lead the desperate veteran to the ED in search of immediate relief. Veterans often have "entrenched" distress marked by "failure, betrayal, alienation, and estrangement" [16]. Veterans often live in a state of hyperarousal, can be mistrustful of others' motives, and can be easily provoked. Given these factors, the doctor–patient relationship is fraught with potential conflict. Thus, the ED clinician steps into this situation with very high stakes: Relief must come quickly, or disappointment, further frustration, and agitation can erupt into demanding and even aggressive outbursts, seemingly without warning.

Veterans may withhold their military history because of a sense of isolation and shame. For example, the soldier above might be thoroughly ashamed that he ended up in the stench of the enemy's abdomen. It does not matter that it was not his fault; in his mind, he has disgraced himself and his unit. He hides what happened from everyone, including doctors. When he goes to the doctor, he is on the defensive against feeling humiliated. Doctors also have a sensitivity to humiliation [17], and issues of control can quickly become the main focus, especially when the veteran has a lot of anger and irritability, and the clinician is attempting to assert his own authority to deal with his own anxiety. Lack of trust, anger, irritability, sensitivity to humiliation, and decreased physical ability can all be reenacted in the medical encounter.

Military Culture

Learning about military culture can assist the clinician in understanding his or her own counter-transference and biases, as well as help give care in a way that preserves the veteran's dignity, honor, and respect. There are different cultural issues for each war. For example, the longest running wars have been Iraq and Afghanistan, while perhaps the most controversial war was Vietnam. World War II veterans were traditionally considered immune to PTSD [10].

There have been more female soldiers in the Iraq and Afghanistan wars than in any other theatre. Some wars consist of enlisted soldiers, while others have a predominance of draftees. Conscription and voluntary enlistment each have their own cultural meanings. In addition, the branch that one goes into may have great symbolism, often reflecting family values and traditions.

More recent wars required multiple deployments, with both enlisted service members and reservists called up for active duty. Reservists tend to be older, are often forced to suddenly uproot from family and work, and can experience both the stress of coming home while simultaneously anticipating future deployments at a moment's notice. Culturally, there may be internal conflicts between the desire to be with family and the sense of loyalty and allegiance to one's unit. In Vietnam, for instance, single entry and exit from theatre often contributed to isolation and estrangement. Each of these factors may have an impact on the soldier's adjustment to both military and civilian life. Veterans typically say that they come back from military "changed," and this may be true for both them and their families. Such an intense experience frequently changes people, but that change does not necessarily have to be devastating. Perhaps no family can stay static while their loved one is away, but each change in their own way at their own rate. When these changes are nonsynchronous, conflict may arise.

Compounding these changes, military boot camp purposely dismantles the individual's identity and replaces it with the identity of the unit. Personalization is stripped: Hair is cut and there is uniformity in dress, living arrangements, meals, and hygiene. One individual is often indistinguishable from the other. Yet, many soldiers, particularly those from troubled homes, find comfort and meaning in the military, which becomes a new and sometimes better family.

The military's central purpose is to train and deploy warriors. To that end, military service is composed of ingrained skills that may not be easily unlearned once the soldier comes home. Soldiers learn to behave "on automatic" in their reactions and to do so with precision and accuracy. There are no second chances in combat, and failing to be perfect puts oneself and others in jeopardy. Soldiers learn that the unit and the mission are what matters beyond all else. Responsibility, respect, fidelity, and commitment are all values instilled in the military. One's unit and one's men are more important than the self, and self-sacrifice to serve and protect is the highest value. Carefully honed skills of precision, intense observation, decisive actions requiring hypervigilance, and rapid response to even subtle changes in one's environment (which might indicate danger) become exaggerated and inappropriate in civilian life. One's fellow soldiers ("buddies") become brethren, with bonds even more profound than civilian loved ones. These intimate bonds are imprinted on the soldier's psyche for life.

Branches

Each branch of the military distinguishes their members differently: airman (Air Force), soldier (Army), sailor (Navy), guardian (National Guard), and marine. A marine, for instance, typically wishes to be referred to as marine even years after discharge. Infantry are "grunts," and noninfantry are "pouges." Pouges may feel (and may be made to feel) inferior to their brethren who are combatants. Rank and title indicate a hierarchy in the level of responsibility, experience, and skill, all of which may cause conflict during interactions with the medical profession, which has its own levels of experience and authority.

Differences exist between noncommissioned and commissioned officers. In Vietnam, noncommissioned officers were highly respected because they demonstrated their competence by coming up "through the ranks," while commissioned officers were considered "green" and often put their men at risk because of naiveté or inexperience. In Vietnam, the stakes became so high that sometimes these officers were "fragged" (literally blown into fragments by a detonating device such as a grenade) by their own men because they were considered gravely dangerous to the unit. In such extreme cases, authority figures may be disdained, and such interactions can spill over into the medical encounter, where the authority of the physician is resented.

Military Ethos

Yet, despite the horror of war, the sense of honor, autonomy, importance, mission, and fidelity are so strong that even some of the most traumatized of veterans would "go back in a heartbeat" to rejoin their units. Veterans are passionately patriotic and want to serve and protect. During the height of our recent wars, many Vietnam veterans yearned to sign up again; Iraq and Afghanistan veterans ached to return to duty. This is the reason that many veterans say that the military was "the best years of my life" and why veterans seek out missions to assist in natural disasters, become missionaries, go into the medical field, or become police officers and firefighters. Many veterans feel that civilian life pales in comparison to the stimulation and purpose of the military and this can lead to feelings of being insignificant and useless.

Intense grief over what one has lost by leaving the military can lead to an inability to make the mundane meaningful, and these factors can further lead to an edgy, irritable, and demoralized state with interpersonal, career, or social consequences.

In terms of healthcare, veterans have a difficult time caring for themselves because of their strong service ethic. They may pride themselves in self-sufficiency, not unlike many healthcare professionals. In this regard, there may be similarities between soldiers and healthcare professionals that can interfere with the doctor–patient relationship. These similarities will be discussed later in this chapter but may involve perceptions of both illness and emotional strength. Illness, for instance, may be perceived as a sign of "weakness," which signifies that their role as a protector has forever ended. Emotional strength on the other hand is often viewed as being inured to strong emotions with the ability to "take it."

Veterans and Guns

Veterans tend to value firearms, perceiving them as a part of who they are. Beliefs such as "firearm ownership is a right" and "guns make you safer" are common. As stated by a veteran, "[B]eing a good soldier means having confidence in yourself and in your weapon." When a health professional believes that a patient should not possess a firearm, this can lead to severe conflict in the doctor–patient relationship. An example of a difficult yet typical case is that of an elderly veteran with mild cognitive impairment whose wife reports on his recent suicidal thinking. Even if the patient has never made a suicide attempt and does not have a clear plan, his ownership of a gun is nonetheless worrisome. In such a situation, it is important for the clinician to understand what gun ownership means to the patient. While gaining this understanding, as well as communicating the fears of the family, the clinician can better negotiate a safety plan that involves restricting access to lethal means. Often, clinicians may be able to arrange for a trusted friend to safeguard the weapon, which allows the patient both to save face and have some control. Thus, when approaching the subject of guns with a veteran, clinicians should avoid asking, "Do you have guns at home?" This can put the patient on the defensive. Instead, clinicians should consider using the following phrasing: "Lots of veterans have firearms at home. What some people in your situation do is store their firearms away from home until they're feeling better. … If you have firearms at home, have you thought of any strategies like that?" [18].

Soldiers protect and serve others. If the veteran can understand that keeping his gun safe is also a way of protecting others, he is more likely to agree to give up the gun, at least temporarily.

Injury in Combat

Injury in combat can be perceived as having deserted one's buddies and having failed the mission. There may be guilt if others died. The injured person may not feel like a hero, and medal recipients often soften the sense of shame and loss by accepting their honors "for my buddies."

The clinician needs to be mindful to approach the veteran in a manner that preserves the veteran's dignity and honor. Veterans want to be remembered for "who they were" [19]. Consider, for example, a recent case of a demanding 65-year-old patient who was dressed in a T-shirt and hat labeled "Vietnam Veteran." This patient was particularly upset about an encounter with a physician and struggled to get up from his chair, finally standing as tall as he could on the walking sticks that he used as canes. Although once burly, the now physically weak patient waved one cane in the air and then threw it to the floor, exclaiming, "I'm a Vietnam veteran!" Such behavior is typical when veterans feel disrespected, often manifesting as defensive and paradoxically undignified attempts to assert their honor. Such behavior may be mitigated by the presence of healthcare team members with military experience. For example, consider another case of a female veteran who was both disruptive and unable to cooperate with the exam. However, she immediately took her position on the stretcher when a former career Army nurse commanded, "Soldier! Attention!"

Military Sexual Trauma

When the very people who are supposed to care cause harm, there are two traumas: the physical act and the permanent mark of betrayal. Such traumas may be experienced when a higher-ranking soldier abuses another soldier or when a commander tacitly condones this behavior among the ranks.

According to the Department of Defense (DOD), 4.3% of active-duty female and 0.9% of active-duty male members report having experienced some form of unwanted sexual contact [19]. However, there is likely under-reporting because of fears of retaliation. The vast majority of perpetrators are male, older, and generally higher ranking, while the majority of victims tend to be women.

Moral Injury

Moral injury occurs when the methods of engagement or service raise moral and ethical concerns [20]. Examples of moral injury come from Vietnam and Iraq where soldiers who were forced to fight a war that many considered to be morally wrong. Symptoms of moral injury can present similarly to PTSD, with intrusive thoughts, avoidance, and numbing, but unlike PTSD, additional symptoms such as guilt, shame, demoralization, self-sabotage (e.g., of relationships), and self-injurious behavior are also present.

Coming Home

Even though veterans are geographically back home, the veteran's body may still be "on automatic" and in theatre. Soldiers are typically not trained in how to reverse their now-ingrained warrior skills. They no longer have the familiar rituals and customs of "military strong," and no longer feel a sense of mission or purpose. Although they may still feel like a warrior, this identity has been suddenly and completely stripped from them. Many feel that they have lost their identity and have to find for themselves a new one. Civilians, even families, do not understand this, because they have not had the same experience of being a warrior. The resulting isolation is in sharp contrast with military life. As one veteran noted, "I wish they would just send me back [to combat]. I'm useless here—I'm useless as a father, I'm useless as a worker, as a man."

Many veterans talk about being "broken" and damaged—that "a piece of my soul is gone." Risk-taking activities such as driving recklessly, getting into fights, or sky-diving help discharge their physiologic hyperarousal. Danger is fascinating and seductive. Veterans need to integrate who they were with a new identity as a civilian. Medical providers may need to respond to these emotions and needs, as well as help reintegrate the veteran into civilian life.

The Veteran as Patient

As noted previously, there can be much shame in being injured, and this is challenging during a medical encounter. Chronically frustrated veterans may have high expectations and a low tolerance for further frustration, and an uncaring bureaucratic process may cause troubling encounters. According to a recent congressional report, 40% of veterans do not trust health care professionals and have only "marginal confidence" in their abilities. Veterans may believe that they "can tell" in the first meeting whether or not the doctor will help, and will not return if they do not feel that it is worth their time [16].

If a physician is rushed and has many acute patients, negative counter-transference can lead to empathic failures. Examples of empathic failures include misstatements during attempts *to be* empathic, such as "I understand what you went through," which can demean the unique individuality and experience of the person. Even subtle messages that it is more important to take care of oneself than it is to serve others can be infuriating. Other common examples of empathic failures include not reading records beforehand, long wait times, inflexibility with treatment plans, not being punctual or organized, acting like an "expert" without relating specifically and uniquely to the patient, appearing indifferent, conveying biases about combat or killing, or discomfort while hearing veterans' stories. Responses to such empathic failures may be aggression, hostility, mistrust, or what appears to be entitlement or otherwise inappropriate behavior.

Veterans and Suicide

Male veterans are twice as likely as their civilian peers to die by suicide and are 58% more likely to use a firearm to end their lives [21]. Female veterans also have a higher rate of suicide than the civilian population and die more frequently from firearms, most likely because they are trained to use them [22]. Risk factors for suicide in veterans include race (Caucasian); age (younger and older vets have a higher rate than middle-aged); being single, divorced, or widowed; having had an inpatient psychiatric hospitalization in the previous year; having a diagnosis of depression with comorbid substance use; living in the southern or western United States; and being without service-connected disabilities (the latter may indicate not only a financial burden but also a lack of recognition by the Veterans Affairs [VA] and society of the veteran's sacrifice) [22, 23].

It is estimated that 20 veterans die by suicide each day. Fourteen of those twenty are veterans who do not utilize the VA for their care [21]. These veterans may be using private hospitals and clinics, necessitating a thorough military history in the medical interview.

Conclusion: Approaching Veterans

The first way to approach those thought to be veterans is to determine if they are, in fact, veterans. If yes, find out where they served, when they served, and whether any injuries, illnesses, or other unusual events occurred, even if the veteran did not serve in combat (see Table 30.2). Respectfully, ask questions and explain that while you do not know about military life, you would like to learn. Self-reflection on one's feelings about war and killing is crucial. Asking questions about how others are adapting to the situation (e.g., "How has your family adjusted to your being home?") is a way for the veteran to focus the conversation on others who they want to protect and care for.

Table 30.2 Taking a military history

Basic questions:
Did you see combat, enemy fire, or casualties?
Were you or a buddy wounded, injured, or hospitalized?
Did you ever become ill while you were in the service?
Do/did you have any concerns about returning to civilian life since you've been back?
How has your family adjusted to your being home?

Adapted from the US Department of Veterans Affairs Pocket card. Available at https://www.va.gov/oaa/pocketcard/m-index.asp

A Message from the Author

The views and opinions expressed are those of the author and do not necessarily reflect the official policy or position of Veterans Health Administration.

This work is based on my 30+ years of experience working as a civilian in the Veterans Affairs (VA) health care system. In writing this chapter, I am aware that any attempt to overgeneralize the veteran population is fraught with bias and the potential to offend. Neither is my intent. Treating veterans is an honor. Veterans have an integrity, immediacy, and presence that I find particularly compelling. There is no pretense when interacting with veterans; they are and expect their clinicians to be "real." My only goal is to educate colleagues about veterans and share what I have learned that makes my work with veterans meaningful.

References

1. Schlenger WE, Corry NH, Williams CS, Kulka RA. A prospective study of mortality and trauma-related risk factors among a Nationally Representative Sample of Vietnam Veterans. Am J Epidemiol [Internet]. 2015;182(12):980–90.
2. Ebner C, Krull H, Brown K, Cefalu M. Current and Projected Characteristics and Unique Health Care Needs of the Patient Population Served by the Department of Veterans Affairs. Available from: https://www.rand.org/pubs/periodicals/health-quarterly/issues/v5/n4/13.html.
3. A Product of the CMS Alliance to Modernize Healthcare Federally Funded Research and Development Center Centers for Medicare & Medicaid Services (CMS) https://www.va.gov/opa/choiceact/documents/assessments/Assessment_A_Demographics.pdf: Rand Corporation; 2015 [Prepared for CAMH under: a. Prime Contract No. HHS-M500–2012-00008I; b. Prime Task Order No. VA118A14F0373]. Available from: https://www.va.gov/opa/choiceact/documents/assessments/Assessment_A_Demographics.pdf.
4. Lohr JB, Palmer BW, Eidt CA, Aailoboyina S, Mausbach BT, Wolkowitz O. M,, et al. is post-traumatic stress disorder associated with premature

senescence? A review of the literature. Am J Geriatr Psychiatry. 2015;23(7):709–25.
5. VA Homeless Veterans 2016 by the Numbers Fact Sheet. 2016. [cited 2016 October]. webpage]. Available from: https://www.va.gov/homeless/docs/HomelessGeneralFactSheet-1610.pdf.
6. Doukas WC, Hayda RA, Frisch HM, Andersen RC, Mazurek MT, Ficke JR, et al. The military extremity trauma amputation/limb salvage (METALS) study: outcomes of amputation versus limb salvage following major lower-extremity trauma. J Bone Joint Surg Am. 2013;95(2):138–45.
7. Marmar CR, Schlenger W, Henn-Haase C, Qian M. Course of posttraumatic stress disorder 40 years after the Vietnam war: findings from the National Vietnam Veterans Longitudinal Study. JAMA Psychiatry [Internet]. 2015;72(8):871–81.
8. Solomon Z, Mikulincer M. Combat stress reactions, posttraumatic stress disorder and somatic complaints among Israeli soldiers. J Consult Clin Psychol. 2007;75(2):316–24.
9. Solomon Z, Shklar R, Singer Y, Mikulincer M. Reactions to combat stress in Israeli veterans twenty years after the 1982 Lebanon war. J Nerv Ment Dis. 2006;194(12):935–9.
10. Richmond JS, Beck J. Posttraumatic stress disorder in a world war II veteran. Am J Psychiatry. 1986;143(11):1485–6.
11. Kardiner AT, Spiegel H. The traumatic neuroses of war. New York: Paul B. Hoeber, Inc.; 1941.
12. Grinker RR, Spiegel JP. Men Under Stress. Philadelphia: Blackiston; 1945.
13. American Psychiatric Association. Diagnostic and statistical manual of mental disorders. In: Association AP, editor. DSM-5. 5th ed. Washington DC: The American Psychiatric Association; 2013.
14. American Psychiatric Association. Diagnostic and statistical manual of mental disorders. 3rd ed: American Psychiatric Association; 1980.
15. Rivers W. The repression of war experience. 1918. Available from: http://net.lib.byu.edu/estu/wwi/comment/rivers.htm.
16. Brim W, Watson P. Health seeking in military and veteran populations. 2015. Available from: www.deploymentpsych.org/military-culture.
17. Lazare A. Shame and humiliation in the medical encounter. Arch Intern Med. 1987;147(9):1653–8.
18. Barber C. Means Matter. 2017. Available from: https://www.hsph.harvard.edu/means-matter/recommendations/clinicians/.
19. Wain H. The psychiatry consult service in a hospital at war APA annual meeting. San Francisco; 2013.
20. Litz BT, Stein N, Delaney E, Lebowitz L, Nash WP, Silva C, et al. Moral injury and moral repair in war veterans: a preliminary model and intervention strategy. Clin Psychol Rev. 2009;29(8):695–706.
21. Male Veterans Have Double the Suicide Rate of Civilians. Available from: https://www.nimh.nih.gov/news/science-news/2007/male-veterans-have-double-the-suicide-rate-of-civilians.shtml.
22. Kaplan MS, McFarland BH, Huguet N. Firearm suicide among veterans in the general population: findings from the national violent death reporting system. J Trauma [Internet]. 2009;67(3):503–7.
23. Zivin K, Zivin AH, Kim M, McCarthy JF. Suicide mortality among individuals receiving treatment for depression in the veterans affairs health system: associations with patient and treatment setting characteristics. Am J Public Health. 2007;97(12):2193–8.

31 Mental Health Issues in Children

Margaret A. Cashman and Jagoda Pasic

Introduction

Children and adolescents who come to the emergency department (ED) with a psychiatric crisis are a concern for all ED professionals. Their visits tend to absorb more prehospital and ED resources than other classes of a pediatric patient, as well as leading to higher rates of admission from the ED [1, 2]. Some studies suggest their numbers may be growing [3, 4].

Children and adolescents present to the ED with certain predictable crises involving mental health problems. One set of concerns arises from deliberate self-injury or the imminent threat of such injury. Another set of concerns arises from the acute emergency of psychosis. Children and adolescents may have become out of control, directing hostility and aggression at the people in their lives. Some youth may be brought in with "internalizing" conditions such as depression or anxiety, in which the youngster's distress is turned inward, rather than being expressed through acting out on the child's environment or family. Substance abuse creates a number of scenarios that may bring a teen or a child into the ED.

Some conditions are beyond the scope of this chapter. For example, eating disorders can cause a medical crisis leading to an adolescent or child being brought to the ED. (See related chapter on eating disorders.) Some children and teens come to the ED because they have been the victims of abuse or neglect. Most emergency departments have established protocols for identifying and managing these children. Additionally, some children and adolescents arrive at the ED with acute and serious physical injury or illness but are at high risk to develop a secondary acute stress disorder from their experience. These youngsters, too, may require emergency psychiatric assessment. Finally, children and adolescents with developmental disorders that impact their coping capacity to tolerate distress can arrive in crisis at the ED, not uncommonly accompanied by their distressed caregiver. For example, ED staff recognize that adolescents with autism spectrum disorder are coming to the ED in greater numbers with mental health crises [5] (Table 31.1).

Psychiatric evaluation of the child or adolescent patient requires particular emphasis on gathering information from multiple sources. Collection and integration of these collateral sources of information frequently lead to longer lengths of stay in the ED for pediatric behavioral

M. A. Cashman (✉) · J. Pasic
Department of Psychiatry and Behavioral Sciences, University of Washington School of Medicine, Seattle, WA, USA
e-mail: cashman@uw.edu

L. S. Zun et al. (eds.), *Behavioral Emergencies for Healthcare Providers*,
https://doi.org/10.1007/978-3-030-52520-0_31

Table 31.1 Common presentations of the child or adolescent in the psychiatric ED

Self-injury or threat of self-injury (suicidal or non-suicidal)
Psychosis
Out of control (the "wild child")
Internalizing disorders (depression, anxiety, OCD)
Substance abuse
Eating disorders
Catastrophic distress in the developmentally disordered child or teen (i.e., innate coping capacities overwhelmed)
Traumatization by abuse, accident, or medical/surgical interventions

health visits, compared with adult psychiatric ED visits.

The emergency department setting available to children and adolescents varies substantially from facility to facility. Children's hospitals may or may not have a specific section dedicated to mental health emergencies with environmental adaptations appropriate for this purpose. General hospital emergency departments similarly may or may not have a dedicated psychiatric emergency service section, let alone a dedicated pediatric psychiatric emergency service section. As much as possible, try to limit the young patient's exposure to the overwhelming sights, sounds, and odors of the busy adult ED, as these stimuli can become associated with a stressful and potentially traumatizing ED experience.

The sequence in which interviewing is conducted is arbitrary. Some experts suggest speaking prior to the child interview with parents or guardians in the case of the *prepubertal child*, while speaking initially to *adolescents* prior to talking with their parents, guardians, or accompanying staff. However, in some circumstances, you may choose to conduct an initial interview with both patient and adults present. Bear in mind the importance of interviewing the young patient individually at some point, in case sensitive information needs to be shared that the adults' presence might squelch.

Hospitals typically will have protocols in place determining the management of pediatric psychiatric patients in EDs. We are at a transition between reliance upon ED staff to recognize pediatric mental health problems using the current informal array of assessment approaches and implementation of screening instruments as a standard of care [4, 6–14]. States vary in their regulations pertaining to such issues as age of consent, privacy of clinical information from parents or guardians, and involuntary treatment practices. Fortunati and Zonana [15] have provided a helpful discussion of the legal concepts pertinent to address this population's needs in the ED. The availability of specialty care, such as inpatient child psychiatric units, also varies from one locality to another. Some counties provide a backup level of crisis-based resources that either can or must be utilized before considering psychiatric hospitalization. Telepsychiatry consultation is being explored to strengthen the capacity of more rural EDs to assess and manage children and adolescents with psychiatric problems, and this trend is likely to grow with acceptance of that model of care integration [16].

The Wild Child: Out-of-Control Children and Adolescents

The child or teen who is aggressive, hostile, and disruptive may be brought to the ED at any hour of the day or night. Establish how the current offending behavior fits into the young patient's typical behavior patterns. Collateral information is essential in such a case. The more convergence there is in information from different sources, the more confident you can be in the current assessment. Try to obtain an immediate history from the child or teen individually, and observe how reactive the young patient is to the people who brought the child or teen in. Most often, the wild teen will be a male [17].

The raging child may arrive in an uncooperative state of mind, but collateral information can be sought during this stage of the visit. Children's aggression can be characterized as proactive or reactive, with differing trajectories for subsequent behavior [18, 19]. The *proactively aggressive* child deliberately engages in aggression for identifiable external goals. Youngsters with conduct disorders typically utilize proactive aggression on a frequent basis [20].

In contrast, youngsters with *reactive aggression* have difficulties with emotional dysregulation, peer rejection, and peer victimization [21]. Reactively aggressive girls, in particular, are at heightened risk for suicidal behavior, especially if they also are depressed. Reactive aggression can erupt when a developmentally disabled youth, who already has increased vulnerability toward becoming overwhelmed, faces changing environmental demands. Children and adolescents with bipolar disorder display elevated levels of reactive aggression and verbal aggression [22]. Delaney [23] suggests reducing the youth's reactive aggression in the hospital by addressing the emotional dysregulation from which this aggression stems: (1) provide structure; (2) buffer unexpected changes to reduce frustration; (3) maintain a positive tone to interactions; (4) reduce perceived threat by establishing ground rules that elicit cooperation and encourage choice; and (5) set expectations appropriate to the youngster's information-processing capacities.

The ED tasks with such children include the following.

1. *Establish current safety for the youngster and those around the youngster.* If the child or teen is agitated or menacing in the ED setting, first utilize verbal and behavioral interventions to reassure the youngster. For example, establish basic expectations and reduce aversive or excessive environmental stimuli. Orient the youngster to the ED environment and make it clear that you will obtain the youngster's side of the story as part of the evaluation.
   a. If the young patient continues to be out of control, some degree of seclusion, physical restraint, or chemical restraint may be necessary. Numerous practice guidelines, as well as institutional guidelines, are available to guide (and restrict) the use of seclusion and restraint in children and adolescents [24–27].
   b. As with much of child psychiatric practice, medication use in such circumstances is largely off-label [28–30]. See Table 31.2 for a list of commonly employed medications for the child and adolescent emergency patient. Marzullo [29] has reviewed the use of pharmacotherapy for managing agitated children and adolescents.
2. *Establish the narrative of what led to the out-of-control behaviors that precipitated a trip to the ED, using multiple sources of information.* What has happened in the past when similar behaviors erupted? What made today's events different from past events that did not lead to an ED visit?
3. *Establish whether important comorbid conditions are present (and if they are, address accordingly):*
   a. Drug or alcohol intoxication
   b. Psychosis
   c. Mood disorder or anxiety disorder
   d. Established pattern of oppositional-defiant behavior or conduct disorder
   e. Significant level of intellectual disability and a recent overwhelming challenge the youngster cannot master
   f. Acute traumatization (e.g., sexual assault)
4. *Determine if there is a significant acute risk for this youngster to harm self or others.* This will influence the type of disposition plan that is appropriate (i.e., whether hospitalization is indicated).
5. *If available, consider enlisting a child crisis intervention response team at this point.* Such teams can provide options for emergency temporary placement or rapid intensive outreach to the home. When out-of-control children go home, the family will need assistance with how to manage future behavior problems.

Use of restraints (physical, pharmacologic, or both) with children and adolescents undergoing a psychiatric evaluation in the ED is associated with the symptoms of visual hallucinations, out-of-control behavior, and hyperactivity, and with the outcome of hospitalization [27].

Table 31.2 Medication options in child and adolescent psychiatric emergencies

Medication	Dose range	Target symptoms	Comments	Adverse effects
Aripiprazole (Abilify)	<25 kg, 1 mg/day 25–50 kg, 2 mg/day 51–70 kg, 5 mg/day >70 kg, 10 mg/day	Severe irritability; psychosis; mania		Sedation, akathisia, NMS. Lower risk of metabolic adverse effects than most atypical antipsychotics
Clonazepam (Klonopin)	<30 kg or age 10, 0.01–0.03 mg/kg/day, divided into 2–3 doses. Do not exceed 0.05 mg/kg/day	Panic and severe anxiety; extreme agitation	Can use as adjunct with antipsychotic	Sedation, confusion, ataxia, paradoxical agitation, respiratory depression
Diazepam (valium)	Oral: 1–2.5 mg, 3–4 times a day	Panic and severe anxiety; extreme agitation	An oral liquid is available	Sedation, confusion, ataxia, paradoxical agitation, respiratory depression
Haloperidol (Haldol)	Oral: Initial dose 0.5 mg/day, divided into 2–3 doses Target dose for psychosis: 0.05–0.15 mg/kg/day Target dose for nonpsychotic disorders: 0.05–0.075 mg/kg/day	Extreme agitation, psychosis, mania, irritability	Considered second-line to atypical antipsychotic medications	Extrapyramidal symptoms (dystonia, akathisia), hypotension, NMS, QTc prolongation
Hydroxyzine (Vistaril, Atarax)	Under age 6: 50 mg/day, divided into 4 doses. Age 6 and older: 50–100 mg/day, divided into 4 doses	Anxiety, pruritis		Sedation, anticholinergic symptoms
Lorazepam (Ativan)	0.05–0.1 mg/kg/day, divided into 3–4 doses PO, IM, and IV administration routes	Panic and severe anxiety; extreme agitation	Can use as adjunct with antipsychotic	Sedation, confusion, ataxia, paradoxical agitation, respiratory depression
Lurasidone	Do not use below age 13 years Initial dose: 20 mg/day bipolar depression; 40 mg/day bipolar mania or schizophrenia	Psychotic agitation; mania; bipolar depression	Atypical antipsychotic medication. In use for schizophrenia and bipolar disorder	Sedation, akathisia, NMS. Lower range among atypical antipsychotics for sedation, metabolic adverse effects. Must administer with food (at least 350 Cal.)

Olanzapine (Zyprexa)	5–20 mg/day, divided into 2 doses	Extreme agitation, psychosis, mania, irritability See Cole et al. [30] for review on use Approved for schizophrenia and manic/mixed episodes (ages 13 and older)	IM formulation not yet studied in children. The soluble tablet absorbs nearly as quickly as IM and is highly useful in ED. Must separate IM olanzapine dose from benzodiazepine dose by at least 90 minutes	Hypotension, bradycardia, NMS
Quetiapine (Seroquel)	Schizophrenia: Start at 50 mg/day, divided into 2 doses. May increase daily dose by 25–50 mg each day until at 400 mg/day Bipolar mania: Start at 100 mg/day, divided into 2 doses. May increase daily dose by 100 mg each day until at 400–800 mg/day	Extreme agitation, psychosis, mania, irritability Approved for schizophrenia (ages 13 and older) and manic/mixed episodes (ages 10 and older)	Oral. Lower dose range can be more sedating than mid-dose range	Sedation, NMS
Risperidone (Risperdal)	Oral: 0.5–4.0 mg/day, divided into 2 doses	Approved for schizophrenia (ages 13 and older), mania/mixed episodes (ages 10 and older), and irritability associated with autism (ages 5–16)	Most commonly used atypical antipsychotic in children and adolescents in the USA	Dystonia, akathisia, hyperprolactinemia, NMS
Ziprasidone (Geodon)	Oral: Initially, 80 mg/day, divided into 2 doses. On day 2, may increase to 120 mg/day, divided into 2 doses. Give oral doses with food IM: 5 mg IM; may repeat after 90 min	Not approved for patients under 18, but clinical data suggest it appears safe and effective in children and adolescents	For agitation target, IM takes effect within 30 minutes. Lower doses are often more activating than higher doses	Nausea, QTC prolongation, NMS. Lower risk of metabolic adverse effects than most atypical antipsychotics

Self-Injury and Suicidality

Interestingly, patients aged 9–17 years at pediatric EDs are least likely to be engaged in current mental health treatment if their current problem is a suicide attempt, compared with young patients who present with behavior problems. Children and teens who present with both existing behavior problems and a suicide attempt fall into an intermediate group in terms of their likelihood already to be engaged in care [31]. The squeaky wheel of the out-of-control child tends to demand attention more compellingly.

Always Ask

Self-injury in the young patient can arise out of a spectrum of intention, ranging from a pure accident with no intent to kill oneself at one extreme, to clear and planned intent to kill oneself at the other extreme. Ask the child or teen with self-injury whether the injury represents the result of an effort to harm or kill himself or herself. Inquire about the degree of suicidality without the parent or guardian is present at some point in the evaluation. Ask the young patient if he/she has made a suicide attempt in the past or has contemplated suicide. Positive responses should be explored further. To date, there is no evidence that asking a young person about suicide heightens the subsequent risk of a suicide attempt, "putting it into the mind" of the patient. The only way to discover which children or teens are at heightened present risk for suicide is to ask directly. One can start with a lead-in query such as "Sometimes, kids just don't want to be alive anymore. Do you feel that way sometimes?" Then move into greater specificity from there. Wintersteen and colleagues [32] suggest a two-question algorithm to identify adolescents with imminent risk for a suicide attempt: (1) "In the past week, including today, have you felt like life is not worth living?" and (2) "In the past week, including today, have you wanted to kill yourself?"

Follow-up screening questions for youngsters endorsing recent suicidal ideation include "Have you ever tried to kill yourself?" and "In the past week, including today, have you made plans to kill yourself?"

Much is made of risk factors for suicidality. For example, the presence of psychotic symptoms places the patient in a higher risk category. These evidence-based risk factors aid in knowing when to suspect heightened suicide risk. However, only a direct inquiry will tell you if the teen or child you are dealing with in the ED is *imminently* suicidal.

Establish the Behavioral Chain

As with the adult patient, one can learn much by inquiring into the concrete events, thoughts, and feelings that immediately preceded the injurious act ("And what was happening just before that?"). Take the events back in time stepwise and then forward from the self-injury's occurrence, until a clear picture emerges of (1) the context for the self-injury, (2) the degree of planning (and intent) involved, and (3) the young patient's expectations for what would happen next. Decide where to place the current suicidal act along the continuum from ambivalent rolling-of-the-dice to clearly lethal intent.

Focus on Means Restriction as Part of Making a Safety Plan, and Use This as an Opportunity to Educate the Family

Presence of firearms in the home clearly represents a risk for subsequent completion of a suicide attempt, and one *must* inquire about the presence of firearms in the homes that the patient will frequent after discharge from the ED [33, 34]. The guns used in four-fifths of adolescent suicides by firearm were found in the victims' homes, and most of these were owned by their parent [35]. If weapons are present, a plan for their safe removal should be explored. Decreasing access to firearms clearly decreases rates of suicide among adolescents [36, 37]. Similarly, review the degree to which family members' medications are secure and address this accordingly. Explore with the patient and adults how to make the suicide method's paraphernalia unavailable. *Means restriction* does not prevent a subsequent attempt, but it affords the patient an opportunity to revisit the question of suicidal intent (whether the suicide act really is what the patient wants to enact): Barriers provide thinking time.

The disposition plan for the suicidal child or teen should include mental healthcare referral. Often, this may mean psychiatric hospitalization. If an outpatient treatment disposition was made, the risk of subsequent suicidal behavior may be reduced by such measures as a follow-up call to verify that the youngster has connected with care [38].

Non-suicidal Self-Injury

It has become clear that, by adolescence, a number of young people engage in a non-suicidal self-injuring behavior. This usually represents a maladaptive effort to modulate internal emotional states, rather than being an interpersonal message aimed at coercing desired responses from the people around them. A typical non-suicidal, self-injuring behavior is superficial self-cutting, initiated to shift from one emotional state to another. There is a self-reinforcing aspect to such behavior that makes it habit-forming. Specific types of psychotherapy, including specialized cognitive-behavioral therapy (CBT) and dialectic behavioral therapy (DBT), appear to be effective in treating repetitive non-suicidal self-injury. A challenge for the ED clinician is to avoid indulging in undue frustration toward the young patient who comes in with the results of non-suicidal self-injury. It is helpful to address the injury and its commission with a matter-of-fact approach, steering the patient toward appropriate treatment.

Management of the non-suicidal self-injuring patient is complicated by the fact that this group of patients does overlap the group of young patients who harbor suicidal ideation and engage in suicidal action, as well; these are not mutually exclusive groups [39].

Substance Use

By adolescence, drug and alcohol use is common, although there has been a modest decline in drug use in adolescence in recent years [40, 41]. Recent trends (years 2013–2016) among youth in grades 8, 10, and 12 for substance use prevalence suggest a high prevalence for alcohol and marijuana use, and the appearance of e-cigarettes and "vaping" of tobacco, cannabis, and other substances. Diversion of prescription drugs, such as oral opioids, also is of concern [42]. Recurrent substance use often is a comorbid condition with other behaviors of concern, such as conduct problems and risky sexual behavior [43, 44]. As such, it can serve as a flag, indicating a young patient who may be more likely to have been exposed to traumatic experiences. The substance use may represent an incidental finding in the ED, or the substance use can directly cause a youth's presentation in the ED, due to symptoms of intoxication. The substance use also can be a secondary part of the clinical picture when, for example, an intoxicated teen has a motor vehicle accident and the resulting injuries lead to ED presentation.

Boys are more likely to engage in illicit substance use, with the exception of Ecstasy (MDMA), which girls more frequently use, particularly the younger adolescent age group [45]. It may be that girls are also more vulnerable to hallucinations while intoxicated with Ecstasy, compared with boys [46].

Some experts note that youths with substance use who have dropped out of school before graduation are particularly prone to risky sexual behavior, so that both the substance use and the risky sexual behavior should be addressed [47].

Some clinicians argue against the clinical utility of routinely using an emergency qualitative urine drug screen in pediatric ED patients who have a psychiatric presentation. The drug screen rarely appears to impact ED management of the patient [48, 49]. A drug screen may be useful in the initial presentation of a psychiatric disorder or for legal purposes such as documentation for commitment or in medical child abuse. Note that the vast majority of novel psychoactive substances, including novel opioids (e.g., many fentanyl analogues, U-47700), synthetic cannabinoids (e.g., "K2" and "Spice"), and hallucinogenic amphetamines (e.g., 2C compounds, 25i-NBOMe) are not detectable on the vast majority of urine drug screens, further limiting the utility of drug screens.

Refer to the chapter on substance abuse emergencies for a broader discussion of assessment and emergency treatment of the substance-abusing patient.

Psychosis

Schizophrenia and bipolar disorder, two common and severe psychiatric disorders arising in young adulthood, can occur with an earlier onset if there is strong familial genetic loading for the condition. Presence of psychotic features in a clinical picture of depression in adolescence appears to be a marker for more likely evolution into bipolar disorder over time, compared with depression without psychotic features [50].

The psychotic child or adolescent may or may not show paranoia. The degree of disorganization in thinking may be subtle, so that the child simply has not been able to process information as effectively in school and the child's grades have dropped. The degree of thought disorganization may also be so florid that the child cannot express ideas clearly in the ED. Inquire about the child's baseline level of function and note the degree of current deviation from that baseline. If the child suddenly stops in midsentence and appears blank, inquire about the child's thoughts: Is this an ictal event or an instance of thought "blocking" (where the mind was blank), or was the child's train of thought derailed by the intrusion of bizarre or irrelevant other thoughts?

Hallucinations in the prepubertal child may represent normative experiences (including the familiar "imaginary friend") [51]. Visual hallucinations are often present in youngsters with childhood-onset schizophrenia [52]. Just as with adult ED patients, hallucinations can arise from an array of toxidromes, as well as from primary psychiatric disorders. Edelsohn provides a practical discussion of evaluating hallucinations in children and adolescents [53].

Always explore the presence of suicidal and homicidal ideation in the psychotic child or teen.

Bipolar Disorder

A definitive diagnosis of pediatric bipolar disorder may occur after initial contact in the ED so as to allow for additional examination of the pattern of symptoms over months and across various settings. Most children and adolescents with rapidly shifting moods and high energy turn out to have conditions other than bipolar disorder [54]. Complicating diagnosis further, attention-deficit/hyperactivity disorder (ADHD) can be a comorbid condition with bipolar disorder, and it can be challenging to distinguish symptoms generated by the one from the other. Doerfler and colleagues note that manic children and adolescents without ADHD are more verbally aggressive and argumentative, and more prone to reactive aggression (angry responses when frustrated), compared with ADHD children and adolescents without bipolar disorder [55].

Children and teens with bipolar disorder appear to be more responsive to atypical antipsychotic medications than to lithium and other mood-stabilizing agents, compared with bipolar adults [56, 57]. The choice and titration of a mood stabilizer may be deferred until the patient is in an appropriate inpatient psychiatric treatment setting. Therefore, ED management of the acutely psychotic or bipolar manic child or teen should consist of the following tasks:

- Assure the immediate safety of the patient
- Reduce environmental stimulation
- Evaluate for other conditions (substance abuse mimicking psychosis; metabolic abnormalities)
- Initiate an atypical antipsychotic, which can be augmented by a benzodiazepine (see Table 31.2) and
- Establish a disposition plan (either hospitalization or discharge home with timely and intensive outpatient support)

Internalizing Disorders in the ED

Anxiety Disorders

Anxiety-related visits to the ED by children younger than fifteen years have increased in recent years [58]. Youngsters with early-onset anxiety and mood disorders suffer a significant disability, as well as psychological distress [59]. The child with severe separation anxiety may manifest impressive rages when forced to experience the separation (e.g., leaving home for school), which the child is dreading and wishing to avoid. Such children should be directed rapidly into outpatient treatment, which includes intensive behavioral or cognitive-behavioral treatment. Similarly, the child or adolescent who is paralyzed functionally by severe obsessive-compulsive disorder should receive appropriately intensive and specific cognitive-behavioral treatment as soon as possible. In both conditions, antidepressants (rather than anxiolytic medications) play an adjunctive role in treatment, but medications alone do not treat the conditions adequately.

Simple phobias are fairly common during childhood, yet rarely do these precipitate emergency room visits. Panic attacks can begin during childhood, and youngsters suffering from these may arrive in the ED. Just as with adults, one often can provide some immediate relief with behavioral interventions in the ED visit. This can provide an empowering sense that there are tools the child (and supportive caregivers, as coaches) can utilize. The youngster with panic disorder should be referred to outpatient treatment, which includes a cognitive-behavioral intervention. The role of medication in the ED should be secondary, but in severe cases, a modest oral lorazepam dose (e.g., 0.5 mg with a repeat if needed, once, after a few minutes, or 1 mg straight off) can be of help so that the young patient can focus on the behavioral intervention.

Depression

Children with depression may go substantially longer than adult-onset depressed people between the onset of major depressive disorder and entry into treatment [59]. Compared with the adult-onset form of major depression, children have longer episodes, higher rates of comorbid psychiatric disorders, and increased suicidality [60]. Case finding for these young depressed patients must be a priority in the ED, so that appropriate referral into treatment can commence and the protracted morbidity associated with this condition can be reduced. Rutman and colleagues [61] suggest using a two-question screening for depression in the busy ED to identify youth who merit further evaluation and referral for care, for positive responses to one or both of the following questions: (1) (pervasive mood) "During the past month, have you often been bothered by feeling down, depressed, or hopeless?" and (2) (anhedonia, amotivation) "During the past month, have you often been bothered by little interest or pleasure in doing things?"

It rarely is appropriate to initiate antidepressant medication treatment in the ED. Most children and adolescents with depression should receive a trial of appropriately specific and intensive psychotherapy for depression (cognitive-behavioral or interpersonal therapy for depression) if they have no prior history of treatment. Children and adolescents who do go on antidepressant treatment must be monitored frequently (e.g., weekly) in the first month of treatment in order to monitor for signs of untoward activation or suicidality. Therefore, decisions regarding medication choice usually are deferred to the outpatient prescriber who will monitor the patient.

As mentioned above, the presence of psychotic symptoms in a depressed child or adolescent is suggestive, though not diagnostic, of the possibility that the depression is part of an emerging bipolar disorder. Presence of bipolar disorder in family members also raises concern for this evolution over time. Particular care should be taken in exposing such patients to antidepressants without first prescribing an atypical antipsychotic or a mood stabilizer.

Trauma

Post-traumatic stress may emerge in children and teens who are exposed to overwhelming experiences: accidental trauma; physical or sexual abuse; repeated or prolonged medical or surgical hospitalizations with difficult procedures to endure; and/or trafficking. At ED presentation, the young person who just experienced such trauma will not have developed post-traumatic stress disorder (PTSD) but may be manifesting acute stress. The National Child Traumatic Stress Network (http://www.nctsn.org/) and the National Center for PTSD have developed a useful resource that is available online: Psychological First Aid: Field Operations Guide (Second Edition) (http://www.ptsd.va.gov/professional/manuals/psych-first-aid.asp). Although the guide is directed toward helping people in the immediate aftermath of disaster or terrorism, many of its principles apply to more individually experienced traumas as well. The chief intervention for post-traumatic stress disorder is a specialized form of cognitive-behavioral therapy for trauma. Typically, there will be a family component, as well as a child-specific component to the treatment.

EDs often must provide the initial screening and evaluation of young people whose trauma will require forensic investigation. The US Department of Justice's Office for Victims of Crime website provides helpful resources (http://www.ojp.usdoj.gov/ovc/publications/infores/sane/saneguide.pdf) for the sexual assault nurse examiner (SANE) and the sexual assault response team (SART) models, which have become prominent over the past 40 years. The ChildAbuseMD.com website (http://childabusemd.com/index.shtml) provides an efficient resource for reviewing the evaluation and management of child and adolescent abuse. One must remember that, along with providing an assessment in the ED, reporting the suspected abuse to the state child abuse hotline or to the police is mandatory.

Conclusion

Youngsters in the ED with psychiatric difficulties can be managed safely, with attention to reducing ED environmental demands which challenge their capacity for emotional regulation. The assessing clinician *must* obtain collateral information beyond what is available from the young patient directly—a suggestion which could benefit the evaluation of patients of any age. A systematic approach to conceptualizing the youth's presenting problems, considering the eight categories listed in Table 31.1, enables the ED clinician to focus more efficiently on the essential concerns demanding attention during the current ED visit.

References

1. Majahan P, Alpern ER, Grupp-Phelan J, Chamberlain J, Dong L, Holubkov R, Jacobs E, Stanley R, Tunik M, Sonnett M, Miller S. Foltin GL, and pediatric emergency care applied research network (PECARN). Epidemiology of psychiatric-related visits to emergency departments in a multicenter collaborative research pediatric network. Pediatr Emerg Care. 2009;25(11):715–20.
2. Santiago LI, Tunik MG, Foltin GL, Mojica MA. Children requiring psychiatric consultation in the pediatric emergency department: epidemiology, resource utilization, and complications. Pediatr Emerg Care. 2006;22(2):85–9.
3. Holder SM, Rogers K, Peterson E, Ochonma C. Mental health visits: examining socio-demographic and diagnosis trends in the emergency department by the pediatric population. Child Psychiatry Hum Dev. 2017;48(6):993–1000.
4. Dolan MA, Fein JA. Pediatric and adolescent mental health emergencies in the emergency medical services system. Pediatrics. 2011;127(5):1356–66.
5. Liu G, Pearl AM, Kong L, Leslie DL, Murray MJ. A profile on emergency department utilization in adolescents and young adults with autism spectrum disorders. J Autism Dev Disord. 2017;47(2):347–58.
6. Newton AS, Soleimani A, Kirkland SW, Goikiert RJ. A systematic review of instruments to identify mental health and substance use problems among

children in the emergency department. Acad Emerg Med. 2017;24(5):552–68.
7. Newton AS, Hartling L, Soleimani A, Kirkland S, Dyson MP, Cappelli M. A systematic review of management strategies for children's mental health care in the emergency department: update on evidence and recommendations for clinical practice and research. Emerg Med J. 2017;34(6):376–84.
8. Nager AL, Pham PK, Grajower DN, Gold JL. Mental health screening among adolescents and young adults in the emergency department. Pediatr Emerg Care. 2017;33:5–9.
9. Cappelli M, Gray C, Zemek R, Cloutier P, Kennedy A, Glennie E, Doucet G, Lyons JS. The HEADS-ED: a rapid mental health screening tool for pediatric patients in the emergency department. Pediatrics. 2012;130(2):321–7.
10. Cappelli M, Zemek R, Polihronis C, Thibedeau NR, Kennedy A, Gray C, Jabbour M, Reid S, Cloutier P. The HEADS-ED: evaluating the clinical use of a brief, action-oriented, pediatric mental health screening tool. Pediatr Emerg Care. 2017. Epub ahead of print.
11. Horowitz LM, Bridge JA, Teach SJ, Ballard E, Klima J, Rosenstein DJ, Wharff EA, Ginnis K, Cannon E, Joshi P, Pao M. Ask suicide-screening questions (ASQ): a brief instrument for the pediatric emergency department. Arch Pediatr Adolesc Med. 2012;166(12):1170–6.
12. Ballard ED, Cwik M, Van Eck K, Goldstein M, Alfes C, Wilson ME, Virden JM, Horowitz LM, Wilcox HC. Identification of at-risk youth by suicide screening in a pediatric emergency department. Pediatr Emerg Care. 2015;31(8):555–9.
13. Downey VA, Zun LS. Identifying undiagnosed pediatric mental illness in the emergency department. Pediatr Emerg Care. 2017. Epub ahead of print.
14. Spirito A, Bromberg JR, Casper TC, Chun TH, Mello MJ, Dean JM, Linakis JG. Pediatric emergency care applied research network. Reliability and validity of a two-question alcohol screen in the pediatric emergency department. Pediatrics. 2016;138(6). Epub ahead of print.
15. Fortunati FG Jr, Zonana HV. Legal considerations in the child psychiatric emergency department. Child Adolesc Psychiatr Clin N Am. 2003;12(4): 745–61.
16. Roberts N, Hu T, Axas N, Repetti L. Child and adolescent emergency and urgent mental health delivery through telepsychiatry: 12-month prospective study. Telemed J E Health. 2017;23(10):842–6.
17. Kennedy A, Cloutier P, Glennie JE, Gray C. Establishing best practice in pediatric emergency mental health: a prospective study examining clinical characteristics. Pediatr Emerg Care. 2009;25(6):380–6.
18. Greening L, Stoppelbein L, Luebbe A, Fite PJ. Aggression and the risk for suicidal behaviors among children. Suicide Life Threat Behav. 2010;40(4):337–45.
19. Fite P, Stoppelbein L, Greening L. Proactive and reactive aggression in a child psychiatric inpatient population. J Clin Child Adolesc Psy. 2009;38:199–205.
20. Card NA, Little TD. Proactive and reactive aggression in childhood and adolescence: a meta-analysis of differential relations with psychosocial adjustment. Internat J Behav Dev. 2006;30:466–80.
21. Dodge KA, Coie JD. Social information-processing factors in reactive and proactive aggression in children's peer groups. J Personality and Social Ps. 1987;53:1146–58.
22. Doerfler LA, Connor DF, Toscano PF Jr. Aggression, ADHD symptoms, and dysphoria in children and adolescents diagnosed with bipolar disorder and ADHD. J Affective Disorders. 2011;131:312–9.
23. Delaney KR. Reducing reactive aggression by lowering coping demands and boosting regulation: five key staff behaviors. J Child Adolesc Psychiatric Nursing. 2009;22(4):211–9.
24. Hilt RJ, Woodward TA. Agitation treatment for pediatric emergency patients. J Am Acad Child Adolesc Psy. 2008;47(2):132–8. Erratum in J Am Acad Child Adolesc Psy. 2008;47(4):478.
25. Hamm MP, Osmond M, Curran J, Scott S, Ali S, Hartling L, Gokiert R, Cappelli M, Hnatko G, Newton AS. A systematic review of crisis interventions used in the emergency department: recommendations for pediatric care and research. Pediatric Emerg Care. 2010;26(12):952–62.
26. Master KJ, Bellonci C, Bernet W. Practice parameter for the prevention and management of aggressive behavior in child and adolescent psychiatric institutions, with special reference to seclusion and restraint. J Amer Acad Child Adolesc Psy. 2002;41(Suppl. 2):4S–25S.
27. Dorfman DH, Mehta SD. Restraint use for psychiatric patients in the pediatric emergency department. Pediatr Emerg Care. 2006;22(1):7–12.
28. Adimondo AJ, Poncin YB, Baum CR. Pharmacological management of the agitated pediatric patient. Pediatric Emerg Care. 2010;26(11):856–60.
29. Marzullo L. Pharmacologic management of the agitated child. Pediatr Emerg Care. 2014;30:269–78.
30. Cole JB, Klein LR, Strobel AM, Blanchard SR, Nahum R, Martel ML. The use, safety, and efficacy of olanzapine in a level 1 pediatric trauma center emergency department over a 10-year period. Pediatr Emerg Care. 2017. Epub ahead of print.
31. Frosch E, McCulloch J, Yoon Y, DosReis S. Pediatric emergency consultations: prior mental health service use in suicide attempters. J Behav Health Serv Res. 2011;38(1):68–79.
32. Wintersteen MB, Diamond GS, Fein JA. Screening for suicide risk in the pediatric emergency and acute care setting. Curr Opin Pediatr. 2007;19(4): 398–404.
33. Brent DA. Firearms and suicide. Ann of the New York Academy of Sciences. 2001;932:225–40.
34. Brent DA, Perper JA, Goldstein CE, Kolko DJ, Allan MJ, Allman CJ, et al. Risk factors for ado-

lescent suicide: a comparison of adolescent suicide victims with suicidal inpatients. Arch Gen Psy. 1988;45:581–8.
35. Johnson RM, Barber C, Azrael D, Clark DE, Hemenway D. Who are the owners of firearms used in adolescent suicides? Suicide Life Threat Behav. 2010;40(6):609–11.
36. Lubin G, Werberloff N, Halperin D, Shmushkevitch M, Weiser M, Knobler HY. Decrease in suicide rates after a change of policy reducing access to firearms in adolescents: a naturalistic epidemiological study. Suicide Life Threat Behav. 2010;40(5):421–4.
37. Grossman DC, Mueller BA, Riedy C, Dowd MD, Villaveces A, Prodzinski J, et al. Gun storage practices and risk of youth suicide and unintentional firearm injuries. JAMA. 2005;293:707–14.
38. Newton AS, Hamm MP, Bethell J, Rhodes AE, Bryan CJ, Tjosvold L, Ali S, Logue E, Manion IG. Pediatric suicide-related presentations: a systematic review of mental health care in the emergency department. Ann Emerg Med. 2010;56(6):649–59.
39. Cloutier P, Martin J, Kennedy A, Nixon MK, Muehlenkamp JJ. Characteristics and co-occurrence of adolescent non-suicidal self-injury and suicidal behaviours in pediatric emergency crisis services. J Youth Adolesc. 2010;39(3):259–69.
40. US Department of Health and Human Services, Centers for Disease Control and Prevention, and National Center for Health Statistics. Health, United States, 2016. DHHS Publication No. 2017-1232. 2017. Trend Tables.
41. McDonald MG, Hsiao RC, Russo J, Pasic J, Ries RK. Clinical prevalence and correlates of substance use in adolescent psychiatric emergency patients. Pediatr Emerg Care. 2011;27(5):384–9.
42. Johnston LD, O'Malley PM, Miech RA, Bachman JG, Schulenberg JE. Monitoring the future: National Survey Results on drug use: 1975–2014: overview, key findings on adolescent drug use. Ann Arbor, MI: Institute for Social Research, University of Michigan; 2015.
43. Wu J, Witkiewitz K, McMahon RJ, Dodge KA. A parallel process growth mixture model of conduct problems and substance use with risky sexual behavior. Drug Alcohol Depend. 2010;111:207–14.
44. Armstrong TD, Costello EJ. Community studies on adolescent substance use, abuse, or dependence and psychiatric comorbidity. J Cons Clin Psy. 2002;70:1224–39.
45. Wu P, Liu X, Pham TH, Jin J, Fan B, Jin Z. Ecstasy use among US adolescents from 1999 to 2008. Drug Alcohol Depend. 2010;112:33–8.
46. Wu LT, Ringwalt CL, Weiss RD, Blazer DG. Hallucinogen-related disorders in a national sample of adolescents: the influence of ecstasy/MDMA use. Drug Alcohol Depend. 2009;104:156–65.
47. Latkin C, Sonenstein F, Tandon SD. Psychiatric disorder symptoms, substance use, and sexual risk behavior among African-American out of school youth. Drug Alcohol Depend. 2011;115:67–73.
48. Tenenbein M. Do you really need that emergency drug screen? Clin Toxicol (Phila). 2009;47(4):286–91.
49. Fortu JM, Kim IK, Cooper A, Condra C, Lorenz DJ, Pierce MC. Psychiatric patients in the pediatric emergency department undergoing routine urine toxicology screens for medical clearance: results and use. Pediatr Emerg Care. 2009;25(6):387–92.
50. Ratheesh A, Davey C, Hetrick S, Alvarez-Jimenez M, Voutier C, Bechdolf A, McGorry PD, Scott J, Berk M, Cotton SM. A systematic review and meta-analysis of prospective transition from major depression to bipolar disorder. Acta Psychiatr Scand. 2017;135(4):273–84.
51. Askenazy FL, Lestideau K, Meynadier A, Dor E, Myquel M, Lecrubier Y. Auditory hallucinations in pre-pubertal children: a one-year follow-up, preliminary findings. Eur Child Adolesc Psy. 2007;16(6):411–5.
52. David CN, Greenstein D, Clasen L, Gochman P, Miller R, Tossell JW, Mattai AA, Gogtay N, Rapoport JL. Childhood onset schizophrenia: high rate of visual hallucinations. J Am Acad Child Adolesc Psy. 2011;50(7):681–6.
53. Edelsohn GA. Hallucinations in children and adolescents: considerations in the emergency setting. Am J Psy. 2006;163(5):781–5.
54. Findling RL, Youngstrom EA, Fristad MA, Birmaher B, Kowatch RA, Arnold E, Frazier TW, Axelson D, Ryan N, Demeter CA, Gill MK, Fields B, Depew J, Kennedy SM, Marsh L, Rowles BM, Horwitz SM. Characteristics of children with elevated symptoms of mania: the longitudinal assessment of manic symptoms (LAMS) study. J Clin Psy. 2010. Epub 2010 Oct. 5.
55. Doerfler LA, Connor DF, Toscano PF Jr. Aggression, ADHD symptoms, and dysphoria in children and adolescents diagnosed with bipolar disorder and ADHD. J Affect Disord. 2011;131(1–3):312–9.
56. Stepanova E, Findling RL. Psychopharmacology of bipolar disorders in children and adolescents. Pediatr Clin N Am. 2017;64(6):1209–22.
57. Scheffer RE, Tripathi A, Kirkpatrick FG, Schultz T. Guidelines for treatment-resistant mania in children with bipolar disorder. J Psychiatr Pract. 2011;17(3):186–93.
58. Smith RP, Larkin GL, Southwick SM. Trends in U.S. emergency department visits for anxiety-related mental health conditions, 1992–2001. J Clin Psy. 2008;69(2):286–94.
59. Naismith SL, Scott EM, Purcell S, Hickie IB. Disability is already pronounced in young people with early stages of affective disorders: data from an early intervention service. J Affective Disorders. 2011;131:84–91.
60. Korczak DJ, Goldstein BI. Childhood onset major depressive disorder: course of illness and psychiatric comorbidity in a community sample. J Pediatr. 2009;155(1):118–23.
61. Rutman MS, Shenassa E, Becker BM. Brief screening for adolescent depressive symptoms in the emergency department. Acad Emerg Med. 2008;15(1):17–22.

Mental Health Issues in Geriatrics

32

Michael Ward, Brian Strickland, and James Ahn

Introduction

The recent induction of the baby boomer generation into the geriatric population will greatly expand the number of geriatrics with psychiatric conditions. Psychiatric workers are ill prepared to manage this demand for mental health services, with only 0.9 geriatric psychiatrists per 10,000 Americans over the age of 75 [1]. Primary care providers, advanced practice providers, and others will need to bridge the gap in mental health resources for our increasingly senescent population.

While geriatric patients represent a small portion of emergency psychiatric patients, they are more likely to require admission [2]. Mental status in the elderly is affected by many factors, (organic illness, polypharmacy, cognitive disorders, substance abuse, and elder abuse), which makes distinguishing between these etiologies difficult. Also, providers may interpret them as normal responses to natural stressors of aging, instead of recognizing them as abnormal and initiating an intervention.

Elderly psychiatric emergencies carry significant morbidity and mortality, and are rarely isolated to a specific psychiatric condition. They are often influenced by an interplay of psychiatric, medical, and social factors, which complicates their care. This chapter will cover key emergent geriatric psychiatric conditions, including depression, suicide, psychosis, agitation, and substance abuse.

Depression

Case Example 1

An 80-year-old female is brought in by her daughter because she has not been herself lately. She recovered from a viral illness 4 weeks ago but continues to have decreased energy and misses her weekly card games with friends.

Geriatric depression is associated with disability, hastened functional decline, increased risk of hospitalization, diminished quality of life, and risk of suicide [3–7]. Elderly patients also present to emergency departments (EDs) more frequently and have longer lengths of hospitalization [8, 9]. Providers must be prepared for geriatric depression, as greater than one in three geriatric patients will screen positive for this

M. Ward (✉)
Department of Emergency Medicine, University of Wisconsin School of Medicine and Public Health, Madison, WI, USA
e-mail: maward@medicine.wisc.edu

B. Strickland
Department of Emergency Medicine, Massachusetts General Hospital, Boston, MA, USA

J. Ahn
Department of Emergency Medicine, University of Chicago, Chicago, IL, USA

L. S. Zun et al. (eds.), *Behavioral Emergencies for Healthcare Providers*,
https://doi.org/10.1007/978-3-030-52520-0_32

disease [10]. Disability, poor social support, new medical illness, poor health status, sleep disturbances, prior depression, bereavement, and cognitive impairment are all risk factors for geriatric depression and may aid in its recognition and treatment [11].

Psychiatric and medical illnesses often share clinical features, including fatigue, insomnia, appetite changes, and alterations in mental status. Depressed geriatric patients more frequently experience somatic and cognitive symptoms than affective ones, described as "depression without sadness," which makes the diagnosis more difficult [6]. Therefore, the majority of geriatric depression diagnoses are missed, as are physician referrals or interventions specific to depression [6, 12, 13].

The Diagnostic Manual of Mental Disorders-V-TR (DSM-V) provides criteria to make a clinical diagnosis of major depression, irrespective of age [14]. A quick tool, the emergency department depression screening instrument (ED-DSI), may screen elderly patients for depression in an emergent setting (Table 32.1) [15]. However, the provider must realize that this tool has 79% sensitivity and excludes patients who have altered mental status or dementia. Other tools, such as the Patient Health Questionnaire (PHQ-9), the Geriatric Depression Scale (GDS), and the Center for Epidemiological Studies Depression–Revised (CESD-R), are more sensitive and specific to the elderly population but may take up to 15 minutes to perform [17–20].

Signs and symptoms of depression in the elderly may not fall under the formal diagnosis of major depressive disorder (MDD); thus, minor depression, medical illness, and cognitive disorders must be considered (Table 32.2). Minor depression occurs in patients with significant depressive symptoms without fulfilling all criteria for MDD. While not described in the DSM-V, this is the most common form of depressive disorder in the elderly [14, 21]. Minor depression affects patients similarly to MDD, and 25% of cases will progress to MDD within 2 years.

Table 32.1 Emergency department depression screening instrument (ED-DSI) [15]

1. Do you often feel sad or depressed?	Yes	No
2. Do you often feel helpless?	Yes	No
3. Do you often feel downhearted or blue?	Yes	No

A "Yes" response to any of the three questions is considered a positive screen.* Table 32.2 should be referenced for all negative screens
aThis scale should be limited to elderly patients without acute medical illness, dementia, or acute changes in mental status

There are several medical disorders and medications with causal and reversible links to depression. However, many providers misattribute signs and symptoms of depression to medical etiologies and miss the diagnosis of depression. Best practices suggest an inclusive approach to these situations: assuming that all depressive symptoms contribute to the depression syndrome, regardless of the underlying medical illness [12]. As depression can be frequently missed, this approach to assess for depression can improve the detection rate of depression in the elderly [12].

Depression is common in individuals with cognitive disorders like Alzheimer's disease (AD) and presents more typically with motivational symptoms and delusions, and less commonly with core symptoms of depression such as sadness, sleep disturbances, and appetite loss. The Provisional Diagnostic Criteria for Depression in Alzheimer's Disease (PDC-dAD) is similar to the DSM-V criteria for major depression but provides a less restrictive set of criteria while being more sensitive and specific for detection of depression with AD. This substitutes affective symptoms for verbally expressive symptoms, decreased positive affect for loss of pleasure, and tearfulness for depressed mood. Social isolation and irritability are included as novel criteria [16].

As noted above, the diagnosis of depression in the geriatric patient may present significant challenges. A reasonable approach is to apply the ED-DSI for relatively healthy, non-demented geriatric patients and strongly consider other factors related to depression, as summarized in Table 32.2 Further, the provider should maintain a high index of suspicion and an inclusive approach to not misattribute symptoms to medical illness in all types of geriatric patients.

Table 32.2 Special considerations in assessing geriatric patients for depression: minor depression, medical illness, dementia

	Comparison to major depression[a]	Special considerations
Minor depression	Increased somatic complaints: Fatigue, sleep issues, vague pain, psychomotor retardation, weight loss Irritability, social withdrawal, apathy, and diminished self-care are increased	Often without affective symptoms Many progress to major depression and should be treated similarly
Medical illness	Similar to minor depression: Increased somatic complaints, etc. Symptoms common to medical illness are very similar to that of depression Medical illness worsens depression, and depression worsens illness	Medical symptoms overlapping with depressive symptoms should be considered at least partially secondary to depression Vitamin deficiency, thyroid dysfunction, corticosteroid use are known to be associated with depression
Dementia	PDC-dAD more sensitive and specific for depression in demented patients; accounts for decreased communication ability and includes social isolation and irritability [16] Motivational symptoms and delusions more prevalent than core symptoms	Flat affect, tearfulness, social isolation, and delusions are hallmark signs of depression in the demented patient Up to 50% of patients with cognitive disorders will develop depression Caretakers of demented patients have an increased risk of depression

[a]Differences are compared to DSM-V criteria for major depression [14]
PDC-dAD Provisional Diagnostic Criteria for Depression in Alzheimer's Disease, *DSM-V* Diagnostic Manual of Mental Disorders-V-TR

Table 32.3 Indications for inpatient admission for depression in elderly patients [22][a]

1. Attempted suicide or expressed suicidal ideations with intent
2. Compliance issues, leading to insufficient management and decompensation of depression
3. Depression with new-onset psychotic features
4. Self-neglect to the degree that patient is inadequately cared for
5. Need for removal from hostile environment
6. Medical illness that would complicate the outpatient treatment of depression
7. Distress or agitation that requires skilled nursing

[a]This table was developed based on recommendations listed by MacDonald with several modifications

Proper disposition is paramount for the depressed elderly patient and may be the most important intervention offered. Most providers will not have the required specialized training to provide definitive treatment and will have to determine whether the patient is appropriate for inpatient or outpatient management. A set of developed criteria is generally accepted for admission of the depressed elderly (Table 32.3). All other patients should be referred to their primary doctor, psychiatric professionals, or partial hospitalization programs.

Case Example 1, Continued

The patient's medical evaluation does not show any abnormalities, and the ED-DSI screen is positive, answering "Yes" to two out of three questions. She denies suicidal ideation. She is started on a selective serotonin reuptake inhibitor (SSRI) and referred to a geriatric psychiatrist for follow-up. Her daughter is given instructions to closely monitor her behavior.

Suicide

Case Example 2

An 87-year-old male presents to the emergency department with a gunshot wound to the left shoulder. He states he was trying to clean his rifle when it accidentally discharged. When his family arrives, they report that he has talked about joining his deceased wife and was started on escitalopram for depression two weeks ago.

Compared to other age groups, elderly patients are at the greatest risk for suicide, with white males over 85 being the highest risk [5]. Elderly patients' attempts are also more likely to succeed, with a 4:1 attempts-to-suicide ratio versus 8–40:1 in the general population. This increased lethality is thought to be due to frailty of patients, increased chance of living alone, and more lethal means of attempting suicide. Geriatric patients are also more reluctant to talk about emotional problems and, therefore, less likely to report suicidal ideation [23, 24].

Suicide risk factors are common among the elderly; advanced age is a strong predictor of suicide and increases risk beyond these individual risk factors alone [24]. Between 71 and 95% of elderly suicide victims have a diagnosable Axis 1 condition, MDD being the most common, with psychotic or medical illness playing a smaller role. HIV/AIDS, multiple sclerosis, renal disease, spinal cord injury, and malignant neoplasms have been shown to increase suicide risk. Pain, fear of illness progression, and familial dependence are the main contributors, and a single episode of depression can precede suicide in these patients. Substance abuse, when coupled with depression, also increases risk [24]. Elderly patients' life stressors, such as bereavement, retirement, family discord, and financial strain, increase risk for suicide as well. These individuals are more apt to visit a physician prior to death, emphasizing a high priority for recognition and an opportunity for intervention [25].

Because of significant financial barriers, older patients tend to rely on primary care during times of great psychiatric need [26]. Retrospective studies indicate that 43–70% of elderly suicide victims visit primary physicians 1 month prior to their deaths, so prevention may be possible in the time preceding the development of the suicidal state [23]. While elderly patients often present with atypical psychiatric symptoms, they will often admit to suicidal ideation when the topic is broached by physicians [27]. Providers should have a low threshold to assess for suicidal thoughts, intentional self-harm, and access to weapons or potentially harmful medications [28].

With rare exception, elderly patients admitting to suicidal ideation require inpatient evaluation and treatment (Table 32.3). Prior to death, suicide victims often share their ideations with a significant other, despite occasionally denying this to their physician [27]. Therefore, discussion with caretakers may uncover suicidal ideation that a patient denied. During evaluation of the suicidal patient, evidence of intentional overdose, toxic ingestion, or self-inflicted wounds should be viewed as potential suicide attempts.

Case Example 2, Continued

The patient recovers well without operative intervention. He screens positive for depression and is transferred to an inpatient psychiatric facility, given his elevated repeat suicide risk.

Psychosis

Case Example 3

An 82-year-old female with a history of Parkinson's disease presents from a nursing home due to altered mental status. Staff states that her confusion has worsened recently, and she has been heard talking aloud in her room at night, though she has no phone or roommate. She had one episode of urinary incontinence today …

Psychosis is defined as the disorganization of mental capacity, characterized by defective contact with reality, as evidenced by delusions, hallucinations, or disorganized speech or behavior. While this may be due to primary psychiatric conditions, psychosis is more often secondary to a medical illness, cognitive disorders, iatrogenic causes, and substance abuse. Approximately, 23% of the elderly will experience psychotic symptoms associated with aggressive or disruptive behavior, which increases the risk of caretaker abuse or institutionalization. While psychotic disorders are reported in less than 5% of elderly patients, psychotic symptoms are present in 10–63% of nursing home residents [29]. Psychosis can be organized into three categories: (1) with dementia; (2) without dementia; (3) secondary to medical and social factors.

Dementia is the most common cause of psychosis in the elderly. Psychosis is pathognomonic in some forms of dementia (e.g., Lewy body dementia) but can be present in all forms of dementia. In particular, vascular dementia patients are at high risk for psychosis. Nearly half of Alzheimer's disease (AD) patients experience delusions or hallucinations within 3 years of clinical onset, and greater than 50% of demented patients develop paranoia or hallucinations [28, 30]. The AD with psychosis is associated with more rapid cognitive decline and is often complicated by aggression and danger to self and others.

Primary psychiatric disorders are a less common cause of psychosis in the elderly. Schizophrenia typically develops in early adulthood, but occasionally occurs as a late-onset variant, in which the patient possesses mostly positive symptoms (delusions, hallucinations, and disorganized speech). Symptoms of brief psychotic episodes and schizophreniform disorder are similar to schizophrenia, but often the onset is more acute and occurs with shorter disease time courses. Depression with psychotic features is most common in patients who develop depression late in life. These patients often demonstrate somatic delusions, such as the belief they have incurable or mistreated diseases, and a higher suicide risk than those without psychotic features [30].

Psychosis may also develop in the elderly secondary to a medical illness, substance use, medications, or stressful situations. The brain deteriorates with age, causing individuals to possess less "cognitive reserve," referring to the ability of the brain to function appropriately while compensating for neuropathic insults. This can explain the increased onset or exacerbation of dementia, risk for schizophrenia and depression, and susceptibility to delirium with age [31]. Even with mild stressors, such as a UTI or medication change, the maladaptive brain may allow for confusion or psychosis. However, the provider should be vigilant of other potential stressors, as asymptomatic bacteriuria increase dramatically with age. Delirium, an acute decline in cognition, is associated with altered consciousness, sleep-wake-cycle disturbance, confusion, and psychosis [30]. Delirium is common among the elderly, as 56% of the elderly develop delirium during hospital admission. Additionally, delirium is associated with functional decline, nursing home placement, and death, with a 33% in-hospital mortality rate [31, 32]. Psychotic symptoms may also occur in substance intoxication and withdrawal [33]. Corticosteroids, anti-inflammatories, angiotensin-converting enzyme (ACE) inhibitors, opioids, dopamine agonists, and drugs with anticholinergic properties such as antihistamines and some antidepressants (such as cyclic antidepressants) contribute to delirium [32]. Further, psychosocial stressors in the elderly increase the risk of psychotic symptoms [34].

The provider's role includes the stabilization of the patient's behavior, delineation of psychotic etiology, initiation of treatment when appropriate, and disposition [28]. Delirium is often confused with primary psychiatric disease or dementia, due to their similarities. However, they have distinct features, as highlighted in Table 32.4. Temporal traits differentiating dementia from delirium may be difficult, and given elderly patient's multiple comorbidities, they may exhibit traits from more than one category. Providers must use information regarding psychiatric illness, substance abuse, elder abuse, medication changes, and psychosocial conditions to consider diagnoses of delirium, dementia, and psychosis.

The assessment of psychosis in elderly patients should include medical clearance and neurologic evaluation, including consideration of head trauma, malignancy, infection, and seizures [30]. A medical psychosis screen may include a complete blood count, comprehensive medical panel, vitamin B12 and folate levels, thyroid function tests, urinalysis, and electrocardiogram, but testing should remain judicious [28, 32]. Lumbar puncture, HIV, and rapid plasma reagin (RPR) testing should be considered, given the high mortality of CNS infections [35]. Medication levels (e.g., antiepileptics and digoxin) and drug screens may help differentiate a toxicologic cause of psychosis [30, 32].

Disposition of the psychotic elderly patient depends on the specific etiology. The high mortality risk associated with delirium should lower the threshold for medical admission. For the elderly with dementia or primary psychiatric illness, medical providers should use criteria in Table 32.3, as well as assess the patient for homicidal ideation, when considering admission to a psychiatric facility [22].

Table 32.4 Presenting characteristics in the psychotic elderly patient to help differentiate underlying illness such as delirium, dementia, and/or primary psychiatric illness[a] [30]

Characteristics	Delirium	Dementia	Psychiatric illness
General traits	Acute onset of confusion with signs and symptoms of medical illness	History of dementia; commonly short-term memory deficit, but also may include CVA and PD traits	Psychiatric history; commonly on psychotropic medications
Onset	Sudden	Insidious	Variable
Alertness	Fluctuating	Normal, except in late or severe disease	Normal
Duration	Hours to weeks	Typically lifetime deficits	Variable, depending on response to treatment
Orientation	Disoriented	Increasingly disoriented with worsening disease	Normal
Hallucinations	At onset	Usually only with late or severe disease or comorbid illness	Dependent on psychiatric illness and compliance with medications
"Sundowning"	Present	Present	Absent
Course	Usually reversible	Irreversible	Usually partially to fully reversible
Special considerations	Initiate workup and treatment; strongly consider encephalitis	Consider medical illness as precipitant for acute decompensation	Critical to assess for suicidal ideation; consider medical illness as exacerbating factor

[a]This table is adapted and modified in reference to the original table by Khouzam and Emes [30]
CVA cerebrovascular accident, *PD* Parkinson's disease

Case Example 3, Continued

The patient was noted to have a UTI that was complicated by an excited delirium. Given the high risk associated with the patient's symptoms, she was started on antibiotics and admitted to the hospital with a sitter.

Agitation

Case Example 4

A 78-year-old female with a history of AD presents from an assisted-living facility with confusion. She reportedly has not slept for 3 days since starting a prednisone course for an asthma exacerbation and assaulted a staff member today …

Agitation is a common manifestation of geriatric psychosis and includes hyperactivity, assaultiveness, verbal abuse, physical destructiveness, and excessive verbalizations of distress [28]. There are three main reasons to initiate treatment of the elderly patient suffering from psychiatric illness: (1) improve patient cooperation; (2) reduce the risk of injury to the patient and the staff; (3) begin the therapeutic process [36]. The management of agitation, especially in severe cases, will be essential to move forward with any disposition in the elderly psychiatric patient.

Noninvasive strategies greatly improve agitation of elderly patients and may reduce the need for chemical or physical restraints. In addition to correcting reversible medical factors, providers can consider environmental modifications: (1) family member involvement; (2) movement of patients to a location of best observation; (3) prevent access to means that may harm patients, including windows, balconies, cords, and coat hangers; (4) employ fall prevention strategies; (5) place devices and catheters in inaccessible or not noticeable areas; and (6) employ one-to-one sitters [37]. Medical staff should communicate with elderly patients in a calming voice, redirecting them away from agitating topics or factors.

Chemical restraint is a common approach in the management of the agitated patient. Scant evidence supports the use of chemical restraint; recommendations include the use of high-potency antipsychotics, benzodiazepines (especially in the setting of alcohol withdrawal), or a combination of both [36, 38]. Certain pitfalls must be considered: (1) treating agitation without considering the cause; (2) "as needed" (PRN) dosing resulting in under- or overdosing; and (3) aggressive sedation causing falls, respiratory depression, or death. While typical antipsychotics, including haloperidol and droperidol, have shown efficacy in reducing agitation in the elderly, atypical antipsychotics have been recommended in the elderly over typical antipsychotics [28, 32, 38]. Atypical antipsychotics, such as olanzapine and quetiapine, have lesser anticholinergic properties and therefore, fewer complications of dystonia and extrapyramidal symptoms; they have also shown efficacy equivalent to typical antipsychotics and benzodiazepines [36, 39]. While studies have shown an increased rate of adverse events and mortality with their use in the demented elderly, these studies were specific to several weeks to months of use [40, 41]. Benzodiazepines are efficacious in decreasing agitation and have increased efficacy when used in combination with haloperidol. While not associated with extrapyramidal symptoms, benzodiazepines risk respiratory depression, excess sedation, and occasionally, a paradoxical increase in agitation. Because of these adverse effects, recommendations are to start cautiously at lower doses [36, 38]. Additionally, the duration of therapy should be limited as much as possible [39].

Physical restraints should be considered when the patient becomes a danger to themselves or to the hospital staff after pharmacologic and nonpharmacologic methods have failed or are not available. Limb, wrist, and vest restraints should be available, in addition to mittens and bed rails, as methods to restrain the patient [36]. Anecdotal evidence has shown that restraints are fraught with complications, including aspiration pneumonia, circulatory obstruction, cardiac stress with cardiovascular collapse, dehydration, and skin breakdown. Seclusion, in which a patient is typically placed in a locked room, has been used in substitution for physical restraints for patients who are imminently violent. Complications with seclusion include assaultiveness toward staff, self-injury, destruction of seclusion room, and deterioration of physical and mental status [36].

Case Example 4, Continued

The patient's delirium and agitation were attributed to her prednisone. After a brief inpatient admission and discontinuation of prednisone, the patient returned to baseline.

Substance Abuse

Case Example 5

A 76-year-old male with chronic pain is found unconscious in his kitchen. When paramedics arrive, he is breathing slowly, groans with a painful stimulus, and awakens after given intranasal naloxone …

Substance abuse within geriatrics has been identified as the fastest-growing health problem in the United States, and existing diagnostic criteria significantly underestimate the prevalence of substance abuse among the elderly [28, 42]. Specifically, studies on alcohol misuse show rates between 2–4%, and 17% of elderly men and 7% of elderly women were found to use excessive amounts of alcohol [43]. Illicit drug use is relatively rare among elderly patients, with a rate of 1–2%, but is expected to rise and is higher in psychiatric and urban populations. Additionally, one out of every four elderly patients uses prescribed psychoactive medications, and 11% of elderly women abuse these medications [44]. The misuse of alcohol, illicit drugs, and prescribed medications may have deleterious medical consequences and psychiatric effects that should be investigated.

Elderly patients are more susceptible to adverse effects of substance use secondary to decreased lean body mass, cognitive reserve, and hepatic and renal function [28, 31, 45].

Specifically, alcohol use is associated with mood disorders, anxiety, cognitive impairment, personality disorders, and schizophrenia, and increases the risk of developing a host of medical conditions, predisposing one to psychiatric illness [28]. Benzodiazepine and opiate use is prevalent and may be associated with increased sedation, impairment of motor coordination, depression, cognitive impairment, and constipation [44]. The adverse effects of cocaine use specific to the elderly are not well described, but cardiovascular complications, seizures, agitation, anxiety, and psychosis have been documented across all age groups [46].

Substance abuse is under-detected by medical personnel [28]. A study employing a mock clinical scenario found that only 1% of primary physicians correctly identified substance abuse as the underlying issue for an elderly patient [44]. Diagnosis is obscured by elderly comorbidities, such as psychiatric disorder, cognitive impairment, chronic pain, and hepatic/renal disorders [44]. The CAGE questionnaire, summarized in Table 32.5, has been adopted as a screening tool for both drug and alcohol abuse, and has been validated in elderly patients [47]. A drug screen may be helpful in management and disposition of the undifferentiated patient, especially when a reliable history is lacking [48]. However, the global use of a drug screen should be discouraged, as it is costly and this information can typically be obtained via history [49].

After the determination of abuse has been made, the appropriate management and disposition are vital to the safety of the patient. The type, amount, and frequency of the abused substance, co-ingestions including current prescriptions, and medical and psychiatric comorbidities will dictate the management. In the alcoholic patient, important historical components include prior complicated detoxifications, history of withdrawal seizures or delirium tremens, or other comorbid factors that would require hospital admission [28]. Clinicians should be aware of the kindling phenomenon, where patients develop increasingly severe withdrawal symptoms with repeated alcohol detoxification attempts [50]. The elderly patient not admitted for further medical or psychiatric management should receive a timely outpatient referral.

Table 32.5 CAGE screening for alcohol and drug abuse in the elderly [47]

1. Have you ever felt you needed to cut down on your drinking or drug use?
2. Have people annoyed you by criticizing your drinking or drug use?
3. Have you ever felt guilty about drinking or drug use?
4. Have you ever felt you needed a drink or to use drugs first thing in the morning (eye-opener) to steady your nerves or to get rid of a hangover?

The screen should be considered positive if the patient answers "Yes" to any of the above questions. This screening questionnaire becomes more specific for abuse for each additional "Yes" answer. This table is adapted from Hinkin et al. [47]

CAGE acronym using the capitalized letters from the above four questions

Case Example 5, Continued

The patient is brought to a local ED and monitored for several hours. He admits to buying heroin to treat his pain since he cannot afford his prescription medications …

References

1. American Geriatrics Society and the Association of Directors of Academic Geriatric Center's Geriatric Workforce Policy Studies Center. 2010.
2. Walsh PG, et al. Psychiatric emergency services for the U.S. elderly: 2008 and beyond. Am J Geriatr Psy. 2008;16(9):706–17.
3. Ganguli M, Dodge HH, Mulsant BH. Rates and predictors of mortality in an aging, rural, community-based cohort: the role of depression. Arch Gen Psy. 2002;59(11):1046–52.
4. Huang BY, et al. Impact of depressive symptoms on hospitalization risk in community-dwelling older persons. J Am Geriatr Soc. 2000;48(10):1279–84.
5. Waern M, et al. Mental disorder in elderly suicides: a case-control study. Am J Psy. 2002;159(3):450–5.
6. Meldon SW, et al. Depression in geriatric ED patients: prevalence and recognition. Ann Emerg Med. 1997;30(2):141–5.
7. Pederson JL, et al. Depressive symptoms are associated with higher rates of readmission or mor-

tality after medical hospitalization: a systematic review and meta-analysis. Journal of Hospital Med. 2016;11(5):373–80.
8. Thienhaus OJ, Piasecki MP. Assessment of geriatric patients in the psychiatric emergency service. Psychiatr Serv. 2004;55(6):639–40, 642.
9. Unutzer J, et al. Depressive symptoms and the cost of health services in HMO patients aged 65 years and older: a 4-year prospective study. JAMA. 1997;277(20):1618–23.
10. Abrams RC, et al. Psychiatric assessment and screening for the elderly in primary care: Design, implementation, and preliminary results. J Geriatrics. 2015.
11. Cole MG, Dendukuri N. Risk factors for depression among elderly community subjects: a systematic review and meta-analysis. Am J Psy. 2003;160(6):1147–56.
12. Alexopoulos GS, et al. Assessment of late life depression. Biol Psy. 2002;52(3):164–74.
13. Arias SA, et al. Disparities in treatment of older adults with suicide risk in the emergency department. Journal of the American Geriatrics Soc. 2017;65(10):2272–7.
14. American Psychiatric Association. Diagnostic and statistical manual of mental disorders: DSM-V. Amer Psychiatric Pub Incorporated; 2013.
15. Fabacher DA, et al. Validation of a brief screening tool to detect depression in elderly ED patients. Am J Emerg Med. 2002;20(2):99–102.
16. Olin JT, et al. Provisional diagnostic criteria for depression of Alzheimer disease. Am J Geriatr Psy. 2002;10(2):125–8.
17. Eaton WW, et al. Center for Epidemiologic Studies Depression Scale: review and revision (CESD and CESD-R). In: The use of psychological testing for treatment planning and outcomes assessment: instruments for adults. Volume 3. 3rd ed. Mahwah, NJ: Lawrence Erlbaum Associates Publishers; 2004. p. 363–77.
18. Yesavage JA, Sheikh JI. Geriatric depression scale (GDS): recent evidence and development of a shorter version. Clin Gerontol. 1986;5(1–2):165–73.
19. Phelan E, et al. A study of the diagnostic accuracy of the PHQ-9 in primary care elderly. BMC Fam Pract. 2010;11(1):63.
20. Costa MV, et al. Accuracy of three depression screening scales to diagnose major depressive episodes in older adults without neurocognitive disorders. Rev Bras Psiquiatr. 2016;38:154–6.
21. Fischer LR, et al. Treatment of elderly and other adult patients for depression in primary care. J Am Geriatr Soc. 2003;51(11):1554–62.
22. Macdonald AJ. ABC of mental health: mental health in old age. BMJ. 1997;315(7105):413–7.
23. Conwell Y. Suicide in later life: a review and recommendations for prevention. Suicide Life Threat Behav. 2001;31(Suppl):32–47.
24. Conwell Y, Van Orden K, Caine ED. Suicide in older adults. Psychiatr Clin N Am. 2011;34(2):451–68.
25. Duberstein PR, Conwell Y, Cox C. Suicide in widowed persons: a psychological autopsy comparison of recently and remotely bereaved older subjects. Am J Geriatr Psy. 1998;6(4):328–34.
26. Conwell Y, Thompson C. Suicidal behavior in elders. Psychiatr Clin North Am. 2008;31(2):333–56.
27. Waern M, et al. Suicidal feelings in the last year of life in elderly people who commit suicide. Lancet. 1999;354(9182):917–8.
28. Piechniczek-Buczek J. Psychiatric emergencies in the elderly population. Emerg Med Clin North Am. 2006;24(2):467–90. viii
29. Mintzer J, Targum SD. Psychosis in elderly patients: classification and pharmacotherapy. J Geriatr Psychiatry Neurol. 2003;16(4):199–206.
30. Khouzam HR, Emes R. Late life psychosis: assessment and general treatment strategies. Compr Ther. 2007;33(3):127–43.
31. Jones RN, et al. Aging, brain disease, and reserve: implications for delirium. Am J Geriatr Psy. 2010;18(2):117–27.
32. Patkar AA, Mago R, Masand PS. Psychotic symptoms in patients with medical disorders. Curr Psychiatry Rep. 2004;6(3):216–24.
33. Diagnostic and Statistical Manual of Mental Disorders. 4thWashington, DC.: American Psychiatric Association. 2000.
34. van Winkel R, Stefanis NC, Myin-Germeys I. Psychosocial stress and psychosis: a review of the neurobiological mechanisms and the evidence for gene-stress interaction. Schizophr Bull. 2008;34(6):1095–105.
35. Mace SE. Central nervous system infections as a cause of an altered mental status? What is the pathogen growing in your central nervous system? Emerg Med Clin North Am. 2010;28(3):535–70.
36. Zun LS. Evidence-based treatment of psychiatric patient. J Emerg Med. 2005;28(3):277–83.
37. Zun LS. Evidence-based evaluation of psychiatric patients. J Emerg Med. 2005;28(1):35–9.
38. Peisah C, et al. Practical guidelines for the acute emergency sedation of the severely agitated older patient. Intern Med J. 2011;41(9):651–7.
39. Sturm AS, et al. Efficacy and safety of atypical antipsychotics for behavioral symptoms of dementia among patients residing in long-term care. Int J Clin Pharm. 2018;40(1):135–42.
40. Yildiz A, Sachs GS, Turgay A. Pharmacological management of agitation in emergency settings. Emerg Med J. 2003;20(4):339–46.
41. Yan J. FDA extends black-box warning to all antipsychotics. Psychiatr News. 2008;43:1):1–27.
42. Patterson TL, Jeste DV. The potential impact of the baby-boom generation on substance abuse among elderly persons. Psychiatr Serv. 1999;50(9): 1184–8.
43. O'Connell H, et al. Alcohol use disorders in elderly people: redefining an age-old problem in old age. BMJ. 2003;327(7416):664–7.
44. Simoni-Wastila L, Yang HK. Psychoactive drug abuse in older adults. Am J Geriatr Pharmacother. 2006;4(4):380–94.

45. Borja B, Borja CS, Gade S. Psychiatric emergencies in the geriatric population. Clin Geriatr Med. 2007;23(2):391–400, vii.
46. Devlin RJ, Henry JA. Clinical review: major consequences of illicit drug consumption. Crit Care. 2008;12(1):202.
47. Hinkin CH, et al. Screening for drug and alcohol abuse among older adults using a modified version of the CAGE. Am J Addict. 2001;10(4):319–26.
48. Fabbri A, et al. Comprehensive drug screening in decision making of patients attending the emergency department for suspected drug overdose. Emerg Med J. 2003;20(1):25–8.
49. Perrone J, et al. Drug screening versus history in detection of substance use in ED psychiatric patients. Am J Emerg Med. 2001;19(1):49–51.
50. Malcolm RJ. GABA systems, benzodiazepines, and substance dependence. J Clin Psy. 2003;64(Suppl. 3):36–40.

Disaster and Terrorism in Emergency Psychiatry

33

Lynn Barkley Burnett

Introduction

During morning rush hour, five members of the Aum Shinrikyo doomsday cult boarded five cars on three lines of the Tokyo subway system. At a prearranged time, they proceeded to puncture 13 bags of sarin with the sharpened ends of umbrellas. Over the next few days, a total of 5500 people received medical attention [1]. Of those, there were 12 deaths [2], fewer than 20 patients who required critical care in an ICU, and 1046 who required admission to the hospital [1]. Most of the patients who sought medical care were thus psychological casualties.

Oncologists in Goiânia, Brazil, closed their medical clinic, abandoning a radiation therapy unit. Scavengers removed 20 g of Cesium 137 from the machine, giving material to friends and family in the immediate vicinity because the material glowed in the dark. Two hundred forty-nine people were contaminated, externally or internally, and there were four deaths [3]. A total of 125,800 individuals sought screening at the local Olympic Stadium in fear they had been contaminated with the radioactive material—placing an immense strain on the public health system [4].

While the primary focus of most disaster and terrorism medical response is on the management of physical injury and illness, the emotional and psychological effects in the affected population are quite often overlooked [5]. The incidents discussed above are exemplifications of the challenges that such situations may present to disaster and terrorism emergency psychiatry.

Context

The World Health Organization (WHO) defines a disaster as "a severe disruption, ecological and psychosocial, which greatly exceeds the coping capacity of the affected community" [6]. Disasters may be natural (e.g., earthquakes, floods) or technological (man-made, either the result of human error or via intentional action) [5, 6].

Ursano, Fullerton, and Norwood (2007) state that terrorism represents a certain type of disaster, employing "a threat or action that creates terror or horror and is undertaken to achieve a political, ideological, or theological goal." Terrorism is psychological warfare [7].

Terrorist incidents and disasters challenge our beliefs [8]. Ordinarily, we make three fundamental assumptions:

- The world is fundamentally a good place.
- Life and events have meaning and purpose.
- One's self is valuable and worthy.

L. B. Burnett (✉)
Department of Clinical Specialties, Community Regional Medical Center, Fresno, CA, USA
e-mail: drlbburnett@sbcglobal.net

L. S. Zun et al. (eds.), *Behavioral Emergencies for Healthcare Providers*,
https://doi.org/10.1007/978-3-030-52520-0_33

How do terrorists go about achieving their goals [4]?

a. Creating mass anxiety, fear, and panic
b. Creating helplessness, hopelessness, and demoralization
c. Destroying our assumptions about personal security
d. Disruption of the infrastructure of a society, culture, or city and
e. Demonstrating the impotence of authorities to protect the ordinary citizen and his/her environment

We typically think of agents employed by terrorists as weapons of mass destruction (e.g., chemical, biological, radiological). Since the primary goal of terrorism is to create terror [3], however, mass casualties are not necessary to fulfill terrorists' objectives; death and physical damage *are*, but as a means to an end, not an end in itself [4].

Differences in Responses to Natural Disasters Versus Terrorism

DiGiovanni (1999) maintains that disasters do not usually produce panic, because they involve familiar phenomena that are time-limited and discernible. For example, people in fires generally act responsibly, even altruistically, because they know about fires and receive sensory cues that enable them to assess the threat and to plan their escape.

A chemical, biological, or radiological incident poses a sudden, unanticipated, and unfamiliar threat to health that may lack sensory cues, may be prolonged or recurrent, and perhaps is contagious. These are factors that historically have spawned fear and panic [7].

The Ratio of Ill or Injured Versus Psychological Patients

Following an attack, patients may present with symptoms of exposure to the chemical, radiologic, or biological agent, even though they have not been affected by the same. The Centers for Disease Control and Prevention advise that the ratio of ill/injured patients compared to those with primary psychological etiology will be on the order of 6–9:1. In the Goiânia incident, 11% of those screened exhibited classic presentation of radiation exposure (nausea, reddened skin, etc.) before being assessed; after being given a clean bill of health, their signs and symptoms dissipated within a few hours [3].

After a terrorist attack or disaster, a clinician may see patients with symptoms that are impossible to explain medically [9]. The term MUPS (multiple unexplained physical symptoms) is seen in the literature [10], as is "medically unexplained symptoms," physical symptoms that have no clinically determined pathogenesis [11]. Identification of patients with unexplained symptoms is important to prevent potentially harmful interventions that are inappropriate and that would draw limited resources away from patients who needed the same [12].

Mass sociogenic illness, also referred to as mass psychogenic illness and epidemic hysteria, is a social phenomenon in which two or more people share beliefs about symptoms for which no identifiable etiology can be found [3]. Such phenomena have been termed as OMUS (outbreaks of medically unexplained symptoms) [10, 11].

Although the term "worried well" is frequently used, such a term is inaccurate and unhelpful [4]. A dismissive approach to medically unexplained physical symptoms may result in a debate between patient and medical staff over "contested causation," with patients' ever-increasing efforts to convince physicians of the reality of their symptoms [4].

The Danger of "Complaint" Fatigue

A risk to patient safety well-known in critical care units is "alarm fatigue"; repeatedly heard monitor and equipment alarms result in reduced attention by medical personnel. Clinicians should guard against the potential for a similar phenomenon of "complaint fatigue" after a terrorist attack. During the anthrax letters incident in 2001, an employee at the Brentwood Post Office in Washington, D.C [13, 14]., presented to an emergency department with worsening nausea, vomiting, abdominal pain, diaphoresis, and lightheadedness—signs and symptoms of inhalational anthrax listed in a warning letter sent by the US Postal Service. After symptomatic treatment, he was discharged home with a diagnosis of gastroenteritis. He died. Did the necessity to assess the high volume of patients presenting with concerns about anthrax infection and "complaint fatigue" associated with the multitude of patients who were not infected play a role in the failure to diagnose?

Psychological Triage

Triage means "to sort," and it is applied classically to those with physical injuries or illnesses. Including behavioral and psychiatric considerations in assessment increases the efficacy of overall management [12]. A psychiatric screening examination [12] may be conducted along with a history and physical examination if the number of personnel and other exigencies permits the same. Those findings facilitate the differential diagnosis of psychiatric symptoms in the medical-surgical and trauma settings. Often, the presence or absence of fever is the only reliable early differentiator between those exposed to a biological agent and those not [9].

Assessment of the patient's mental status begins with their level of consciousness, employing the AVPU approach (alert, responds to voice, responds to pain, unresponsive). Following this, the classical four legs of orientation are person, place, purpose, and time (the latter by asking the year and month, or who is the president of the United States). Periodically insert nonsense questions to determine if the patient is confused, such as "Do catfish fly?" or "Do beagles yodel?" If the patient looks surprised at those questions, confusion is not present [12].

The presence of behavioral signs and significant physical findings complicate differential diagnosis (as per the below charts). Never lose sight that multiple disorders may be present [12].

Differential Diagnosis of Psychological Versus Physical Problems

Psychological causes presenting as physical problems

Psychological cause	Physical problem impression
Depressed mood or resignation	Malaise and lassitude often are seen after employment of biochemical terrorism agents [12]
Dissociation	Unresponsiveness or diminished neurological responsiveness secondary to head injury [12]
Substance withdrawal syndromes	Physiologic depression or hyperstimulation may be confused with exposure to nerve agents or cyanide
Anxiety or panic attacks	Nerve agent or cyanide toxicity [12]
Pharmacological agents (e.g., neuroleptics and benzodiazepines) used to manage agitation	Physiologic depression secondary to hypovolemia, hypoxia, or head injury

Physical causes presenting as psychological problems

Physical cause	Psychological problem impression
Nerve agents	Have the highest potential among toxic agents for causing diagnostic confusion. May present with impaired concentration, memory deficits, slowing of information processing, delayed speech, and word-finding difficulty. Psychological findings may be more prevalent than physical results, especially in early stages of exposure [7]. Persistent long-term neuropsychiatric effects can be seen, as well, including drowsiness, memory impairment, depression, fatigue, and increased irritability [12] Should not be mistaken for anxiety or panic attacks. Vital in the differential diagnosis is the history of nerve agent use and the presence of early cholinergic symptoms such as lacrimation, salivation, and rhinorrhea [12] Poisoning with nerve agents at a sublethal level may cause or mimic psychiatric disturbances such as anxiety disorders, mood disorders, and delirium These should not be treated with highly anticholinergic antipsychotic agents, as they may worsen the syndrome [12]

Physical causes presenting as psychological problems	
Physical cause	Psychological problem impression
Cyanide	Early symptoms of cyanide exposure are anxiety, confusion, giddiness, and hyperventilation. These symptoms are difficult to distinguish from situational anxiety [12]
Lacrimating agents (e.g., tear gas)	May be confused with lacrimation (tearing) produced by nerve agents and lead to inappropriate treatment with anticholinergic medication [7, 12]
Vesicants	Blister agents such as mustard gas and lewisite have been reported to produce long-term psychological symptoms such as apathy and depression. Acutely, blister agents can also cause delirium [12]
Hypovolemia, hypoxemia, central nervous system mass effect (e.g., hemorrhage (brain bleed), foreign bodies), infection, and adverse effects of resuscitative medications [12]	Delirium (clouded consciousness, agitation, diminished responsiveness, disorientation) A prodrome of confusion, restlessness, irritability, and insomnia may portend a full syndrome, which includes short-term memory deficit, distractibility, difficulty abstracting, disorganized thinking, dysarthria, reduced comprehension, illusions, visual hallucinations, sleep-wake-cycle disturbance ("sundowning"), and either hypoactivity or hyperactivity [12]
Botulism	Autonomic complications may include dry mouth, ileus, and urinary retention. Patients who fear of being exposed, but have not been, could report similar symptoms due to anxiety and worry [12]
Biological agents including anthrax, botulinum toxin, tularemia, plague, brucellosis, Q fever, smallpox, the viral Encephalitides, and staphylococcal B enterotoxin	Delirium [7]
Viral Encephalitides (e.g., viral hemorrhagic fevers)	Delirium. Long-term cognitive impairment and alterations in mood may also be seen [7]
Atropine	Has the most potential for serious alterations in mental status. Causes neuropsychiatric effects, which may be worse than the nerve agent itself in some cases. Doses necessary for treatment may cause significant drowsiness, concentration disturbance, hyperactivity, hallucinations, and stupor or coma [12] Atropine causes significant anxiety, and itself can cause psychosis effects Increases heart rate
Epinephrine	Causes blood pressure and heart rate elevations, and patients to feel anxious or panicky [12]
Morphine	Causes sedation and impairs orientation and responsiveness [12]

Regardless of etiology, delirium must be addressed rapidly, because the mortality rate from all underlying causes increases when delirium goes unaddressed. The resolution requires treating the underlying metabolic abnormality caused by the insult [12].

It is important to find out which medications an injured patient has received, in what amounts, and over what time period, as well as what substances the patient has not been exposed to [12].

PsySTART (simple triage and rapid treatment) [15] is an approach to rapid mental health triage and includes the use of a rapid triage tag that may be employed in the field by first responders who do not have mental health expertise.

After initial triage and treatment of victims, it is important to create a "holding environment" where persons developing symptoms can be observed and monitored. This area should be sufficiently removed so as not to disrupt the ongoing triage and stabilization of life-threatening physical injuries, but close enough to allow reevaluation and further medical intervention, should symptoms worsen [12].

Psychological First Aid (PFA)

The essential elements of PFA are as follows:

a. Providing survivors with physical and psychological comfort
b. Protecting them from further harm
c. Providing accurate information
d. Reestablishing a sense of order and control (e.g., by restoring public utilities)
e. Involving survivors, where necessary, in purposeful activities
f. Developing or reestablishing, where appropriate, links with family, friends, and other survivors
g. Providing information about helping agencies
h. Conducting triage to identify individuals at most risk of adverse psychological reactions

Detailed information may be obtained by referring to the text Psychological First Aid: Field Operations Guide [16] that is available free online via the URL in the references section below.

Reactions to a Disaster or Terrorist Incident

Necessary interventions such as barrier environments, mass immunization, decontamination, the destruction of personal clothing and property, and disposal of dead bodies may give rise to psychological problems. Restrictions on travel, quarantine, and isolation of contaminated individuals may have adverse effects on family and social networks, the first line of support for those affected [4].

The majority of persons experiencing disaster or terrorism get better spontaneously [11]. Responses such as anger, disbelief, sadness, anxiety, fear, and irritability are normal, anticipated, and usually transitory [3]. This normal distress responds well to meeting basic needs. Resilience may be promoted by re-achieving simple structure and schedule (to the degree possible), time spent with family and friends, participating in recreational activities, engaging in spiritual/religious activities, and rebuilding [6].

Adverse consequences of stressors are pronounced when individuals lack: (1) control; (2) predictability; (3) direction; and (4) social support [11]. Patients with preexisting medical or psychiatric illnesses are at risk for idiosyncratic or unusual presentations. This is especially true of the chronically mentally ill with severe psychiatric disorders such as schizophrenia and bipolar disorder [11]. Of particular importance is the potential worsening of symptoms because of an inability to obtain medication or the development of an abstinence syndrome (withdrawal) [6].

Stress is the combination of an event (stressor) plus its meaning, which is affected by an individual's background, life experiences, coping strategies and abilities, culture, and the psychological environment before, during, and after the event. The development and resolution of a stress reaction is a function of meaning to the individual [9]. Of those with an acute stress response, some will rapidly improve by talking about their experiences, whereas others may recover more slowly [6].

Distress may be experienced by direct victims, witnesses to the event, family members and friends of victims, and those who watch the incident online or TV with repetitive replaying of the traumatic episode [4]. Children and those who have previously experienced trauma are at increased risk [6]. Distress also results from concern about another attack [3].

Panic is an individual's loss of rational thought due to overwhelming terror, paralyzing them by fear. The term also applies to contagious fear among groups. Group panic is not seen following a disaster because of the modifying effect of pro-social behavior. Following a terrorist attack, however, there may well be inadequate resources, insufficient personnel, and overall poor experience in responding to such events. Factors such as these, especially when combined, could result in group panic [17].

Post-Incident Psychological Problems

Post-disaster psychiatric sequelae	Comments
Acute stress disorder	Interferes with function; presents 1 day to 1 month after the event. Manifestations include re-experiencing the event (distressing dreams, flashbacks); hyperarousal; avoidance of situations that resemble the original trauma, even if only symbolically; and dissociative phenomena (e.g., derealization, numbing)
Post-traumatic stress disorder (PTSD)	Manifestations similar to those of acute stress disorder; excessive stress lasting greater than 1 month; impairs social, occupational, and other critical functions; previous trauma increases the risk of a more severe stress response Physical symptoms may also be seen, including difficulty with sleep and impaired concentration [11]
Anxiety disorders	Generalized anxiety disorder manifests excessive anxiety plus apprehension about events or activities; constant worry, restlessness, irritability, trembling, twitching, and sleep disturbance. New disorders may emerge. Preexisting disorders increase the risk of a pathological stress response
Panic disorder	Recurrent, unexpected panic attacks followed by worry and behavioral changes secondary to the attacks
Hypochondriasis	Includes somatic symptom disorder (fear or belief that one has a serious illness, accompanied by significant symptoms), and illness anxiety disorder (similar fear or belief, despite the lack of significant symptoms). Patients with preexisting hypochondriasis may have problems managing anxiety and beliefs. New cases may appear. Sub-syndromal hypochondriacal fears may be widespread and amenable to reassurance
Psychotic disorders	Brief psychotic reactions may be more common in women, children, and members of non-Western cultures
Normal bereavement	Present in most disasters. An essential element is an ability to retain a sense of self and purpose
Complicated grief	Mourning to such an extent that normal life cannot be resumed
Substance abuse	High risk of abuse of alcohol and other drugs to cope with stress and loss following a disaster; risk shared by those with and without a preexisting history of substance abuse. May be a particular problem with first responders and health professionals, given their exposure
Dissociative disorders	Disruption of integrated functions of consciousness, memory, identity, or perception of the environment. Includes amnesia, fugue states, depersonalization, and derealization. Situational dissociation does not meet the diagnostic criteria for dissociative disorder; it is very prevalent in any traumatic or terrorist incident. Dissociation may be an adaptive response that may prevent dangerous behaviors (e.g., fleeing a scene and being exposed to further danger)

Adapted from Ritchie et al. [6]; Source: Wynn et al. [12]

Sight should not be lost of the potential positives that can develop after a catastrophe, including a more united community or country; closer bonding of relationships; identification of new strengths within individuals; and reevaluation of life's priorities and values [4]. Such positive reframing may promote resiliency [6]—one need only look at what happened in the United States after the attacks on 9/11.

Interventions

Injured and frightened survivors should not be left alone, and parents should reunite with their children. Providing survivors with blankets and food helps reassure them that someone is concerned about them. Survivors should be encouraged to verbalize their experiences; they may be able to do this better in a group setting than one-on-one. Individuals with significant psychiatric disorders should get referred for hospitalization. As soon as possible, disaster survivors should be encouraged to participate in useful but straightforward tasks [7].

Critical incident stress debriefing is debated; some experts believe it could be detrimental to recovery and may cause re-traumatization, whereas others disagree. It may still be useful in first responders who have an operational debriefing as part of their routine [6].

Cognitive-behavioral therapy may be valuable. It involves education about the nature and universality of symptoms, examination of the precipitants of symptoms (mainly cognitive distortions), and development of reframing and interpretive techniques to minimize further symptoms. Even brief interventions may reduce immediate symptoms and diminish the development of long-term morbidity [17].

If necessary, symptoms of anxiety may be treated with the short-term use of long-lasting benzodiazepines. If these symptoms are only experienced episodically, shorter acting benzodiazepines can be used on an as-needed basis. Care should be taken to screen for present and past substance misuse or abuse; with such a history, supervision and close follow-up should be provided whenever possible [6].

Screening, assessing, and treating alcohol and opioid withdrawal is essential [6]. Alcohol withdrawal can be life-threatening if not adequately treated with benzodiazepines, and opioid withdrawal is extremely uncomfortable if not adequately treated. Benzodiazepines can be prescribed on a tapering schedule to manage alcohol withdrawal, though laws vary and steps should be taken to properly observe local laws for the outpatient management of withdrawal from a controlled substance. Supportive treatment for nausea, vomiting, and muscle cramping resulting from opioid withdrawal is helpful.

Antidepressants (e.g., selective serotonin reuptake inhibitors (SSRIs)) and serotonin-norepinephrine reuptake inhibitors (SNRIs) can be used for the treatment of acute stress disorder, depression, and generalized anxiety disorder, and are commonly used to treat symptoms of post-traumatic stress disorder (PTSD) [6]. Pharmacotherapy is effective in reducing post-traumatic symptoms. While much of the initial emotional response may resolve without such intervention, it is important to note that delay in instituting mental health diagnosis and treatment may increase long-term morbidity [17].

For patients with unexplained symptoms, non-pharmacologic (e.g., cognitive behavioral therapy, aerobic exercise) and pharmacologic (non-opioid analgesics and antidepressants, including tricyclic drugs) treatments are useful. Early (optimally primary care) intervention is important, because unexplained symptoms can become increasingly refractory to treatment the longer they have lasted [11].

Care must be taken to avoid drug/drug interactions between medications that can affect the metabolism and subsequent blood levels of the therapeutic agents used in the treatment of biological or chemical terrorist attack victims [17]. Clinical pharmacists or a poison center (1-800-222-1222) may aid in minimizing interactions. A conservative approach that reduces the initial use of psychotropic medications is warranted [12]. However, patients with mental illness should be maintained on their medication regimen and may require higher doses of antipsychotics, anxiolytics, and antidepressants, because stress and fear may worsen psychosis, anxiety, and depression [6].

Care of Self and Colleagues

Medical professionals and first responders [6] in the US have little experience in managing terrorist incidents. They are therefore not exempt from the psychological sequelae of disasters; they may experience fear, shock, anger, helplessness, and worries about their families and friends, and may not seek (and even resist) therapeutic intervention [7]. While work, activity, and provision of aid are often healthy coping techniques, it is essential to watch for symptoms of fatigue, burnout, and traumatization, particularly in the intermediate to late phases of a disaster.

References

1. Pagni R. Consequence management in the 1995 Sarin attacks on the Japanese Subway system. BCSIA discussion paper 2002–4, ESDP discussion paper ESDP-2002-01. Harvard University: John F. Kennedy School of Government; 2002.
2. TEEX Texas A&M Engineering Extension Service, National Emergency Response and Rescue Training Center (NERRTC), US Department of Homeland Security, Federal Emergency Management Agency, National Preparedness Directorate, and National Education and training division. Medical Management of Chemical, Biological, Radiological, Nuclear, and Explosive (CBRNE) Events: Instructor Guide; 2013.
3. Ursano RJ, Fullerton CS, Norwood AE. Terrorism and disaster: individual and community mental health interventions. Cambridge: Cambridge University Press; 2003. Available at assets.cambridge.org/052182/6063/sample/0521826063WS.pdf.
4. Alexander DA, Klein S. Biochemical terrorism: too awful to contemplate, too serious to ignore. Br J Psy. 2003;183:491–7.
5. McCormick LC, Tajeu GS, Klapow J. Mental health consequences of chemical and radiologic emergencies: A systematic review. Emerg Med Clin N Am. 2015;33:197–211.
6. Ritchie EL, O'Brien KM, Chanoff M, Stewart SA. Disaster psychiatry. In: Stern TA, Fava M, Wilens TE, Rosenbaum JF, editors. Massachusetts General Hospital Comprehensive clinical psychiatry. 2nd ed. London: Elsevier; 2016.
7. DiGiovanni C. Domestic terrorism with chemical or biological agents: psychiatric aspects. Am J Psy. 1999;156:1500–5.
8. Williams R, Alexander D. Psychosocial resilience and distress in the face of adversity, conflict, terrorism, or catastrophe. In: Adriaan PCC, Burna H, Burris DG, Hawley A, Ryan JM, Mahoney PF, editors. Conflict and catastrophe medicine: a practical guide. 2nd ed. London: Springer-Verlag; 2009.
9. Palmer IP. Mental health: part A—practical psychological aspects of humanitarian aid. In: Burma AH, editor. Conflict and catastrophe medicine. 2nd ed. London: Springer; 2009.
10. Greenstone JL. The elements of disaster psychology: managing psychosocial trauma. Springfield, IL: Charles C. Thomas Publisher Ltd; 2008.
11. Clauw DJ, Engel CC Jr, Aronowitz R, Jones E, Kipen HM, Kroenke K, Ratzan S, Sharpe M, Wessely S. Unexplained symptoms after terrorism and war: an expert consensus statement. J Occup Environ Med. 2003;45:1040–8.
12. Wynn GH, Rundell JR, Benedek DM. Military psychiatry. In: Stern TA, Fava M, Wilens TE, Rosenbaum JF, editors. Massachusetts general hospital comprehensive clinical psychiatry. 2nd ed. London: Elsevier; 2016.
13. Borio L, Frank D, Mani V, Chiriboga C, Pollanen M, Ripple M, Ali S, Diangelo C, Lee J, Arden J, Titus J, Fowler D, O'Toole T, Masur H, Bartlett J, Inglesby T. Death due to bioterrorism-related inhalational anthrax: report of 2 patients. JAMA. 2001;286:2554–9.
14. UCLA Fielding School of Public Health Department of Epidemiology. American Anthrax Outbreak of 2001. Available at http://www.ph.ucla.edu/epi/bioter/detect/antdetect_case16.html.
15. Schreiber M. The PsySTART mental health triage and incident management system. 2010. Available at http://pdfs.semanticscholar.org/f81d/383085aa8b113541d7ccc5360fdb66a1d469.pdf.
16. Brymer M, Jacobs A, Layne C, Pynoos R, Ruzek J, Steinberg A, Vernberg E, Watson P, National Child Traumatic Stress Network, and National Center for PTSD. Psychological first aid: field operations guide. Second ed. July 2006. Available at http://www.nctsn.org; www.ncptsd.va.gov.
17. Benedek DM, Grieger TA. Psychosocial management of bioterrorism events. In: Lutwick LI, Lutwick SM, editors. Beyond Anthrax: the Weaponization of infectious diseases. New York: Humana Press; 2009.

34 Mental Health Issues in the Homeless

Linda Ronquillo

Introduction

There is limited research on behavioral emergencies in the homeless population. The number of individuals who are homeless has become increasingly overwhelming and continues to be a public concern. Many of the homeless population have a mental health or substance use disorder [1, 2]. As medical and mental health professionals working in the field, it is increasingly important that steps are taken to improve the care and treatment of this population.

Case Example 1

Bob was a 45-year-old homeless Caucasian male. Bob presented to the local emergency department (ED) stating he was actively suicidal. He was discharged after 2 hours in the ED. Upon leaving the hospital, Bob walked half a mile from the hospital and died by suicide by overdosing on his psychiatric medication.

Case Example 2

Nick is a 39-year-old homeless Caucasian male who receives SSI benefits. He has a history of significant alcohol use and unstable housing. Nick has completed over ten rehabilitation programs but is unable to stay sober for more than 2 months due to his chronic homelessness.

Homelessness in the United States

The number of people in the United States who are classified as homeless continues to be significant. In 2016, over 549,900 people were homeless on any given night, with more than 176,357 of these individuals living on the street, in a car, or in an abandoned building [3, 4].

There are associated risks that can impact the health of this population, particularly from infectious diseases. Moreover, the homeless population is at risk for chronic medical conditions [2, 5]. For example, San Diego, California, has recently experienced a Hepatitis A outbreak that has taken the lives of 17 people [6]. This is concerning, as homeless individuals may be less likely to seek physical and mental health care on a regular basis [2, 7].

It is important to recognize personal bias and stigma associated with the homeless population. A study found that emergency medicine

L. Ronquillo (✉)
Alliant International University, San Diego, CA, USA

L. S. Zun et al. (eds.), *Behavioral Emergencies for Healthcare Providers*,
https://doi.org/10.1007/978-3-030-52520-0_34

physicians may be more likely to hold the belief that people choose to be homeless [8]. Moreover, medical school students may hold more negative beliefs toward this population at the end of clinical rotations rather than at the beginning of medical school [9]. Understanding personal beliefs and potential biases can help to ensure that patient care is not negatively impacted.

Homelessness in the Veteran Population

In 2016, almost 40,000 veterans were homeless on a single night [3]. The majority of these veterans were male [3]. Research has demonstrated that being a veteran may be associated with a higher risk of homelessness [10]. Similar to the general homeless population, substance use and mental illness were found to be significant risk factors for homeless veterans [11]. There are also important safety considerations for this population as suicide is a significant cause of premature death among veterans [12]. In addition, a study found that suicidality was associated with a longer period of homelessness within this population [13].

Mental Health and Co-occurring Disorders

Mental illness continues to be a national public health problem. In 2015, over 43 million adults in the United States were identified as having mental illnesses [14]. Moreover, 9.8 million adults have a serious mental illness [15]. On any given night, there are over half a million homeless individuals. Of that number, over 200,000 have a serious mental illness or chronic substance use disorder [4]. This is consistent with research that indicates people with a substance use disorder spend less time in stable housing [16].

While every person's presentation differs, it is not uncommon to see both mental health and substance use disorders together in the homeless population [2, 16]. Depression is a common mental health disorder comorbid with a substance use disorder among the homeless population, specifically with women [17]. Moreover, there may be a strong association with psychiatric disorders and suicide in homeless individuals [18].

Research has shown that homeless individuals with mental health concerns have increased emergency department visits [19, 20]. Although the homeless population utilizes the ED, there is a lack of treatment engagement in follow-up care through outpatient providers or alternative community referrals [19, 21]. Given that many homeless individuals have limited support and limited community engagement, having an interdisciplinary team available to meet the needs of this population likely maximizes the chance of successful therapeutic interventions [7, 21]. Full-service partnerships and Housing First programs have also been shown to be effective in this population in obtaining stable housing [21, 22]. Research has shown that suicidality can, in fact, be reduced with Housing First programs [23].

Issues in the Emergency Department Presentation

Homeless patients have been shown to have increased ED visits [24]. As the number of visits increase, homeless patients may initially be misidentified as "medication-seeking" or wanting a hot meal and/or shelter for the night. It is important to conduct thorough risk assessments for all patients presenting to the ED and to any crisis walk-in centers as a serious mental health problem or imminent risk may actually be the presenting problem. Environmental concerns play a role as well; extreme temperatures should factor into medical evaluations of homeless patients. Thus far, over 400,000 ED visits a year are a result of suicidal behavior such as suicide attempts [25].

If a patient is not determined to be at acute risk, referrals should always be given to crisis hotlines, short-term residential programs, crisis walk-in centers, and outpatient treatment for both mental health and substance use. Bob's case illustrates the need for complete and thorough risk assessments and appropriate referrals, despite initial presentations and possible provider perceptions.

Many homeless patients often use alcohol and other drugs to help them survive life on the street. In the case of Nick, he reports that he cannot remain sober if he is homeless because he cannot handle always being on alert at all hours of the night. This case is a reminder of the importance of providing referrals in the community that not only include mental health follow-up but also housing resources. It is important to note that, oftentimes, homeless shelters are in neighborhoods surrounded by readily available illicit substances and paraphernalia. Therefore, including multiple shelters and housing resources upon discharge is crucial for individuals who want to remain clean and sober.

Conclusion

Since the rate of homelessness in the United States continues to increase, it is important for emergency providers to complete thorough assessments and provide appropriate intervention and/or referrals as the ED is often the main point of contact for this population. If immediate contact cannot be made with members of a multidisciplinary team, a warm handoff is recommended. For example, a follow-up appointment scheduled or specific treatment provider recommendation could be more beneficial than simply handing a patient a list as they are walking out of the facility.

References

1. Opalach C, Romaszko J, Jaracz M, Kuchta R, Borkowska A, Buciński A. Coping styles and alcohol dependence among homeless people. Plos ONE (serial online). 2016;11(9):1–14. Ipswich, MA: Academic Search Premier. Accessed 29 Sept 2017.
2. Fazel S, Geddes JR, Kushel M. The health of homeless people in high-income countries: descriptive epidemiology, health consequences, and clinical and policy recommendations. Lancet. 2014;384(9953):1529–40. https://doi.org/10.1016/S0140-6736(14)61132-6.
3. U.S. Department of Housing and Urban Development, Office of Community Planning and Development. The 2016 Annual Homeless Assessment Report to Congress (AHAR). 2016. Available at https://www.hudexchange.info/resources/documents/2016-AHAR-Part-1.pdf. Accessed 20 Sept 2017.
4. Substance abuse and mental health services administration (SAMHSA). Homelessness and housing. 2017. Available at https://www.samhsa.gov/homelessness-housing. Accessed 20 Sept 2017.
5. Stenius-Ayoade A, Haaramo P, Erkkilä E, Marola N, Nousiainen K, Wahlbeck K, Eriksson JG. Mental disorders and the use of primary health care services among homeless shelter users in the Helsinki metropolitan area, Finland. BMC Health Serv Res. 2017;17:428.
6. NBC San Diego. San Diego County Hepatitis A Outbreak 2017. 2017. Available at http://www.nbcsandiego.com/news/health/Hepatitis-A-Outbreak-CDC-San-Diego-448021043.html. Accessed 29 Sept 2017.
7. Lamanna D, Stergiopoulos V, Durbin J, O'Campo P, Poremski D, Tepper J. Promoting continuity of care for homeless adults with unmet health needs: the role of brief interventions. Health & Social Care In The Community (serial online). 2017. Ipswich, MA: PsycINFO. Accessed 30 Sept 2017.
8. Morrison A, Roman B, Borges N. Psychiatry and emergency medicine: medical student and physician attitudes toward homeless persons. Acad Psychiatry (serial online). 2012;36(3):211–5.
9. Masson N, Lester H. The attitudes of medical students towards homeless people: does medical school make a difference? Med Educ. 2003;37:869–72.
10. Fargo J, Metraux S, Byrne T, et al. Prevalence and risk of homelessness among US veterans. Prev Chronic Dis. 2012;9:E45.
11. Tsai J, Rosenheck RA. Risk factors for homelessness among US veterans. Epidemiol Rev. 2015;37:177–95.
12. Katz I. Homelessness and premature mortality among veterans. Psych Serv (serial online). 2013;64(7):605.
13. Harris T, Kintzle S, Wenzel S, Castro C. Expanding the understanding of risk behavior associated with homelessness among veterans. Military Med (serial online). 2017;182(9):e1900–7.
14. The National Institute on Mental Health (NIMH). Any Mental Illness (AMI) Among U.S. Adults. 2016. Available at https://www.nimh.nih.gov/health/statistics/prevalence/any-mental-illness-ami-among-us-adults.shtml. Accessed 20 Sept 20, 2017.
15. The National Institute on Mental Health (NIMH). Serious Mental Illness (SMI) Among U.S. Adults. 2016. Available at https://www.nimh.nih.gov/health/statistics/prevalence/serious-mental-illness-smi-among-us-adults.shtml. Accessed 20 Sept 2017.
16. Urbanoski K, Veldhuizen S, Goering P, et al. Effects of comorbid substance use disorders on outcomes in a housing first intervention for homeless people with mental illness. Addiction (serial online). 2017. Ipswich, MA: PsycINFO. Accessed 27 Sept 2017.
17. Upshur C, Jenkins D, Weinreb L, Gelberg L, Orvek E. Prevalence and predictors of substance use disorders among homeless women seeking primary care: an 11 site survey. Am J On Addictions (serial online). 2017. Ipswich, MA: PsycINFO. Accessed 27 Sept 2017.

18. Feodor Nilsson S, Hjorthoj CR, Erlangsen A, Nordentoft M. Suicide and unintentional injury mortality among homeless people: a Danish nationwide register-based cohort study. Eur J Pub Health. 2014;24(1):50–6.
19. Lam CN, Arora S, Menchine M. Increased 30 day emergency department revisits among homeless patients with mental health conditions. West J Emerg Med. 2016;17(5):607–12.
20. Cherner R, Aubry T, and Ecker J. Predictors of the physical and psychological integration of homeless adults with problematic substance use. J Comm Psychiatry (Serial Online). 2017;45(1):65–80. Ipswich, MA: PsycINFO. Accessed 27 Sept 2017.
21. Gilmer TP, Stefancic A, Ettner SL, Manning WG, Tsemberis S. Effect of full-service partnerships on homelessness, use and costs of mental health services, and quality of life among adults with serious mental illness. Arch Gen Psychiatry. 2010;67(6):645–52.
22. Adair C, Streiner D, Goering P, et al. Outcome Trajectories among Homeless Individuals with Mental Disorders in a Multisite Randomised Controlled Trial of Housing First. Can J Psychiatry (Serial Online). 2017;62(1):30–39. Ipswich, MA: Academic Search Premier. Accessed 28 Sept 2017.
23. Collins S, Taylor E, Nelson L, et al. Suicidality among chronically homeless people with alcohol problems attenuates following exposure to housing first. Suicide Life Threat Behav (serial online). 2016;46(6):655–663. Ipswich, MA: PsycINFO. Accessed 29 Sept 2017.
24. Kushel MB, Perry S, Bangsberg D, Clark R, Moss AR. Emergency department use among the homeless and marginally housed: results from a community-based study. Am J Public Health. 2002;92(5):778–84.
25. Doshi A, Boudreaux ED, Wang N, Pelletier AJ, Camargo CA. National study of US emergency department visits for attempted suicide and self-inflicted injury, 1997–2001. Ann Emerg Med. 2005;46:369–75.

Behavioral and Neurocognitive Sequelae of Concussion in the Emergency Department

35

Andy Jagoda, Arjun Prabhu, and Silvana Riggio

Introduction

A concussion occurs when the brain is subjected to an acceleration-deceleration force or, as in the case of blast injury, to a pressure wave sufficient to disrupt brain function [1]. The 2013 American Academy of Neurology (AAN) guidelines on the evaluation and management of sports-related concussions define concussion as a "pathophysiologic disturbance in neurologic function characterized by clinical symptoms induced by biomechanical forces, occurring with or without loss of consciousness. Standard structural neuroimaging is normal, and symptoms typically resolve over time [1]." The terms "concussion" and "mild traumatic brain injury" (mTBI) are often used interchangeably in much of the literature and will be used, as well, in this chapter. However, an mTBI diagnosed by a Glasgow Coma Scale (GCS) score of 13–15 simply reflects that the patient at the time of measurement is alert; it is well known that patients can have a significant intracranial lesion, for example, subdural or traumatic subarachnoid, and yet have a GCS of 15. Concussion, on the other hand, implies that not only is the patient awake but also has normal head computed tomography (CT). The International Conference on Concussion in Sport 2012 Zurich Consensus Statement, therefore, describes a concussion as a distinct subtype of mild traumatic brain injury [2]. The decision about which patients should obtain emergent brain imaging in the emergency department is outside the scope of this chapter.

There is considerable controversy surrounding the diagnostic criteria needed to validate that a brain injury has occurred, and there is no agreed marker of injury that provides a gold standard [3]. There are a number of neurobehavioral sequelae, also referred to as "post-concussive symptoms," that have been associated with a concussion, encompassing a spectrum of somatic and neuropsychiatric symptoms (see Table 35.1).

The neuropsychiatric symptoms are subdivided into cognitive and behavioral categories. The development, severity, and duration of neurobehavioral sequelae vary; the literature is unclear on the impact of external stressors and conditions on the development and duration of these sequelae, but there is no question that the expression of these symptoms is multifactorial (see Fig. 35.1).

This figure demonstrates the number of factors that must be assessed and collated in the

A. Jagoda (✉) · A. Prabhu
Department of Emergency Medicine, Mount Sinai Health System, New York, NY, USA
e-mail: andy.jagoda@mssm.edu

S. Riggio
Department of Psychiatry and Neurology, Icahn School of Medicine at Mount Sinai, New York, NY, USA

L. S. Zun et al. (eds.), *Behavioral Emergencies for Healthcare Providers*,
https://doi.org/10.1007/978-3-030-52520-0_35

Table 35.1 Neurobehavioral sequelae from concussion

Neuropsychiatric
Cognitive: Deficits in attention, memory, executive function
Somatic: Sleep disturbance, fatigue, dizziness, vertigo, headaches, visual disturbances, nausea, sensitivity to light and sound, hearing loss, seizures
Behavioral
Primary psychiatric disorder
Mood disorder, anxiety
Personality disorder
Other

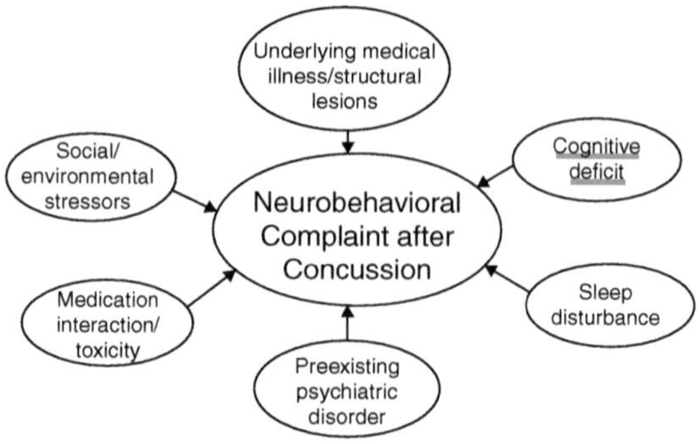

Fig. 35.1 Factors that must be assessed and collated in the evaluation of a patient presenting with a neurobehavioral complaint after a concussion

evaluation of a patient presenting with a neurobehavioral complaint after a concussion. For example, in a patient who complains of difficulty concentrating after a TBI, the clinician must consider the role of a primary injury on cognitive function, plus impact of comorbidities, for example, change in sleep pattern, new medications, and new social stressors since the accident

The DSM-IV-TR, which was released in 2000 as an update to the DSM-IV, proposed criteria for diagnosing "post-concussional disorder," which includes physical fatigue, disordered sleep, headaches, or vertigo/dizziness [4]. ICD-10 uses eight diagnostic criteria to make the diagnosis of post-concussive syndrome: fatigue, dizziness, poor concentration, memory problems, headache, insomnia, irritability, and reduced tolerance to stress, emotional excitement, or alcohol [5]. Few of these criteria are unique to brain trauma, thus making their diagnostic and prognostic significance of questionable value [6]. That said, these neurobehavioral sequelae are reported in the literature, and an awareness of them is important in evaluating, treating, and counseling patients who have sustained a concussion.

Released in 2013, the DSM-5 attempted to clarify diagnostic criteria by defining "major or mild neurocognitive disorder due to traumatic brain injury" as cognitive deficits following "an impact to the head or other mechanisms of rapid movement or displacement of the brain within the skull" associated with varying degrees of loss of consciousness, post-traumatic amnesia, disorientation and confusion, and neurological signs. By DSM-5 criteria, the severity of a TBI is categorized as mild, moderate, or severe based on the Glasgow Coma Scale and on the length of loss of consciousness (LOC) and post-traumatic amnesia (PTA) and disorientation/confusion at initial assessment. The utility of these classifications is limited by the caveat that the severity rating of a TBI does not always correspond to the severity of the resulting neurocognitive disorder.

The DSM-5's definition of a neurocognitive disorder is equally vague. According to the DSM-5, a "neurocognitive disorder" is defined as evidence of cognitive decline not exclusively in the context of delirium and not explained by another mental disorder. A neurocognitive disorder can be the result of vastly different underlying pathology such as Alzheimer's disease, HIV infection, and a TBI, among other causes. Thus, while perhaps more specific than past definitions, the DSM-5's definition of neurocognitive disorder from TBI remains ambiguous as a diagnostic tool for concussion [7].

Identifying clear criteria that define sequelae from a brain injury is encumbered by the lack of a standardized definition of what constitutes an mTBI/concussion. Much of the literature, including the DSM-5, uses the Glasgow Coma Scale (GCS) score for identifying the study population. The GCS was developed to facilitate communication between clinicians caring for patients with a severe TBI. It categorizes patients into three groups: coma, lethargic, and awake. The scale was developed prior to the widespread availability of computed tomography, and its use was never intended to supplant a careful neurologic and neurocognitive evaluation. The GCS score is limited in its ability to provide prognosis related to post-concussive symptoms after an mTBI. Likewise, neither a CT nor an MRI is sufficiently sensitive to diagnose the type of injuries that predispose patients to neurobehavioral sequelae.

Not all mTBI is the same, and sequelae that develop are most likely related to the localization and lateralization of the injury, to the medical and psychiatric comorbidities, and to the pre- and post-psychosocial factors. Neurocognitive testing supports the hypothesis that some types of concussion result in impairment in brain connectivity specifically as it relates to attention. It is the impairment in attention that can then lead to difficulty with concentration, visual tracking, and task performance—impairment in these activities contributes to headaches, difficulty focusing on tasks, and difficulty with sleep, all of which are common complaints in patients after an mTBI. The multiple factors that contribute to behavioral complaints after a concussion require that the clinician ascertain premorbid medical, neurological, and psychiatric conditions, obtain a history of drugs and medications, establish baseline occupational and social function, and identify psychological and social stressors.

Pathophysiology and Chronic Traumatic Encephalopathy

A sudden deceleration or rotational acceleration injury may generate sufficient shearing forces to result in axonal injury and edema, which has been implicated as a contributing factor to the development of some post-concussive symptoms [8]. Concussion was once graded according to the presence or absence of a PTA and/or an LOC; however, studies have failed to demonstrate a correlation between an LOC and a PTA on neurocognitive performance testing after injury [9, 10]. Thus, a brief LOC and duration of post-traumatic amnesia should not be used to predict outcome after a concussion, although the 2012 Zurich Consensus Statement recommends a cautious approach to those with an LOC of greater than 1 minute [2].

A cortical contusion can result in a loss of function served by a given brain area. White matter lesions can result in interruption of information being transmitted between cortical areas within the brain. Diffuse axonal injuries can result in slowed and inefficient information processing. There is also the possibility that head trauma causes traumatic tearing of neuronal connections, impairing cortical and thalamic circuitry, and contributing to cognitive impairment [11]. The impact of injury on neurotransmitter function is poorly defined but clearly could provide a biological explanation for some of the behavioral changes seen after a TBI. Clinical presentations after a TBI may correlate with the area of the brain most injured; for example, injury to the frontal region may result in behavior changes, while injury to the temporal region may result in memory disturbances.

Chronic Traumatic Encephalopathy (CTE)

CTE is a neurodegenerative condition associated with recurrent head injury and is currently diagnosed only by postmortem examination of brain tissue. Incidence and prevalence remain unknown and will likely require in vivo detection and diagnosis, but recent postmortem analysis by Bieniek et al. showed that 32% (21 of 66) of brains of contact sports athletes (primarily football and boxing) with a documented history of repetitive brain trauma (RBT) showed CTE pathology. No cases of CTE were found in control brains without a history of brain trauma or single traumatic brain injury [12]. Prospective clinical trials are underway.

CTE has been associated with both repeat concussion and a genetic predisposition. In boxers, the development of CTE has been associated with the number of years of boxing and the presence of the ApoE4 allele [13]. Male boxers with more than 12 professional bouts and the ApoE4 allele have twice the risk of CTE than matched controls without the allele [14].

While it is established that RBT is associated with CTE, it remains unclear whether clinically significant concussions, repetitive subclinical hits, or both lead to neurodegeneration; nor is it clear what the contribution of other factors are including alcohol, drug and medication use, and genetic predisposition. Regardless, it appears that axonal and cytoskeleton alternations from brain trauma lead to accumulations of abnormal protein aggregates expressed in neurofibrillary tangles, termed "tauopathy." These proteins include synuclein, ubiquitin, progranulin, TAR, DNA-binding protein 43, amyloid precursor protein, and its metabolite Aβ [15].

In 2015, the NINDS/NIBIB published results from the first consensus meeting to define neuropathological criteria for the diagnosis of CTE. The group of neuropathologists defined the pathognomonic lesion of CTE to be an abnormal accumulation of tau in neurons and astroglia distributed around small blood vessels of sulci in the cortex in irregular spatial patterns [16]. While TDP-43 and Aβ plaques are also seen in CTE, these are not unique to the disease, while the pathognomonic tau accumulations identified were not seen in other tauopathies, such as Alzheimer's disease or progressive supranuclear palsy [16]. Interestingly, the dementia of CTE is associated with neurofibrillary tangles and neuropil threads that are distributed in patches throughout the neocortex, but it spares the mesiotemporal region, which is generally affected by Alzheimer's disease. In addition, the neuropathology seen in CTE tauopathy does not have the amyloid plaques seen in Alzheimer's disease.

While advances have been made in postmortem diagnosis of CTE and RBT has been identified as the greatest risk factor for CTE's pathological features, more specific risk factors, premortem diagnosis, nature of onset, constellation of symptoms, and progression of the disease remain unsolved. Research into neuroimaging with structural or diffusion MRI and biomarkers (including PET signals) aims at elucidating diagnosis of CTE in living subjects, but low specificity and need for postmortem validation are limitations. Tau-binding radionuclide PET signal appears to be the most promising biomarker [17]. Diagnosing CTE clinically is equally problematic. Some researchers have attempted to define a "CTE clinical syndrome" but include broad, nonspecific impairment in cognitive function, behavior, and mood, with limited supporting data [18]. Further research will attempt to clarify these important details.

Epidemiology

The true incidence of concussion is unknown since the majority of cases are not recorded in any specific database. It is estimated that up to 4 million Americans sustain a recreational or sport-related concussion annually; approximately 1.5 million Americans have evaluated annually in emergency departments for an mTBI [19]. Post-deployment studies of soldiers fighting in Afghanistan and Iraq report that up to 25% of soldiers sustain a TBI, the majority of which are classified as "mild [20]." The sports medicine literature estimates that concussion represents 9% of all high school athletic injuries; the sports with the highest risk of concussion, in descending order of prevalence, are football, girls' soccer, boys' lacrosse, boys' soccer, girls' basketball, wrestling, and girls' lacrosse [21].

Up to 80% of patients with a concussion experience at least one neurobehavioral symptom for up to 3 months after the injury—most commonly, headache [22]. Up to 45% of mTBI patients meet ICD-10 criteria for the post-concussive syndrome at 5 days post-injury [6]. Use of different study populations and varying definitions contribute to the difference in the reported incidence of symptoms. Some of the risk factors that have been identified for the development of post-concussive symptoms include female gender, advanced age, pain, and prior affective or anxiety diagnoses [23, 24].

In approximately 15% of mild TBI patients, neurobehavioral sequelae persist beyond 3 months and may contribute to long-term social and occupational difficulties [25–27]. Cognitive dysfunction in the form of impaired attention, memory, and executive function has a predominant role in patients who experience persistent symptoms [22]. A meta-analysis of neuropsychologic outcomes after an mTBI reported that the majority of patients are back to baseline by 3 months; however, participants in litigation were reported to have longer-lasting cognitive sequelae, and litigation was associated with stable or worsening of cognitive functioning over time [28].

The sports literature supports the finding that the majority of adult athletes who sustain an mTBI return to baseline by 10 days [10, 29]. Children appear to return to baseline at a slower rate, with 40% in one study not at baseline after 2 weeks and 10% still not at baseline at 6 weeks [9]. Studies have tried to identify risk factors that lead to delayed recovery; however, thus far, no clinical factors, such as length of loss of consciousness or post-traumatic amnesia, have been found to predict which patients will have delayed recovery [30].

Patient Evaluation

Before focusing on the neurobehavioral complaints of the patient who has sustained a concussion, a comprehensive history and physical exam are required. The history focuses on the events preceding the concussion. Though LOS and PTA are important to identify, neither is prognostic in isolation. A careful neurologic exam is indicated to identify subtle deficits that may put the patient at risk for developing post-concussive symptoms or for sustaining another injury. In particular, subtle cranial nerve IV and VI injuries may cause headaches due to the visual disturbances, while postural instability identified on balance testing may result in falls. Deficits identified on attention testing (see neurocognition section below) may put the patient at risk for headaches or for accidents while driving. While specific criteria for concussion remain elusive, the sports community has developed a number of tools that assist in acute evaluations, including the Standardized Assessment of Concussion (SAC), the Balance Error Scoring System (BESS), and the Sports Concussion Assessment Tool 3 (SCAT3) [31]. However, none of these tools can be considered a gold standard for concussion assessment [32]. Research is ongoing to validate more specific clinical criteria for a diagnosis of concussion. A 2014 systematic review of the diagnostic criteria for concussion by Carney et al. found four promising indicators: (1) observed or documented disorientation or confusion, (2) impaired balance within 1 day after injury, (3) slower reaction time within 2 days after injury, and (4) impaired verbal learning and memory within 2 days after injury [33].

Diagnosis of concussion remains a clinical diagnosis at present, but researchers are looking into imaging and biomarker testing to aid in diagnosis. The American College of Emergency Physicians in partnership with the Centers for Disease Control developed guidelines identifying which patients with a concussion require a head CT [34]. Those guidelines do not provide insight into which patients are at risk for developing neurobehavioral sequelae. Magnetic resonance imaging (MRI) is more sensitive than CT for identifying contusions, petechial hemorrhage, and white matter injury; however, there are no clear guidelines on which patients require imaging, its timing, or its prognostic value [35]. Functional imaging (e.g., fMRI, PET, SPECT) looks at metabolic and blood flow changes in the brain, and there is emerging evidence that it may assist in documenting brain dysfunction after an injury. Research into these modalities suggests a complex relationship between cognitive load/attentional demand and neuronal activation, but patient heterogeneity and variations in scan time post-injury represent limitations [36]. Thus, at this time, functional imaging remains a research tool [35].

Diffusion tensor imaging (DTI) is used to study the structural images of white matter tracts in the brain. Studies show that in mTBI, the structural integrity of axons within the genu of the corpus callosum is affected, resulting in misalignment of fibers, edema, and axonal degeneration; this has been correlated with delays in reaction times [37]. At the current time, while DTI has been proven to detect axonal damage, which leads to an increased risk of developing post-concussive syndrome (PCS), there is insufficient evidence supporting any parameter in a specific brain region as a biomarker for diagnosing PCS [38]. Thus, at present, DTI is a research tool but holds the potential to be a diagnostic tool for concussion in the future.

Finally, the biomarker hypothesis of brain injury proposes that traumatic injury to the brain causes cellular damage and disintegration, resulting in a release of cell type-specific proteins into bio fluids (CSF and blood), and that the biomarker levels are associated with pathophysiologic mechanisms initiated by the trauma and correlate with the magnitude of the injury. Proteins that have been studied as potential brain biomarkers include those derived from neurons, ubiquitin C-terminal hydrolase (UCH-L1) and neuron-specific enolase (NSE), and those derived from glial cells, S100B, and glial fibrillary astrocytic protein (GFAP) [39]. While these biomarkers have shown promise, a multi-marker strategy will likely be needed to enhance the accuracy of diagnosis and outcome prediction, and a rigorous validation of brain damage biomarkers in a multicenter clinical trial will likely be necessary due to their limited individual sensitivities and specificities [39].

Post-concussive Cognitive Disorders and the Role of Neuropsychologic Testing

Cognitive dysfunction after a concussion plays a role in many of the symptoms expressed after injury. Cognitive impairment includes problems with information processing, decision-making, motor function, reaction time, and memory. As a consequence of these deficits, patients may become irritable, anxious, apathetic, or depressed. A clinical expression may be misinterpreted as secondary to a primary affective disorder and lead to unnecessary pharmacologic interventions.

The use of neurocognitive testing in athletes before and after injury has contributed to our understanding of post-concussive cognitive performance. The literature is not conclusive on which neurocognitive battery best assesses post-concussive performance; Table 35.2 lists the domains that are tested.

Table 35.2 Domains that can be evaluated in post-concussive cognitive testing

Verbal memory
Visual memory
Reaction time
Visual motor speed/processing speed
Impulse control
Fine motor speed
Working memory
Attention

Limiting much of the literature on cognitive testing are the absence of preinjury performance and the absence of reliable matched control data.

Historically, cognitive function has been assessed using paper and pencil tests such as Digit Symbol Substitution Test and Trail Making Tests. More recently, computerized test platforms—for example, ImPACT—have gained acceptance [31]. ImPACT specifically assesses verbal memory, visual memory, processing speed, and reaction time. A recent study examining the construct validity of ImPACT with traditional neuropsychological measures suggests that ImPACT is a good screening tool but one that must be used carefully with an understanding of its limitations—in particular, it is of more limited value if the premorbid baseline is not known [40].

An evaluation of the post-TBI cognitive function is essential with a focus on assessing attention versus memory. If attention is impaired, there will be difficulty in retaining information with obvious impact on memory and, thus, performance. If the patient has an underlying affective disorder, attention can also be impaired due to lack of interest and/or distractibility. Therefore, the assessment of memory must be placed in a context of attention, and a detailed psychiatric history is warranted to exclude other disorders that may interfere with performance.

Recently, the Department of Defense, Centers for Disease Control, and Brain Trauma Foundation have developed a multidisciplinary task force to assess the use of eye-tracking as a surrogate for attention in order to diagnose a concussion. Eye-tracking devices involve participants tracking a target moved along a circular trajectory; early results indicate that there may be ranges of stimulus frequencies that differentiate the effects of the concussion from normal individuals [41]. However, further research is required.

Cognitive deficits after a sports-related concussion generally resolve within 10 days [42, 43]. It is unclear if this pattern of recovery is followed in other populations, such as the elderly or patients with socioeconomic stressors. Resolving this time course is made more difficult since most patients do not have an established cognitive baseline. Neither an LOC nor a PTA predicts which patients are at risk for cognitive deficits after an mTBI [2]. Performance on neurocognitive testing compared to preinjury baseline, in combination with findings on symptom inventories, has been reported to improve the prognostic ability of either alone; however, the sensitivity of the combined findings in predicting protracted recovery was only 65%, and the specificity, 80% [44]. In an emergency department-based study using ImPACT, 25 mTBI patients were compared to 38 controls [45]. The authors reported a subtle deficit in visual motor speed and reaction time; the verbal and visual memory score did not reflect a deficit. Long-term deficits were not assessed; thus, the study is limited in its ability to offer prognostic information. However, the study does demonstrate that computer-based neurocognitive testing can be performed in the ED and may provide a baseline that is helpful in discharge planning (i.e., return to work) and follow-up (i.e., the need to see a TBI specialist).

Post-concussive Behavioral Disorders

Behavioral manifestations of a concussion may be due to the injury, to underlying psychopathologies, or to medical comorbidities. Symptoms may also be due to an emotional response to the injury, its physical limitations, or fear of the impact on function. Radhakrishnan et al. concluded, based on a careful review of the available literature, that development of post-concussive behavioral disorders is likely due to a combination of factors such as psychological stress, preexisting vulnerabilities, and brain dysfunction [46]. Interestingly, while concussion can lead to these behavioral manifestations, behavior components themselves (such as premorbid psychiatric, cognitive, and personality factors) have also been found to be associated with a greater severity of the post-concussive syndrome [47].

Personality Changes

Affective and behavioral disturbances after a TBI may be expressed as personality changes appreciated by the patient or her family/caregiver. Personality changes may include aggression, impulsivity, irritability, emotional lability, or apathy [48]. Impulsivity and irritability may lead to verbal and physical inappropriateness expressed as verbal outbursts or combativeness. These personality changes may be due to impaired judgment secondary to an underlying structural lesion or the exacerbation of an underlying psychiatric disorder or to an emotional response to trauma. Aggression is a commonly reported behavioral symptom of a TBI but is reported more frequently after a moderate or severe TBI. Risk factors for aggression after a TBI include frontal lobe injury, premorbid psychiatric disorders, and/or alcohol or substance abuse.

Major Depression

Major depression has been reported as a sequela of concussion, both acutely but also long term. The actual prevalence is unknown with considerable variation in studies. An estimated 12–44% of individuals experience some degree of depression within the first 3 months following an mTBI [49, 50]. Additionally, the degree to which a premorbid psychiatric disorder increases the risk for post-concussive major depression is unclear, but studies indicate a positive correlation, especially in the more severe category of TBI. Risk factors for developing major depression after a TBI fall into two categories: premorbid psychiatric pathology and low socioeconomic status. For instance, depression is 43 times more likely if the patient was previously diagnosed with PTSD. The relationship between rates of depression and the severity of a TBI is unclear.

Studies have found a link between a TBI and suicidality, as well as between psychiatric comorbidity in the setting of a TBI and suicidality [51]. In a retrospective study of 5034 patients, Silver et al. reported that a history of TBI with LOC posed a four times greater likelihood of attempted suicide than in those without a TBI: 8.1% versus 1.9% [52]. This risk of suicide attempt remained even after controlling for demographics, quality-of-life variables, alcohol abuse, and any comorbid psychiatric disorders. Interestingly, research to date has not shown an association between CTE and suicidality [53].

Post-traumatic Stress Disorder (PTSD) and Anxiety

Some studies report an increased risk of developing a new anxiety disorder after an mTBI [54]. Other studies have demonstrated a similar incidence of anxiety disorders in mTBI patients and non-head-injured trauma patients, suggesting that the brain injury per se is not responsible for the development of the new behavior disorder [6, 55]. Increased age, a history of post-traumatic stress disorder (PTSD), and an avoidant coping style increase the risk of acute stress symptoms after a TBI [55]. In turn, a diagnosis of acute stress disorder is a risk factor for the development of PTSD after a TBI: In a study of 79 patients with a mild TBI, Bryant and Harvey diagnosed 14% of the patients with acute stress disorder at 1 month, and 24% were diagnosed with PTSD at 6 months post-injury; 82% of the patients diagnosed with acute stress disorder had developed PTSD by 6 months [56].

Qureshi et al. performed a systematic review of the literature, looking at cognition including memory in PTSD patients versus those patients exposed to trauma but without PTSD [57]. The authors reported that there exists a relationship between cognitive impairment in PTSD that is not seen in trauma patients who do not have PTSD. However, the authors emphasize that premorbid conditions and associated socioeconomic factors impact cognitive performance and that more study is required.

The relationship between a TBI and PTSD remains controversial. There is the possibility that the two conditions are not coincidental but rather that a TBI may increase the risk of developing PTSD following a psychological trauma [58]. Physical injury of any type, even if not involving the brain, has been reported to increase the risk of developing PTSD [59]. It remains unknown if a neural insult might alter reactions to psychological stressors and increase the likelihood that PTSD will develop. Current biological models of PTSD postulate that key frontal and limbic structures, including the prefrontal cortex, amygdala, and hippocampus, are involved in the development of PTSD [60].

A growing literature is beginning to address the issue of overlap between PTSD and an mTBI, and the data also is unclear about whether a relationship exists. One recently published structured interview-based study showed no association between an mTBI and PTSD [61], whereas another study found that PTSD was more common in those with an mTBI (46%) compared to those without an mTBI (23%) [62]. Hoge et al. surveyed over 2700 US Army infantry soldiers from two brigades 3–4 months after returning from a 1-year deployment in Iraq [63]. Fifteen percent of the soldiers reported having sustained a TBI; all but four of the 384 TBIs reported were mTBIs. In soldiers who reported an mTBI, complaints of a headache, poor memory, and lack of concentration were frequent, suggesting that a persistent post-concussive syndrome was present. Of those reporting a TBI with a LOC, 44% met criteria for PTSD, while PTSD was present in 27% of those reporting altered mental status without an LOC. In addition, major depression was present in 23% and 8%, respectively. This high coincidence of PTSD and depression led the authors to perform a covariate analysis for the two disorders, and interestingly, after adjusting for the coexistence of PTSD and depression, an mTBI history was no longer significantly associated with adverse physical health outcomes or symptoms, except for a headache. More recent data also suggest that PTSD and depression are significantly associated with most other mental health diagnoses post-concussion, and depression itself is more likely to occur post-concussion in individuals who have PTSD [61].

Substance Use Disorders

A review of the literature by van Reekum et al. reported a 22% prevalence of substance abuse in TBI patients versus a 15% lifetime prevalence in the general population [49]. A review of subsequent studies by Rogers et al. in 2007 showed a prevalence of 12% [64]. Premorbid substance use has been found to be strongly associated with post-TBI drug use, and multiple studies have cited substance abuse as a risk factor for a TBI rather than the other way around. A 30-year longitudinal study by Koponen et al. showed that 71% of TBI patients who were using drugs currently also had done so pre-TBI [65]. Interestingly, the co-occurrence of a TBI, substance abuse, and other mental health disorders appears to exacerbate symptoms of each and may have additive effects on self-regulation [66].

Post-concussive Somatic Symptoms

Prevalence of post-concussive headache varies greatly by study, ranging from 25% to 90% of patients, making it the most common post-concussive symptom [67]. Post-concussive headaches are classified as acute or chronic. According to the International Headache Society, acute post-traumatic headaches begin within 2 weeks of the injury and resolve within 2 months; chronic post-traumatic headaches begin within 2 weeks and persist for more than 8 weeks [68]. A headache often presents concomitantly with other post-concussive symptoms. Up to one-third of post-concussive headache patients may have depression, and about one-quarter may have insomnia, while anxiety and cognitive issues are also common [69]. One study reported that 53% of patients with a post-concussive headache had at least one other somatic complaint (fatigability, sleep disturbance, dizziness, or alcohol intolerance), 49% had at least one cognitive complaint (memory dysfunction or impaired concentration/attention), 26% had at least one psychiatric complaint (irritability, aggressiveness, anxiety, depression, or emotional labiality), 17% had all three types of complaints, and 17% had none [70].

A history of a headache before the TBI increases the risk of post-traumatic headaches, though in the majority of these cases, the headaches resolve within 3–6 months [70]. An age of less than 60 is also a risk factor for the development of a post-traumatic headache [69]. The presence of a post-traumatic headache has not been consistently correlated with the severity of the injury; in fact, some authors have reported that mild TBI patients have higher rates of a headache during the initial post-traumatic phase than patients with the more severe injury [71].

Dizziness/Nausea

Dizziness is the second most commonly reported somatic symptom after a concussion [72]. Most studies do not differentiate post-traumatic dizziness from vertigo, though the pathophysiology may be greatly different. Vertigo, characterized by the appearance of movement of the environment around oneself, may be peripheral or central in etiology. Peripheral etiologies include cupulolithiasis, perilymphatic fistula, post-traumatic Meniere's disease, damage to the vestibular nerve, and use of ototoxic medications. Central etiologies include damage to the brain stem involving the vestibular nucleus. Dizziness/vertigo is reported in 67–77% of mild TBI patients acutely—significantly higher than the prevalence in non-TBI patients in the community [72, 73]. Dizziness following a concussion has also been implicated as a risk factor for prolonged recovery [73].

Fatigue

Fatigue is a commonly reported, potentially debilitating sequelae after a concussion [74]. The presence of fatigue is associated with poorer social integration, decreased level of productive activities, and decreased overall quality of life [48]. In a recent prospective cohort study of patients 11–22 years old presenting with an acute concussion, 59.8% of patients had persisting fatigue after 1 week and 21.6% after 1 month

[75]. When fatigue persists, it may present a barrier to recovery [76]. Severity of a TBI and age have not been found to be predictors of severity of fatigue. Post-TBI fatigue is most likely the result of a combination of etiologies. Studies have shown that fatigue can be associated with a number of other post-concussive symptoms [77]. Hypopituitarism, with resultant neuroendocrine abnormalities such as growth hormone deficiency and cortisol deficiency, may also be associated with post-TBI fatigue [78]. Other possible contributing factors to fatigue include vertigo, diplopia, insomnia, and iatrogenic causes, such as psychotropic or analgesic medications.

Sleep Disturbance

Sleep disturbances include difficulties in initiating sleep, maintaining sleep, or attaining restful sleep, as well as excessive daytime somnolence and, less commonly, parasomnias. Sleep disturbances are reported in up to 70% of post-TBI patients, which is greater than the 32–35% prevalence reported in the general population [79, 80]. A retrospective cohort study showed that compared to healthy controls, 49% of TBI patients had significantly poorer sleep quality and 24% had higher levels of daytime sleepiness [81, 82]. Additionally, individuals with preexisting sleep problems may have more severe cognitive impairment and headaches following concussion [83]. Sleep disturbance has not been clearly linked to severity of a TBI, with a headache, anxiety, and depression being higher risk factors for insomnia than the severity of the TBI [84, 85]. Abnormalities on polysomnography in mild TBI patients with chronic sleep disturbance have been shown, and as with all the other somatic symptoms, the etiology is complex and therefore takes more than a prescription to solve.

Seizures

A convulsion immediately after a concussion can occur, and the best available evidence suggests that these convulsions are benign and not associated with any adverse clinical, cognitive, or neuroimaging outcomes [86]. In fact, the 2012 Zurich Consensus Statement specifically states that "impact seizures do not reliably predict outcome after concussion [2]." Post-traumatic seizures developing in the days to years after a concussion are relatively rare but can occur and can present as focal or generalized, motor, or nonmotor (e.g., complex partial). Complex partial seizures and other nonmotor convulsions present with a spectrum of behavioral changes ranging from inattention to psychosis; these events generally have a sudden onset and relatively sudden change back to baseline behavior, with or without a significant postictal period. For the clinician, nonconvulsive seizures are in the differential of patients with atypical changes in behavior that cannot be explained; a past history of brain injury, even an mTBI, may be the key to pursuing the diagnosis.

Balance

Of all the physical findings after a concussion, balance has emerged as the most sensitive and specific in the identification that an injury has occurred. The Balance Error Scoring System (BESS) is the most frequently used tool in sports. It tests a combination of three stances on various footing surfaces; each stance is observed with eyes closed and hands on hips, and error points are given for various responses, for example, opening eyes or lifting hands off the hips [37]. Studies in college football players report that 36% of concussed players have an impaired BESS score, compared to 5% in controls; 24% of those impaired remained impaired at 2 days and 9% at 7 days. Transient impairments in balance have been found to typically last between 3 and 10 days post-injury [73].

Post-concussive Symptoms in Nonconcussed Patients

In a provocative study, Iverson and McCracken studied the prevalence of post-TBI symptoms in patients with non-TBI chronic medical conditions. They reported that 94% of these patients met criteria for commonly ascribed post-concussive symptoms [87]. They reported disturbed sleep, fatigue, and/or irritability in 81% of patients and one or more cognitive problems in 42% of patients. Other authors have reported similar findings [88, 89]. Meares et al. performed a prospective study at a Level 1 trauma center. Ninety patients with a mild TBI were compared to 85 with non-brain injury trauma; both groups had the same incidence of symptoms with the strongest predictor of symptoms in either group being a previous affective disorder [6]. Though this study questions the existence of a unique neurobehavioral sequelae of an mTBI, a limitation of its design assigned MVA patients with a non-LOC or PTA to the control group, while indeed by mechanism alone, they would have been subject to a cranial acceleration/deceleration injury.

A correlation between pain and post-concussive symptoms has been reported, and pain has been associated with the persistence of symptoms [89]. Hart et al. reported that pain after a TBI was associated with cognitive impairment, including deficits in attention, memory, processing speed, and reaction time. The occurrence of cognitive complaints in non-TBI chronic pain patients has been demonstrated, once again questioning the relationship between a TBI per se and NBS [88].

Discharge Planning and Return to Full Activities

The key in the diagnosis and management of post-TBI complaints is to avoid premature closure on a diagnosis, to coordinate care through a multidisciplinary team, and to involve the patient and her family in decision-making. There is evidence to support the benefit of education and reassurance after TBI on an outcome. Ponsford et al. studied 202 mTBI patients and reported that patients who were given an information booklet on mTBI and coping strategies for symptoms were significantly less symptomatic at 3 months than those who were not provided education [25]. An extensive review of articles on early intervention after a mild TBI by Borg et al. showed that early educational information reduces long-term complaints [90].

Cognitive and physical rest have long been thought to be key components of recovery. The American Academy of Pediatrics recommends that children who have sustained a concussion be provided an environment conducive to recovery, which may include temporary leave of absence from school, shortened school days, a reduction in work, and elongated time to complete tasks and exams [31]. In general, it is recommended that physical exertion is minimized initially and then gradually increased as tolerated. A return of symptoms with a physician or mental stress is an indication that recovery is not complete and that more time is needed. The 2012 Zurich Consensus Guidelines state that an initial period of rest in the acute symptomatic period after injury (24–48 hours) may be of benefit, with a gradual return to low-level exercise, but concede that there is an absence of evidence-based recommendations. The sports community recommends a strict resolution of symptoms before return to play. The 2012 Zurich Consensus Guidelines indicate that return to play should not occur on the day of concussive injury with a stepwise return to play from no activity to light aerobic exercise, sport-specific exercise, noncontact training drills, full-contact practice, and, finally, return to play. If any post-concussive symptoms occur while in the stepwise program, the patient should drop back to the previous asymptomatic level and try to progress again after a further 24-hour period of rest has passed [2]. Alcohol is contraindicated during the recovery phase.

Despite being key components of treatment, cognitive and physical rest are supported by limited research. An alternate hypothesis has emerged that physical activity can be helpful, particularly in patients with symptoms persisting beyond 1 month after initial injury. In a 2017 systemic review and meta-analysis, Lal et al. analyzed 14 studies, including five randomized control trials, studying the effect of physical exercise after a concussion and found that physical exercise appears to improve the post-concussion symptom scale

Table 35.3 Components of the concussion symptom inventory

Headache
Nausea
Balance problems/dizziness
Fatigue
Drowsiness
Feeling like "in a fog"
Difficulty concentrating
Difficulty remembering
Sensitivity to light
Sensitivity to noise
Blurred vision
Feeling slowed down

Modified from Randolph et al. [60]

(PCSS) score and symptoms [91]. Further research is required to validate treatment of concussion.

In sports, Randolph et al. have developed the "Concussion Symptom Inventory" (CSI), which may be useful in monitoring recovery and determining return to play [92]. This inventory was derived from 27 symptom variables, and the final 12 symptoms that comprise the inventory are listed in Table 35.3.

At a minimum, the CSI provides a framework for clinicians to use following patients after a concussion. The scale is not validated, nor has it been correlated with long-term prognosis.

Recognizing the possibility of an mTBI patient developing neurobehavioral sequelae, education is a key component of the discharge process. The CDC has collaborated with the American College of Emergency Physicians (ACEP) to develop sample discharge instructions that inform patients when to return to the ED versus when to seek follow-up care with a clinician experienced in sequelae of TBI [93]. A key component of those discharge instructions includes information about post-concussive symptoms and recommendations on when to return to work/school/sports.

Conclusion

Neurobehavioral sequelae after concussion may have both somatic and neuropsychiatric components. The neuropsychiatric symptoms are divided into cognitive and behavioral. Expression of the sequelae is multifactorial, and there is evidence of a genetic contribution. The clinical presentations must be placed in the context of the patient's premorbid state. The evaluation consists of a history, physical, neurologic, and psychiatric examination. A careful assessment of attention and cognition and of cranial nerves and balance may identify subtle indicators that an injury has occurred. The role of neuroimaging is of limited value in the evaluation of a patient who has sustained a concussion; functional imaging and serum biomarkers may have a future role. Management strategies are based on placing the findings on an exam in context of the patient's premorbid state and social context. An education intervention is an important part of the patient's care plan, allowing the patient and family to understand the course of recovery.

Minimizing physical and mental stress immediately after injury and then allowing for a gradual return to full activity have been thought to maximize outcomes, but some recent research suggests benefits of physical exercise. Caution against driving and using alcohol until symptoms resolve is advised; pharmacotherapy, in general, is not indicated. Referral to a specialist with expertise in traumatic brain injury should be provided for those cases in which symptoms have not resolved within 2 weeks post-injury. Finally, CTE is a neurodegenerative disease diagnosed by postmortem pathologic analysis associated with repetitive brain trauma with genetic factors also playing a role. Further research is required to elucidate more specific risk factors, diagnosis in living patients, a constellation of symptoms, and diagnostic or clinical tools to monitor the progression of a disease.

References

1. Elder G, Mitsis E, Ahlers S, Cristian A. Blast-induced mild traumatic brain injury. Psych Clin No Amer. 2010;33:757–82.
2. McCrory P, Meeuwisse WH, Aubry M, Cantu RC, Dvorak J, Echemendia RJ, et al. Consensus statement on concussion in sport: the 4th International Conference on Concussion in Sport held in Zurch. Br J Sports Med. 2013;47:250–8.
3. Ruff R, Iverson G, Barth J, Bush SS, Broshek DK, NAN Policy and Planning Committee. Recommendations

for diagnosing a mild traumatic brain injury: a National Academy of Neuropsychology education paper. Arch Clin Neuropsychol. 2009;24:3–10.
4. American Psychiatric Association. Diagnostic and statistical manual of mental disorders (text revision). Washington, DC: American Psychiatric Association; 2000.
5. World Health Organization. The ICD-10 classification of mental and behavioral disorders: clinical descriptions and diagnostic guidelines. Geneva: World Health Organization; 1992.
6. Meares S, Shores E, Taylor A, Batchelor J, Bryant RA, Baguley IJ, et al. Mild traumatic brain injury does not predict acute postconcussion syndrome. J Neurol Neurosurg Psychiatry. 2008;79:300–6.
7. American Psychiatric Association. Diagnostic and statistical manual of mental disorders. 5th ed: American Psychiatric Publishing; 2013. p. 592–627.
8. Zink B, Szmydynger-Chodobska J, Chodobski A. Emerging concepts in the pathophysiology of traumatic brain injury. Psych Clin No Amer. 2010;33:741–56.
9. Thomas D, Collins M, Saladino R, et al. Identifying neurocognitive deficits in adolescents following concussion. Acad Emerg Med. 2011;18:246–54.
10. McCrory P, Meeuwisse W, Johnston K, Dvorak J, Aubry M, Molloy M, et al. Consensus statement on concussion in sport: the third International Conference on concussion in Sport held in Zurich, November 2008. Physc Sports Med. 2009;37:141–59.
11. DeKosky S, Ikonomovic M, Gandy S. Traumatic brain injury: football, warfare, and long-term effects. New Engl J Med. 2010;363:1293–6.
12. Bieniek KF, Ross OA, Cormier KA, Walton RL, Soto-Ortolaza A, Johnston AE, et al. Chronic traumatic encephalopathy pathology in a neurodegenerative disordered brain bank. Acta Neuropathol. 2015;130:877–99.
13. McCrory P. Sports concussion and the risk of chronic neurological impairment. Sport Med. 2011;21:6–12.
14. Jordan B, Reikin N Ravdin L, Jacobs AR, Bennett A, Gandy S. Apolipoprotein E episolon4 associated with traumatic brain injury in boxing. JAMA. 2007;278:136–40.
15. McKee A, Cantu R, Nowinski C, Hedley-Whyte ET, Gavett BE, Budson AE, et al. Chronic traumatic encephalopathy: progressive tauopathy after repetitive head injury. J Neuropathol Exp Neurol. 2009;68:709–735.17.
16. McKee AC, Cairns NJ, Dickson DW, Folkerth RD, Keene CD, Litvan I, et al. The first NINDS/NIBIB consensus meeting to define neuropathological criteria for the diagnosis of chronic traumatic encephalopathy. Acta Neuropathol. 2016;131:75–86.
17. Sparks P, Lawrence T, Hinze S. Neuroimaging in the diagnosis of chronic traumatic encephalopathy: a systematic review. Clin J Sport Med. 2017. Epub ahead of print
18. Asken BM, Sullan MJ, DeKosky ST, Jaffee MS, Buaer RM. Research gaps and controversies in chronic traumatic encephalopathy: a review. JAMA Neurol. 2017;74:1255–62.
19. Division of Injury and Disability Outcomes and Programs, National Center for Injury Prevention and Control, Centers for Disease Control and Prevention, and Department of Health and Human Services. Traumatic Brain Injury in the United States: Emergency Department Visits, Hospitalizations, and Deaths. October 2004.
20. Terrio H, Brenner L, Ivins B, Cho JM, Helmick K, Schwab K, et al. Traumatic brain injury screening: preliminary findings in a US Army brigade combat team. J Head Trauma Rehabil. 2009;24:14–23.
21. Lincoln A, Caswell S, Almquist J, Dunn RE, Norris JB, Hinton RY. Trends in concussion incidence in high school sports: a prospective 11 year study. Am J Sports Med. 2011;20:1–6.
22. Lundin A, de Boussard C, Edman G, Borg J. Symptoms and disability until 3 months after mild TBI. Brain Inj. 2006;20:799–806.
23. Meares S, Shores EA, Taylor AJ, Batchelor J, Bryant RA, Baguley IJ, et al. The prospective course of postconcussion syndrome: the role of mild traumatic brain injury. Neuropsychol. 2011;25:454–65.
24. King NS. A systematic review of age and gender factors in prolonged post-concussion symptoms after mild head injury. Brain Inj. 2014;28:1639–45.
25. Ponsford J, Willmott C, Rothwell A. Impact of early intervention on outcome following mild head injury in adults. J Neurol Neurosurg Psychiatry. 2002;73:330–2.
26. Ruff RM, Camenzuli L, Mueller J. Miserable minority: emotional risk factors that influence the outcome of a mild traumatic brain injury. Brain Inj. 1996;(8):61–5.
27. Moran B, Tadikonda P, Sneed KB, Hummel M, Guiteau S, Coris EE. Postconcussive syndrome following sports-related concussion: a treatment overview for primary care physicians. South Med J. 2015;108:553–8.
28. Belanger H, Curtiss G, Demery J, Lebowitz BK, Vanderploeg RD. Factors moderating neuropsychological outcomes following mild traumatic brain injury: a meta analysis. J Internat Neuropsychol Soc. 2005;11:215–27.
29. Zuckerman SL, Lee YM, Odom MJ, Solomon GS, Forbes JA, Sills AK. Recovery from sports-related concussion: days to return to neurocognitive baseline in adolescents versus young adults. Surg Neurol Int. 2012;3:130.
30. Makdissi M. Is the simple vs. complex classification of concussion a valid and useful differentiation? Br J Sports Med. 2009;43(Suppl. 1):i23–7.
31. Halstead M, report WKC. Sport-related concussion in children and adolescents. Pediat. 2010;126:597–615.
32. Echemendia RJ, Iverson GL, McCrea M, Macciocchi SN, Gioia GA, Putukian M, et al. Advances in neuropsychological assessment of sport-related concussion. Br J Sports Med. 2013;47:294–8.
33. Carney N, Ghajar J, Jagoda A, Bedrick S, Davis-O'Reilly C, du Coudray H, et al. Executive summary

of concussion guidelines step 1: systematic review of prevalent indicators. Neurosurgery. 2014;75:S1–2.
34. Jagoda A, Bazarian J, Bruns JJ Jr, Cantrill SV, Gean AD, Howard PK, et al. Clinical policy: neuroimaging and decision-making in adult mild traumatic brain injury in the acute setting. Clin Ann Emerg Med. 2008;52:714–48.
35. Jantzen K, Anderson B, Steinberg F, Kelso J. A prospective functional MRE imaging study of mild traumatic brain injury in college football players. Am J Neuroradiol. 2004;25:738–45.
36. Mayer AR, Bellgowan PS, Hanlon FM. Functional magnetic resonance imaging of mild traumatic brain injury. Neurosci Biobehav Rev. 2015;49:8–18.
37. Davis G, Iverson G, Guskiewicz K, Ptito A, Johnston KM. Contributions of neuroimaging, balance testing, electrophysiology, and blood markers to the assessment of sport related concussion. Br J Sports Med. 2009;43:36–45.
38. Khong E, Odenwald N, Hashim E, Cusimano MD. Diffusion tensor imaging findings in post-concussion syndrome patients after mild traumatic brain injury: a systematic review. Front Neurol. 2016;7:156.
39. Mondello S, Schmid K, Berger RP, Kobeissy F, Italiano D, Jeromin D, et al. The challenge of mild traumatic brain injury: role of biochemical markers in diagnosis of brain damage. Med Res Rev. 2014;34:503–31.
40. Maerlender A, Flashman L, Kessler A, Kumbhani S, Greenwald R, Tosteson T, et al. Examination of the construct validity of ImPACT computerized test, traditional and experimental neuropsychological measures. Clin Neuropsychol. 2010;24:1309–25.
41. Maruta J, Jaw E, Modera P, Pajashekar U, Spielman LA, Ghajar J. Frequency responses to visual tracking stimuli may be affected by concussion. Mil Med. 2017;182:120–3.
42. Bleiberg J, Cernich AN, Cameron K, Sun W, Peck K, Ecklund PJ, et al. Duration of cognitive impairment after sports concussion. Neurosurgery. 2004;54:1073–80.
43. McCrea M, Guskiewicz KM, Marshall SW, Barr W, Randolph C, Cantu RC, et al. Acute effects and recovery time following concussion in collegiate football players: the NCAA concussion study. JAMA. 2003;290:2556–63.
44. Lau B, Collins M, Lovell M. Sensitivity and specificity of subacute computerized neurocognitive testing and symptom evaluation in predicating outcomes after sports related concussion. Am J Sports Med. 2011;20:1–8.
45. Peterson S, Stull M, Collins M, Wang H. Neurocognitive function of emergency department patients with mild traumatic brain injury. Ann Emerg Med. 2009;53:796–803.
46. Radhakrishnan R, Garakani A, Gross L, Goin MK, Pine J, Slaby AE, et al. Neuropsychiatric aspects of concussion. Lancet Psych. 2016;3:1166–75.
47. Morgan CD, Zuckerman SL, King LE, Beaird SE, Sills AK, Solomon GS. Post-concussion syndrome (PCS) in a youth population: defining the diagnostic value and cost-utility of brain imaging. Childs Nerv Syst. 2015;31:2305–9.
48. Tateno A, Jorge RE, Robinson RG. Clinical correlates of aggressive behavior after traumatic brain injury. J Neuropsych Clin Neurosci. 2003;15:155–60.
49. van Reekum R, Cohen T, Wong J. Can traumatic brain injury cause psychiatric disorders? J Neuropsych Clin Neurosci. 2000;12:316–27.
50. Broshek DK, De Marco AP, Freeman JR. A review of post-concussion syndrome and psychological factors associated with concussion. Brain Inj. 2015;29:228–37.
51. Simpson G, Tate R. Suicidality in people surviving a traumatic brain injury: prevalence, risk factors and implications for clinical management. Brain Inj. 2007;21:1335–51.
52. Silver JM, Kramer R, Greenwald S, Weissman M. The association between head injuries and psychiatric disorders: findings from the New Haven NIMH Epidemiologic Catchment Area Study. Brain Inj. 2001;15:935–45.
53. Manley G, Gardner AJ, Schneider KJ, Guskiewicz KM, Bailes J, Cantu RC, et al. A systematic review of potential long-term effects of sport-related concussion. Br J Sports Med. 2017;51:969–77.
54. Mooney G, Speed J. The association between mild traumatic brain injury and psychiatric conditions. Brain Inj. 2001;15:865–77.
55. Bryant RA. Posttraumatic stress disorder and traumatic brain injury: can they co-exist? Clin Psychol Rev. 2001;21:931–45.
56. Bryant RA, Harvey AG. Relationship between acute stress disorder and posttraumatic stress disorder following mild traumatic brain injury. Am J Psych. 1998;155:635–29.
57. Qureshi S, Long M, Bradshaw M, Pyne JM, Magruder KM, Kimbrell T, et al. Does PTSD impair cognition beyond the effect of trauma. J Neurospych Clin Neurosci. 2011;23:16–28.
58. Gil S, Caspi Y, Ben-Ari IZ, Koren D, Klein E. Does memory of a traumatic event increase the risk of posttraumatic stress disorder in patients with traumatic brain injury? A prospective study. Am J Psych. 2005;162:963–9.
59. Koren D, Norman D, Cohen A, Berman J, Klein EM. Increased PTSD risk with combat-related injury: a matched comparison study of injured and uninjured soldiers experiencing the same combat events. Am J Psych. 2005;162:276–82.
60. Liberzon I, Sripada CS. The functional neuroanatomy of PTSD: a critical review. Prog Brain Res. 2008;167:151–69.
61. Walker WC, Franke LM, McDonald SD. Prevalence of mental health conditions after military blast exposure, their co-occurrence, and their relation to mild traumatic brain injury. Brain Inj. 2015;29:1581–8.

62. Nelson NW, Hoelzle JB, Doane BM. Neuropsychological outcomes of US veterans with report of remote blast-related concussion and current psychopathology. J Int Neuropsychol Soc. 2012;18:845–55.
63. Hoge CW, McGurk D, Thomas JL, Thomas JL, Cox AL, Engel CC, et al. Mild traumatic brain injury in U.S. Soldiers returning from Iraq. N Engl J Med. 2008;358:453–63.
64. Rogers J, Read C. Psychiatric co-morbidity following traumatic brain injury. Brain Inj. 2007;21:1321–33.
65. Koponen S, Taiminen T, Portin A. Axis I and II psychiatric disorders after traumatic brain injury: a 30-year follow-up study. Am J Psych. 2002;159:1315–21.
66. Cernich AN, Chandler L, Scherdell T, Kurtz S. Assessment of co-occurring disorders in veteran diagnosed with traumatic brain injury. J Head Trauma Rehabil. 2012;27:253–60.
67. Uomoto JM, Esselman PC. Traumatic brain injury and chronic pain: differential types and rates by head injury severity. Arch Phys Med Rehab. 1993;74:61–4.
68. Baandrup L, Jensen R. Chronic post-traumatic headache: a clinical analysis in relation to the international headache classification. Second ed. Cephalgia. 2005;25:132–8.
69. Minen MT, Boubour A, Walia H, Barr W. Post-concussive syndrome: a focus on post-traumatic headache and related cognitive, psychiatric, and sleep issues. Curr Neurol Neurosci Rep. 2016;16:100.
70. Packard RC. Epidemiology and pathogenesis of posttraumatic headache. J Head Traum Rehab. 1999;14:9–21.
71. Couch JR, Bears C. Chronic daily headache in the posttrauma syndrome: relation to the extent of head injury. Headache. 2001;41:559.
72. Chamelian L, Feinstein A. Outcome after mild to moderate traumatic brain injury: the role of dizziness. Arch Phys Med Rehab. 2004;85:1662–6.
73. Valovich McLeod TC, Hale TD. Vestibular and balance issues following sport-related concussion. Brain Inj. 2015;29:175–84.
74. Anstey KJ, Butterworth P, Jorm AF, Christensen H, Rodgers B, Windsor TD. A population survey found an association between self-reports of traumatic brain injury and increased psychiatric symptoms. J Clin Epid. 2004;57:1202–9.
75. Eisenberg M, Meehan WP, Mannix R. Duration and course of post-concussive symptoms. Pediatrics. 2014;133:999–1006.
76. Cantor JB, Ashman T, Gordon W, Engmann C, Egan M, Spielman L, et al. Fatigue after traumatic brain injury and its impact on participation and quality of life. J Head Trauma Rehabil. 2008;23:41–51.
77. Ashman TA, Cantor JB, Gordon WA, Spielman L, Egan M, Ginsberg A, et al. Objective measurement of fatigue following traumatic brain injury. J Head Trauma Rehabil. 2008;23:33–40.
78. Popovic V. GH deficiency as the most common pituitary defect after TBI: clinical implications. Pituitary. 2005;8:239–43.
79. Rao V, Rollings P. Sleep disturbances following traumatic brain injury. Curr Treat Options Neurol. 2002;4:77–87.
80. Tkachenko N, Singh K, Hasanaj L, Serrano L, Kothare SV. Sleep disorders associated with mild traumatic brain injury using Sport Concussion Assessment Tool 3. Pediatr Neurol. 2016;57:46–50.
81. Ponsford JL, Parcell DL, Sinclair KL. Changes in sleep patterns following traumatic brain injury: a controlled study. Neurorehabil Neural Repair. 2013;27:613–21.
82. Sumpter RE, Dorris L, Kelly T, McMillan TM. Pediatric sleep difficulties after moderate-severe traumatic brain injury. J Int Neuropsychol Soc. 2013;19:829–34.
83. Sufrinko A, Pearce K, Elbin RJ. The effect of preinjury sleep difficulties on neurocognitive impairment and symptoms after sport-related concussion. Am J Sports Med. 2015;43:830–8.
84. Clinchot DM, Bogner J, Mysiw WJ, Fugate L, Corrigan J. Defining sleep disturbance after brain injury. Am J Phys Med Rehab. 1998;77:291–5.
85. Hou L, Han X, Sheng P, Tong W, Li Z, Xu D, et al. Risk factors associated with sleep disturbance following traumatic brain injury: clinical findings and questionnaire based study. PLoS One. 2013;8:e76087.
86. McCrory P, Bladn P, Berkovic S. Retrospective study of concussive convulsions in elite Australian rules and rugby league footballers: phenomenology, aetiology, and outcome. BMJ. 1997;314:171–4.
87. Iverson GL, McCracken LM. 'Postconcussive' symptoms in persons with chronic pain. Brain Inj. 1997;11:783–90.
88. Hart RP, Martelli MF, Zasler ND. Chronic pain and neuropsychological functioning. Neuropsychol Rev. 2000;10:131–49.
89. McCracken LM, Iverson GL. Predicting complaints of impaired cognitive functioning in patients with chronic pain. J Pain Symp Manag. 2001;21:392–6.
90. Borg J, Holm L, Peloso PM, Cassidy JD, Carroll LJ, von Holst H, et al. Non-surgical intervention and cost for mild traumatic brain injury: results of the WHO Collaborating Centre Task Force on Mild Traumatic Brain Injury. J Rehabil Med. 2004;(43) Suppl:76–83.
91. Lal A, Kolakowsky-Hayner SA, Ghajar J, Balamane M. The effect of physical exercise after a concussion. Am J Sports Med. 2017. Epub ahead of print
92. Randolph C, Millis S, Barr W, McCrea M, Guskiewicz KM, Hammeke TA, et al. Concussion symptom inventory: an empirically derived scale for monitoring resolution of symptoms following sport related concussion. Arch Clin Neuropsychol. 2009;24:219–29.
93. What to expect after a concussion. CDC Heads Up Series. www.cdc.gov/headsup/basics/concussion_symptoms.html.

36 Mental Health in Pregnancy

Eric L. Anderson

Introduction

For many psychiatric illnesses, the onset of symptoms begins during the late teens to the early thirties [1]. This is especially concerning in women, as it coincides with the childbearing years. Pregnancy was once thought to be protective of psychiatric illness. However, as the recent explosion of literature addressing the safety of psychotropic agents in pregnancy illustrates, the puerperal period is not exempt from mental illness [2–4]. The presence of mental illness in pregnancy is associated with poor compliance with prenatal care; increased tobacco, alcohol, and illicit substance use; inadequate maternal nutrition; poor mother–infant bonding; and disruption of the home environment [5].

While the diagnostic criteria are the same as in nonpregnant patients, many symptoms common in mental illness, such as fatigue, low energy, and disrupted sleep, are also normal for pregnancy [6]. Medication treatment is a controversial issue: In the case of the pregnant patient, there are at least two (or more!) patients, mother, and unborn child, and many of the treatments available to address mental illness can potentially harm the fetus [3].

E. L. Anderson (✉)
Luminis Health, J. Kent McNew Family Medical Center, Annapolis, MD, USA

This chapter will present the major mental health topics of concern in pregnant patients and offer guidelines for the management of these patients in the emergency setting.

Self-Injurious Behavior, Suicide, and Violence

Perhaps most concerning is the patient with suicidal or violent ideations. These thoughts may lead to violent actions against one's self, unborn child, or another. In the emergency setting, it is imperative to assess the safety of the pregnant patient by inquiring about these thoughts. Suicidal, homicidal, and violent ideations are the presence of a desire to end one's life, the life of another person, or to do harm to another, respectively. "Passive death wishes" differ from suicidal intent in that the person longs for death but not at her own hands. Regardless, they, too, are a worrisome symptom.

The risk of suicide during pregnancy is lower than in the general US population, with a 2% completion rate in pregnant patients versus a completion rate of 5% in all females of childbearing age [7, 8]. The rate rises in the postpartum period, with up to 20% of female deaths attributable to suicide [9]. Discontinuation of psychotropic medications potentially contributes to this increase, as discontinuation prior to or during

L. S. Zun et al. (eds.), *Behavioral Emergencies for Healthcare Providers*,
https://doi.org/10.1007/978-3-030-52520-0_36

pregnancy is associated with a high rate of symptoms relapse [2, 7, 10]. Unfortunately, the recommendation to discontinue psychotropic medication is usually made before an adequate risk–benefit analysis has been conducted [9].

Suicidal and violent symptoms should be assessed in any patient presenting with emotional, psychological, or social stress. This evaluation is sometimes referred to as the "risk assessment." Direct, nonjudgmental questions are advised: "Do you have any thoughts of wanting to kill yourself? Do you have any thoughts of wanting to hurt someone else, including your baby?" Contrary to popular belief, asking about these symptoms does not increase the likelihood they will occur. On the contrary, the risk often decreases [7]. Any affirmative answer necessitates further exploration: Is there a plan? Is there intent? Is there access to lethal means? Who is the intended target?

If the patient expresses a desire to harm another person, the clinician may be required to warn the intended victim. The duty to warn stems, at least in part, from the now-famous Tarasoff case. In the event there is a duty to warn, a reasonable effort must be made to contact the intended victim. Barring that, law enforcement can be contacted.

Safety is paramount, both for the patient and for her unborn child. The patient may be initially monitored in a safe environment in the emergency department, evaluated by a mental health clinician, and sometimes admitted to an inpatient psychiatric unit, depending on acuity. Further management and disposition of these patients do not differ significantly from non-pregnant patients.

Management of the Agitated Patient

The management of agitation in pregnant patients is similar to nonpregnant patients. Once the etiology is found and addressed, agitation usually resolves. Possible causes of agitation requiring a rule-out include medical problems such as thyrotoxicosis, substance intoxication or withdrawal, and pain. However, there may be instances where either the etiology remains unknown or the agitation persists in spite of management of the presumed etiology. Additional management strategies come in two major forms: medication and nonmedication.

Nonmedication strategies include brief, focused counseling interventions. Emergency-department-based clinicians may be reluctant to employ these techniques, believing it will take too much time or that they have too limited skills in counseling. However, evidence shows that these interventions do not require a great deal of time and can ultimately save time in the patient's acute management. The ability to establish a trusting relationship between clinician and patient matters more than the specific technique used in the emergent setting [11]. Another critical step to this strategy involves discovering the patient's motivation(s). Many times, agitation can be quelled simply by making the effort to meet a patient's perceived need [7]. Recommended techniques for verbal, nonmedication management of agitation include persuasion, coercion, factual and simple language, and attempts to understand the patient's views by inviting their ideas [12].

Despite best efforts, clinicians may find more intensive management is required to keep the patient and her baby safe. Unfortunately, no specific research-based guidelines exist for the pharmacologic management of agitation in pregnancy. While the lowest possible dose of medication is recommended, the American College of Obstetricians and Gynecologists (ACOG) recommends that single agents, at higher doses, be used over multiple medications [5]. Current guidelines recommend the use of oral medications, if possible, before intramuscular (IM) forms are used [13]. The Best Practices in Evaluation and Treatment of Agitation project has also presented guidelines for the management of acute agitation [14]. A collation of these recommendations is presented in Table 36.1.

On rare occasions, it may be necessary to physically restrain a pregnant patient. Special precautions are necessary for pregnant patients after the first trimester; patients should be placed in the left lateral decubitus position to prevent aortocaval compression syndrome [15]. Monitoring should be frequent and include regular monitoring of fetal heart tones and fetal movement [7].

Table 36.1 Treatment of agitation [12, 13, 16]

Medical condition (such as delirium)
Haloperidol 2.5–10 mg (liquid, PO, IM) + lorazepam 2 mg (PO, IM)
Risperidone 2 mg (liquid, PO, ODT) +/– lorazepam 2 mg (PO, IM)
Olanzapine 5–10 mg (PO, ODT)[a]
Intoxication and/or withdrawal
Lorazepam 1–2 mg (PO, IM, IV)
Diazepam 5–10 mg (PO)[a]
Primary psychiatric disturbance (such as psychosis)
Ziprasidone 10–20 mg (PO, IM) +/– lorazepam 2 mg (PO, IM)
Risperidone 2 mg (liquid, PO, ODT) +/– lorazepam 2 mg (PO, IM)
Haloperidol 2.5–10 mg (PO, IM) + lorazepam 2 mg (PO, IM)
Olanzapine 5–10 mg (PO, ODT, IM)[a]
Unknown etiology
Diphenhydramine 25–50 mg (PO, IM, IV)
Lorazepam 1–2 mg (PO, IM)

IM Intramuscular, *PO* By Mouth, *IV* Intravenously, *ODT* Orally Disintegrating Tablets, [a]Second-line options

Mood Disorders

Unipolar disorders (such as major depression) and bipolar disorders comprise the mood disorders. They tend to have an age of onset that coincides with the peak years of childbearing. For many women, psychotherapy is insufficient to control their symptoms, making medication management necessary in order to function. The risk of suicide (2%) is lower than in nonpregnant women in the same age group (5%), but this risk rises dramatically in the postpartum period, especially in patients who have discontinued their medications (up to 20%) [7–9]. Infanticide rates up to 4% have also been reported in symptomatic postpartum patients [15].

Depressive Disorders

The prevalence of depression varies from 12% to 25% in women. Depression is as common in pregnancy as it is in the nonpregnant state. It is estimated that roughly 10–16% of all pregnant women suffer from clinical depression [17–19]. In a study by Flynn et al. 31% of pregnant women screened demonstrated evidence of depressive symptoms, but only 22% of them received treatment [20]. One of the reasons cited for low treatment rates is that depressive symptoms are often similar to the symptoms of normal pregnancy, including sleep problems, appetite changes, low energy, and problems with concentration [15].

Risk factors for depression include a personal or family history of depression, limited social support, history of abuse (especially sexual or physical), environmental stressors (financial, occupational, relationship, health), living alone, and the presence of substance use [17]. The presence of depression during pregnancy is associated with poor outcomes such as miscarriage, inadequate maternal weight gain, underutilized prenatal care, marital discord, inability to care for other children in the home, low birthweight, preterm delivery, neonates that are small for gestational age, developmental delay, and suicide [15, 18, 20, 21].

Screening is similar as in nonpregnant patients. Several tools exist, including the three-item RAND screening instrument [22], the Edinburgh scale [23], and the Beck Depression Inventory [17].

The management of depression in pregnancy depends upon the severity and course of illness, the presence of depression prior to pregnancy, treatment prior to or during pregnancy, available resources, and the patient's level of support. Treatment options include psychotherapy, medications, partial or full hospitalization, electroconvulsive therapy (ECT), and repetitive Transcranial Magnetic Stimulation (rTMS).

For patients with mild depression, referral for psychotherapy such as cognitive-behavioral or interpersonal therapy may suffice [1]. A list of referral resources should be kept in the emergency department for such purposes. Emergency department personnel may find it useful to establish a working relationship with local mental health clinicians to expedite the referral process. In moderate to severe depression, medications, hospitalization, TMS, or ECT may be required.

The use of medications in pregnancy is a source of debate, but there is a high risk of symptom recurrence if antidepressant medications are discontinued [1, 2, 6]. Sixty-eight percent of patients who discontinue their medications relapse. This compares to a relapse rate of 26% in those who continued their medications. Half of the patients relapsing did so within the first trimester, and over 90% relapsed by the end of the second trimester [17].

Despite the potential risk of relapse and subsequent complications of continued depressive symptoms for both mother and infant, medication use is not a straightforward decision. Antidepressant medications usually take several weeks to become effective. They must be monitored for side effects.

Medication use carries at least four types of potential risks that must be addressed when used in pregnancy: pregnancy loss, organ malformation, neonatal adaptability, and long-term neurodevelopmental sequelae.

The evidence regarding antidepressant use and spontaneous loss of a pregnancy is conflicting, as some recent studies implicate antidepressants as a general class [6, 17], while other studies do not support such claims [2, 24]. Furthermore, stress and depression themselves are risk factors for premature delivery and spontaneous abortion [21].

The data for organ malformation are also conflicting. Overall, there is not a statistically significantly increased risk of organ malformation when antidepressants as a class are considered [6, 16, 25]. Specific medications have been implicated in increased relative risk. Tricyclic antidepressants (TCA) such as amitriptyline, clomipramine, and nortriptyline are associated with an increased risk of cardiac defects, but no specific pattern has emerged [19]. Diav-Citrin et al. found an increased rate of cardiovascular abnormalities in selective-serotonin-reuptake-inhibitor- (SSRI) exposed infants, although causation could not be determined [26]. Louik et al. found no increased risk of craniosynostosis, omphalocele, or heart defects with SSRI exposure overall. But the authors did find an increased relative risk of septal defects in neonates exposed to sertraline, with an odds ratio (OR) of 2.0 based upon thirteen exposed patients [27]. In a retrospective cohort study, Malm et al. found that fluoxetine was associated with an isolated relative risk of ventricular septal defects (OR 2.03), paroxetine was associated with a relative risk of right ventricular outflow tract defects (OR 4.68), and citalopram was associated with neural tube defects (OR 2.46). While the absolute risk of these defects was small, the authors recommended against paroxetine and fluoxetine as first-line options [25]. These studies contrast with other authors, who have found paroxetine [19] and fluoxetine to be relatively safe in pregnancy [1, 6, 15, 19]. As a class, SSRIs are felt to be safe in pregnancy, with neonatal complications and rates of congenital anomalies falling within the general population rate of 1–3% [19, 21, 28]. Data are lacking for other antidepressants, such as venlafaxine, duloxetine, mirtazapine, and trazodone, but no significant associations with malformations have been reported [2, 3, 19]. Buproprion is not associated with an increased risk of fetal malformations. It is the only antidepressant to date that has a Pregnancy and Lactation Labeling Final Rule (PLLR) rating above other antidepressants [2, 29].

Late pregnancy exposure to SSRIs has been associated with an increase in premature delivery, low birth weight, and lower Apgar scores [3]. Poor neonatal adaptability (PNA) has been reported in up to 30% of newborns exposed to SSRIs [30]. PNA symptoms include irritability, abnormal crying, tremor, respiratory distress, jitteriness, lethargy, poor tone, tachypnea, and, possibly, persistent pulmonary hypertension of the newborn (PPHN) [29, 31]. While paroxetine appears to be the SSRI most associated with these symptoms [32], a study by Lorenzo et al. found the absolute risk of PPHN in SSRI-exposed neonates was less than 1%. The major associative factor was the mode of delivery [19]. Seizures in the newborn have also been noted with exposure to TCAs such as clomipramine [6].

Croen et al. found that prenatal exposure to SSRIs was associated with a modest increase in autism spectrum disorders (ASD). However, the authors concluded that SSRI exposure is very unlikely to be a major risk factor for ASD [33]. Most studies find no adverse neurodevelopmental issues up to the age of two for children exposed to SSRIs in utero and no significant cognitive or behavioral issues [2, 24]. Remission of a mother's depression may have a positive impact on childhood development and behavior [34].

Inpatient treatment may be required for patients with severe depression, especially if psychotic or suicidal features are present. Psychoses and suicidal thoughts are psychiatric emergencies, whether or not a patient is pregnant. Inpatient psychiatric treatment seeks to ensure the safety of the patient and her unborn child.

In some cases, especially where medications may not be desired or appropriate, brain stimulation treatment may be utilized. The two most commonly employed forms are electroconvulsive therapy (ECT) and repetitive transcranial magnetic stimulation (rTMS). rTMS has not been systematically studied in pregnancy, but has been found to be helpful in the treatment of depression [35]. It requires no anesthesia, has no cognitive side effects, and can be conducted on an outpatient basis. ECT is an effective treatment for severe depressive symptoms, but it requires anesthesia and the delivery of a seizure-inducing electric stimulus. Cognitive impairments are common but typically limited to the actual treatment course. In a review of the literature, ECT was found to be safe and effective for the treatment of depression in pregnancy [36].

The choice of antidepressant treatment is dependent upon the patient's symptoms and preferences, a thorough risk–benefit analysis, and the ability to monitor and adjust the medications and clinical course. An algorithm for decision-making is presented in Fig. 36.1 to aid in this decision process.

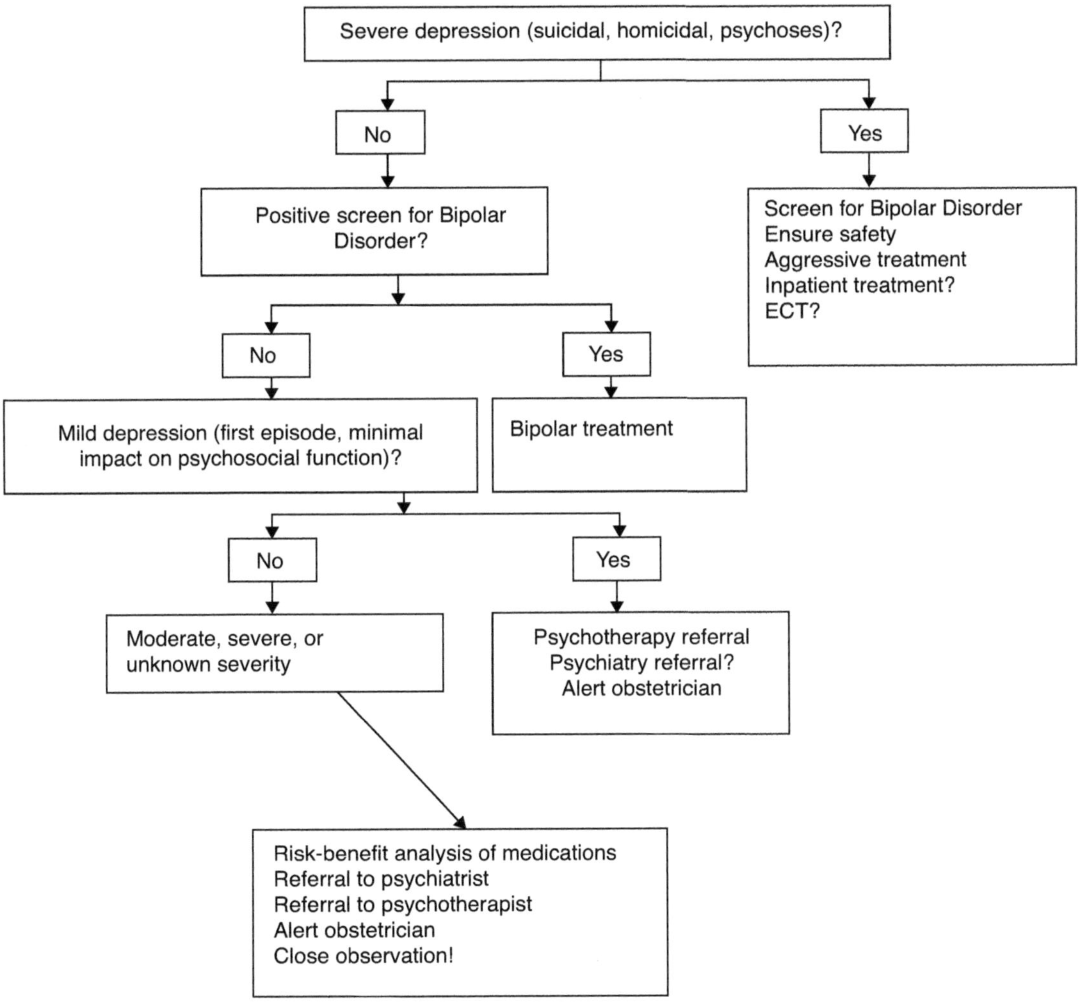

Fig. 36.1 Depression treatment algorithm [18]

Bipolar Disorders

The prevalence of bipolar disorders, sometimes referred to as bipolar affective disorders (BPADs), in the US is 3.9–6.4%. Men and women are equally affected [5]. Treatments for BPAD consist of the traditional mood stabilizers such as lithium, valproic acid, lamotrigine, carbamazepine, and oxcarbazepine, and the second-generation antipsychotic (SGA) medications. First-generation antipsychotics (FGA) and benzodiazepines are also used, but usually as an adjunct to a traditional mood stabilizer or SGA (see Table 36.2). Patients with BPAD run the risk of symptom exacerbation in the prepartum and postpartum periods [37]. Relapse rates up to 71% have been reported if medications have been discontinued [38]. Nearly half of all relapses occur during the first trimester [39].

Most pregnant patients who present acutely manic or hypomanic have a prior history of BPAD. In any pregnant patient presenting with depressive symptoms, screening for BPAD should be conducted. The diagnosis does not differ from non-pregnant states. However, pregnant patients in a manic, hypomanic, or mixed episode should be considered a psychiatric and obstetric emergency due to the risk to both mother and child [2, 39]. Inpatient hospitalization to stabilize the patient's mood is often required. Symptoms of a manic, hypomanic, or mixed episode include poor sleep, abnormally increased energy, agitation, irritability, euphoria, impulsivity, and flights of ideas.

Any pregnant patient with the diagnosis of BPAD should be considered a high-risk pregnancy [40]. Treatment depends upon the severity of illness but usually consists of a mood stabilizer of some kind [40]. Most mood stabilizers carry a teratogenic risk, especially if used in the first trimester [37].

Lithium is the mood stabilizer of choice in pregnancy [15]. Relative to the other traditional mood stabilizers, it is the least problematic. However, lithium's use is associated with Ebstein's anomaly, a downward displacement of the tricuspid valve, in 1:2000 live births [2, 5]. For patients receiving lithium, a high-resolution ultrasound and fetal echocardiogram at 16–18 weeks are advised to assess for cardiac issues [5, 37]. During the last month of pregnancy, lithium levels should be monitored on a weekly basis [3]. Lithium is not associated with intrauterine growth retardation (IUGR) or PNA, although it has been implicated in neonatal hypothyroidism and goiter, nephrogenic diabetes insipidus, and floppy baby syndrome [16]. Floppy baby syndrome is self-limited; infants present with cyanosis and hypotonia immediately postpartum. Conservative management and monitoring are usually all that is required [37]. Some authors advocate decreasing the dose of lithium by 25% or stopping it altogether 2–3 days before delivery in order to prevent neonatal toxicity [3].

Other traditional mood stabilizers such as valproic acid, lamotrigine, carbamazepine, and oxcarbazepine are antiepileptic agents. They carry significant teratogenic risk. Folate (4–5 mg administered daily) is recommended for all pregnant patients taking one of these agents [41, 42].

Valproic acid (VPA) is associated with a neural tube defect rate of 5–9% (ten to twenty times greater than the general population), possible IUGR, craniofacial anomalies, limb abnormalities, and withdrawal symptoms consisting of jitteriness, irritability, feeding difficulties, and poor tone [2, 3, 37]. The risk of teratogenic effects increases if VPA is used in combination with other medications or is at a dose greater than 1000 mg daily [43]. Given these risks, ACOG recommends against VPA use in pregnancy, especially in the first trimester [5]. If VPA is deemed necessary, the first-trimester ultrasound to evaluate for neural tube defects is recommended. Other recommendations include serial ultrasounds to assess for IUGR, a fetal echocardiogram to assess for cardiac anomalies, alpha-fetoprotein at sixteen to eighteen weeks, and a late-pregnancy ultrasound [42, 43]. Postpartum vitamin K (1 mg IM) should be given to the neonate to prevent valproic acid-induced coagulopathies [42].

Carbamazepine is associated with craniofacial defects, fingernail hypoplasia, developmental delay, neural tube defects, cardiovascular abnormalities, and vitamin K deficiency [2, 3, 37]. Concurrent use of valproic acid increases its teratogenic potential. ACOG advises against its use,

Table 36.2 Bipolar and anxiety medications [5, 15, 41, 42]

Medication or risk	FDA classification*	Select reported adverse events and (time of risk conveyance/ incidence, if known)
Lithium	D	Floppy baby syndrome (hypotonia, lethargy) [PP], thyroid abnormalities, cardiac anomalies (Ebstein's anomaly) [1]
Valproic acid	D	NTD (spina bifida) [1], cardiovascular defects [1], IUGR [1–3], fetal anticonvulsant syndrome [1], coagulopathy, developmental delay [NN], risk for neonatal withdrawal [PP]
Carbamazepine	D	NTD (spina bifida) [1], fetal anticonvulsant syndrome, developmental delay [NN], coagulopathy, craniofacial defects [1], risk for neonatal withdrawal [PP]
Lamotrigene	C	Nonspecific congenital malformations reported at 1–2.5% [1]
FGA	C	Nonspecific congenital malformations reported [1], risk for neonatal neuroleptic malignant syndrome [PP]
SGA	C	Nonspecific congenital malformations reported [1], risk for (except clozapine) neonatal neuroleptic malignant syndrome [PP]
Clozapine	B	Nonspecific congenital malformations reported [1], risk for neonatal neuroleptic malignant syndrome [PP]
Diphenhydramine	B	Anticholinergic symptoms
Alprazolam, Chlordiazepoxide, clonazepam, diazepam, Oxazepam, lorazepam	D	Cleft/facial defects [1], risk for neonatal withdrawal (hypotonia, respiratory problems, seizures) [PP]

*Pre-PLLR

NTD Neural tube defects, *IUGR* Intra-uterine growth retardation, *FGA* First-generation antipsychotics, *SGA* Second-generation antipsychotics, 1 First trimester, 3 Third trimester, *PP* Delivery and postpartum period, *NN* Neonatal period, *PLLR* The Pregnancy and Lactation Labeling Rule

and it is therefore reserved for use only if other options are lacking. Its use should be avoided in the first trimester [5, 42].

No clear guidelines exist for lamotrigine and oxcarbazepine. Lamotrigine has been associated with an increased risk of cleft palate [2, 37] but the Lamotrigine Pregnancy Registry reports a less than 2% risk of fetal malformations with first-trimester exposure [3].

Antipsychotic medications are frequently used as solo or adjunct treatments for mood disorders, whether or not psychotic features are present. Given the relative safety of these agents, they are sometimes preferred over even lithium [16]. Unlike many traditional mood stabilizers, antipsychotics have a rapid onset of action that may begin to work in days or even hours [44]. Antipsychotic medications are broadly divided into first-generation antipsychotics (FGAs) and second-generation antipsychotics (SGAs). The FGAs are commonly used for the treatment of acute mania and are felt to be relatively safe in pregnancy [6, 37]. FGAs are associated with neonatal extrapyramidal side effects that can persist for several months. High-potency FGAs, such as haloperidol, are preferred because low-potency FGAs, such as chlorpromazine, have been associated with nonspecific teratogenic effects when used in the first trimester [3].

There are limited data on the safety of SGAs in pregnancy [6, 37], but they do not appear to be associated with an increased risk of major malformations [3]. The major concern with SGA use in pregnancy is the propensity of this class of medications to cause maternal hyperglycemia and excessive weight gain. These agents are associated with gestational diabetes, insulin resistance, and preeclampsia [37].

Benzodiazepines are sometimes used in the treatment of acute mania, especially when agitation is present. Concerns for midline defects such as cleft palate exist, but it is unlikely that limited exposure to benzodiazepines carries an appreciable risk to the developing child. Neonatal withdrawal symptoms are possible, especially if benzodiazepines are administered close to delivery [3, 37].

Anxiety Disorders

Like the mood disorders, anxiety disorders remain problematic during pregnancy; pregnancy is not protective against these disorders. The anxiety disorders encompass a broad range of diagnoses such as social phobia, generalized anxiety disorder, panic disorder (with and without agoraphobia), obsessive-compulsive disorder (OCD), post-traumatic stress disorder, and simple phobias.

Anxiety disorders are not rare in pregnancy and have a prevalence that exceeds the general population. Generalized anxiety is present in up to 10.5% of pregnant patients. Other disorders are also not uncommon, including panic (over 5%), obsessive-compulsive disorder (over 5%), and post-traumatic stress disorder (3%) [45]. Some disorders, such as panic disorder, have a variable course. Others, such as OCD, may be exacerbated by pregnancy [38]. Anxiety disorders appear to have an adverse impact on the developing fetus. For example, a panic disorder in the mother is associated with lower neonatal Apgar scores and increased rates of maternal preterm labor and placental abruption [6]. Anxiety, in general, is associated with an increased incidence of delivery by forceps, prolonged labor, fetal distress, preterm delivery, and decreased neonatal adaptability [5].

One of the most effective forms of treatment for anxiety is cognitive-behavioral therapy (CBT), a structured, duration-limited psychotherapy [46]. While this form of therapy may not be practical in the emergency setting, aspects of CBT may be used effectively to alleviate the patient's suffering. Skills such as deep breathing, guided imagery, and progressive muscle relaxation can be quickly taught to patients, allowing immediate use to combat anxiety symptoms.

Medication management of anxiety symptoms in pregnancy is controversial. Traditional antidepressants, such as the SSRIs, serotonin-norepinephrine reuptake inhibitors (SNRIs), and tricyclic antidepressants (TCAs), are also used to treat anxiety disorders. However, these medications have drawbacks, as illustrated earlier.

Benzodiazepines such as lorazepam are the medication class of choice for acute anxiety symptoms. While some studies demonstrate no association between extended benzodiazepine use and major malformations, other data suggest a small increase in relative risk (0.6%) for malformations such as oral cleft [47]. The use of benzodiazepines near or at delivery may result in floppy infant syndrome: hypotonia, apnea, temperature instability, and neonatal withdrawal symptoms [5, 6, 15]. If benzodiazepines are chosen, there must be a clear risk–benefit completed with the patient and documented in her medical record [12].

Psychotic Disorders

The psychotic disorders include psychotic disorder not otherwise specified, schizophrenia, brief psychotic disorder, and schizoaffective disorder. The general population prevalence of Schizophrenia is roughly 1%. Males and females are equally affected. Recent evidence indicates a prodromal period that may be present as early as late childhood, but for most women, the peak onset of symptoms occurs between the ages of 25–35 [48]. Psychotic symptoms may be found in the presence of severe mood disorders, such as manic episodes in bipolar disorder or severe depression. The course of psychotic disorders and psychosis in pregnancy is not well understood, and the literature is sparse and contradictory [10].

A psychotic, pregnant patient is an obstetric and psychiatric emergency. Psychoses during pregnancy may interfere with a patient's ability to obtain and participate in appropriate prenatal care. The presence of psychotic symptoms may lead to a lack of cooperation at delivery [6]. Psychotic disorders are associated with a higher use of tobacco products and alcohol, lower socioeconomic status, more unplanned pregnancies, low birthweight, preterm labor, placental abnormalities, and poor neonatal health, including postnatal death [5, 10, 48]. As new-onset psychosis in pregnancy is uncommon, a thorough medical evaluation, including laboratory testing, is warranted in such cases [12].

FGAs (such as haloperidol, fluphenazine, chlorpromazine, and perphenazine) and SGAs (such as quetiapine, olanzapine, risperidone, aripiprazole, ziprasidone, lurasidone, asenapine, iloperidone, and paliperidone) are the mainstays of treatment in psychotic disorders. High-potency FGAs such as haloperidol have a greater risk for acute dystonic reactions, akathisia, extrapyramidal symptoms (EPS), and tardive dyskinesia (TD) than do low-potency FGAs. However, low-potency FGAs such as chlorpromazine have a greater risk of sedation, weight gain, and seizures. With the advent of the SGAs, the risks of EPS and TD are lower but still present to a degree. SGAs have the potential to cause metabolic disturbances, such as weight gain, hyperlipidemia, and hyperglycemia [3, 48]. Hyperlipidemia is concerning, as it may lead to gestational diabetes [10].

Few data exist to guide the clinician with respect to antipsychotic use in pregnancy [49]. Some authors advise the use of high-potency FGAs over low-potency FGAs and SGAs [1]. There appears to be an increased risk of teratogenic effects, specifically congenital malformations, with the use of low-potency FGAs [10, 15]. SGAs such as quetiapine and olanzapine can lead to significant weight gain, but there appears to be a minimal risk for major fetal malformations [48]. For patients receiving clozapine, white blood cell counts (WBC) must be obtained every 2 weeks. A screening WBC for the neonate is also advised [42].

The choice of antipsychotic treatment for the long-term is problematic, but in the emergency setting, the same guidelines for acute agitation may be followed (see Table 36.1). Haloperidol is preferred especially during labor, due to its potency, low sedative properties, and intravenous or intramuscular mode of delivery [6].

Substance-Use Disorders

Substance-use (formerly known as substance abuse or substance dependence disorders) disorders are common in the United States, and unfortunately, pregnancy is no exception. It is estimated that 4.5–10.3% of pregnant women drink alcohol to excess; 12.6–22.1% smoke nicotine; and 5.1% use illicit substances such as cocaine, marijuana, or opioids [50]. Substance use is associated with preterm delivery, low birthweight, smaller fetal head circumference, miscarriage, and fetal central nervous system damage [15].

Screening for substance use in the emergency setting should be simple, direct, and nonjudgmental. Some pregnant patients may be hesitant to disclose their substance use for fear of judgment or losing their baby to state custody. Reassuring patients that the focus of the screens is treatment, not punishment, may be necessary to obtain honest answers. Several rapid screening tests are available to assess for alcohol use. These include the T-ACE, CAGE, and TWEAK screens [51].

Management of the intoxicated patient depends upon the substance(s) ingested. Alcohol withdrawal poses a medical and obstetric emergency, due to the risk of withdrawal seizures. Prolonged seizures, especially status epilepticus, can be fatal to the fetus. Benzodiazepines are the preferred treatment. Dosing should proceed as with the nonpregnant patient. Anti-epileptic agents are frequently used along with benzodiazepines to prevent seizures and stabilize the person's mood, but they are not recommended for use in pregnant patients for reasons detailed above [16].

Opioid intoxication and withdrawal may lead to fetal demise. While detoxification can be attempted, maintenance treatment with either methadone or buprenorphine is preferred to prevent withdrawal and relapse of opioid use [14, 16]. Treatment of withdrawal from other substances such as cocaine, marijuana, and phencyclidine tends to be supportive only: it provides a calm, quiet setting with frequent monitoring of both the patient and her baby.

Some states require reporting of pregnant patients with concurrent substance use. State regulations vary from state to state, so emergency clinicians are advised to know the regulations and laws of their state.

Eating Disorders

Eating disorders (EDs), such as anorexia nervosa and bulimia nervosa, have a lifetime prevalence rate of roughly 1% in women over the age of 18 [52].

EDs usually manifest by the patient's late teens, during the beginning and peak years of a woman's reproductive age. They are associated with a high risk of miscarriage, congenital malformations, smaller fetal head circumference, premature delivery, low birthweight, and delivery via cesarean section [53]. There is a greater risk of postpartum depression in women who have an eating disorder during pregnancy [54]. Pregnant patients with a concurrent eating disorder are considered high-risk. Close observation throughout pregnancy is warranted to ensure proper weight gain.

Screening for eating disorders is reasonable in any pregnant patient who appears to be underweight. Questions should be direct, simple, and nonjudgmental: "Do you have any struggles with eating? Are you afraid of getting fat? Do you ever force yourself to throw up? Do you exercise several hours or more a day?" For patients demonstrating poor weight gain, admission to an eating disorders unit may be necessary. At the very least, the patient should be referred to a therapist skilled at treating eating disorders. The National Eating Disorders Association (www.edap.org) maintains a referral hotline: 1-800-931-2237.

Domestic Violence

In the United States, over two million women are assaulted annually, and 50 million over the course of their lifetime [55]. Pregnancy fails to protect against domestic violence, although evidence suggests that pregnancy itself does not increase the rate of violence [55]. A male partner usually perpetrates the domestic violence. Its most common forms include physical abuse, sexual abuse, verbal threats, isolation, and economic abuse, such as withholding of financial resources [56]. Data are limited, but prevalence rates of violence in pregnancy are estimated at 1 to 20.6% [15, 56]. This wide range is likely the result of many factors, such as the method used to screen, the population sampled, and whether or not emotional abuse was counted in the data.

Risk factors for pregnancy-related violence include low socioeconomic status, low levels of social support, no prior parenting experience, unwanted or unexpected pregnancy, extremes of age, single marital status, higher parity, and substance use [55, 57]. Consequences of violence include late entry into prenatal care, depression, anxiety, low maternal weight gain, emotional distress, infection, anemia, short interpregnancy interval, bleeding, low birthweight, uterine rupture, fetal injuries (such as fractures), and maternal or fetal death [55, 56].

Warning signs of domestic violence include repeated visits, recurrent headaches, recurrent vaginitis, irritable bowel syndrome, substance use, a history of depression or anxiety, suicide attempts, a personal history of abuse or assault, and repeated visits for injuries [57]. The patient may demonstrate fright, startle responses, overcompliance, excessive distrust, flat affect, anxiety or depression symptoms, psychic numbing, and dissociation. Warning signs in the partner's behavior may include solicitousness, refusal to leave the patient, monitoring of the patient's responses, answering for the patient, hostility, and excessive demands [57].

Screening questions should be asked in private, away from the patient's partner, family, and friends. Patents should be reminded about confidentiality. The most effective means of screening is done personally in a nonjudgmental, brief, direct manner. For example, "Many women experience violence. Because it can have a negative impact on health and wellness, I ask all my patients about it" [57].

Patients with a positive domestic violence screen should be referred for treatment. Treatment varies from formal domestic violence consultations to safe havens. Accurate medical documentation is important for any future legal cases [15]. In many states, clinicians are required to report acts of domestic violence (whether or not the patient is pregnant) [56, 57]. It is important to know the state and local (if applicable) mandatory reporting regulations. Many clinicians feel powerless and helpless in these situations because they cannot convince the patient to leave her abusive situation. While the emergency clinician's role is to keep the patient and her baby safe as mentioned above, ultimately the woman must make the decision to end the relationship for herself [56].

Postpartum Mood and Anxiety Disorders

The immediate period following labor and delivery is a time of significant physical adjustment for most mothers. Emotional and mental adjustments also occur, and many of these changes are well within the spectrum of normal experience. Some women experience mood or anxiety symptoms in the postpartum period significant enough to warrant further management, especially if the patient has a history of a psychiatric disorder and her medications were discontinued during or prior to pregnancy.

Postpartum "blues" (PPB) are common, occurring in up to 75–85% of women postpartum [58]. Patients with PPB feel irritable and demonstrate mood lability and emotional sensitivity. Symptoms usually begin within 1 week of delivery and resolve within 1 month. The symptoms typically do not impair the patient. Supportive care is the most appropriate treatment option [4].

Postpartum depression (PPD) presents in a fashion similar to MDD. The same risk factors for MDD also exist for PPD, including younger age, lower education level, financial hardships, single parenthood, and low socioeconomic/occupational status [59]. The prevalence of PPD is 10–15%, presenting most frequently within the first 2–3 months following delivery [2]. Unfortunately, many of the symptoms of PPB overlap with PPD, making it difficult to distinguish the two. However, if there is a prior history of depression, PPD should be suspected, since roughly half of all women who stop their antidepressant medications develop recurrence of their depressive symptoms within six months of delivery [38]. In patients with a prior history of MDD or PPD, rates of subsequent PPD are 25% and 50–62%, respectively [1, 15].

Screening tools such as the Edinburgh scale may help to differentiate PPB from PPD [23]. Untreated PPD can have a negative impact on child well-being and development, so prompt recognition and treatment are both critical [2]. For mild-to-moderate PPD, the use of CBT and/or IPT has been studied and found to be effective [2]. In cases of more severe depression, treatment with medications, in addition to therapy, may be warranted [1].

The SSRIs are considered first-line treatment, due to their low side-effect profile and tolerability, followed by bupropion and the tricyclic antidepressants [2]. Fluoxetine and its active metabolite are excreted in breast milk [24]. They have a possible association with colic, poor feeding, constant crying, seizure-like episodes, and irritability. Paroxetine is excreted in breast milk but no adverse impacts have been reported in nursing infants [24]. The lowest exposure to nursing infants appears to be with sertraline, and the highest with citalopram and fluoxetine [23]. rTMS is an option for patients wishing to avoid medications. In severe cases of depression, especially if psychotic symptoms are present, inpatient psychiatric treatment with or without ECT may be necessary to stabilize the patient's symptoms.

The prevalence of manic symptoms following pregnancy is unknown. BPAD has a high rate of recurrence if it remains untreated in the early postpartum period [4], with rates reported as high as 60%. Symptoms often present less than a week following delivery [15]. BPAD should be considered in any new onset PPD.

Symptoms of postpartum mania include precipitous deterioration, insomnia/poor sleep, labile affect, and unhealthy or paranoid preoccupation with the baby's well-being. There are a 5% suicide rate and a 4% infanticide rate for untreated patients with BPAD [15]. Rapid stabilization includes a mood stabilizer and a timely referral to a psychiatrist [15]. There should be a low threshold for inpatient hospitalization.

The choice of a mood stabilizer involves a risk–benefit analysis, especially for breastfeeding mothers. The American Academy of Pediatrics (AAP) advises caution in patients who are breastfeeding if they are concurrently taking lithium, with special attention being paid to potential toxicity in the infant [37]. Lithium is readily excreted into breast milk. Toxic lithium levels in infants manifest as lethargy, cyanosis, hypotonia, and hypothermia. If possible, its use should be postponed until the infant is 5 months old, when infant renal clearance is less of an issue [42]. If its use cannot be avoided, infants should be monitored both clinically and with serum blood counts and lithium levels.

The American Academy of Neurology (AAN) and AAP both endorse the use of valproic acid and carbamazepine in breastfeeding mothers [37]. The AAP advises the monitoring of hepatic function in breastfeeding infants whose mothers take either of these two medications [6, 42]. The additional benefit of valproic acid, especially in the emergency setting, is that it may be loaded as a single dose at 15–25 mg/kg. Subsequent daily dosing is adjusted to 10–15 mg/kg/day. A serum level should be checked in 4–5 days so further adjustments can be made.

Data for lamotrigine are limited. The risk of serious side effects such as Stevens–Johnson syndrome is present for both mother and breastfeeding infant; close monitoring is warranted [42]. Data regarding the use of oxcarbazepine in nursing infants are lacking.

FGAs and SGAs can be used in the emergent treatment of postpartum mania, with the same guidelines as in nonpregnant patients. Data are limited for breastfeeding patients; to date, no serious adverse events have been reported in nursing infants [42].

Data on postpartum anxiety disorders are sparse. Patients presenting with acute anxiety in the postpartum period may be treated using the same treatment guidelines as nonpregnant patients. In patients who are breastfeeding and receiving benzodiazepines, infants should be monitored for clinical signs of intoxication or toxicity, including hypotonia, poor feeding, thermoregulation problems, seizures, lethargy, and irritability [3, 5].

Postpartum Psychotic Disorders

The prevalence of new-onset psychosis in the postpartum period is not known, but estimates have placed the incidence as high as 1–2 in 1000 live births [60]. A history of a prior psychotic or mood disorder is common [6]. In women with a history of postpartum psychosis, the risk of recurrent episodes in subsequent postpartum periods is very high, estimated up to 70% [58]. Risk factors for postpartum psychosis include a history of psychotic symptoms (especially in pregnancy), multiple hospitalizations for psychosis, a history of a mood disorder (especially bipolar disorder), and antipsychotic discontinuation or noncompliance [60].

Postpartum psychotic symptoms start rapidly after delivery, usually within 3 weeks. Some patients may demonstrate signs as early as 72 hours after giving birth [2]. Symptoms include sleep disruption, paranoia, restlessness, agitation, disorganized thinking, impulsivity, risky or reckless behavior, and labile affect [4]. The workup for a woman with postpartum psychosis is as any other patient, with special attention paid to thyroid studies, since up to 9% of all postpartum women experience postpartum thyroiditis [61].

Postpartum psychosis is a psychiatric emergency, due to the risk to both mother and child. Emergency department treatment follows the same guidelines as for acute agitation (see Table 36.1), with the exception of the addition of lithium. Lithium monotherapy is argued to be the ideal initial medication treatment for patients with postpartum psychosis [62]. However, given the time it takes to reach a serum-steady state, lithium may not be the ideal choice for patients in an emergency department setting. Other authors argue that ECT ought to be the treatment of choice [58] or at least as a useful adjunct to lithium treatment [62]. ECT may be necessary to stabilize the patient's condition [2, 4, 15]. Regardless, inpatient psychiatric hospitalization is frequently required.

Conclusion

Pregnancy does not convey protection against mental illness. Pregnant patients with comorbid psychiatric problems are a special challenge to emergency department personnel. From a diagnostic standpoint, pregnant patients differ little from nonpregnant patients. However, acute management differs because one must also take the developing child's safety and well-being into consideration. The information and guidelines presented in this chapter will aid the emergency department clinician in evaluating and treating this special population of psychiatric patients.

References

1. Altshuler LL, Cohen LS, Moline ML, et al. Treatment of depression in women: a summary of the expert consensus guidelines. J Psychiatr Pract. 2001;7:185–208.
2. Cohen LS, Wang B, Nonacs R, et al. Treatment of mood disorders during pregnancy and postpartum. Psychiatr Clin N Am. 2010;33:273–93.
3. Jain AE, Lacy TL. Psychotropic drugs in pregnancy and lactation. J Psychiatr Pract. 2005;11:177–91.
4. Chaudron LH. Critical issues in perinatal psychiatric emergency care. Psychiatr Times. 2006;23:36–8.
5. ACOG Practice Bulletin. Use of psychiatric medications during pregnancy and lactation. Obstet Gynecol. 2008;111:1001–20.
6. Cohen LS, Nonacs R, Viguera AC. The pregnant patient. In: Stern TA, Fricchione GL, Cassem NH, et al., editors. Massachusetts General Hospital handbook of general hospital psychiatry. Fifth ed. Philadelphia: Mosby; 2004. p. 593–611.
7. Mills MD, Berkowitz P. Psychiatric emergencies in pregnancy. In: Foley MR, Strong TH, Garite TJ, editors. Obstetric intensive care manual. 3rd ed. New York: McGraw-Hill Companies, Inc; 2011.
8. Marzuk PM, Tardiff K, Leon AC, et al. Lower risk of suicide during pregnancy. Am J Psy. 1997;154:122–3.
9. Dell DL, O'Brien BW. Suicide in pregnancy. Obstet Gynecol. 2003;102:1306–9.
10. Patton SW, Misri S, Corral MR, et al. Antipsychotic medication during pregnancy and lactation in women with schizophrenia: evaluating the risk. Can J Psychiatr. 2002;47:959–65.
11. Horvath AO, Symonds BD. Relation between a working alliance and outcome in psychotherapy: a meta-analysis. J Couns Psychol. 1991;38:139–49.
12. Wilson MP, Nordstrom K, Shah AA, et al. Psychiatric emergencies in pregnant women. Emerg Med Clin N Am. 2015;33:841–51.
13. Ladavac AS, Dubin WR, Ning A, et al. Emergency management of agitation in pregnancy. Gen Hosp Psy. 2007;29:39–41.
14. Wilson MP, Pepper D, Currier GW, Holloman GH, Feifel D. The psychopharmacology of agitation: consensus statement of the American Association for Emergency Psychiatry Project BETA psychopharmacology workgroup. West J Emerg Med. 2012;13(1):26–34.
15. Henshaw E, Marcus S. Psychiatric emergencies during pregnancy and postpartum and review of gender issues in psychiatric emergency medicine. In: Glick RL, Berlin JS, Fishkind AB, Zeller SL, editors. Emergency psychiatry: principles and practice. Philadelphia: Lippincott Williams & Wilkins; 2008. p. 317–43.
16. Aftab A, Shah AA. Behavioral emergencies. Special considerations in the pregnant patient. Psychiatr Clin N Am. 2017;40:435–48.
17. Muzik M, Marcus SM, Heringhausen JE, et al. When depression complicates childbearing: guidelines for screening and treatment during antenatal and postpartum obstetric care. Obstet Gynecol Clin N Am. 2009;36:771–88.
18. Yonkers KA, Wisner KL, Stewart DE, et al. The management of depression during pregnancy: a report from the American Psychiatric Association and the American College of Obstetricians and Gynecologists. Gen Hosp Psy. 2009;31:403–13.
19. Lorenzo L, Byers B, Einarson A. Antidepressant use in pregnancy. Expert Opin Drug Saf. 2011;10(6):883–9.
20. Flynn HA, Davis M, Marcus SM, et al. Rates of maternal depression in pediatric emergency department and relationship to child service utilization. Gen Hosp Psy. 2004;26:316–22.
21. Gelenberg AJ, Freeman MP, Markowitz JC, et al. (Work Group on Major Depressive Disorder). APA Practice Guideline for the Treatment of Patients with Major Depressive Disorder. Third ed. APA. 2010. Available at http://www.psychiatryonline.com/pracGuide/pracGuideTopic_7.aspx. Accessed 13 Oct 2018.
22. Kemper KJ, Babonis TR. Screening for maternal depression in pediatric clinics. Am J Dis Child. 1992;146:876–8.
23. Cox JL, Holden JM, Sagovsky R. Detection of postnatal depression: development of the 10-item Edinburgh postnatal depression scale. Br J Psy. 1987;150:782–6.
24. Hallberg P, Sjoblom V. The use of selective serotonin reuptake inhibitors during pregnancy and breast-feeding: a review and clinical aspects. J Clin Psychopharmacol. 2005;25:59–73.
25. Malm H, Artama M, Gissler M, et al. Selective serotonin reuptake inhibitors and risk for major congenital anomalies. Obstet Gynecol. 2011;118:111–20.
26. Diav-Citrin O, Shechtman S, Weinbaum D, et al. Paroxetine and fluoxetine in pregnancy: a prospective, multicentre, controlled, observational study. Br J Clin Pharmacol. 2008;66:695–705.
27. Louik C, Lin AE, Werler MM, et al. First-trimester use of selective serotonin-reuptake inhibitors and the risk of birth defects. N Engl J Med. 2007;356:2675–83.
28. Hendrick V, Smith LM, Suri R, et al. Birth outcomes after prenatal exposure to antidepressant medication. Am J Obstet Gynecol. 2003;188:812–5.
29. Food and Drug Administration. Fed Regist. 1980;44:37434–67. Accessed October 17, 2011.
30. Koren G, Matsui D, Einarson A, et al. Is maternal use of selective serotonin reuptake inhibitors in the third trimester of pregnancy harmful to neonates? CMAJ. 2005;172:1457–9.
31. Chambers CD, Hernandez-Diaz S, VanMarter LJ, et al. Selective serotonin-reuptake inhibitors and risk of persistent pulmonary hypertension of the newborn. N Engl J Med. 2006;354:579–87.
32. Sanz EJ, De-las-Cuevas C, Kiuru A, et al. Selective serotonin reuptake inhibitors in pregnant women and

neonatal withdrawal syndrome: a database analysis. Lancet. 2005;365:482–7.
33. Croen LA, Grether JK, Yoshida CK, et al. Antidepressant use during pregnancy and childhood autism spectrum disorders. Arch Gen Psy. 2011;68(11):1104–12.
34. Wickramaratne P, Gameroff MJ, Pilowsky DJ, et al. Children of depressed mothers 1 year after remission of maternal depression: findings from the STAR*D-child study. Am J Psy. 2011;168:593–602.
35. George MS, Lisanby SH, Avery D, et al. Daily left prefrontal transcranial magnetic stimulation therapy for major depressive disorder. A sham-controlled randomized trial. Arch Gen Psy. 2010;67:507–16.
36. Anderson EL, Reti IM. ECT in pregnancy: a review of the literature from 1941 to 2007. Psychosom Med. 2009;71:235–42.
37. Yonkers KA, Wisner KL, Stowe Z, et al. Management of bipolar disorder during pregnancy and the postpartum period. Am J Psy. 2004;161:608–20.
38. Altshuler LL, Hendrick V, Cohen LS. An update on mood and anxiety disorders during pregnancy and the postpartum period. Primary Care Companion J Clin Psy. 2000;2:217–22.
39. Viguera AC, Whitfield T, Baldessarini RJ, et al. Risk of recurrence in women with bipolar disorder during pregnancy: prospective study of mood stabilizer discontinuation. Am J Psy. 2007;164:1817–24.
40. Viguera AC, Cohen LS, Baldessarini RJ, et al. Managing bipolar disorder in pregnancy: weighing the risks and benefits. Can J Psy. 2002;47:426–36.
41. Marcus SM, Barry KL, Flynn HA, et al. Treatment guidelines for depression in pregnancy. Int J Gynaecol Obstet. 2001;72:61–70.
42. Ernst CL, Goldberg JF. The reproductive safety profile of mood stabilizers, atypical antipsychotics, and broad-spectrum psychotropics. J Clin Psy. 2002;63:s42–55.
43. Diav-Citrin O, Shechtman S, Bar-Oz B, et al. Pregnancy outcome after in utero exposure to valproate. CNS Drugs. 2008;22:325–34.
44. Goodwin GM, Consensus Group of the British Association for Psychopharmacology. Evidence-based guidelines for the treatment of bipolar disorder: revised second edition—recommendations from the British Association for Psychopharmacology. J Psychopharmacol. 2009;23:346–88.
45. Bar-Shai M, Gott D, Kreinin I, et al. Atypical presentations of pregnancy-specific generalized anxiety disorders in women without a previous psychiatric background. Psychosomatics. 2015;56:286–91.
46. Otto MW, Smits JA, Reese HE. Cognitive-behavioral therapy for the treatment of anxiety disorders. J Clin Psy. 2004;65:S34–41.
47. Dolovich LR, Addis A, Régis-Vaillancourt JM, et al. Benzodiazepine use in pregnancy and major malformations or oral cleft: metaanalysis of cohort and case-control studies. BMJ. 1998;317:839–43.
48. McKenna K, Koren G, Tetelbaum M, et al. Pregnancy outcome of women using atypical antipsychotic drugs: a prospective comparative study. J Clin Psy. 2005;66:444–9.
49. Webb RT, Howard L, Abel KM. Antipsychotic drugs for non-affective psychosis during pregnancy and postpartum. Cochrane Database Syst Rev. 2004;(2):1–14.
50. SAMHSA, Office of Applied Studies. National Survey on Drug Use and Health. Available at http://www.oas.samhsa.gov/nsduh/2k8nsduh/2k8Results.pdf. 2005, 2006, 2007, 2008. Accessed 17 Oct 2011.
51. Russell M. New assessment tools for drinking during pregnancy, T-ACE, TWEAK, others. Alcohol Health Res World. 1994;18:55–61.
52. National Institute of Mental Health. Statistics. Available at https://www.nimh.nih.gov/health/statistics/eating-disorders.shtml. Accessed 13 Oct 2018.
53. Kouba S, Hallstrom T, Lindholm C, et al. Pregnancy and neonatal outcomes in women with eating disorders. Obstet Gynecol. 2005;105:255–60.
54. Franko DL, Blais MA, Becker AE, et al. Pregnancy complications and neonatal outcomes in women with eating disorders. Am J Psy. 2001;158:1461–6.
55. Jasinski JL. Pregnancy and domestic violence: a review of the literature. Trauma Violence Abuse. 2004;5:47–64.
56. Espinosa L, Osborne K. Domestic violence during pregnancy: implications for practice. J Midwifery Womens Health. 2002;47:305–17.
57. US Department of Health and Human Services Centers for Disease Control and Prevention. Intimate partner violence during pregnancy: a guide for clinicians. 2011. Available at https://www.cdc.gov/ViolencePrevention/intimatepartnerviolence/index.html. Accessed 13 Oct 2018.
58. Focht A, Kellner CH. Electroconvulsive therapy (ECT) in the treatment of postpartum psychosis. J ECT. 2012;28:31–3.
59. Fisher SD, Wisner KL, Clark CT, et al. Factors associated with onset timing, symptoms, and severity of depression identified in the postpartum period. J Affect Disord. 2016;203:111–20.
60. Harlow BL, Vitonis AF, Sparen P, et al. Incidence of hospitalization for postpartum psychotic and bipolar episodes in women with and without prior prepregnancy or prenatal psychiatric hospitalizations. Arch Gen Psy. 2007;64:42–8.
61. Bokhari R, Bhatara VS, Bandettini F, et al. Postpartum psychosis and postpartum thyroiditis. Psychoneuroendocrinology. 1998;23:643–50.
62. Bergink V, Rasgon N, Wisner KL. Postpartum psychosis: madness, mania, and melancholia in motherhood. Am J Psy. 2016;173:1179–88.

37 Cultural Concerns and Issues in Emergency Psychiatry

Suzanne Bruch

Introduction

The increasing diversification of the population in the United States and other countries has placed increased demands on health-care systems to treat patients of different cultural backgrounds. A person's ethnic background, race, religion, values, beliefs, customs, and language can affect not only the symptoms with which a psychiatric illness may present but also the manner in which that person may seek help. Culture in the United States has been heavily influenced by Euro-American Protestant values, including independence, autonomy, and self-sufficiency [1]. However, the complexion of the population in this country has changed dramatically over the past several decades. Between 1980 and 2010, the population of Asians in the United States increased by 319%, Hispanics by 246%, American Indians by 106%, and African Americans by 47% in comparison to a 9% increase in the non-Hispanic White population [2].

S. Bruch (✉)
Psychiatry, Northern California, CA, USA

Culture, Cultural Competence, and Cultural Formulation

The Department of Health and Human Services defines culture as a common heritage or set of beliefs, norms, and values [3]. Culture encompasses race, ethnic background, spirituality, gender, age, sexual orientation, marital status, socioeconomic status, and education. Cultural competence refers to the set of skills needed to provide care that respects the patient's ethnocultural beliefs, values, attitudes, and conventions [4]. Cultural competency aligns with the trend toward evidence-based medicine as both represent a focus on providing effective treatment for each individual patient. Currently, scientific evidence to guide treatment of patients belonging to a minority culture is limited.

The charge to provide culturally competent care in the United States is rooted in the civil rights movement of the 1960s and reflects an interpretation of the Declaration of Independence to extend basic civil rights to all citizens and to outlaw discrimination [5]. Title VI of the 1964 Civil Rights Act mandated service providers receiving federal financial assistance to provide meaningful and equal access to services for people with limited English proficiency (LEP), which has been defined as "limited ability to listen, speak, read, and write in English, and speak[ing] English less than very well" [6].

L. S. Zun et al. (eds.), *Behavioral Emergencies for Healthcare Providers*,
https://doi.org/10.1007/978-3-030-52520-0_37

Transcultural psychiatry was recognized by the American Psychiatric Association as a specialty in 1969 [7]. In the 1980s, the biopsychosocial model of case formulation took hold in psychiatry. By the 1990s, states including California and New York enacted legislation to ensure the provision of culturally and linguistically appropriate health care. At the same time, the American Psychiatric Association included an outline for cultural formulation in the Diagnostic and Statistical Manual of Mental Disorders Fourth Edition and reference to cultural factors in its published practice guidelines for adults, providing a framework for culturally competent evaluations of psychiatric patients. In 2000, President Bill Clinton signed Executive Order 13166, requiring recipients of federal funding to take "reasonable steps to ensure meaningful access" for LEP persons [8].

Section 1557 of the Affordable Care Act of 2010 (ACA) extends nondiscrimination protection to health care and health coverage, including the health insurance exchanges [9]. Several sections of the ACA require that patient communication be provided in "plain language" [9]. Furthermore, providers and health-care entities must offer "qualified" interpreters and translators at no cost to LEP patients [10]. In Australia, the department of social services provides free translating and interpreting services for medical providers and pharmacists. Unfortunately, in the United States, the cost of interpreter services, coupled with the lack of comprehensive reimbursement practices, operates as a disincentive for clinicians to see LEP patients [11].

Despite the government mandate for equal access to health care and the increased focus on cultural competency, progress has been slow. The United States Surgeon General's report on Mental Health: Culture, Race, and Ethnicity and the Institute of Medicine's Unequal Treatment report concluded that ethnic minority patients have less access to services, are less likely to receive mental health treatment, receive a lower quality of care both in terms of medical and psychiatric treatment, and are underrepresented in mental health research [3, 5, 7]. Yet migrant populations exhibit a higher incidence of mental illness compared with native populations, and ethnic minorities experience a greater disability burden from mental illness than do non-Hispanic Whites [12, 13]. While one in five Americans experiences mental illness, the majority of people with diagnosable disorders do not receive treatment, regardless of race or ethnicity [3]. As a result of this report, the US Surgeon General declared that cultural competence should be a core component of any service [5]. Unfortunately, 80% of psychiatric staff feel that their professional training prepares them "very little" or "not at all" for cross-cultural clinical work [12].

A culturally competent evaluation of the psychiatric patient includes assessment of the cultural identity of the individual, the role of culture in the expression and evaluation of psychiatric symptoms, and the effect of cultural differences on the relationship between patient and clinician. In assessing a patient's cultural identity, it is helpful to assess the degree of involvement with both the culture of origin and the host culture, identifying areas of cultural conflict pertinent to the patient's presentation. Goals of cultural formulation include increased understanding of patients' perceptions of illness, more accurate diagnosis, more appropriate treatment, and improved access to care.

Explanatory Models of Illness

A patient's explanatory model of illness reflects his own cultural background. Each culture regulates its own patterns of emotional expression, determining which are socially acceptable and which are deviant. Culture influences the sources of distress, the illness experience, the symptomatology and interpretation of these symptoms, coping mechanisms and help-seeking behaviors, and family and community support, as well as the social response to distress and disability [3, 14]. The cultures of the clinician and system of care influence diagnosis, treatment, and delivery of care. The stigma associated with mental illness appears to be universal cross-culturally, and alternative conceptualizations of illness may mitigate this stigma [15].

In many cultures, mood and anxiety disorders may be viewed as moral or social defects rather than illness. The United States is unique in the open expression of interpersonal conflict. Many other cultures value the suppression of both internal and interpersonal conflict, prioritizing nonconfrontational interaction and social harmony.

Understanding the patient's own view of illness promotes collaboration between clinician and patient, enabling the clinician to more successfully develop and implement a viable treatment plan and leading to improved outcomes and greater patient satisfaction. When the clinician shares the patient's model of understanding distress and treatment, patient satisfaction is greatest [16]. Conflicting explanatory models may result in poor rapport, nonadherence to treatment, and dropout of treatment. The clinician should attempt to implement an evidence-based treatment that does not conflict with the patient's cultural beliefs. The conflict between patient and family explanatory models leads to family discord, shame, and an impaired support system. When the patient's explanatory model differs from that of his community, he may suffer social isolation and stigmatization [1].

Language

According to the American Community Survey 2011, over 300 languages are spoken in the United States [17]. Of the 291.5 million people aged 5 and over in this country, more than 60.5 million (over 20%) speak a language other than English at home [17]. Thirty-one million patients speak primary languages that differ from those of their health-care providers [18]. Communication barriers adversely impact access to health-care services, health outcomes, and patient satisfaction [19]. The National Healthcare Disparities Report found that 47% of LEP patients do not have a usual source of care, and 6% have a usual source of care that does not provide language assistance [20]. LEP patients are less likely to have regular health providers or to receive routine preventive treatment [11, 19, 21–23]. Language barriers contribute to the poor understanding of a diagnosis and treatment plan, including medication instructions and follow-up recommendations, increased risk of adverse events, and lower patient satisfaction [23]. As a result, LEP patients typically experience reduced clinical encounter time, increased risk of medication nonadherence, increased frequency of medical complications, and increased risk of patient safety events, and they are less satisfied with both clinician communication and overall health care [21, 22]. Language concordance between patient and provider promotes increased patient comprehension, compliance, and satisfaction [23].

Language barriers prove particularly problematic for patients presenting with psychiatric symptoms. Patients experiencing acute psychiatric illness may lose their ability to communicate freely in an acquired language. Whether more psychopathology is evident when a patient is interviewed in his native tongue or a second language is debated in the literature [24, 25].

Interpreters, Translation, and Communication

Interpretation is of critical importance in the evaluation of behavioral emergencies. As the mental status exam is more subjective than the physical exam, many symptoms are elicited only by self-report, and any distortion may lead to misdiagnosis or misunderstanding of treatment. Interpreters have reported that differences in illness perspective between patient and clinician are especially common when psychiatric diagnoses are involved [26]. Some patients consider such diagnoses to be disbelief on the part of the clinician—or rejection. Language discordance between patient and provider interferes with assessing disorders of speech and thought processes, in particular. For example, clinicians who tend to use closed-ended questions when evaluating LEP patients may incorrectly conclude that the patient is guarded or withdrawn or that his thought process is impoverished. LEP patients or providers speaking in a second language may make tense errors, leading to confusion regarding whether the symptoms are current or were experienced in the past. In emergency situations, health-care providers are forced to complete an evaluation in a limited period of time. Yet it is important that sufficient time is devoted to the interview to allow the patient to present his own narrative describing symptoms and illness, which can be particularly challenging when interpretation is required.

In addition to the notion of cultural competence, we must also consider the concept of communication competency in medical interviews [27]. A translator provides a more literal interpretation of a patient's report, while an interpreter provides a cultural context. When using interpreters, health-care professionals must work to maintain basic principles of medical ethics, including patient rights, patient autonomy, patient confidentiality, and informed consent. Upholding these principles can be particularly difficult when the health-care provider is dependent on an informal or ad hoc interpreter. Utilization of a layperson as interpreter provides for potential distortions based on the interpreter's attitudes toward both patient and clinician. Untrained interpreters may feel uncomfortable with the personal nature of the clinician's questions or overwhelmed by the responsibility of the task, and they are more likely to make errors and violate confidentiality [28]. Family and friends interpreting are not desirable due to their lack of objectivity and tendency to respond to clinicians' questions without input from the patient. Use of professional interpreters appears to facilitate increased disclosure of sensitive information, including psychological and physical symptoms and traumatic events [29]. Errors committed by untrained interpreters may critically compromise patient safety and can even prove life-threatening [22]. Patients who depend on untrained, ad hoc interpreters report less satisfaction with their patient-provider relationship [6]. Language competency, interpretative skills, and cultural knowledge are critical components in the successful evaluation of a patient presenting with a behavioral emergency.

The psychiatric interview is highly dependent on the interpreter, who has the power to control the information being exchanged. The accuracy of meaning may be diminished when an unskilled interpreter simply translates. The effectiveness of communication essential for an accurate psychiatric diagnosis and treatment plan may be altered by the dynamic of using an interpreter. In addition to the clinician-patient relationship, there now also exist relationships between patient and interpreter and between clinician and interpreter. Anxious or paranoid patients may find the presence of the interpreter problematic.

The following table illustrates common errors of interpretation [12]. In addition to those errors noted, studies have shown cases of interpreters dissuading patients from disclosing information deemed stigmatizing in their culture [12]. Errors in interpretation are more common when the patient is speaking than the clinician and are more common when a patient is acutely ill or psychotic [29] (Table 37.1).

Table 37.1 Common errors of interpretation

Omission	Information is partially or completely deleted by the interpreter More likely when discussing sensitive personal issues, such as substance use or sex, or when the interpreter has a personal conflict of interest (e.g., when a family member is acting as an informal interpreter)
Addition	The interpreter includes information not expressed by the patient
Condensation	A long or complicated response is simplified. Particularly problematic in the psychiatric evaluation of a patient with disorganized or incoherent responses, or when a response is shortened such that critical information is deleted
Substitution	The interpreter rephrases the question in a manner that changes the concept
Role exchange	The interpreter takes over the interview, replacing the interviewer's questions with his own
Closed/open	The interpreter alters the way the question was asked. The interpreter may elaborate with his own series of questions, delivering results of this exchange, rather than an accurate response to the original question
Normalization	The interpreter attempts to make sense of the patient's response Particularly problematic in evaluating a behavioral emergency

Adapted from Farooq and Fear [12]

Psychiatric evaluation is further hindered by interpretation as speech content is temporally separated from facial expression and psychomotor activity. The interpreter may focus on what the patient is saying, rather than how he is saying it, yet meanings of both verbal and nonverbal expressions are integral components of the psychiatric exam. During a psychiatric interview, many questions could be considered presumptuous and adversely affect rapport if asked without appropriately empathic expression. Looking at the patient and addressing the patient directly, rather than addressing the interpreter, will facilitate better rapport. Affect, thought process, and ambivalence can be particularly subject to distortion, in part due to difficulty conveying the meaning of paralinguistic cues [30]. To prevent misunderstandings and misinterpretation, the clinician is advised to speak in short, clear sentences, avoiding slang and medical jargon, and to pause frequently to check on the patient's level of understanding.

While time is limited in the emergency setting, meetings between clinician and interpreter both before and after interviewing the patient have proven effective in minimizing distortions [12, 30]. A preinterview meeting allows the clinician to discuss the goals of the interview, including specific areas of focus and any potentially sensitive topics, and allows the clinician to assess the interpreter's attitude toward both patient and subject matter. Interpreters should be encouraged to ask both clinician and patient for clarification when needed and should be counseled not to attempt to make sense of the patient's statements. The clinician should request a verbatim translation if the response is still unclear. A post-interview meeting provides the opportunity for clarification of both interview content and dynamics of the interaction, including discussion of paralinguistic cues. The interpreter may also benefit from the opportunity to discuss and process his or her own feelings and reaction to the interview.

Interpreter services improve health-care experiences and outcomes [21]. Despite the use of interpreters, LEP patients are less likely to express concerns or ask questions. High-quality health care for LEP patients depends on high-quality interpreter services when language-concordant clinicians are not available as patients who rate their interpreter highly are more apt to rate the health care received highly [21]. Patient satisfaction depends on the ability of the patient to convey information to the health-care provider, the expertise of the physician, and the emotional tone of the encounter [27]. Enhanced communication leads to a stronger doctor-patient relationship and increased patient autonomy, allowing the patient to better understand his condition, more effectively participate in treatment planning, and make informed decisions. Therapeutic alliance is a positive prognostic indicator of treatment [31]. Using professional interpreters, whether in person or remotely, increases patient satisfaction, strengthens adherence, improves outcomes, and lessens adverse events [28].

Despite the benefits of using qualified medical interpreters, clinicians tend to underutilize available interpreter services and to perceive a compromised quality of care, even when an interpreter is used [22]. There is some concern that clinicians may project their discomfort in treating LEP patients onto the patients themselves, preventing them from acknowledging the patient's feeling of being helped and desire for continued care [29]. Clinicians who have received interpreter training are more satisfied with their ability to communicate with LEP patients [23]. Physicians and interpreters have shown a strong preference for in-person interpreters, in comparison to remote interpreting via telephone or video, whereas patients have shown no preference [11, 22, 32]. Clinicians appear to have a better understanding of a patient's cultural beliefs when an in-person professional interpreter is used [11]. In the emergency department (ED), using professional interpreters has been correlated with an increased intensity of services, reduced return ED visits, and lower cost, while non-interpreted non-English-speaking patients had the shortest length of ED stay and fewest tests and medications [33].

Language barriers influence the authenticity of the informed consent process. A patient's understanding of both illness and proposed treatment and their ability to voluntarily make treatment decisions form the basis for informed consent. The clinician must attend to the patient's perspective, attempt to understand it, avoid declarations, and recognize the social context within this exchange [34]. He has the responsibility of ensuring that the patient has an accurate understanding of the totality of information required to make the decision. Recognition of an individual's autonomy, avoidance of coercion, and voluntary patient participation are essential elements of the informed consent process.

In acknowledging the benefits that professional medical interpreters provide, it is also important to recognize the limitations in comparison to language-concordant physician-patient encounters. Patients typically feel less understood by their physicians, and they themselves have difficulty understanding physicians' explanations and follow-up instructions when interpreters of any kind are used [19].

Minority Populations

Increasing awareness and understanding of different cultures will aid in more accurate assessment and diagnosis. At present, patients with psychiatric illnesses are diagnosed according to the Diagnostic and Statistical Manual of Mental Disorders, Fifth Edition (DSM-5). However, this classification system is based on Western concepts of mental health and illness and can potentially lead to patients from minority populations being misunderstood and misdiagnosed. To that end, increasing understanding of specific populations may prove useful for clinicians, particularly when evaluating for potential underlying psychiatric illness in an emergency setting.

Ethnic and racial minorities in the United States experience an environment of social and economic inequality plagued by greater exposure to racism, discrimination, poverty, and violence. People in the lowest socioeconomic strata are two to three times more likely to suffer mental illness than those in the highest strata [3]. Racism and discrimination adversely affect mental health and place minorities at increased risk of such illnesses as depression and anxiety. Mistrust of mental health services deters minorities from seeking treatment and is reinforced by clinician bias and stereotyping. Providing evidence-based treatment for minority populations is challenged by the tendency of conventional psychiatric research to reduce the complexity of illness narratives to a checklist of symptoms [14].

Education about other cultures and belief systems is an important starting point in the provision of culturally competent care. Overall, Euro-Americans align with professional disease-oriented perspectives on mental illness, seeking treatment when needed and viewing psychotropic medication as a necessary component of treatment [15]. In contrast, psychiatric patients of non-Western origin abandon treatment against medical advice far more often [35]. While the following discussion is neither complete nor exhaustive, it does provide a basic framework for understanding other cultures. Each patient must still be evaluated individually as these generalizations are not meant to invoke stereotypes or dismiss pathology as a cultural phenomenon. Even clinicians of the same ethnicity as the patient must be careful to consider each patient individually in order to avoid overidentification and assumptions.

According to federal classification, the four most recognized racial and ethnic minority groups in the United States are Hispanic Americans/Latinos, African Americans/Blacks, Asian Americans and Pacific Islanders, and American Indians and Alaska Natives.

Hispanic Americans

Hispanics are the largest ethnic minority population in the United States, and this population is rapidly growing, with a 43% increase between 2000 and 2010 [2]. Their ancestry may trace to Africa, Asia, Europe, the Middle East, the Caribbean, or the Americas [3, 19]. Latino groups experience high levels of stress and distress, which can exacerbate preexisting conditions or increase the risk of developing substance use and psychiatric disorders [19]. Their resilience and coping skills promote mental health. Hispanic American youth experience higher rates of depression, anxiety, suicidal ideation, and suicide attempts as compared to White youth [3]. Interestingly, rates of mental illness are lower for Mexican Americans than other Hispanics [13].

Limited availability of ethnically or linguistically compatible providers and lack of health insurance have limited access to psychiatric services such that Hispanic Americans are less likely than White Americans to receive needed psychiatric services [3, 11]. Contributing factors include stigma associated with mental health services, cultural and linguistic barriers, poverty, discrimination, and lack of empirically based treatments [31]. Lack of culturally appropriate care contributes to premature dropout from treatment [31]. Limited outcome data suggest that Hispanic Americans are less likely to receive treatment in accordance with evidence-based guidelines [3]. For example, Latino and African Americans with co-occurring depression and substance abuse have less access to treatment with selective serotonin reuptake inhibitors in comparison to European Americans with the same co-occurring conditions [36].

Cultural factors including language, family, and beliefs about health can impact the assessment and treatment of Hispanic patients presenting with behavioral emergencies. Latinos tend to use non-biomedical interpretations of emotional, cognitive, and behavioral problems [15]. They tend to downplay their symptoms and normalize their illness experience [15]. Hispanics are less accepting of mental illness and view depression as a sign of weakness or madness. Psychiatric labels have the potential to be socially damaging in this population [15]. Hispanics may somatize their symptoms and may prefer alternative treatment options, such as spiritual healers. Increased frequency of somatic complaints has been noted in Mexican American and Puerto Rican patients [24]. When depressed, Hispanics are more likely to endorse appetite or weight disturbances [37]. Hispanic patients may present with atypical psychotic symptoms, including auditory and visual hallucinations, but have an otherwise unremarkable mental status exam. Hispanics tend to believe in predetermination and that a higher power is in control. Typical gender roles dictate that men are strong, loving providers for their families and that woman are spiritually superior, deferring their own needs for children and family. Deviation from these roles may lead to depression [38]. As family provides primary social support, involving relatives in treatment can be beneficial.

Incorporating cultural constructs can increase the effectiveness of service delivery to Hispanic patients. *Familismo* (family orientation) emphasizes the importance of family, loyalty, and solidarity, as well as the focus on the greater good of the family over individual needs, and it highlights the importance of family involvement in treatment [31]. *Personalismo* (personal relationship) highlights the importance of relating on a personal level, which helps patients develop rapport and establish trust. Otherwise, the clinician may be perceived as cold or unpleasant, which can adversely affect treatment compliance [31]. *Respeto* (respect, mutual and reciprocal deference) refers to the adherence to hierarchical structure, in which individuals defer to those with more seniority or higher status. For example, when speaking Spanish, the patient should be addressed using the formal pronoun *usted* in place of the informal *tu* until given permission to do otherwise as disrespect or offensive gestures could adversely affect treatment outcomes [31]. *Confianza* (trust and intimacy in a relationship) is an essential component in establishing a therapeutic treatment alliance and typically develops in relationships based on *personalismo* and *respeto* [31]. *Fatalismo* (fatalism) encompasses the belief that outcomes may not be entirely under one's control and that fate, luck, or a higher power may play a role [31]. Patients may refer to *Dios quiere* (God's will) or *el destino* (destiny). Exploring a patient's contributions to the achievement of his goals may be an effective means of empowering the patient and strengthening the therapeutic alliance without questioning the patient's religious or spiritual beliefs. *Contralarse* (self-containment or conscious control of negative affect) and *aguantarse* (ability to withstand stressful situations, particularly during difficult times) reflect inner strength in times of adversity [31]. *Sobreponerse* (self-suppression) refers to a particular mindset needed to overcome challenges, though the clinician must not appear to be minimizing or dismissive of the presenting issues [31]. Incorporating these cultural constructs during assessment and treatment of Hispanic patients may enhance therapeutic alliance and improve treatment outcomes.

Latinos are generally amenable to treatment with psychotropic medication but tend to utilize psychosocial interventions less frequently [15]. Latino men tend to view clinicians as a means to obtaining medication, whereas women are more likely to utilize psychosocial interventions such as groups and therapy [15].

African Americans

While the majority of African Americans trace their ancestry to slaves brought from Africa, this population is diversifying with the influx of immigrants and refugees from African nations and the Caribbean. The legacy of slavery, racism, and discrimination continues to affect this population. Nearly one-quarter of African Americans suffers from poverty [3]. Mortality rates are disproportionately high. Resilience is a strength of this population. Prevalence rates of mental illness for African Americans are similar to those for non-Hispanic Whites [3]. Yet African Americans are less likely to use and receive mental health care, and they are overrepresented in high-need populations, including the homeless, the incarcerated, and children in foster care [3, 15]. Availability of services is limited due to reliance on safety net providers and lack of African American clinicians specializing in mental health. Access to treatment and utilization of services are limited by lack of insurance and less inclination to take advantage of available services. African Americans are more likely to delay treatment until their symptoms are severe and to receive psychiatric treatment in emergency rooms and psychiatric hospitals [3]. Errors in diagnosis are more common for African Americans than Whites, and African Americans are less likely to receive care directed by evidence-based treatment guidelines. When treated appropriately, African Americans respond as favorably as Whites [3].

African Americans are more likely to use non-biomedical interpretations of behavioral, emotional, or cognitive problems [15]. They may attribute symptoms to supernatural or demonological forces, or they may formulate characterological explanations [15]. African Americans with mental illness tend to downplay their symptoms and normalize their illness experience [15]. Those with depression are more likely to present with somatic and neurovegetative symptoms than with mood or cognitive disturbances, and they are more likely to endorse appetite or weight disturbances [37]. African Americans find mental illness stigmatizing and consider it private family business. Diagnostic labels may have damaging social consequences, including ridicule, disparagement, and retaliation [15]. The perception that individuals with mental illness are dangerous persists in this population [15].

From a treatment perspective, African Americans are more critical of mental health services and of psychotropic medication, sensing that medication compliance is the clinician's primary concern [15]. They may become frustrated with dosing changes, feeling that they are being experimented on [15]. They tend to feel that treatment providers do not listen, care, or help solve problems [11]. They may feel treatment providers are trying to control them [15]. Difficulty communicating with clinicians constitutes a significant barrier to seeking services and engaging in treatment [15].

Asian Americans and Pacific Islanders

Over 17 million Asians reside in the United States, and this population is rapidly growing, with a 43% increase between 2000 and 2010 [2]. This minority population is remarkably diverse, accounting for 43 ethnic groups speaking over 100 different languages and dialects and representing a range of educational and socioeconomic backgrounds [3]. With this diversity, expectations may vary concerning when to seek medical treatment, the role of a physician, the roles of the patient and family, and privacy issues, including disclosure to patient and family.

Asian Americans use fewer mental health services than any other minority group, tending to access services only in crisis and to drop out prematurely [39]. Availability of services is limited due to the limited English proficiency of nearly half this population and lack of providers with compatible language skills [3]. Stigma and shame associated with mental illness further limit utilization of services. Asians may experience trepidation when navigating an unfamiliar health-care system, frustration when unable to effectively communicate their symptoms, and anger when feeling they are being viewed with mistrust or suspicion by hospital staff. Of those who utilize available services, the severity of presentation is high, suggesting that Asians delay treatment until the condition is serious.

In general, strengths of the Asian population include family cohesion and motivation for upward mobility and educational achievement. In contrast to the Western focus on the patient as an individual, Asian culture emphasizes family, and understanding religious and social support systems may prove invaluable in formulating a diagnosis and treatment plan. Family structure is patriarchal and hierarchical. Japanese Americans, in general, are highly successful, attaining high rates of educational achievement and income and low rates of mental illness, alcoholism, and juvenile delinquency. One theory is that the highly structured role relationships in the family, with their stability and predictability, protect family members from outside stressors and form the basis for an individual's ability to adapt and adjust [13].

In Asian culture, there is a belief that avoiding bad thoughts can lead to mental health. Expression of feelings, particularly negative ones, and emotional distress are taboo, disgracing individual and family. Suppression of negative affect is valued. Mental illness may be indicative of character weakness or lack of self-control and can shame the family. Family members may fear they are at risk for genetic inheritance of these traits. Self-control, desire to save face, need to protect a family, lack of available language to describe symptoms, and stigma associated with mental illness have led to somatization of psychiatric symptoms, which is both culturally acceptable and less stigmatizing [40]. The Asian conceptualization of mind and body as a whole has also contributed to the somatization of mental illness. In fact, somatic presentations of mental illness are seen in most patients from non-Western cultures [38]. An Asian person with depression may present to the emergency department with a chief complaint of a headache, a backache, some muscle pain, a stomachache, dizziness, low energy, or insomnia. He may be inclined to deny depressed mood in order to preserve his own self-image and avoid negative reflection on his family. Asian patients tend to minimize symptoms and underreport suicidal ideation and suicide attempts [37, 38]. Careful history-taking may identify a trauma or loss precipitating onset of physical symptoms.

Treatment interventions should be problem-focused and include psychotropic medication; supportive, cognitive, or behavioral therapy; and family therapy, particularly with inclusion or support of the identified family leader. Instillation of hope is important. Patients from Asian cultures traditionally show tremendous respect toward clinicians and expect this person to be authoritative and directive once rapport has been established. Failure to provide instructions to the patient could lead the patient to conclude that the clinician is uncaring or incompetent. Traditionally recommended treatments for substance use disorders, including group therapeutic interventions such as Alcoholics Anonymous, can prove problematic due to the cultural taboo associated with public expression of emotions and group confrontation.

Asians with psychotic disorders are more likely to experience visual, olfactory, or tactile hallucinations than the auditory hallucinations typically experienced by Western patients [40]. Misdiagnosis of mental illness is common in this patient population with atypical nature of presenting symptoms, language barriers, lack of knowledge of Asian cultures, and lack of cultural sensitivity contributing [40].

In evaluating patients from southeast Asia, the clinician must be cognizant of the following cultural beliefs: preference for group interest over individual interest; harmonious family relationships; respect for elders; control of emotions, including those which may be undesirable; and confrontation avoidance [41]. Relevant history may include migration history and refugee status, which may provide an opening for discussion of possible past trauma. Southeast Asian refugees are at increased risk of post-traumatic stress disorder related to pre-immigration trauma. Southeast Asians may use moral, religious, magical, or medical models to explain the illness. The moral model links the medical or psychiatric condition to such negative traits as laziness, selfishness, and low morality and posits that correction of such behaviors is necessary for symptom resolution. Supernatural factors underlying mental illness are the central tenet of the religious model, and appeasing God or angered spirits is an essential treatment component. In the medical model, traditional Eastern therapies including local healers, acupuncture, meditation, herbs, yoga, and dietary modification may be preferred to Western medicine. An Asian typically turns to family for support before seeking treatment outside the home. Families may try to protect those with psychotic symptoms to save face and avoid stigma and shame [40]. Often, symptoms are quite severe by the time a patient presents for treatment. Mistrust of the mental health system, conflicting Eastern and Western values, discomfort with Western treatment methods, and medication side effects impede engagement in psychiatric treatment and lead to early dropout [40].

Filipino Americans are the second fastest growing Asian immigrant group in the United States behind the Chinese [39]. They believe happiness and health result from balance and that rapid temperature changes can cause illness [39]. They have a fatalistic and passive attitude and underutilize existing mental health services, which are culturally, socially, and linguistically incompatible [38, 39]. Stigma and preference for traditional healing methods, such as faith healers, inhibit Filipinos from seeking treatment. Depression may manifest with classical symptoms, somatization, or the incongruous smiling depression [39]. Suicide rates are lower, likely reflecting the influence of Catholicism, as well as extended family and social support systems [39]. Some Filipinos believe that persons with mental illness are dangerously unpredictable [39]. Filipino women are at increased risk of physical and mental health problems as they are expected to work outside the home while maintaining primary responsibility for childcare and domestic duties [39]. Filipinos will express their feelings toward health-care providers who are respectful, approachable, and accommodating but will otherwise interact in a formal, superficial, and reticent manner, concealing emotion [39]. Filipino patients may look down to convey respect. Respect or embarrassment may prevent the asking of questions due to desire to save face and mask any lack of understanding. Filipinos often attempt to gain familiarity with the treatment provider and are often more comfortable in the presence of family. They typically accept medications as a means of treatment.

Japanese refer to doctors using the title *sensei*, which means "master," "teacher," or "doctor" and which is shared by other professionals deemed to be morally and socially responsible public figures [18]. Doctors with greater expertise and those physicians seen as saving lives are held in higher regard. Japanese patients typically comply with their physicians' treatment recommendations. It is important to them that their physicians convey respect. Regardless of religious affiliation, there are three types of Japanese religious practices which may affect treatment [18]. The first emphasizes wish fulfillment through the power of prayer and may place greater emphasis on religious and magical prayers than on medical treatments, potentially leading to treatment refusal [18]. The second religious practice is akin to determinism and emphasizes self-control [18]. Followers seek to live their lives in accordance with the will of God, gods, or spiritual principles and accept their illnesses as an unavoidable fate, living their lives within these constraints [18].

The third religious practice involves the cultivation of mind through universal truth [18]. For example, Buddhism teaches patients to recognize the state of their illness in an objective manner as part of a natural reality and to seek new paths to fulfillment by transcending states of suffering [18]. Japanese avoid conversations with direct eye contact. Given that suppressing feelings of anger and sadness is considered a virtue, Japanese patients often do not want to hear the name of their illness directly from their doctor, but rather they wish to be informed indirectly so that they can be prepared [18]. Japanese patients typically present for treatment with family members. Because of stigma and potential embarrassment, Japanese patients have difficulty openly discussing mental illness. A clinician inquiring directly about personal information deemed irrelevant to the presenting illness would be considered rude and inappropriate. Japanese are frustrated by the inability to adequately explain symptoms in English, and this tenet holds true even when the individual appears to have very good command of the English language [18].

Most Koreans will not seek medical treatment unless seriously ill, and even then, they are apt to first consult with a physician in the family or close social circle, or with a pharmacist [18]. Koreans view doctors as masters accorded absolute authority, holding specialists in higher regard [18]. They feel large hospitals have greater credibility than individual doctors [18]. Koreans trust their doctors regarding treatment choice. When illness is severe, family members will accompany the patient. Koreans may experience tension between respect for modern medicine and fundamentalist tendencies to eschew medical treatment. While Korean Protestantism emphasizes the healing power of the Holy Spirit, religious leaders do typically encourage medical attention [18]. Only the most conservative branches preach reliance on the healing power of God. Shamanism is also practiced in Korea, and shaman-nesses are thought to have magical and miraculous healing abilities. Koreans tend to view their constitution as unique and question whether Western medicine is able to effectively treat their illnesses [18]. If conventional medical treatments fail, Koreans may devote themselves to prayer [18]. Regardless of religion, Koreans believe in destiny according to cosmic providence [18].

Indians tend to utilize both traditional and Western approaches to medicine. Indians trust their primary care physicians and typically consult them first rather than go directly to a hospital or specialist [18]. They are accustomed to having significant personal interaction with their physicians and expect to be able to spend time with them [18]. Indians are highly respectful of physicians, particularly specialists, and tend to comply with proposed treatment [18]. Wealthier members of Indian society go to the doctor with even minor complaints, whereas poorer Indians are more apt to attempt a home remedy and go to the doctor only if it fails [18]. Ayurvedic practice is also popular. Ayurvedic medicines called *bhasmas* are composed of heavy metals, such as lead, arsenic, mercury, or cadmium, that are mixed with herbs or spices. Ingestion of these compounds has the potential to cause heavy metal toxicity, which may manifest with such symptoms as confusion, memory loss, insomnia, and tremor. Indians may practice Hinduism, Christianity, Islam, or other religions, but religion plays a less prominent role in health-care ideology [18]. Family members typically accompany patients to medical visits and are privy to the patient's medical information. Indians want to feel that clinicians are trying to understand them and their culture and that their lifestyle choices are respected as this personal interest contributes to a sense of belonging [18]. Indian women tend to be shy in front of male doctors and may prefer female doctors or the presence of female nursing staff [18]. Suicide is the leading cause of death for Indians aged 15–24 years old [40].

American Indian and Alaska Natives

Five hundred and sixty-one tribes are represented by the Bureau of Indian Affairs [3]. This minority group is the most impoverished, with over one-quarter living in poverty [3]. Availability of mental health services is limited by geographic location due to the distance from treatment centers and lack of available specialists [3]. Lack of health insurance limits access [3]. Utilization of mental health services, appropriateness of treatment, and outcomes are not well understood due to lack of research.

Prevalence rates of mental illness for American Indians and Alaska Natives are higher than the general population, with individuals reporting higher rates of frequent distress [3, 13]. American Indians and Alaska Natives are five times more likely to die of alcohol-related causes than Whites [3, 13]. Both youth and adults experience increased mental illness, and the suicide rate is 50% higher than the national rate [3]. Suicide is the second leading cause of death among American Indians and Alaska Natives aged 10–34 years old [42]. Concern about suicide clusters necessitates a community-based, culturally competent response strategy [42].

Establishing trust with patients from American Indian and Alaskan Native communities may prove difficult as many tribal communities were destroyed by the introduction of European infectious diseases, and many treaties established by the US government with tribal nations were broken [42]. Casual conversation may aid the development of rapport. Showing respect is important, in part by allowing time for patients to express their opinions without interruption. Admitting limited knowledge of the patient's culture is acceptable, particularly while inviting the patient and his family or friends to educate you about specific cultural protocols in their community. Most American Indians and Alaska Natives have learned to "walk in two worlds," observing the cultural practices of the setting they are in at the time [42]. Many practice organized religion and have strong faith-based communities. They have a holistic worldview centered on the balance between mind, body, spirit, and environment. Social and health problems are often seen as spiritually based, and most use traditional and spiritual healing practices to complement Western medicine [42]. Recognizing and identifying strengths in the patient's community can provide insight for developing culturally appropriate treatment interventions. Examples of such strengths include extended family, shared sense of collective community responsibility, physical resources, survival skills and resiliency when encountering challenges, and ability to adapt to fit in with both one's traditional culture and the dominant culture [42].

American Indians and Alaska Natives communicate meaningfully using nonverbal gestures, requiring careful observation on the part of the clinician to avoid miscommunication [42]. Like Asians, they may look down as an act of deference to show respect. They may ignore someone to express disagreement or displeasure [42]. They tend to use humor when discussing difficult subjects, and smiles and jokes may mask pain [42]. American Indians are likely to endorse somatic symptoms when depressed [37]. Consultation with local cultural advisers should be considered for questions about symptomatology and treatment options.

Immigration, Acculturation, and Mental Illness

Acculturation is a process that reflects a balance of stress and resilience, and mental health reflects a complex interplay of racism, adaptation strategies, and cultural resources. Learning a new language, reconciling cultural conflicts, formation of identity, alienation from culture or family, and loss of resources are potentially stressful events associated with immigration. Overcoming these obstacles and adapting require resilience. Processes of adaptation, adjustment, and incorporation into society are not uniform, and different immigrant groups face different challenges in negotiating acculturation [43]. Some immigrants experience better mental health than individuals born in the United States, but as they become more integrated with American culture, values, and lifestyles, their mental health worsens and becomes more comparable to that of those born in the United States [43].

Acculturation in Asian Americans is inversely related to prevalence rates of mental illness and to reporting symptoms, and Asian American immigrants who moved to the United States at an earlier age experience few difficulties adjusting [13]. In contrast, prevalence rates of mental illness in Mexican Americans are directly related to a level of acculturation and increase with length of time in the United States [13]. Mexican Americans born in the United States experience higher rates of mental illness than those born in Mexico, and place of birth appears to be a more important variable in determining mental illness than age, gender, or social class [13, 44]. One possible explanation is an erosion of family networks, which provide support and resources, exerting a protective or preventive effect. Alternatively, expectations may differ depending on place of birth, such that Mexican Americans born in the United States may have higher expectations for educational attainment and wealth, and may feel more demoralized when they fail to achieve these goals [13].

Association between immigrant status and suicidality is unclear. Lack of social integration, low assimilation, and the high stress accompanying the immigrant experience may contribute to increased suicide risk [45]. Immigrants leave behind customs, norms, and relationships in their home country, only to experience pressure to integrate and assimilate culturally, socially, linguistically, and economically with the dominant population, often at a rapid pace and with limited emotional and economic support. On the other hand, the "healthy immigrant thesis" postulates that immigrants have above-average physical and mental health and are thus at lower risk for suicide [45].

Religion

Patients of different spiritual backgrounds may have different conceptualizations of their illnesses and treatment needs. Clinicians responsible for evaluating behavioral emergencies in the United States are typically trained to view religion as a protective factor in terms of suicide risk; however, this is a Western notion rooted in Christianity. It is important for the clinician to determine whether a patient's religious beliefs provide for coping skills that are positive or negative. For example, a patient who attributes his illness to God's will may be less likely to adhere to treatment recommendations. He may not disclose his beliefs to the clinician, fearing shame and ridicule.

Hinduism

According to Ayurvedic beliefs, mental health depends on the actions, air, and personal nature of the individual. Hindus believe that mental illness may result from disrespect toward the creator, the Brahmins, and teachers. They believe that neglecting duty to God, cruelty to others, and such vices as lust and extortion lead to possession by spirits and that such fate can be avoided by keeping themselves clean, observing social obligations, and giving to charity [41].

Buddhism

Buddhism teaches that nothing is permanent and that everything is interdependent. Buddhists believe that mental health results from knowing and following the Four Noble Truths and the Eightfold Path while renouncing worldly attachments. Mental illness may be caused by misdeeds of the patient or ancestors or may result from being overly ambitious or having too much desire. Therapeutic healing requires the following four components: the physician, the attendant(s), the patient, and the drug, which must come from local herbs. Kindness and consideration are of particular importance to the Buddhist patient. Buddhists believe that possessed individuals may be aided by worship or prayer, burning of a specific incense, and following certain rituals and that meditation can lead to a tranquil state of mind [41]. Charity work may also provide benefit. Jodo Shinshu Buddhists are more willing to seek medical treatment as they believe that illness comes from causes and conditions and that eradication comes through medications and treatments [18].

Chinese Spiritual Beliefs

Chinese beliefs are heterogeneous, often reflecting a mix of principles based on Buddhism, Taoism, and ancestor worship. In general, there is a holistic view of mind and body as one with mental health dependent on physical health. Unbalanced, undisciplined, or excessive emotions form the primary basis for any kind of illness [41]. Taoists believe that mental illness results from an imbalance between yin and yang. Chinese patients may believe in deities, devils, and spiritual beings and that certain rituals may relieve suffering. For example, schizophrenia may be explained as possession of one's spirit by angry ancestors, and symptoms may include auditory and visual hallucinations of being tormented or raped by ghosts [40]. Animism is the belief that humans, animals, and inanimate objects have souls or spirits, and followers believe that mental illness is caused by the loss of one's soul or possession by evil or vengeful spirits. Chinese healing methods include herbal medicine, acupuncture, and qigong, among many others.

Islam

Islamic faith tends to view people as being made up of body and soul, and it is this unity that forms the psyche and reflects itself in one's behaviors [41]. Mental health is indicative of closeness to God and reflects ongoing purification of thought and deeds. Neglect of religious duties, failure to read the Qur'an, or deviation from inherent goodness may allow evil to take hold and may result in psychiatric symptoms. The belief in predestination may prevent patients from seeking medical or psychiatric treatment. Muslims may prefer folk and traditional practices to alleviate mental distress [41].

Cultural Concepts of Distress

The DSM-5 defines cultural concepts of distress as "ways that cultural groups experience, understand, and communicate suffering, behavioral problems, or troubling thoughts and emotions" [46]. The three central concepts include cultural syndromes, cultural idioms of distress, and cultural explanations or perceived causes. Cultural syndromes refer to clusters of symptoms that reflect the interaction of cognitive schemata and bodily processes as interpreted in an ethnophysiologic and ethnopsychological context. They may seem bizarre to the clinician from an outside culture. Cultural idioms of distress refer to manners of expressing distress, which are relatable to others in one's community without necessarily involving specific symptoms. Understanding cultural concepts can help prevent misdiagnosis, establish rapport, and improve therapeutic efficacy [46].

Neurasthenia is a Chinese syndrome of physical and emotional weakness attributed to anxiety or neurological weakness or exhaustion and characterized by the physical symptoms of a headache, pain, fatigue, gastrointestinal symptoms, and sexual dysfunction and the psychiatric symptoms of irritability, excitability, dyssomnia, poor concentration, and memory loss.

Cultural concepts of distress in Hispanic populations include *nervios* (nerves), *ataque de nervios* (attack of nerves), and *susto* (fright or soul loss). *Nervios* is common in Latinos in the United States and Latin America and represents instability of mood similar to general anxiety disorder. The term *nervios* may refer to a general state of vulnerability to stressful life experiences or a syndrome brought on by difficult life circumstances. Patients may present with physical and emotional symptoms, including affective instability, restlessness, inability to function, and feeling out of control. They may report headaches, gastrointestinal distress, dyssomnia, nervousness, or tearfulness. Typically, this condition is chronic with a fluctuating degree of disability. *Ataque de nervios* is primarily seen in Latinos from the Caribbean but is recognized by many people of Latin American and Latin Mediterranean descent. Like *nervios*, this syndrome is characterized by a feeling of being out of control but is more analogous to a panic attack, only without fear. Episodes are often accompanied by violent behavior and may include crying, screaming, shouting, trembling, palpitations, and seizure-like episodes. Typically, they are precipitated by a specific event, often involving family. This condition is often associated with other psychiatric conditions, including depression and anxiety.

Approach to Treatment

Clinicians should adopt open, interested, and respectful attitudes toward their patients and attempt to understand each individual's illness within a cultural context. Care must be taken to investigate unexplained symptoms and to perform a complete diagnostic medical workup rather than dismiss symptoms as somatization. Attention to precipitating, aggravating, and ameliorating factors should be paid. Review of systems will allow the clinician to screen for psychiatric symptoms. As the interview progresses and the patient engages, more sensitive topics may be broached, including psychiatric symptoms, personal or family problems, and trauma history. Clinicians should inquire about stressors as patients may not make the connection between stressors and physical symptoms. Inquiry about herbal medications is merited, given that 42% of patients in the United States use some type of complementary or alternative medical treatment [38]. Common stressors, including failure to live up to one's own and familial expectations, threats to competence (such as failure at work or school), familial conflict, recent immigration, and poor acculturation, may result in feelings of guilt or shame, isolation, and decreased functioning [38]. The more persistently a patient rejects any link between psychosocial factors and physical symptoms, the less likely the clinician recognizes and treats psychiatric illness [14].

Biological, psychological, and social methods can be utilized to overcome the stigma associated with mental illness and engage patients in treatment. Explaining illness in physiologic terms can dispel feelings of guilt and shame. Medication education, with a discussion of dosing, duration of treatment, and potential side effects, promotes compliance. A psychological approach based on principles discussed in the DSM-5 cultural formulation incorporates the patient's traditional beliefs and explanation of illness. Using the patient's own explanatory models of illness facilitates understanding and engagement. Involving family and spiritual or religious leaders in treatment can be beneficial. Family therapy utilizing a psychoeducational approach is particularly helpful when treating patients from non-Western countries. Eliciting the patient's point of view and resistance to proposed treatment allows alternative options to be discussed and a viable treatment plan formulated. The clinician must convey hope and optimism regarding illness and recovery.

Treatment noncompliance rates are much higher in intercultural environments, reflecting inadequate communication and cultural differences in expectations [14]. Patients may be reluctant to question or disagree with clinicians due to etiquette, deference to authority, or desire to be viewed as a good patient [14]. Patients from ethnocultural populations dominated or marginalized by European or American powers or affected by racism may experience difficulty expressing their own concerns due to potential conflict. Concern about the strength of prescribed treatment, side effects, and social stigma contributes to noncompliance [14].

Ethnicity and Psychopharmacology

In addition to differences in beliefs and traditions, there are biological differences in ethnic populations. Polymorphic variability among ethnic groups may account for different responses to drugs. Mutations in cytochrome P450 enzymes affect the metabolism of psychotropic medications, including selective serotonin reuptake inhibitors, selective norepinephrine reuptake inhibitors, tricyclic antidepressants, and antipsychotics. Alcohol consumption, nicotine use, and diet may also affect metabolism.

African Americans are at risk for overtreatment both in terms of the number of medications used and the doses prescribed, despite pharmacokinetic data that indicate that lower doses should be used [38]. African Americans receive more antipsychotic medications regardless of diagnosis, but fewer antidepressant medications, and they are often treated with older medications [38].

In general, Asians have difficulty metabolizing psychotropic medications [40]. Thus, lower doses are required to achieve a therapeutic effect, and risk of side effects may be greater. Starting with half the recommended dose of an antidepressant or neuroleptic medication has been recommended [38].

If a patient experiences side effects, the medication dose should be lowered, and the possibility of using a medication metabolized through an alternative pathway should be considered. The lack of minority participation in research studies has complicated efforts to apply culturally appropriate evidence-based treatment algorithms to these populations.

Conclusion

Individualized treatment is essential. The **LEARN** principle can be used as a model when training clinicians to perform a culturally appropriate assessment [38, 41]. They should:

- **L**isten to understand the patient's perception of the problem.
- **E**xplain their perception to the patient.
- **A**cknowledge and discuss similarities and differences.
- **R**ecommend and **N**egotiate an agreed-upon treatment plan [38, 41].

Clinicians need to verify that patients understand the information discussed. The National Healthcare Disparities Report noted that 26% of hospitalized patients reported communication problems pertaining to medications and that 21% experienced problems with discharge information [20].

In order to develop evidence-based treatment guidelines that are culturally appropriate, research must include minority populations. Since 1994, the National Institutes of Health have required the inclusion of ethnic minorities in all research studies that they fund [3]. The development of culturally appropriate behavioral health interventions has the potential to reduce bias in the formulation of diagnosis and treatment plans, improve treatment compliance, and increase the efficacy of treatment.

Improving geographic availability of mental health services, increasing access to mental health care and utilization, and decreasing barriers to treatment are essential to prevent behavioral emergencies. Community education to increase awareness of psychiatric illness and integration of mental health services with primary care clinics will decrease stigmatization. Providing linguistically compatible care will ensure the necessary communication for evaluation of a patient presenting with a behavioral emergency, accurate diagnosis, and comprehensive discussion of treatment. Promoting an environment that appreciates diverse cultures will be more attractive to patients seeking treatment. People who receive quality health care are more likely to stay in treatment and have better outcomes [3].

Clinicians evaluating patients experiencing behavioral emergencies must be trained to perform culturally competent interviews, identifying the patient's cultural beliefs, explanatory model of illness, and view of potential treatments, so that they may tailor treatment to an individual patient based on assimilation of this information rather than rely solely on assessments standardized to the majority of population. The clinician must also be aware of his own cultural identity and how these similarities and differences may affect communication, rapport, transference, countertransference, and the overall therapeutic alliance. A primary goal of treatment should be symptom relief, not changing core beliefs.

References

1. Lim RF. Clinical manual of cultural psychiatry. Arlington, VA: American Psychiatric Publishing; 2006.
2. US Census Bureau. Table 1: United States: race and hispanic origin: 1790 to 1990. Washington, DC, US Census Bureau. 2002 [cited 2011 September 30]. Available from: http://www.census.gov/population/www/documentation/twps0056/tab01.pdf.
3. Department of Health and Human Services, US Public Health Services. Mental health: culture, race, and ethnicity: a report of the Surgeon General. 2001

[cited 2017 September 16]. Available from: http://www.surgeongeneral.gov/library/mentalhealth/cre/execsummary-1.html.
4. Whitley RW. Cultural competence, evidence-based medicine, and evidence-based practices. Psychiatr Serv. 2007;58(12):1588–90.
5. Lim RF, Luo JS, Suo S, Hales RE. Diversity initiatives in academic psychiatry: applying cultural competence. Acad Psychiatry. 2008;32:283–90.
6. Gany F, Kapelusznik L, Prakash K, Gonzalez J, Orta LY, Tseng CH, Changrani J. The impact of medical interpretation method on time and errors. J Gen Intern Med. 2007;22(2):319–23.
7. Lim RF, Lu FG. Culture and psychiatric education. Acad Psychiatry. 2008;32(4):269–71.
8. Exec. Order No. 13166, 3 C.F.R. 2000. [cited 2017 October 1]. Available from: https://www.gpo.gov/fdsys/pkg/FR-2000-08-16/pdf/00-20938.pdf.
9. Patient Protection and Affordable Care Act. Pub. L. No. 111–148, 124 Stat. 119. 2010 [cited 2017 October 1]. Available from: http://housedocs.house.gov/energycommerce/ppacacon.pdf.
10. Meaningful access for individuals with limited English Proficiency, 45 C.F.R. Sect. 92.201. 2016.
11. Nápoles AM, Santoyo-Olsson J, Karliner LS, O'Brien H, Gregorich SE, Pérez-Stable EJ. Clinician ratings of interpreter mediated visits in underserved primary care settings with ad hoc, in-person professional, and video conferencing modes. J Health Care Poor Underserved. 2010;21(1):301–17.
12. Farooq S, Fear C. Working through interpreters. Adv Psychiatr Treat. 2003;9:104–9.
13. Sue S, Chu JY. The mental health of ethnic minority groups: challenges posed by the supplement to the Surgeon General's report on mental health. Cult Med Psychiatry. 2003;27:447–63.
14. Kirmayer LJ. Cultural variations in the clinical presentation of depression and anxiety: implications for diagnosis and treatment. J Clin Psychiatry. 2001;62(Suppl. 13):22–8.
15. Carpenter-Song E, Chu E, Drake RE, Ritsema M, Smith B, Alverson H. Ethnocultural variations in the experience and meaning of mental illness and treatment: implications for access and utilization. Transcult Psychiatry. 2010;47(2):224–51.
16. Bhui K, Bhurga D. Explanatory models for mental distress: implications for clinical practice and research. Br J Psychiatry. 2002;181:6–7.
17. Ryan C. American Community Survey Reports: Language Use in the United States: 2011. Washington, D.C.: US Census Bureau. 2013 [cited 2017 October 1]. Available from: https://www.census.gov/prod/2013pubs/acs-22.pdf.
18. Andresen J. Cultural competence and health care: Japanese, Korean, and Indian patients in the United States. J Cult Divers. 2001;8(4):109–21.
19. Gany F, Leng J, Shapiro E, Abramson D, Motola I, Shield DC, Changrani J. Patient satisfaction with different interpreting methods: a randomized controlled trial. J Gen Intern Med. 2007;22(2):312–8.
20. Agency for Healthcare Research and Quality. Key themes and highlights from the National Healthcare Disparities Report. 2006 [cited 2011 June 21]. Available from: http://www.ahrq.gov/qual/nhdr06/highlights/nhdr06high.htm.
21. Green AR, Ngo-Metzger Q, Legedza AT, Massagli MP, Phillips RS, Iezzoni LI. Interpreter services, language concordance, and health care quality: experiences of Asian Americans with limited English proficiency. J Gen Intern Med. 2005;20:1050–6.
22. VanderWielen LM, Enurah AS, Rho HY, Nagarkatti-Gude DR, Michelsen-King P, Crossman SH, Vanderbilt AA. Medical interpreters: improvements to address access, equity, and quality of care for limited-English-proficient patients. Acad Med. 2014;89(10):1324–7.
23. Masland MC, Lou C, Snowden L. Use of communication technologies to cost-effectively increase the availability of interpretation services in healthcare settings. Telemed J E Health. 2010;16(6):739–45.
24. Marcos LR, Alpert M, Urcuyo L, Kesselman M. The effect of interview language on the evaluation of psychopathology in Spanish-American schizophrenic patients. Am J Psychiatry. 1973;130(5):549–53.
25. Del Castillo JC. The influence of language upon symptomatology in foreign-born patients. Am J Psychiatry. 1970;127(2):242–4.
26. Hudelson P. Improving patient-provider communication: insights from interpreters. Fam Pract. 2005;22(3):311–6.
27. Bezuidenhout L, Borry P. Examining the role of informal interpretation in medical interviews. J Med Ethics. 2009;35:159–62.
28. Juckett G, Unger K. Appropriate use of medical interpreters. Am Fam Physician. 2014;90(7):476–80.
29. Bauer AM, Alegria M. Impact of patient language proficiency and interpreter service use on the quality of psychiatric care: a systematic review. Psychiatr Serv. 2010;61(8):765–73.
30. Marcos LR. Effects of interpreters on the evaluation of psychopathology in non-English-speaking patients. Am J Psychiatry. 1979;136:171–4.
31. Añez LM, Paris M, Bedregal LE, Davidson L, Grilo CM. Application of cultural constructs in the care of first generation Latino clients in a community mental health setting. J Psychiatr Pract. 2005;11(4):221–30.
32. Locatis C, Williamson D, Gould-Kabler C, Zone-Smith L, Detzler I, Roberson J, Maisiak R, Ackerman M. Comparing in-person, video, and telephonic medical interpretation. J Gen Intern Med. 2010;25(4):345–50.
33. Bernstein J, Bernstein E, Dave A, Hardt E, James T, Linden J, Mitchell P, Oishi T, Safi C. Trained medical interpreters in the emergency department: effects on services, subsequent charges, and follow-up. J Immigr Health. 2002;4(4):171–6.
34. Fulford B, Mordini E. Informed consent in psychiatry: cross-cultural and philosophical issues. Bull Med Eth. 1994:22–4.

35. Kortmann F. Transcultural psychiatry: from practice to theory. Transcult Psychiatry. 2010;47(2):203–23.
36. Hernandez M, Nesman T, Mowery D, Acevedo-Polakovich ID, Callejas LM. Cultural competence: a literature review and conceptual model for mental health services. Psychiatr Serv. 2009;60(8):1046–50.
37. Uebelacher LA, Strong D, Weinstock LM, Miller IW. Use of item response theory to understand differential functioning of DSM IV major depression symptoms by race, ethnicity, and gender. Psychol Med. 2009;39:591–601.
38. Lim RF, Lu F. Clinical aspects of culture in the practice of psychiatry: assessment and treatment of culturally diverse patients. Medscape. 2005 [cited 2017 Oct 1]. Available from: http://www.medscape.org/viewarticle/507208.
39. Sanchez F, Gaw A. Mental health care of Filipino Americans. Psychiatr Serv. 2007;58(6):810–5.
40. Herrick C, Brown HN. Mental disorders and syndromes found among Asians residing in the United States. Issues Ment Health Nurs. 1999;20:275–96.
41. Haque A. Mental health concepts in Southeast Asia: diagnostic consideration and treatment implications. Psychol Health Med. 2010;15(2):127–34.
42. Substance Abuse and Mental Health Services Administration. Culture card: a guide to build cultural awareness: American Indian and Alaska Native. 2009 [cited 2011 August]. Available from: http://store.samhsa.gov/shin/content/SMA08-4354/SMA08-4354.pdf.
43. Takeuchi DT, Alegria M, Jackson JS, Williams DR. Immigration and mental health: diverse findings in Asian, Black, and Latino populations. Am J Public Health. 2007;97(1):11–2.
44. Escobar JI. Immigration and mental health: why are immigrants better off? Arch Gen Psychiatry. 1998;55:781–2.
45. Duldulao AA, Takeuchi DT, Hong S. Correlates of suicidal behaviors among Asian Americans. Arch Suicide Res. 2009;13(3):277–90.
46. American Psychiatric Association. Diagnostic and statistical manual of mental disorders. 5th ed. Washington, D.C.: American Psychiatric Publishing; 2013.

Emergency Psychiatry in Rural Versus Urban Settings

38

Alicia Romeo

Introduction

The prevalence of mental illness and what defines a psychiatric emergency is similar in rural and urban settings [1]. Constraints on mental health services in both environments provide unique challenges to the delivery of care. The unique characteristics of rural and urban mental health populations are in the early stages of being described in research. The following chapter describes the history of mental health treatment in emergency departments (EDs), as well highlights unique attributes in rural and urban patient populations. A greater understanding of care needs in a given geographic location may help to focus resources in the setting of increasing demand.

Background

Emergency medicine and psychiatry share a long relationship. The first emergency psychiatric care in the United States dates back to the 1920s. Psychiatry residents worked in metropolitan medical emergency departments to help evaluate challenging psychiatric cases and provide disposition planning [2]. Usually, treatment planning included long-term containment of the most severely ill psychiatric patients in free-standing private or government hospitals. Two pieces of legislation formally established a need for psychiatric emergency management. The Community Mental Health Services Act of 1963 sought to provide community-based treatment alternatives, including short-term hospitalization and outpatient treatment [3]. A decade later, the Emergency Medical Services Act provided federal support to establish comprehensive delivery of emergency care to patients in an appropriate geographical area [4].

In the last 50 years, a dwindling number of inpatient psychiatric beds and a lack of outpatient mental health resources led to a shrinking system left to meet the needs of an increasing number of patients. The number of community short-term hospitals with psychiatric units declined from 1571 in 1990 to 1149 in 2014 [5]. Although health policy experts concluded the minimum number of psychiatric beds per 100,000 people is 50, fifteen states have 10 psychiatric beds per 100,000 [6]. Meanwhile, approximately 1 in 5 adults, or 43.8 million people, experiences a mental illness in a given year. Only 41% of people with a mental health diagnosis receive treatment [1].

Given the discrepancy between services and need, the number of patients with mental health

A. Romeo (✉)
Department of Psychiatry, Atrium Health Behavioral Health Charlotte, Charlotte, NC, USA
e-mail: alicia.romeo@atriumhealth.org

L. S. Zun et al. (eds.), *Behavioral Emergencies for Healthcare Providers*,
https://doi.org/10.1007/978-3-030-52520-0_38

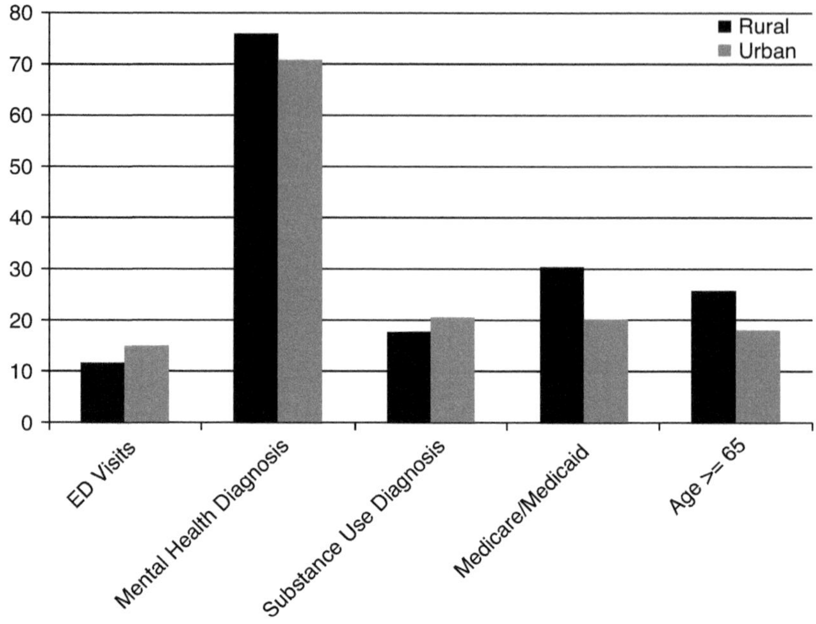

Fig. 38.1 Key characteristics in rural versus urban emergency psychiatry patient populations [1]

diagnoses treated in emergency departments has been on the rise. Approximately 140 psychiatric emergency departments or psychiatric emergency services operate in the United States. The majority of these programs are located in major metropolitan areas. Meanwhile, over 5000 emergency medical departments provide a safety net of care for patients in all geographic settings [7]. In 2013, 14.6% of all emergency department visits were for a primary psychiatric diagnosis [5].

The following case examples taken from emergency departments intend to highlight some of the unique attributes of rural versus urban patients in need of psychiatric care. Figure 38.1 provides an overview of some of the characteristics specific to each geographic setting.

Case Example 1: A Rural Emergency Department Patient

Mr. A. is a 65-year-old single male residing in an assisted-living facility (ALF) in a rural town with a population of 1444 residents. He had numerous inpatient psychiatric hospitalizations since he was diagnosed with schizophrenia in his 20s. The patient presented to the emergency department brought in by ambulance due to worsening agitation at his ALF. The closest emergency department is in the town serving as the county seat. It has a population of 5509.

Mr. A. stated he came to the emergency department for medication refills. When approached by a female emergency physician, the patient reported, "Are you one of my children? Are you a composite of my children? Can I watch a sitcom?" He refused to speak to the physician further, stating, "I am already spoken for."

Staff at his ALF stated the patient runs up and down the hallway at night. He spits and cusses at other residents. They have heard him talking and yelling to himself while he is alone in his room. The patient refused all psychotropic medications for the past month. His mental health provider and the date of his last visit were not known. His recent hospitalization was 7 months earlier, after presenting to the same emergency department with a similar clinical picture. At that time, he was hospitalized at a psychiatric facility 68 miles from the community ED.

Discussion

The discrepancy between rural and urban mental-health-provider supply has been well documented. In addition, rural communities utilize less emergency department care than urban communities for mental health care [1]. Since the illness burden is similar in rural and urban populations, an explanation may be that patients do not recognize that mental illness can be effectively treated. In this case, the distance to both the closest emergency department and the closest inpatient psychiatric unit may hinder accessibility.

Mr. A.'s severe mental illness would be a treatment challenge in any clinical setting. His presentation to this small community ED illustrates several patterns identified among patients who go to rural EDs with symptoms of mental illness. First, rural patients are more likely to present with primary psychiatric diagnoses, as opposed to a primary substance-use complaint. One explanation for this finding may be that substance-use treatment admissions in rural areas are more likely to be referred through the criminal justice system directly to specific treatment programs [8].

In general, patients aged 18–44 make up the largest proportion of mental health ED visits in all settings. A higher proportion of rural residents with mental health symptoms presenting to the ED were aged 65 and older [1]. Although not an acute symptom in the case described above, previous research suggested that suicide rates are higher in rural areas compared to urban areas [9]. Older adults, particularly men, are known to have a higher risk for completed suicide [10, 11]. Thus far, no known research exists to suggest more elderly men present to rural or urban emergency departments with intentional self-harm compared to the rest of the population. The lack of data may be due to high lethality of suicide attempts in this group, resulting in death prior to the opportunity for a treatment intervention in an emergency department.

Rural emergency departments are more likely to treat patients publically insured, including by Medicaid and Medicare. Medicaid patients have increased difficulty accessing primary care, a greater frequency of ED visits, and higher readmission rates that privately funded peers [1]. When it is available, stigma about mental health treatment may prevent patients from discussing psychiatric symptoms in a primary care setting. One care model developed to address these concerns is telemedicine. State Medicaid policies and rules continue to evolve. Medicaid in 48 states currently reimburses some telepsychiatry services. Medicare will reimburse for telepsychiatry in rural areas [12].

As in the majority of community hospitals, the ED in the case described above did not have a psychiatrist on call. A 2016 poll of emergency physicians found only 17% reported having a psychiatrist to respond to psychiatric emergencies [12]. However, this emergency department did have access to telepsychiatry. Substantial evidence exists that telepsychiatry is equivalent to in-person care in diagnostic accuracy, treatment accuracy, quality of care, patient satisfaction, and privacy [13].

An emergency psychiatry consultant provided a virtual examination of Mr. A. over HIPAA-compliant video and audio lines. Mr. A. was assessed to require inpatient psychiatric hospitalization, and medication recommendations were made. An inpatient psychiatric bed was not available for the patient immediately; he was boarded in the ED until one became available at the closest appropriate hospital 93 miles away from the community hospital ED. In the interim, the telepsychiatry consultant was available for recommendations related to medication changes and management of agitation.

Case Example 2: An Urban Emergency Department Patient

Mr. B. is a 43-year-old divorced, undomiciled male with a history of unspecified psychosis and depression, as well as substance use. He went to the ED of a tertiary-care academic medical center in a city with a population of over 800,000 people. Mr. B. told the emergency physician he was hearing voices telling him to kill himself. His urine drug screen was positive for cocaine, and his blood alcohol level was 37 mg/dL at the time of arrival.

Mr. B. had presented to the same ED 10 days earlier with similar complaints. The emergency psychiatrist had evaluated Mr. B. and recommended psychiatric hospitalization. Mr. B. then spent two nights in the hospital's psychiatric observation area, where he was monitored for alcohol withdrawal and treated for his mental illness symptoms. Then he transferred to an inpatient psychiatric facility 45 miles away for an additional four nights. Mr. B. reported he was offered a referral to a long-term substance treatment program at discharge, but he declined it.

Mr. B. did not continue his psychiatric medications after discharge, because he could not afford them. He did not follow up with referrals to outpatient community mental health and substance-use treatment centers. One day after discharge, he relapsed on cocaine and started drinking up to 13 beers daily. During his psychiatric exam, he continued to endorse suicidal thoughts, stating, "I will drink something I mixed up." Mr. B. reported a previous suicide attempt by caustic ingestion, as well as several family members who died by suicide.

Discussion

Mr. B.'s clinical presentation demonstrated characteristics prevalent in the urban ED patient population with mental health complaints. In addition to treating a higher number of patients overall per year due to higher populations, urban EDs also treat a higher percentage of patients with mental health and substance-use complaints compared to rural counterparts [1]. Mr. B.'s age is consistent with the most substantial proportion of patients treated in EDs for mental health complaints. Urban residents like Mr. B. are more likely to present with psychiatric complaints related to substance use, with cocaine use being the primary substance of abuse [8]. However, opioid use, previously considered a substance of abuse relegated to the rural population, has been shown to be of similar magnitude across urban and rural settings [14]. Future data will be needed to assess the impact of the opioid crisis on emergency services. Urban substance-use treatment admissions are more likely to be self- or individual-referred [8]. Self-referrals for substance-use treatment often begin with ED visits, where a patient may access social services and treatment information. As might be expected, the number of public and private substance treatment programs within Mr. B.'s county of residence exceeds those available in the rural county described in the first case example.

Mr. B.'s presentation to the ED resulted in the transfer to a psychiatric observation area. In this hospital, patients awaiting admission are held in a quieter environment separate from the main medical and trauma areas. Research has suggested patients have worse outcomes with increased boarding times in emergency department [6]. Psychiatric observation areas do require adequately trained staff and appropriate patient supervision to maximize patient safety.

As opposed to patients in rural communities, the urban ED mental health patient is more likely to be uninsured or privately insured [1], but that may not guarantee access to care. While private insurance can increase the options for psychiatric hospitalization, the number of psychiatrists accepting a given private insurance provider for outpatient care may vary throughout metropolitan areas across the nation. Mr. B. was both uninsured and unemployed, increasing his difficulty in accessing outpatient mental health treatment. Generally, free or low-cost mental health services are available in most urban areas. In Mr. B.'s city, two mental health clinics offer free or sliding scale services for the uninsured. An additional community service provided housing resources and vouchers for free medications. While these resources would suggest easier access to care, the public low-cost/free services in the city were overburdened. Intake visits usually required long waiting time in walk-in clinics. An appointment with a psychiatrist or advanced clinical practitioner (a nurse practitioner or physician assistant) may take several months after the initial intake is completed. In the interim, a patient on psychotropic medications may be left with no alternative than to seek prescription renewals from an emergency department. These obstacles can contribute to a patient's inability to engage in sustained outpatient mental health treatment. Patients like Mr. B. may be left to conclude that an emergency department visit may be the only way to get their psychiatric needs met in a comprehensive and timely fashion.

Conclusions

In the most general of terms, a psychiatric emergency may be defined as dangerousness to self, dangerousness to others, or grave disability. However, given the strain on mental health services, the current availability of psychiatric services is inadequate to manage the increasing number of patients requiring both acute and long-term mental health care. As a result, emergency departments have served as both the safety net and initial point of contact, connecting patients requiring specialty care. To most effectively utilize available services, identification of characteristics of rural and urban patients presenting to emergency departments with psychiatric needs can permit care models to be tailored to geographic needs. For example, rural communities may devise health initiatives intended to screen elderly populations in assisted living and skilled nursing centers for psychiatric needs. Community outreach can reduce the stigma of seeking mental health care. In combination with mental health workforce initiatives and telepsychiatry services, specialty care can be provided promptly. Additionally, utilization of telepsychiatry services in the urban setting may also decrease the wait time required for a patient to be evaluated or treated with psychiatric medications in community clinics, thus limiting the need to turn to the emergency department for primary mental health care. Telepsychiatry currently requires a physician to be licensed in the state where patients will be treated. Innovative workforce initiatives and telepsychiatry exposure at the training program level may provide highly skilled professionals to the areas with the greatest need. An urban setting may also consider outreach programs to connect patients with substance-use treatment programs. For the most severely ill, prompt access to an emergency psychiatric consultant is needed to ensure the safety of the patient and the emergency department staff.

In summary, limitations of mental health care access and increasing demands for care require a comprehensive understanding of the communities being served, as well as potential advantages and obstacles of novel care delivery in rural and urban settings.

References

1. Shroeder S, Leigh-Peterson M. Rural and urban utilization of the emergency department for mental health and substance abuse. Grand fork (ND): CRH: Supported by the Federal Office of Rural Health Policy, Health Resources and Services Administration; 2017. p. 6.
2. Wellin E, Slesinger DP, Hollister D. Psychiatric emergency services: evolution, adaptation and proliferation. Soc Sci Med. 1987;24(6):475–82.
3. Gerson S, Bassuk E. Psychiatric emergencies: an overview. Am J Psy. 1980;137:1):1–11.
4. Harvey J. The emergency medical service systems act of 1973. JAMA. 1974;230(8):1139–40.
5. Nami.org. National Alliance on Mental Illness. 2017. Available at http://www.nami.org. Accessed on 27 Sep 2017.
6. Treatmentadvocacycenter.org. Treatment Advocacy Center. 2015. Available at http://www.treatmentadvocacycenter.org. Accessed on 12 Sep 2017.
7. Emnet-usa.org. Emergency Medicine Network. 2013. Available at http://www.emnet-usa.org/nedi/nedi_usa.htm. Accessed on 9 Sep 2017.
8. Substance Abuse and Mental Health Services Administration. National Survey of substance abuse treatment services (N-SSATS): 2016—data on substance abuse treatment facilities. BHSIS series S-93, HHS publication no. (SMA) 17–5039. Rockville, MD: Substance Abuse and Mental Health Services Administration; 2017.
9. Neufeld E, Hirdes JP, Perlman CM, Rabinowitz T. A longitudinal examination of rural status and suicide risk. Health Manage Forum. 2015;28(4):129–33.
10. Hawton K, van Heeringen K. Suicide. Lancet. 2009;373(9672):1372–81.
11. Conwell Y, Duberstein PR, Caine ED. Risk factors for suicide in later life. Biol Psy. 2002;52(3):193–204.

12. American Psychiatric Association Committee on Telepsychiatry. What is telepsychiatry? 2017. Available at https://www.psychiatry.org/patients-families/what-is-telepsychiatry. Accessed on 8 Sep 2017.
13. Hilty DM, Yellowlees PM, Parish MB, Chan S. Telepsychiatry: effective, evidence-based and at a tipping point in healthcare delivery. Psych Clin N Amer. 2015;38(3):559–92.
14. Humphreys K. Opioid abuse started as a rural epidemic. It's now a national one. In: Washington post. Washington, D.C.: WP Company LLC; 2017. Available at https://www.washingtonpost.com/news/wonk/wp/2017/07/31/opioid-abuse-started-as-a-rural-epidemic-its-now-a-national-one/?utm_term=.8fd87b0fb906. Accessed 22 Sep 2017.

Part VII

Administration of Psychiatric Care

Coordination of Care with Psychiatry

39

Benjamin L. Bregman and Seth Powsner

Introduction

No one can win a relay race alone, but anyone can lose it by dropping the baton. Care of chronically ill patients, medical or psychiatric, frequently involves passing a patient from one treatment setting to the next. The complexity of caring for psychiatric patients in emergency departments (ED) described in previous chapters suggests that a closer alignment of psychiatric and emergency departments would be beneficial to both clinicians and patients. Developing and maintaining a means of coordinating care and communicating between clinicians may present a unique challenge to each practice environment. The goal of this chapter is to outline general themes that arise in the coordination of care between emergency and psychiatry practitioners and to articulate the non-patient care-related benefits of having working relationships with liaison psychiatrists, including staff well-being, multidisciplinary research initiatives, joint training opportunities, quality improvement endeavors, and patient safety activities.

This chapter will address three themes relevant to the coordination of care between the emergency medicine and psychiatry clinicians. These include (1) Who is involved in the coordination of care; (2) Creating a coordination team; and (3) The benefits of nonclinical interdisciplinary collaboration. These themes were chosen to highlight differences in culture, training, or approach, and may provide providers with the clarity to decrease interdepartmental frustrations and improve patient outcomes.

Who Is Involved in the Coordination of Care

Coordinating care with mental health professionals implies the challenge of understanding who is who—and who is likely to be doing what. Because there are so many kinds of mental health professionals, below is a list arranged as an outline of organizational services.

Clinics

Mental health clinics are more likely to be government operated or government funded, as compared with their private or academic medical

B. L. Bregman (✉)
Department of Psychiatry and Behavioral Health, George Washington University of Medicine, Washington, DC, USA

S. Powsner
Department of Psychiatry, Yale University School of Medicine, New Haven, CT, USA

L. S. Zun et al. (eds.), *Behavioral Emergencies for Healthcare Providers*,
https://doi.org/10.1007/978-3-030-52520-0_39

counterparts. Even though some look and run just like any medical clinic, there is less of a tradition of around-the-clock care, and there may be no fee for service incentive. As such, their patient volume may not support an answering service outside of regular business hours.

Individual Treaters

Often called "therapists" and "counselors" by their patients, they are often generically labeled "mental health professionals." Individual treaters may have their own office, may share an office complex, and very frequently work in a clinic (if only to share clerical and billing overhead).

Psychiatrists

These are physicians (MD or DO) who have completed four or more years of training after medical school: training specifically focused on mental illness. They would normally be licensed by their state government as physicians able to prescribe medication and be board-eligible (i.e., completed their psychiatric training in good standing) or board-certified (i.e., passed examination by the ABPN, the American Board of Psychiatry and Neurology). Though psychiatric residency training is broad in scope and nationally regulated, individual practitioners may only accept a limited type of patient or only offer limited types of treatment (e.g., primarily medication, psychotherapy, addiction treatment, or electroconvulsive therapy).

Nonpsychiatric Physicians

Some internal medicine, family practice, and pediatric physicians will prescribe psychiatric medications in cooperation with nonphysician mental health specialists. They may be affiliated with a mental health clinic proper, or they may be helping one or two nonphysician mental health professionals working in a traditional medical clinic. It is common in some communities to find a patient's internist or pediatrician prescribing an antidepressant on the recommendation of the patient's therapist who is a psychologist or social worker without a medical degree. Moreover, internists are able to prescribe buprenorphine-naloxone, which offers a private practice alternative to methadone maintenance, a clinic treatment.

APRN, NP, PA Clinicians

There are practitioners who do not have an MD or DO but are allowed to prescribe medication, usually in collaboration with a physician. Advanced practice registered nurses, nurse practitioners, and physician assistants have various privileges determined by the regulatory agencies in their locale. Patients may refer to them as a "doctor," if only because they write prescriptions. They typically graduate with less direct clinical experience than a board-eligible psychiatrist. However, they can easily become seasoned clinicians, as they are often 100% occupied with clinical care.

Psychologists (PhD, PsyD, MA)

There are many different kinds of psychologists: clinical, industrial, research, and others. To further complicate matters, a psychologist may or may not have doctoral-level training and may or may not have a clinical license. If they have been licensed after receiving their doctoral degree, they have likely received more training in evaluation and psychotherapy than provided for a physician in a psychiatry residency. Psychologists usually do not prescribe medication; psychologist prescribing is only allowed in five states: New Mexico, Louisiana, Illinois, Idaho, and Iowa, as well as in the US Public Health Service (Indian Health Services and National Health Service Corps), US military, and Guam.

Social Workers (MSW, LCSW)

There are a variety of different kinds of social workers. They may or may not be licensed. They may or may not be specifically trained to do psychotherapy or treat psychiatric patients. And depending on their clinical environment, they may have a variety of different assignments. Some function as a patient's regular treater, meeting with their patient every week or so to provide counseling and psychotherapy. Other social workers may be assigned to help patients navigate the social services system (e.g., apply for welfare benefits and Medicaid). Social workers may be designated case managers, implying that they keep tabs on their patients, and coordinate their overall care.

Counselors (Psychological, Substance Abuse)

Counselors are a very varied group. To further complicate matters, patients are not reliable about using the term "licensed professional counselor," which implies advanced training and licensure. Some patients use the term generically like a therapist. In any case, the demand for lower cost mental health and addiction services has to lead to a growing number of clinic staff who meet routinely with patients to provide guidance, support, and therapy. It is hard to be specific about an individual counselor's qualifications without asking or knowing more about their practice setting.

Outreach Operations

The motto for outreach programs is "If patients won't come to treatment, then take treatment to the patients: That is the motto for outreach programs." A simple approach is to provide brief psychiatric sessions and dispense medications from a van that operates as a clinic on wheels. Unfortunately, paranoid patients may avoid even the friendliest clinic staff, and among the severely mentally ill patients, even outreach cannot overcome their medication nonadherence.

Assertive Community Treatment (ACT) Teams

These teams drive out to find patients, encourage them to take their medication, and help with whatever practical problems may arise (e.g., arrange housing, welfare benefits, and medical clinic visits). It turns out that a significant number of patients will accept medication and other help when the team's persistent efforts demonstrate that someone cares. It is difficult and sometimes thankless working with a collection of these patients. Although inefficient by usual clinic metrics (visits per hour or visits per day, the total number of patients carried by each clinician, etc.), ACT teams can reduce hospital readmissions and incidents in their community.

Inpatient Psychiatric Units

Inpatient services tackle the challenge of treating patients who are so disturbed that they could hurt themselves or someone else. Such cases can profoundly affect the operation and design of a ward: There must be staff available at all times to monitor dangerous patients, prevent any violent actions, and yet still perform routine functions of patient care (e.g., check vital signs, administer medications, and conduct therapy sessions). So inpatient services are usually staffed by the same professionals that staff psychiatric clinics, but with additional nurses, aides, and security.

Inpatient services usually have ancillary support services such as physical therapy, occupational therapy, phlebotomy, and a chaplain. These staff may be shared with other wards. They are less likely to be points of contact for emergency department collaboration.

Inpatient staff frequently focus their attention on protocols, rules, and regulations governing patient admission (or discharge). Inpatient psychiatric care is subject to legal constraints and regulatory review beyond that of medical-surgical units, which generally reflect society's fears about loss of patient autonomy, risk assessments within legal protections, and perceived potential dangerousness of the mentally ill. Additionally, American inpatient psychiatric services have also been shaped by pernicious cost-cutting efforts since the late 1970s (decades longer than other hospital services). This has led to a shortage of psychiatric beds, and consequently, it has led to a backup of psychiatric patients in general emergency departments. Admitting patients for inpatient psychiatric care is more complex than admitting medical or surgical patients.

Partial Hospital Programs (PHP)/ Intensive Outpatient Programs (IOP)

These facilities serve as "step-down" settings for patients who need additional supervision or support following inpatient psychiatric hospitalization. (They can also serve as a "step-up" setting for clinics or emergency department referrals). These facilities are typically staffed only during work hours and provide patients who aren't ready to return to their daily routine with a structured, therapeutic environment where they can access psychotherapeutic and medication management services. The expectation for one of these programs would be that patients attend daily for the work-week and return home at night and on weekends. Patients typically participate in these programs for at least 1 week and often longer, depending on their individual needs. These facilities are typically for-profit and are often affiliated with inpatient facilities where the majority of their referrals originate.

Residential Facilities

When, due to the severity of their symptoms, patients are unable to reintegrate into their lives following an inpatient or partial hospital stay, residential facilities provide a setting where they are able to have longer periods of structured and supervised care. These facilities offer around-the-clock services (though psychiatrists may only be physically present during business hours) and provide their patients with a variety of services including, but not limited to, medication management, individual psychotherapy, group psychotherapy, social skills training, and vocational training. There are few public facilities of this nature still in existence, and those that do exist are typically reserved for the most recalcitrant cases. There are, however, a growing number of privacy settings that provide these services to individuals who are able to afford them with or without the use of insurance.

Substance Rehabilitation Facilities

Patients seeking treatment for substance abuse have limited options in the outpatient setting. Rehabilitation facilities meet this need by providing inpatient, residential, and intensive outpatient services to people who are unable to remain abstinent on their own. These facilities are staffed by psychiatrists, substance-abuse and mental-health counselors, and community support individuals who may be recent graduates from the treatment program and have maintained sobriety for an extended period of time). Though not all facilities provide "detoxification" services, most offer medication management, psychotherapy, social skills, and vocational training. These facilities are often privately funded but may also take insurance.

Visiting Nurses

Often called VNA, it is important to know that not all visiting nurses are part of a visiting nurse association (which may or may not be a member of Visiting Nurse Associations of America). In some locales, there are many agencies that provide home services by registered nurses, nurse aides, and other related staff. Visiting nursing staff can provide very helpful information about a patient's baseline level of function at home and can communicate the time course of a recent change. Occasionally, they can serve as care coordinator because they are in contact with a patient's regular prescriber. Unfortunately, newly assigned staff or temporary covering staff may send a patient for emergency evaluation simply because they are not familiar with poor baseline function.

Housing Supervisors

A number of the seriously, persistently mentally ill (SPMI) live in settings that include some sort of housing supervisor. In a boarding home that accepts the mentally ill, the landlord often provides supervision. Likewise, homeless shelters may employ or designate a supervisor. There are many other arrangements, including rest homes and retirement homes. These supervisors can be very helpful, but be aware that they are unlikely to be clinically trained or selected for their clinical ability.

Low-cost housing meant for the SPMI is now more likely to include an on-site supervisor with clinical training or experience. Likewise, "crisis and respite" facilities will likely have staff on site around the clock (temporary halfway house/group home). Though they may not be licensed clinical professionals, these staff members tend to be self-selected for this kind of work; they can often provide information about a patient's recent behavior, and they can sometimes help assure a patient is directed to treatment.

Case Managers

Outpatient case managers handle challenges much like traditional hospital social workers. They try to assure that patients are registered for care and benefits, and have housing. Unlike a medical ward social worker, they are assigned to patients for months or years, following them through emergency visits, admissions, discharges, clinical changes, and the like. With phone calls and outings to transport patients to critical appointments, they can become a source of valuable patient observations. *They may also know more than any individual treater about a patient's course.* Unlike ACT team members, they do not usually pursue patients into the community or push them into treatment.

Family and Court-Appointed Guardians/Conservators

Family are often overlooked as clinical collaborators. Family can often help ensure that patients attend treatment, or they can alert 911 if there are signs of violence after skipping medication. They can often recount the time course of a patient's behavior, including stressors a patient might not report such as drug use or arguments with friends.

Specific information relevant to deterioration and safety should be elicited and factored into the evaluation. However, it is not useful to ask the family if their loved one "needs to be admitted." Moreover, asking "Is Mr. Jones suicidal?" may be like asking "Is Mr. Jones having a heart attack?" In other words, most family members will translate all of these into "Do you want Mr. Jones admitted today?" They may answer yes or no based on nonclinical considerations. Nonprofessionals are more reliable in answering simple, open-ended questions like "What has your family member done that worries you the most?"

Legal Officers

Police and parole officers are not traditionally considered collaborators. However, for some patients, only law enforcement personnel demonstrate a long-term interest. For some patients, only law enforcement agencies have any way to ensure treatment. (There is no outpatient commitment in most locales, aka Kendra's Law or Laura's Law.)

The challenge in collaborating with law enforcement is to reasonably maintain confidentiality. Some clinicians feel this is impossible; they refuse to contact police or to even review a patient's legal record (e.g., online police blotter or court records). Other clinicians feel it is mandatory; they often cite Tarasoff and state laws requiring physicians to report gunshot wounds, child abuse, and such. Consultation with legal staff is recommended so that both staff and the hospital are in a defensible position.

In summary, the successful coordination of the diverse team of caretakers involved in the life of one patient could be an overwhelming task. Recognizing the training and role of each individual contributor and drawing on their strengths and abilities can create a collaborative care environment that can help patients in the short and long term. Conversely, not understanding the role of each player could contribute to frustrations and problematic communication that could ultimately worsen a patient's condition and long-term prognosis.

Creating a Cohesive Coordination Team

In the previous section, we described many of the players involved in the coordination of care for psychiatric patients. Unfortunately, as is often the case, simply having such resources does not mean that they work together in an efficient way. Creating an effective team requires additional steps, including (1) assessing the availability of willing resource partners, (2) recognizing the abilities and liabilities of those resource partners, and (3) designing a model for coordinating care.

The Availability of Psychiatric Resources

Though it is more than likely that each community has many of the players listed above, whether or not they are available is a different question. The process of identifying participating partners may be as easy as transferring a patient in-house or as difficult as calling nearby hospitals and outpatient providers to ask whether they are currently taking patients. Local "bed-boards" offer one solution for this problem, specifically for inpatient beds. These (mostly) state-government-run services query psychiatric administrators at local hospitals daily to identify the number of psychiatric beds available and their available services (i.e., male/female, voluntary/involuntary, substance abuse/detoxification, dual-diagnosis, adolescent, child, and full fee/Medicaid). When a hospital receives a patient that they are unable to treat, they are able to call this service and quickly discover whether another regional hospital is able to care for their patient and efficiently arrange for transfer to that institution. These services offer an elegant solution to identifying the availability of psychiatric resource partners.

Some states have a similar system to access social services. Called by a variety of names (e.g., core service agency, community service board), these organizations are central clearinghouses for any of a number of services provided by the state, county, or municipality for individuals with public insurance or without insurance. Services offered by these organizations include case management, psychiatric services, substance abuse and dependence treatment, free medication services, counseling, low-income housing, food stamps/food bank/soup kitchens, homeless shelters, medical care, dental care, partial hospitals, day programs, halfway homes, and ACT teams. In addition, these organizations often have access to medical and psychiatric information on patients that can be accessed if the patient is hospitalized, including diagnosis, recent hospitalizations, a recent medication list, and the phone numbers of team members associated with their care. For areas where many people access community services, having easy access to the phone number of the agency could reduce confusion over medications and time spent in the ED (i.e., the ACT team could pick the patient up), among other things.

Unfortunately, a similar system does not exist for outpatient resources for those people who do not qualify for social services. As a result, finding a psychiatrist or a therapist for a patient not requiring inpatient admission can be complex and cumbersome. This is especially true if the person requiring care does not have health insurance, has health insurance without a mental health rider, or has a language barrier. Moreover, even if a patient is able to access psychiatric care or therapy, the professional they find may not match their needs. As such, having an updated list of local resources could give patients the direction they need to access mental-health-care choices. Some recommendations for such a list include:

- Resident clinics at local psychiatry and psychology programs (low-fee by trainees)
- Psychoanalytic institutes (low-fee by trainees)
- Religious organizations (especially helpful for non-English-speaking patients)
- Veterans administrations/vet centers
- Low-fee clinics (especially helpful for non-English-speaking patients)
- The mental-health-care phone number for common local insurances (e.g., BCBS, Aetna)

If these inpatients, social services, and outpatient options do not exist, it may be valuable to reach out to internal and external resources to design an ad-hoc system. In such a situation, identifying and coordinating with local hospitals and mental health professional groups such as local clinics may help to start a collaborative endeavor that could help both partners involved. Moreover, these local mental health resources may be more informed of other available mental healthcare settings, further increasing potential transfer and referral points.

Recognize Each Party's Strengths and Limitations

Beyond knowing who is available and how to access them, being aware of the strengths and limitations of each partner is vital. Certain requests for collaboration may not succeed, simply because they are beyond the scope of practice for one party or the other. It is easy for each partner not to recognize critical differences between the way they and their counterpart operate. These differences do not equate to dysfunction. Indeed, as mentioned above, understanding that a family member can recognize and report behaviors, though not necessarily symptoms, or that one type of treatment facility may be better equipped to care for one type of patient over another, may save time, frustration, and money, and may even prevent negative outcomes. Consequently, in order to create an efficient coordination effort, identify what each player can contribute and how they may be a liability if not used appropriately.

Medical and Psychiatric Clearance

One example of this centers on the expectation of the treatment capacities of referring and receiving facilities. For example, psychiatric inpatient facilities are much better equipped to handle medical conditions than a rest home and probably better than a skilled nursing home. However, most psychiatric wards will not try to maintain IV fluids, oxygen, or tube feedings and may or may not have easy access to blood testing or to an internist. No one argues that this is a good or necessary state of affairs. Although the American Psychiatric Association makes recommendations about the level of medical care that a psychiatric hospital should be able to provide, implementation is variable and unreimbursed costs are a factor.

This particular limitation is best seen in the need for medical clearance. Medical clearance was first addressed in Weisberg's paper [1] where, among the articulated concerns, he reviewed the use and misuse of extensive preadmission workups, identifying that they are often done for the purpose of placating a psychiatrist's feelings of inadequacy when addressing the medical care of a psychiatric patient. Since that time, other papers [2–5] have addressed the role and validity of medical clearance. The American College of Emergency Physicians (ACEP) has issued a consensus opinion that emergency physicians need not perform a reflexive set of laboratory tests as part of the medical clearance of psychiatric patients [6], though it is common practice for emergency departments to order laboratory and imaging studies to rule out potential medical conditions underlying psychiatric presentations. This consensus was echoed by an American Association for Emergency Psychiatry task force [7, 8].

Though not as well characterized, the converse of this limitation is true, as well: medical and surgical subspecialists are often uncomfortable caring for psychiatrically ill patients without psychiatric clearance. This is understandable, given the potential complications (financial, safety, and otherwise) that accompany psychiatric patients. This limitation can be manifested as a reluctance to start a psychiatric medication due to lack of familiarity with treatment indications or psychiatric medications themselves, or as an incomplete assessment of patients with substance abuse due to negative countertransference.

In both cases, recognizing and playing to the strengths of the provider can significantly improve patient care, decrease costs to the system, and save providers from unneeded stress in providing services they feel ill-equipped to render.

Designing a Coordination of Care Model

When a situation arises that necessitates a concerted, coordinated effort of the available partner resources, just like running a code, having a clear protocol for who does what and when before anything happens can be invaluable. Consider the unique milieu of each institution (i.e., demographic, legal, financial, academic affiliation, etc.). It also helps to have a clear picture of the extramural limitations superimposed upon each organization (i.e., state-specific legal restrictions pertaining to restraints, involuntary hospitalization, isolation, involuntary administration of medications, transfer, and boarding). Are there laws that block coordinated efforts between two institutions? In designing such a model, considerations should include:

- Which institution is responsible for arranging transportation? And who maintains the patient's safety during a transfer?
- What are the inter- or intrastate transfer laws of the jurisdiction where the patient is seen?
- What care protocols exist for patients who must wait before a psychiatric bed becomes available (i.e., visitation, in-hospital mobility, cell phone access, food)?
- Can the treatment be initiated prior to transfer to an accepting facility?
- Can a patient be re-evaluated for admission and discharged if deemed safe?
- Is the patient admitted voluntarily or involuntary?
- Who arranges for post-discharge follow-up? What are the steps that need to be taken to ensure that a patient receives the correct referral?
- Are the financial burdens disproportionately felt by some members of the collaboration more than another?
- How does one measure and monitor the efficacy of a coordinated care program?

Asking and attempting to answer these questions may help improve patient care, in addition to reducing financial, temporal, and stress burdens on a system.

Nonclinical Collaboration Between the Psychiatry and Emergency Departments

In addition to coordinating patient care, collaborations between psychiatry and emergency services can be helpful for departments in a number of ways, including educational programs, research initiatives, and improving well-being and morale.

Education

Though patients with mental illness are common visitors to acute care settings, nurses, ED technicians, residents, and attending physicians may have limited training or experience in dealing with psychiatric emergencies. The reverse is also true: Psychiatrists often feel unfamiliar with current treatments for common medical illnesses encountered in inpatient and outpatient settings. Engaging both emergency physicians and psychiatrists to provide frequent lectures/training can reframe care for psychiatric patients in acute care settings, improve familiarity and comfort in dealing with psychiatric patients, and communicate the importance of attending to psychiatric issues for the ED staff. In addition, updates on nonpsychiatric medications and treatment protocols, refresher courses on medical codes, and conversations about treatment protocols for psychiatric patients in the ED can help psychiatrists feel more comfortable with patients who might have previously been subjected to unnecessary testing and consults under the care of the psychiatry team.

Educational seminars have been implemented at the supporting institution of one of the authors (BB). Three separate seminars were provided on a weekly-to-monthly basis for ED staff, including one for nurses and technicians, one for residents, and one for medical students. In addition to going over role-specific information and talking about the psychiatric concepts of transference and countertransference, these seminars provided the opportunity for the learners to talk about their experiences with psychiatric patients. This aspect of the seminar served both to allow the students to learn from each other and to provide an informal "psychiatric supervision" that has been reported to be helpful in mitigating the negative feelings elicited by working with psychiatric patients.

Some emergency medicine residency training programs include explicit lectures and rotations in psychiatry. This is not yet common, but the other author's (SP) department of emergency medicine provides lectures on topics in emergency psychiatry for trainees and attending physicians. For trainees, there is a required two-week PGY-3 rotation in a locked psychiatric emergency service. This department also supports psychiatric trainees by requiring a full month PGY-2 rotation in a locked psychiatric emergency service and then night rotations in their PGY-3 year.

Research

Organizations such as the American Academy of Emergency Psychiatry (AAEP) and the Society for Academic Emergency Medicine (SAEM) have spearheaded efforts to improve research in the interdisciplinary intersection between emergency medicine and psychiatry; however, more research needs to be done. In addition to examining psychopharmacological interventions, research on ultra-brief psychotherapy, psychiatric trauma, first-break psychosis, access to care, somatization, psychiatric and medical comorbidities in the ED, and recidivism are just a few potential topics in this rich, untapped research field.

Morale and Well-being

Caring for patients can be physically and emotionally taxing. This is especially true for psychiatric patients, who often contribute to the overall level of tension in the ED. In such settings, psychiatrists can play an additional role in the coordination of care, specifically that of caring for the caretakers.

A psychiatric liaison can help to reframe, resolve, and prevent the impact of negative patient interactions in several ways. First, through interactive educational modules, such as the one described above, ED staff can discuss their experiences with psychiatric patients, thereby providing a forum for peer learning and offering a time for psychiatric supervision. In addition to education, these classes allow for time to deal with potentially harmful negative feelings that arise between ED providers and patients with psychiatric issues. Second, asking for a psychiatrist to be available to participate in the debriefing of difficult cases can help to resolve frustration with other staff members and patients by shedding light on intra-psychic conflicts that patients bring to and foist upon ED staff. Clarifying these patient-system conflicts can be comforting to staff members, who may be exhausted from dealing with complicated patients or traumatized by poor outcomes. Finally, having a psychiatrist on ED committees can provide a different and possibly beneficial perspective on an administrative level. Having a psychological perspective on potential staff and patient interpersonal dynamics may give committees information that can raise awareness of potential flash points before they become active problems. Tasks could include the creation of interdisciplinary plans for problem patients and protocols for safe and effective management of agitated and aggressive patients. Including a psychiatrist in these functions can build resilience in the ED staff, as well as improve morale and ideally prevent staff burnout.

The Economics of Coordinated Care

Given the importance of reimbursement on models of coordinated care, the authors would be remiss not to comment on how different economic scenarios can strongly affect the ways in which healthcare systems organize and prioritize coordination of care. At the time of the revision of this chapter (Autumn 2020), there appears to be uncertainty in the way the American healthcare system will be funded moving forward. There appear to be three potential outcomes to the current debate over how public health care is funded: (1) a single-payer system, where healthcare systems receive the bulk of healthcare dollars from a coordinated state–federal partnership in a capitated fashion; (2) a pure fee-for-service, where services rendered are the primary source of payment; and (3) a multi-payer system, where both private and public insurance providers are equal sources of healthcare revenue through both fee-for-service and capitated models. As one might imagine, these approaches to healthcare economics incentivize coordination of care differently.

In a single-payer healthcare system that uses a capitated model, the overall *quality* of care is prioritized over the *amount* of care offered. As the total dollar amount offered to care for an individual is limited and poor outcomes are penalized, healthcare systems will likely incentivize robust efforts to develop coordinated care models that can provide evidence-based services to the majority of the lives they cover. In this approach to care, the weight of patient care falls on primary care providers, who will be expected to coordinate basic services for their patient panels. As such, systems will have an incentive to develop a strong infrastructure of ancillary services to take some of the burden off physicians and other highly paid professionals. Unfortunately, in this model, patients who require a higher level of care or have unique needs may find that they are unable to access specialty care as easily as in the other two models.

In a pure fee-for-service model, the *amount* of care is implicitly prioritized over the (overall) *quality* of care rendered. In this approach, each patient encounter is reimbursed based on its complexity, regardless of the outcome. This incentivizes providers to see patients more frequently and offer them more complex services. Here, the individual is responsible for coordinating their own care, accessing services that they believe are essential. As such, healthcare systems will likely not have a financial inducement to develop services that streamline patient care or coordinated care. In this scenario, all patients will be able to access all levels of care—that is, until they are unable to afford it.

In the current mixed system, some care is reimbursed on a fee-for-service basis (private physicians in private hospitals), some care is salaried (physicians in government hospitals/clinics), and some care is capitated (HMO style). And the underlying financing is also mixed: Some money comes from out-of-pocket payments (co-pays, cosmetic surgery, or discretionary vision-correction procedures), some comes from private insurance coverage, and some comes from governmental insurance coverage (Medicaid, Medicare, Veterans Administration). In such an environment, efforts at clinical care coordination compete with organizational efforts at cost reduction and cost shifting. For example, clinics directly supported by state funds might restrict their services to patients with no benefits whatsoever, directing patients with Medicaid or Medicare to go to private, low-cost clinics, which can "bill" the government for reimbursement. This might seem inefficient, but it shifts part of the state's cost to the federal government, which provides some money for Medicaid and all the money for Medicare. Private clinics might refuse to accept Medicaid or Medicare patients to avoid low reimbursement rates. Private insurance companies may refuse to cover preexisting conditions to avoid covering certain costs. Each organization is tempted to pursue maneuvers to "game the system," none of which help coordinate care.

There have been some government efforts that encourage some aspects of care coordination. HBIPS (hospital-based inpatient psychiatric services) from CMS (the Centers for Medicare and Medicaid Services) did include:

[t]he transition record measures [that focus] on effective and timely communication of specified elements with patients and between treatment settings, thereby promoting care coordination and enhancing continuity of care.

It would include

Contact Information/Plan for Follow-up Care

- 24-hour/7-day contact information, including a physician for emergencies related to inpatient stay

- Contact information for obtaining results of studies pending at discharge
- Plan for follow-up care
- Primary physician, other health care professional, or site designated for follow-up care [9, 10]

However, these measures do not directly apply to EDs (patients are considered outpatients, not inpatients), and CMS changes its reporting requirements over time. Readers can get a sense of how coordination of care is abstracted from the distant vantage point of national agencies.

In conclusion, as the healthcare economics landscape changes in the context of political efforts to change the current law, coordination of care will be valued differently.

Conclusion

Given the high volume of psychiatric patients seen in acute-care settings, creating and sustaining a relationship between the psychiatry and emergency medicine departments can decrease patient length of stay, increase safety for patients and ED staff, increase awareness of mental illness in patients and staff, and improve patient outcomes. As there are differences in clinical training and approaches to patient care, improving communication and developing an awareness of expectations can improve overall interdepartmental coordination of patient care.

As the American medical landscape continues to adapt to new political and economic pressures, interdisciplinary collaborations will be vital to maintaining excellent, safe, and cost-effective health care. In addition, having an awareness of the mental health of one's staff and an informed approach to maintaining their morale can help maintain patient care excellence in acute-care settings.

References

1. Weissberg MP. Emergency room medical clearance: an educational problem. Am J Psy. 1979;136(6):787–90.
2. Dolan JG, Mushlin AL. Routine laboratory testing for medical disorders in psychiatric patients. Arch Intern Med. 1985;145:2085–8.
3. Riba M, Hale M. Medical clearance: fact or fiction in the hospital emergency room. Psychosomatics. 1990. Fall;31(4):400–4.
4. Korn CS, Currier GW, Henderson SO. "Medical clearance" of psychiatric patients without medical complaints in the emergency department. J Emerg Med. 2000;18(2):173–6.
5. Pinto T, Poynter B, Durbin J. Medical clearance in the psychiatric emergency setting: a call for more standardization. Healthc Q. 2010;13(2):77–82.
6. Lukens TW, Wolf SJ, Edlow JA, Shahbuddin S, Allen MH, Currier GW, Jagoda AS. Mental health emergencies/Clinical policy: critical issues in the diagnosis and Management of the Adult Psychiatric Patient in the emergency department. Ann Emerg Med. 2006;47(1):79–99.
7. Anderson EL, Nordstrom K, Wilson MP, et al. American Association for Emergency Psychiatry Task Force on medical clearance of adults part I: introduction, review and evidence-based guidelines. West J Emerg Med. 2017;18(2):235–42.
8. Wilson MP, Nordstrom K, Anderson EL, et al. American Association for Emergency Psychiatry Task Force on medical clearance of adult psychiatric patients. Part II: controversies over medical assessment, and consensus recommendations. West J Emerg Med. 2017;18(4):640–6.
9. Inpatient Psychiatric Facility Quality Reporting Program Manual. Washington, D.C.: Centers for Medicare & Medicaid Services. 2016. Available at http://www.qualityreportingcenter.com/wp-content/uploads/2016/02/IPF_NewMeasuresPt2_20160119_FINAL.2508.pdf. Accessed on 16 Oct 2017.
10. Hospital-Based Inpatient Psychiatric Services (HBIPS). Oakbrook Terrace, IL: The Joint Commission. 2015. Available at https://manual.jointcommission.org/releases/TJC2015A1/HospitalBasedInpatientPsychiatricServices.html. Accessed on 16 Oct 2017.

Integration with Community Resources

40

Jennifer M. Peltzer-Jones

Introduction: Integration with Community Resources

In the United States, emergency departments (EDs) have become primary sites for emergent psychiatric evaluations and crisis intervention. These types of ED visits have been steadily increasing per year and have been found to have significantly longer lengths of stay than for non-mental-health-related visits [1–4]. Recent data demonstrate a discrepancy in disposition options for mental-health-related complaints as compared to nonmental illness presentations in the ED, with presentations due to mental illness having disproportionately higher rates of hospital admission (Figs. 40.1 and 40.2) [1, 2, 5]. ED staff treat acute medical emergencies (e.g., cardiac arrest, stroke, and pulmonary embolism), diagnose and manage new-onset illnesses, and evaluate exacerbations for chronic diseases (congestive heart failure, diabetes, and chronic obstructive pulmonary disorder), understanding that not all sickness requires inpatient medical admission. As the number of mental health presentations continues to increase, ED staff need an understanding of and access to alternative community resources to avoid the exclusive use of hospitalization as the disposition choice for mental health crises. Lack of safe, non-hospital interventions leaves ED staff to over-rely on inpatient levels of care [6]. This, in turn, contributes to the decreased availability of inpatient beds for significant crises, subsequently increasing psychiatric boarding [7–10].

Case Example

Greg, a 20-year-old single African-American male, is brought into the emergency department (ED) by his parents. His parents have noticed odd behaviors, but Greg denies any, as he reports he is a god and can push goodness into the world. He hears the "whispers of the wind," urging him to "connect with the universe." Family are concerned because he has left school, spends large amounts of time isolated on his computer, and has not been eating or caring for himself. Tonight, they entered his room, and he was sitting in his closet in the dark because he was fearful the devil was coming to the house to battle him. He agreed to come to the ED to be checked for dehydration. Greg denies having thoughts to harm himself or others. His family wants to have him drug-tested and believes he may just have "dehydration." They don't think he has any mental illness, and they don't think he needs to go into a hospital. They just want to have a doctor see Greg and treat him so they can bring him home.

J. M. Peltzer-Jones (✉)
Department of Emergency Medicine, Henry Ford Health System, Detroit, MI, USA
e-mail: jpeltze1@hfhs.org

L. S. Zun et al. (eds.), *Behavioral Emergencies for Healthcare Providers*,
https://doi.org/10.1007/978-3-030-52520-0_40

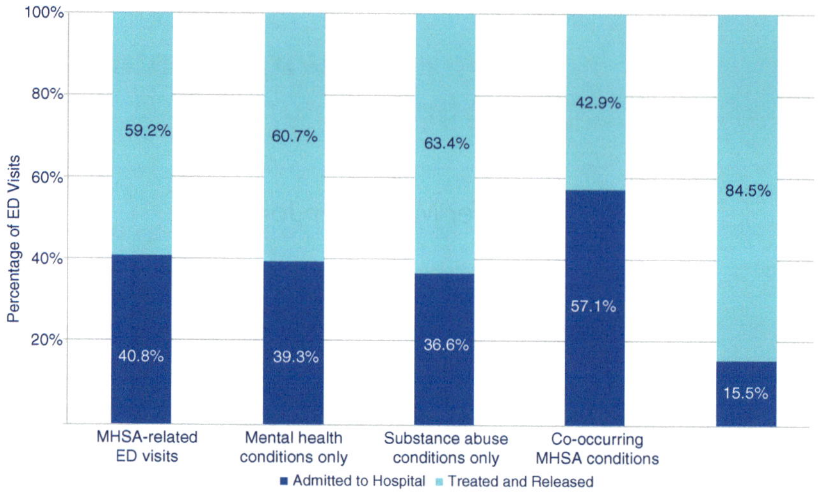

Fig. 40.1 MHSA-related ED visits were three to four times more likely to result in hospitalization than other types of ED visits, 2007.(Owens et al. [1])

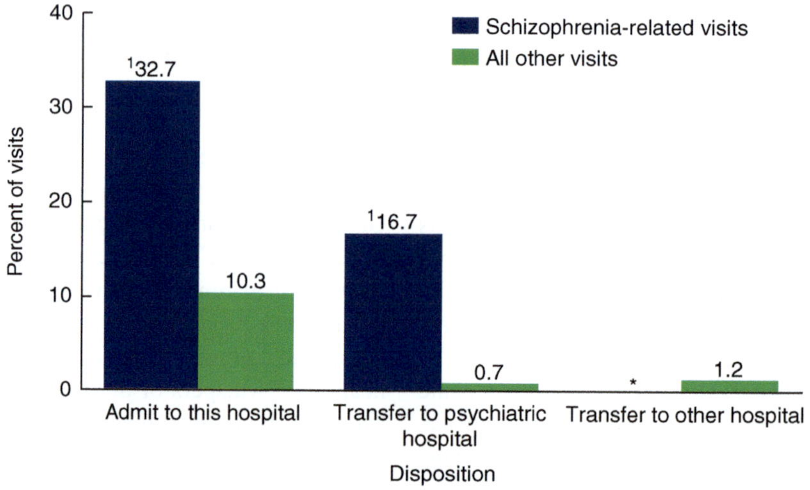

Fig. 40.2 Selected dispositions of emergency department visits made by adults aged 18–64 by schizophrenia diagnosis: United States, 2009–2011. Available at https://www.cdc.gov/nchs/data/databriefs/db215_fig 4.png. (*Figure does not meet standards of reliability or precision. [1]Percentage is significantly different ($p < 0.05$) for schizophrenia-related visits compared with all other visits, based on a two-tailed t test. Notes: Figure is based on 3-year annual averages. Emergency department visits related to schizophrenia are defined as code 295 of the *International Classification of Diseases, Ninth Revision, Clinical Modification* for any of the up to three collected visit diagnoses. Source: CDC/NCHS, National Hospital Ambulatory Medical Care Survey, 2009–2011)

Improving management of the psychiatric crisis is complicated by several factors. First, the United States lacks a standardized delivery model of emergency mental health care. Patients who present to an ED in crisis may or may not speak with a mental health professional. While a mental health professional may instruct a patient to "go to the nearest ED in the event of a crisis," there may not be a psychiatrically trained professional providing consultation to the ED staff. If there is a consultant, training backgrounds vary (social workers, psychiatric residents, psychiatric nurse practitioners, psychologists, psychiatrists), as do hours of availability. ED physicians are not universally trained during residency to manage psychiatric crises [11, 12]. Thus, variable knowledge and limited access to clinical resources contribute to variance in treatment and disposition recommendations from one emergency department to the next [13–16].

In reading Greg's case example scenario, it's clear that he will need additional assistance; however, the reality is the assistance he's offered will rely on the resources his ED can access. Becoming familiar with the community resources can improve patient care. The second benefit of having educated ED staff is to create a space in which ED providers can align with mental health providers in advocacy. This chapter is a brief introduction to various alternative levels of care available to treat psychiatric crises.

Legacy of Deinstitutionalization

To discuss community resources, it is critical for ED staff to understand why community-based treatment is historically important. Deinstitutionalization has often been cited as the single most important factor contributing to the current mental health system crisis. What is not well understood is that it wasn't the actual drive to deinstitutionalize that led to challenges in organizing mental health care; it was the lack of funding to support deinstitutionalization that has led to the continued mental health system crisis. In the mid-twentieth century, large numbers of patients were in state institutions receiving sub-par/harmful/no care. There was little thought of recovery for the institutionalized; rather, large state institutions were warehouses for the mentally ill and developmentally disabled. Proponents of deinstitutionalization advocated for humane treatment for patients instead of locking away these people without any hope of achieving some type of quality of life. Several legal precedents were important in the deinstitutionalization process.

The National Mental Health Act of 1946 was the first major federal law supporting community-based care as the recommended treatment for mentally ill patients. Under this act, the National Institute for Mental Health was formed to help distribute grants to fund outpatient care [17]. As a result, by 1955, over 1000 outpatient mental health clinics were open and receiving state assistance to care for patients in the community [17]. The Joint Commission on Mental Illness was formed under the Mental Health Study Act of 1955 and came to three conclusions: (1) more mental illness research was needed, (2) more mental health providers were needed (recommendations specifically proposed one mental health clinic for every 50,000 people), and (3) "spending for public mental health services should be greatly expanded—doubled in the next 5 years, tripled in the next 10 years" [18].

Throughout the 1960s, despite the discovery of antipsychotic medication and the increased legal pressures for change, there were still between 500,000 and 600,000 patients hospitalized in state institutions across the country. In 1963, President Kennedy proposed the Community Mental Health Centers Act (CMHC). This act called for increase funding for mental health care, with a focus on decreasing the number of institutionalized patients by 50% over the next one to two decades [18]. Federal grants and research monies would shift from state legislatures to local hospitals and nonprofit care organizations [18–20]. When the CMHC Act was passed in 1963, the transition to outpatient community care was sorely underfunded—the federal monies promised in this act were less than 10% of existent costs for treating the institutionalized patients. Thus, patients were to be moved from the most intense level of care to new programs in community care, but community care would receive only one-tenth of the money needed for inpatient care [17]. With the passage of the CMHC Act, deinstitutionalization as a national agenda was born, but from the beginning, community-based care was never funded appropriately to take on the demand.

Before deinstitutionalization, psychiatric crises were sent to state-based settings. As deinstitutionalization occurred, many state facilities closed, leaving communities to find their ways to develop care. In response, psychiatric units were developed within general medical hospitals and free-standing psychiatric facilities. These hospital settings were meant to assist with the temporary crisis in the community, as a person's family/support system could be more involved in the crisis care. Treatment within a person's community continues to be a guiding principle in the structure of today's mental health-care system: "The new priorities of psychiatric hospitalization focus on ameliorating the risk of danger to self or others. Inpatient units are seen as short-term intensive settings to contain and resolve crises that cannot be resolved in the community" [21]. However, the lack of adequate funding in creating true community resources has led to decreased wrap-around resources, leading back to an over-reliance on inpatient hospital care for the psychiatric crisis.

Community Mental Health Organization

The Substance Abuse and Mental Health Services Administration (SAMHSA) designates state mental health agencies (SMHAs) as responsible for "assuring the provision of mental health services to persons with mental illnesses and emotional disturbances" within each state. The SMHA sets programmatic state goals for care, ensures the quality of care, and distributes federal monies to state-based programs. In sum, SMHAs are the organizers of community mental health [22]. The number of people served in these community mental health programs has steadily risen. In 2009, 6,401,613 people received some service that was partially or wholly funded by an SMHA—an increase from 2007 by 300,000 patients [23]. Unfortunately, funding to these organizations continues to receive cuts, stretching the capacity of programs and limiting services [23].

Since large numbers of patients obtain mental health intervention through safety net resources, large numbers of patients seen in the ED are already connected with local community mental health centers (CMHCs). CMHCs can be contacted by each state's department of mental health or department of health and human services, or by contacting the SMHA. CMHCs may be organized under regional authorities or may be directly managed by individual counties. Thus, given the wide range of services and the increasing population CMHCs serve, EDs must develop strong partnerships with their area CMHCs or SMHA to understand specific crisis services and outpatient programs available for patients.

Non-hospital-Based Services

As stated above, the goal of the deinstitutionalization movement was to help people with mental illness try to function within their communities actively. As such, a core principle of mental health treatment is to treat a patient in the least restrictive environment that is recovery oriented and in collaboration with the patient and their supports. Payment barriers aside, the work of the last 50-plus years has driven the advent and management of various models of care developed to meet the needs of patients in the community. The following types of program interventions aim to provide patient-centered care in the community.

Mobile Crisis Teams

Mobile crisis teams (MCTs) consist of trained mental health and law enforcement personnel organized to respond to psychiatric crises in a variety of locations. These programs may be community-based through local police department partnerships with the mental health community, through community mental health centers, or through community mental health insurance providers. Dependent upon the team structure, a crisis team may be called to meet with a patient via accessing a crisis hotline or may be called to respond in conjunction with an emergency management system (EMS) call through local emergency dispatch. Some mobile teams are used as screening agents to conduct assessment and provide authorizations for the level of care requests for county mental health organizations or SMHAs [24]. Mobile crisis teams may also offer the availability of follow-up, postincident visits by the team. Because many mobile crisis teams are linked through local suicide hotlines and "warmlines" (suicide prevention resources staffed explicitly by patients in mental health recovery themselves), patients form strong connections and relationships with their contacts. A CIT, or crisis intervention team, is a specific MCT model that spreads mental health crisis response expertise to police responders of psychiatric crises, which are linked with the EMS system and therefore often the first responders for mental health crises. When a crisis occurs, departments with a CIT send out at least one trained officer to help problem-solve the situation. In establishing a CIT response effort, local resources establish predetermined access to a variety of disposition options, including a designated single point of entry for emergency care. This type of program requires investment from both the community (mental health providers and hospitals) and police departments [25]. MCT outcome studies have reviewed outpatient follow-up for suicidal patients (no benefit), follow-up attendance at subsequent outpatient treatment (improved follow-up), and lower inpatient referrals rates when MCT was utilized [24, 26, 27]. CIT program outcomes have included decreases in the arrests of mentally ill individuals, reduction in police officer stigma toward the mentally ill, and decreased officer and patient injuries [28–30]. While further large-scale research is needed to address the determination of appropriate measures of success and funding justification, providing patients with the information how to access local mobile crisis teams can serve as an additional resource for ED staff.

Residential Services

Crisis residential services, respite services, and transitional housing programs are all community levels of care that may be available from an ED at time of discharge. Crisis residential services can vary from organizing and insurance-reimbursed settings to consumer-run levels of care. Crisis residential residences are unlocked facilities to which patients voluntarily agree to treatment. Like mobile crisis teams, there is not a uniform definition, criteria for admission, or standard admission process. Insurance coverage also varies. This level of care may focus on providing a stable place for people whose housing instability is affecting their mental health stability, or it may target people who have stable housing but need temporary respite to focus on stabilizing their mental health outside of their home environment.

The START model, or short-term acute residential treatment model, in San Diego has demonstrated improved quality of life, with symptom reduction equal to that seen in hospitalized patients [31]. In the START model, the average length of stay in the program was 9 days. Patients lived in a remodeled home that housed 10–12 patients. The program structure included two community meetings, two group sessions, individual counseling, medication meetings run by psychiatrists, recreational activities, and participation in chore and meal preparation for participating patients. There was a low patient-to-staffing ratio, and the staff consisted of master's- and doctoral-level clinicians. At the time of discharge and 2-month follow-up, there were no significant differences on selected symptom measures between the groups in START versus hospitalized patients, despite an almost equal number of days in each program setting. These findings and those of similar studies [32, 33] suggest that patients in acute crisis can be safely and effectively managed in residential crisis services.

Day Treatment Programs

Day treatment programs, partial hospital programs (PHPs), and intensive outpatient (IOP) services are full or half multiday (4–9 hours) programs for patients. These programs provide a structure similar to an inpatient milieu, as patients have group therapy, meet with psychiatrists, and engage in individual therapy, all while also being able to return to home at night and continue to work during the day. These programs may or may not be used in conjunction with a crisis residential program as a step down from an inpatient psychiatric admission or an alternative for inpatient care [34]. Because patients do not live at the site of care and transportation can be a barrier to obtaining care, transportation may be offered by the program site. These programs may focus on primary mental health, substance abuse, or comorbid mental health/substance-use disorders. Day treatment programs may be based at the site of a hospital or outpatient clinic. These programs are not restricted to Medicaid patients, as private insurance companies and Medicare also typically reimburse this level of care. Several agencies set minimum standards or provide accreditation for day treatment models, including the Association for Ambulatory Behavioral Healthcare and Commission on Accreditation of Rehabilitation Facilities (CARF). Patients who present to the ED in crisis may benefit from this intense level of care as an alternative to hospitalization, though reviews of efficacy are mixed, due in large part to methodologic problems in their evaluation [35].

Case Management

Several agencies define the expectations of effective case management. The Commission on Accreditation of Rehabilitation Facilities (CARF) defines case management as a level of care that "provide(s) goal-oriented and individualized support focusing on improved self-sufficiency for the persons served through assessment, planning, linkage, advocacy, coordination, and monitoring activities. Successful service coordination results in community opportunities and increased independence for the persons served. Programs may provide occasional supportive counseling and crisis intervention services when allowed by regulatory or funding authorities" [36]. The National Association of State Mental Health Program Directors (NASMHPD) further states that case management "is a range of services provided to assist and support patients in developing their skills to gain access to needed medical, behavioral health, housing, employment, social, educational, and other services essential to meeting basic human services; linkages and training for patient served in the use of basic community resources; and monitoring of overall service delivery" [37]. In practice, case management typically refers to a level of care in which a mental health professional, usually a clinically trained psychiatric social worker, provides individualized assistance and treatment planning for patients. Case managers may assist patients with clinical care, as well as navigation of the complex mental health systems. They may provide crisis counseling and access social services such as housing, food assistance, or job training/referral to supported employment programs. Case management philosophies focus on meeting patients at their current level of function to set goals and create plans to achieve these goals within the community. This is different from the classic idea of psychotherapy, in which patients examine intrapersonal barriers to achieving goals.

Intense case management strategies, such as the assertive community treatment (ACT) model or programs of assertive community treatment (PACT), are highly standardized, intense service delivery models targeting patients who experience more crises and need increased support. SAMHSA considers ACT programs to be evidenced-based, best-practice models of care, as the ACT has repeatedly been shown to decrease inpatient acute hospitalization and incarceration for patients with the severe mental illness. Essential features of the ACT model include low patient-to-psychiatric-staff ratios; the availability of 24-hour crisis coverage; multidisciplinary teams; and comprehensive patient-centered planning (with medication management, supportive therapy, and rehabilitative support). Peer support, transportation, and community outreach are additional basic tenets of the model [38]. ACT teams have very distinct admission criteria for patients but are not time-limited. Despite the many studies that demonstrate the positive outcomes of an ACT model, many insurance companies are reluctant to fund this level of care, and the lack of an "end" may overshadow the long-term financial benefits to fund such a plan. Regardless, EDs may not be aware that the patients they are evaluating have these services, may not ask patients for their ACT team contact information, and may not recognize ACT teams will often deploy teams directly to the ED to assist with crises. EDs would benefit from reaching out to local ACT programs to obtain contact information and engage in joint crisis planning for patients who may frequently use the ED. Local ACT teams are usually found through local CMHCs or can be located through the SMHA.

Family Resources

Recent research indicates that early, multimodal interventions such as medication management, family psychoeducation, social skills training, and supported employment/education programs for patients with first episodes of psychosis are superior to treatment as usual [39, 40]. It is not clear how often ED staff have discussions with families of patients who are suffering with first episodes of psychosis or with an episode of psychiatric crises regarding available resources. Organizations such as the National Alliance on Mental Illness (NAMI) can provide educational information and support information for families who are caring for individuals with mental illness. As with our case example of Greg, there may continue to be a delay in accessing mental health resources if his family does not recognize the severity of his symptoms, possibly leading to dangerous outcomes. NAMI can provide information for local families and groups. Additional sources of education and support for families include Mentalhealth.gov, the American Psychiatric Association, and the American Psychological Association.

Nontraditional Community Resources

Untreated mental health problems can lead to negative consequences in medical health, work, or school, in addition to the negative impact on patient quality of life. People may not have symptoms that warrant immediate safety interventions (such as inpatient care) but may have daily stressors negatively affecting life. It is important for ED physicians to be aware of additional resources in the community that are not found in "traditional" outpatient clinic settings.

Just as EDs have increasingly become the sites of care for psychiatric crises, primary care physicians are increasingly treating mental health disorders in their clinics. Numerous studies have demonstrated that poor mental health management contributes to poor medical outcomes with chronic medical conditions such as diabetes and congestive heart failure. Patients may feel stigmatized going to primary mental health clinics, so alternatively, they meet only with their primary care physicians. In response, there has been an increase in the number of integrated behavioral-health/primary-care collaborative models, which have demonstrated positive outcomes for mental health treatment engagement and other behavioral outcomes [41, 42]. These programs may include colocated mental health practitioners, embedded mental health practitioners, or telepsychiatry programs. Common problems that may be addressed in the integrated models may include treatment of depression, anxiety, sleep disorders, and substance use, but may also include identification and attention to low health literacy barriers, subtle cognitive disorders, treatment adherence, weight loss counseling, smoking cessation, etc. When patients present to the ED with medical complaints for which the ED staff has determined there may be psychological factors impacting medical behavior, it may be beneficial to discuss with the patient or directly contact the primary care physician to determine what resources may be available at the office site.

An employee assistance program, or EAP, is a "voluntary, confidential program that helps employees work through various life challenges that may adversely affect job performance, health, and personal well-being to optimize an organization's success" [43]. These programs have been in existence since the 1940s, but are not always well known as a resource to patients [44]. Types of problems EAP counselors often treat include marital difficulties, interpersonal difficulties in the workplace between coworkers, substance use, legal challenges, organizational changes, workplace violence events, etc. This assistance is often a service for which the employees seeking care do not pay. When patients report these types of struggles during an ED visit, ED physicians may want to encourage the patient to check with their human resource department to determine what type of program may be offered.

Other nontraditional resources that emergency departments may want to reach out to for partnerships may include the following:

- Clubhouse Psychosocial Rehabilitation Centers are found in 36 states in the United States and are internationally located in 33 countries. These programs are "non-clinical, integrated therapeutic working communities open to anyone with a history of mental illness. … [Goals include] helping members participate in mainstream employment, educational opportunities, community-based housing, wellness or health promotion activities, reduce hospitalizations or involvement with the criminal justice system, and improve social relationships, satisfaction and quality of life" [45]. To find out if there is a Clubhouse in the area, access the Clubhouse International website.
- Supported employment or vocational rehabilitation programs offer training and work assistance for patients with mental illness. Patients can be linked to these programs through local community mental health programs.
- Most local colleges and universities will have university-based counseling clinics specifically for students while enrolled. These clinics can offer assistance with common early adult struggles, including adjustment to college, career counseling, eating disorders, Lesbian, Gay, Bisexual, Transgender, and Questioning (LGBTQ) issues, etc.
- Local doctoral training programs for psychology and counseling often have training clinics to assist students with the psychotherapy skills development. These clinics are generally open to the public, with sliding-scale pay structures. Contact the local psychology/counseling departments for referral information.
- For issues with grieving, funeral homes may have grief therapy for family members. In addition, for patients who are grieving the loss of a loved one from violence, local city/county/state police departments may offer support groups.
- For patients who are victims of crime, there may be free counseling services; every state has compensation funds available. For state-by-state information, ED physicians can refer to the National Association of Crime Victim Compensation Boards.

Conclusion

ED personnel are increasingly treating patients with psychiatric disorders. Not all presentations require inpatient psychiatric intervention, and thus, knowledge of all available referral options may decrease unnecessary hospitalization, increase patient engagement with care, and improve patient quality of life. Reaching out to local programs to develop or improve collaborative relationships can affect patient- and system-level outcomes.

References

1. Owens PL, Mutter R, Stocks C. Mental health and substance abuse-related emergency department visits among adults, 2007. HCUP statistical brief #92. Rockville, MD: Agency for Healthcare Research and Quality; 2010. Available at http://www.hcup-us.ahrq.gov/reports/statbriefs/sb92.pdf.
2. Slade EP, Dixon LB, Semmel S. Trends in the duration of emergency department visits, 2001–2006. Psychiatr Serv. 2010;61(9):878–46.
3. Ting SA, Sullivan AF, Boudreaux ED, Miller I, Camargo CA Jr. Trends in US emergency department visits for attempted suicide and self-inflicted injury, 1993–2008. Gen Hosp Psy. 2012;34:557–65.
4. Nolan JM, Fee C, Cooper BA, Rankin SH, Blegen MA. Psychiatric boarding incidence, duration, and associated factors in United States emergency departments. Journal Emerg Nurs. 2015;41(1):57–64.
5. Albert M, McCraig LF. Emergency department visits related to schizophrenia among adults aged 18–64: United States, 2009–2011. NHCS data brief no. 215. Hyattsville, MD: National Center for Health Statistics; 2015.
6. Stefan S. Emergency department assessment of psychiatric patients: Reducing inappropriate inpatient admissions, August 2006. Available at https://www.medscape.org/viewarticle/541478. Accessed on 12 Nov 2017.

7. Bender D, Pande M, Ludwig M. A literature review: psychiatric boarding. Washington, D.C.: Office of Disability, Aging and Long-Term Care Policy, Office of the Assistant Secretary for Planning and Evaluation, and US Department of Health and Human Services; 2008. Available at http://aspe.hhs.gov/daltcp/reports/2008/PsyBdLR.pdf.
8. Torrey EF, Entsminger K, Geller J, Stanley J, Jaffe DJ. The shortage of public hospital beds for mentally ill persons: A report of the Treatment Advocacy Center. Available at http://www.treatmentadvocacycenter.org. Accessed on 12 Nov 2017.
9. Misek RK, DeBarba AE, Brill A. Predictors of psychiatric boarding in the emergency department. West J Emerg Med. 2015;56(1):71–5.
10. Simpson SA, Joesch JM, West II, Pasic J. Who's boarding in the psychiatric emergency service? West J Emerg Med. 2014;55(6):649–74.
11. Park JM, Park LT, Siefert CJ, Abraham ME, Fry CE, Silvert MS. Factors associated with extended length of stay for patients presenting to an urban psychiatric emergency service: a case control study. J Beh Health Sci Res. 2009;36:3.
12. Smith JL, De Nadai AS, Storch EA, Langland-Orban B, Pracht E, Petrilia J. Correlates of length of stay and boarding in Florida emergency departments for patients with psychiatric diagnoses. Psychiatr Serv. 2016;67(11):1169–74.
13. Olfson M, Marcus SC, Bridge JA. Emergency treatment of deliberate self-harm. Arch Gen Psychiatry. 2012;69(1):80–8.
14. Baraff LJ, Janowicz N, Asarnow JR. Survey of California emergency departments about practices for management of suicidal patients and resources available for their care. Ann Emerg Med. 2006;48(4):452–8.
15. Douglass AM, Luo J, Baraff LJ. Emergency medicine and psychiatry agreement on diagnosis and disposition of emergency department patients with behavioral emergencies. Acad Emerg Med. 2011;18(4):368–73.
16. Bessaha ML, Shumway M, Edmondson-Smith M, Bright CL, Unick GJ. Predictors of hospital length of stay and cost of stay in a national sample of adult patients with psychotic disorder. Psychiatr Serv. 2017;68(6):559–65.
17. Grob GN. Mad, homeless, and unwanted. A history of the care of the chronic mentally ill in America Psychiatr Clin North Am. 1994;17(3):541–59.
18. Rochefort DA. Origins of the "third psychiatric revolution": the community mental health centers act of 1963. J Health Politics, Pol Law. 1984;9(1):1.
19. Prepared by C. Koyanagi from the Judge David Bazelon Center for Mental Health Law, for the Kaiser Commission on Medicaid and the Uninsured. 2007. Learning from history: deinstitutionalization of people with mental illness as precursor.
20. Klerman G. Better but not well: social and ethical issues in the deinstitutionalization of the mentally ill. Schiz Bull. 1977;3(4):617–31.
21. US Department of Health and Human Services. Mental health: a report of the surgeon general—executive summary. Rockville, MD: US Department of Health and Human Services, Substance Abuse and Mental Health Services Administration, Center for Mental Health Services, National Institutes of Health, and National Institute of Mental Health; 1999.
22. Substance Abuse and Mental Health Services Administration. Funding and characteristics of state mental health agencies, 2009. HHS publication no. (SMA) 11–4655. Rockville, MD: Substance Abuse and Mental Health Services Administration; 2011.
23. NAMI. State mental health cuts: a national crisis. A report by the national alliance on mental illness. Changes in Number of People Served By the State Mental Health Authority, March 2011. Available at http://www.nami.org/Template.cfm?Section=state_budget_cuts_report. Accessed on 19 Sep 2011.
24. Guo S, Biegel DE, Johnsen JA, Dyches H. Assessing the impact of community based mobile crisis services on preventing hospitalization. Psychiatr Serv. 2000;52(2):223–8.
25. Dupont R, Cochran S, Pillsbury S. Crisis intervention team core elements. 2007. Available at http://cit.memphis.edu/pdf/CoreElements.pdf. Accessed on 12 Nov 2017.
26. Currier G, Fisher S, Caine E. Mobile crisis team intervention to enhance linkage of discharged suicidal patients to outpatient psychiatric services: a randomized control trial. Acad Emerg Med. 2010;17(1):36–43.
27. Boudreaux JG, Crapanzano KA, Jones GN, Jeider TA, Dodge VH, Hebert MJ, et al. Using mental health outreach teams in the emergency department to improve engagement in treatment. Comm Mental Health. 2016;52:1009–14.
28. NAMI–CIT Toolkit CIT Facts. Available at https://www.nami.org/Law-Enforcement-and-Mental-Health/What-Is-CIT. Accessed on 12 Nov 2017.
29. Lee SJ, Thomas P, Doulis C, Bowles D, Henderson K. Keppich-Arnold S, et a. Outcomes achieved by and police and clinician perspectives on a joint police officer and mental health clinician mobile response unit Int J Mental Health Nurs. 2015;24:538–46.
30. McKenna B, Furness T, Brown S, Tacey M, Hiam A, Wise M. Police and clinician diversion of people in mental health crisis from the emergency department: a trend analysis and cross comparison study. BMC Emerg Med. 2015;15:14.
31. Hawthorne WB, Green EE, Gilmer T, Garcia P, Hough RL, Lee M, et al. A randomized trial of short term acute residential services for veterans. Psychiatr Serv. 2005;56(11):1379–86.
32. Sledge WH, Tebes J, Rakfeldt J, Davidson L, Lyons L, Druss B. Day hospital/crisis respite care versus inpatient care, part 1: clinical outcomes. Am J Psy. 1996;153(8):1065–73.
33. Fenton WS, Hoch JS, Herrell JM, Mosher L, Dixon L. Cost and cost-effectiveness of hospital vs. residential crisis care for patients who have serious mental illness. Arch Gen Psych. 2002;59:357–64.
34. Taube-Schiff M, Ruhig M, Mehak A, Deathe van Dyk M, Cassin SE, Ungar T, et al. Staff perspec-

tives: what is the function of adult mental health day hospital programs? J Psychiatr Mental Health Nurs. 2017;24:580–8.
35. Horvitz-Lennon M, Normand ST, Gaccione P, Frank R. Partial versus full hospitalization for adults in psychiatric distress: a systematic review of the published literature (1957–1997). Am J Psy. 2001;158:5.
36. Commission on accreditation of rehabilitation facilities 2017 behavioral health programs descriptions. Available at http://www.carf.org/WorkArea/DownloadAsset.aspx?id=23988. Accessed on 12 Nov 2017.
37. National Association of State Mental Health Program Directors Research Institute, Inc. Glossary. Available at https://www.nasmhpd.org/node/1394. Accessed on 12 Nov 2017.
38. NAMI fact sheet: assertive community treatment. Available at http://www.namihelps.org/assets/PDFs/fact-sheets/General/Assertive-Community-Treatment.pdf. Accessed on 12 Nov 2017.
39. Byrne P. Managing the acute psychotic episode. BMJ. 2007;334:686–95.
40. Kane JM, Robinson DG, Schooler NR, Mueser KT, Penn DL, et al. Comprehensive versus usual community care for first-episode psychosis: 2-year outcomes from the NIMH RAISE early treatment program. Am J Psy. 2016;173(4):362–72.
41. Miller-Matero LR, Dubaybo F, Ziadni MS, Feit R, Kvamme R, Eshelman A, Keimig W. Embedding a psychologist into primary care increases access to behavioral health services. J Prim Care Comm Health. 2015;6(2):100–4.
42. Unutzer J, Harbin H, Schoenbaum M, Druss B. The collaborative care model: An approach for integrating physical and mental health care in Medicaid health homes. Centers for Medicare & Medicaid Services. 2013 Brief. Available at https://www.medicaid.gov/state-resource-center/medicaid-state-technical-assistance/health-homes-technical-assistance/downloads/hh-irc-collaborative-5-13.pdf. Accessed on 12 Nov 2017.
43. Work-Life: Employee Assistance Programs. Available at https://www.opm.gov/policy-data-oversight/worklife/employee-assistance-programs/. Accessed on 12 Nov 2017.
44. Frauenholtz S. Responding to the affordable care act: a leadership opportunity for social workers in employee assistance programs. Health Soc Work. 2014;30(2):153–60.
45. McKay C, Nugent KL, Johnsen M, Eaton WW, Lidz CW. A systematic review of evidence for the clubhouse model of psychosocial rehabilitation. Admin Pol Ment Health. 2016:1–20.

The Role of Telepsychiatry

41

Zakaria Abdulnabi

Introduction

You are working a busy Friday night in your suburban emergency department (ED), and there has been an unusually high volume of patients presenting with psychiatric complaints this evening. As they are placed into rooms and medically assessed, an increasing number of beds in the department are not turning over as these patients wait for psychiatric consultations; there is no on-call psychiatrist at your hospital. As the night progresses, patients in the waiting room become upset about the wait time, anxious patients grow restless in the noisy environment, and the ED staff begins to feel the rising level of stress. Fortunately, the charge nurse remembers that the ED has recently launched a new telepsychiatry program. She retrieves a mobile telehealth unit comprised of a monitor and camera, and wheels it into a patient's room. Within 10 minutes, the patient is speaking to a board-certified psychiatrist via a secure two-way video connection. The psychiatrist later calls you to discuss the case, give medication recommendations, inform you that the patient requires inpatient admission, and tells you that she will begin the process of finding a bed at an appropriate facility. The mobile unit is wheeled into the next patient's room, and the process is repeated.

Telepsychiatry is a subset of telemedicine, which is the process of providing health care from a distance, typically using a telephone, internet connection, or videoconferencing technology. This modality can be used for a wide range of psychiatric services including clinical assessment, therapy, patient education, and medication management [1]. In the emergency department setting, use of telepsychiatry services is primarily aimed at providing access to mental health specialists in locations that would otherwise not have such access, controlling psychiatric patient boarding times in the ED, and controlling costs [2].

Background

Telepsychiatry is one of the most established areas of telemedicine, dating back to 1959 when it was utilized at the Nebraska Psychiatric Institute. Although telepsychiatry is currently widely used in clinics and correctional facilities, its use in EDs remains more limited [2]. Much of the recent literature into the costs, efficacy, and implementation of telepsychiatry programs has focused on its use in rural settings, where access to trained mental health providers is often limited. The trend in increased use of telepsychiatry

Z. Abdulnabi (✉)
Department of Emergency Medicine, Carle Foundation Hospital, Urbana, IL, USA

L. S. Zun et al. (eds.), *Behavioral Emergencies for Healthcare Providers*, https://doi.org/10.1007/978-3-030-52520-0_41

is not, however, limited to rural areas; many grade schools and colleges have begun to utilize telepsychiatry services, as these programs have proven cost-effective by allowing the school to pay for psychiatric services on an as-needed basis. In emergency departments across the country, remote access to specialized providers via teleconferencing technology allows for more rapid evaluation and disposition of patients with acute psychiatric illnesses, as well as specialist expertise for difficult or rare cases [3].

How It Is Used

Although telemedicine has proliferated greatly in recent decades, use of telepsychiatry in EDs has been slow to develop. Especially when compared to ED use of telemedicine for other clinical fields such as neurology and obstetrics [4]. A review of 43 national and regional telemedicine programs found that only eight (18%) offered ED telepsychiatry services [2]. Like most telemedicine networks, telepsychiatry networks typically operate a system of "hub" and "spoke" sites that communicate with one another remotely. The site where the specialist or psychiatrist is located is called the hub, whereas the site where the patient is physically located is a spoke [2]. In this manner, multiple emergency departments or clinics can maintain as-needed access to specialists at one common regional site that operates 24 hours per day.

In recent years, videoconferencing has come to dominate telepsychiatry, although there are still occasional programs that use other mediums such as telephone and email [2]. Most telepsychiatry programs today use commercially available telemedicine software and equipment, which ranges from simple webcams to fixed monitors and mobile units. Typically, an emergency department provider will first evaluate a patient with a psychiatric complaint; once the patient is medically cleared, the provider uses a simple screen interface to connect to the hub. After providing basic identifying information, a videoconference channel with a specialist provider is established, allowing the specialist to interview the patient and provide recommendations for care in much the same way they could if they were physically on site. In addition to patient evaluation and medication management, the hub can often aid in facilitating acceptance and transfer of a patient to an inpatient psychiatric facility, if deemed necessary (Fig. 41.1).

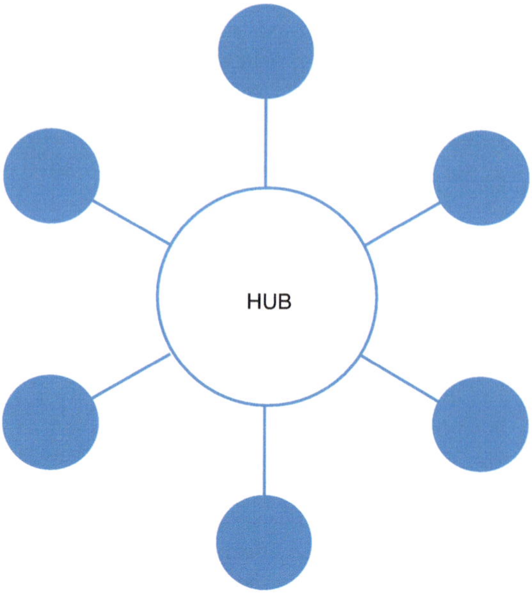

Fig. 41.1 Model of a hub and spoke network

Reliability and Outcomes

Numerous studies have been published regarding the efficacy of telepsychiatry, and the evidence suggests it is equivalent to face-to-face services in terms of reliability of clinical assessment and patient outcome [5]. These studies have generally found a high level of agreement, or inter-method reliability, between assessments done via telepsychiatry and those done face-to-face with regard to DSM diagnoses [5]. This means that a given patient is likely to be conferred the same diagnoses in a given encounter, regardless of whether they are interviewed face-to-face or via telepsychiatry. The studies regarding treatment outcomes are equally promising, with the majority of studies showing telepsychiatry performed at least, as well as the standard face-to-face care with regard to various patient outcomes, including measures of symptom burden associated with depression, PTSD, bulimia, and other psychiatric disorders [5].

Potential Benefits

The problem of long boarding times for psychiatric patients in the ED is one that is very familiar to most ED providers. On average, psychiatric patients spend three times longer in the ED than other medical patients [6]. Theoretically, instant access to mental health specialists 24 hours per day could help alleviate this problem by limiting the amount of time patients have to wait for a specialist to arrive at the bedside. This is especially true for rural emergency departments, where specialists may be fewer in number and farther away.

Cost is another important consideration when comparing telepsychiatry to standard face-to-face care. Estimating the overall costs and savings of ED psychiatry programs is complex and involves assessment of a variety of direct and indirect factors, ranging from the initial cost of equipment to increases in hospital revenue due to faster ED bed turnover. Studies of telepsychiatry as a whole have shown mixed results, but these have largely focused on outpatient settings. Further research is needed to specifically assess the costs and savings associated with emergency department telepsychiatry programs.

Another potential benefit of telepsychiatry is the prevention and mitigation of inappropriate commitments. Many states have civil commitment laws that allow various agents such as police officers and judges to hold patients involuntarily under certain circumstances. Timely access to a telepsychiatrist can decrease the number and length of inappropriate commitments; this not only saves in costs but also alleviates situations that could potentially build distrust between a patient and the mental healthcare system.

Patient and Provider Satisfaction

For any new model of healthcare delivery to succeed, it is vital that both providers and patients are satisfied enough with the experience to buy into its use. Studies overall have shown that patients tend to be highly satisfied with telepsychiatry, whereas providers have more mixed opinions. When assessing patient satisfaction using self-reported questionnaires, most patients rate their experience with telepsychiatry between "good" and "excellent" [5]. Patients tend to specifically enjoy the ease of use and decreased burden of traveling to appointments associate with telepsychiatry, whereas areas of concern reported by patients included privacy concerns and challenges in developing a doctor–patient rapport. Patients generally report that they are comfortable sharing the same information via telepsychiatry that they would share in a face-to-face encounter [5].

Providers, on the other hand, tend to have more varied opinions on the use of telepsychiatry when compared to standard face-to-face care. Concerns expressed by providers included lack of experience using telepsychiatry, technological challenges, and lack of access to training on telepsychiatry [5]. An additional important concern that many providers have expressed is that telepsychiatry can hinder patient–provider interactions and therapeutic rapport [7, 8]. While endorsing many of the same concerns as other providers, ED providers have generally expressed a high level of satisfaction with telepsychiatry in studies [9, 10].

Limits and Drawbacks

There are various limitations and drawbacks to the use of telepsychiatry that are important to discuss. Many of these limitations result from the technology utilized. Like all telecommunications systems, telepsychiatry systems do not operate with 100% success, and there are a litany of possible issues that can arise. Common issues include insufficient bandwidth to transmit a reliable signal, hardware malfunction, and poor interoperability between systems made by different manufacturers. In addition to technological challenges, there are barriers caused by medical licensing laws. Most states currently require providers to be licensed in that state in order to practice there. This can cause issues for telemedicine programs that intend to provide care across state lines, as the process of licensure is often expensive and time-consuming. An additional consideration is the rules regarding reimbursement for telemedicine services. While the Centers for Medicare and Medicaid Services (CMS) has been reimbursing for telemedicine since 1997 [2], there remain some private insurers that do not reimburse such services—or that do so, but at a lower rate than face-to-face encounters. Finally, there are complex privacy issues relating to the use of telepsychiatry. These include ensuring privacy at physical locations, preventing hacks and system breaches, and concerns surrounding the recording and storage of audio or video from patient encounters. It is important for providers to be open and address as many of these concerns as possible prior to beginning a telepsychiatry encounter. The provider at the hub site will often also address privacy concerns prior to beginning the interview.

Looking Forward

As technology continues to pervade and infiltrate every aspect of healthcare provision, telemedicine and other technology-assisted patient care modalities will likely continue to expand. These modalities have great potential to improve care and expand access, but it is important to understand their proper uses and limitations. While much research remains to be done regarding the role of telepsychiatry in the management of mental health emergencies, there is already substantial evidence that this modality can provide comparable outcomes to traditional face-to-face care while expanding geographic access to care and reducing the amount of time psychiatric patients spend in the ED. As we move deeper into the twenty-first century and public awareness of mental health issues grows, there will be greater pressure to address these shortcomings, and telepsychiatry will likely play an expanding role in this endeavor (Fig. 41.2).

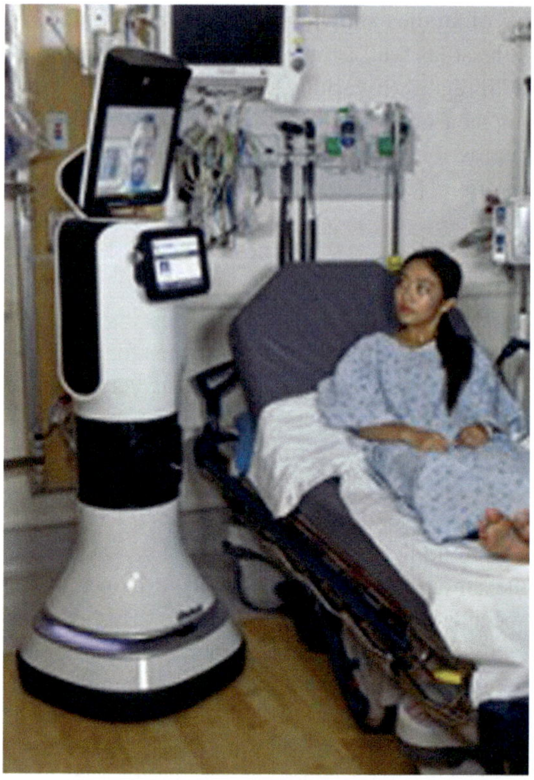

Fig. 41.2 Mobile telemedicine unit. (Image Courtesy of InTouch Health)

References

1. Shore JH. What is telepsychiatry? Available at https://www.psychiatry.org. Retrieved 2017.
2. California Healthcare Foundation. Telepsychiatry in the emergency department: overview and case studies. Available at http://www.chcf.org/publications/2009/12/telepsychiatry-in-the-emergency-department-overview-and-case-studies. Retrieved 2017.
3. Deslich S, et al. Telepsychiatry in the 21st century: transforming healthcare with technology. Perspect Health Inf Manag. 2013;10(Summer):1f.
4. Hilty DM, et al. The effectiveness of telemental health: a 2013 review. Telemed J E Health. 2013;19(6):444–54.
5. Hubley S, et al. Review of key telepsychiatry outcomes. World J Psychiatry. 2016;6(2):269–82.

6. Nicks BA, Manthey DM. The impact of psychiatric patients boarding in emergency departments. Emerg Med Int. 2012;2012:360308.
7. Pangka KR, et al. Exploring the views of emergency department staff on the use of videoconferencing for mental health emergencies in southwest Ontario. Stud Health Technol Inform. 2015;209:114–20.
8. Sinclaire C, et al. Online mental health resources in Australia: clinician perceptions of acceptability. J Med Internet Res. 2013;5(9):e193.
9. Saurman E, et al. No longer 'flying blind': how access has changed emergency mental health care in rural and remote emergency departments, a qualitative study. BMC Health Serv Res. 2015;15:156.
10. Sorvaniemi M, et al. Telepsychiatry in emergency consultations: a follow-up study of sixty patients. Telemed J E Health. 2005;11(4):439–41.

Triage of Psychiatric Patients in the Emergency Department

42

Divy Ravindranath and Mark Newman

Introduction: What Is Triage?

Patients arrive in emergency departments (EDs) with concerns needing rapid assessment and effective clinical management. Providers in the ED have an obligation to rule out any apparent life-threatening presenting conditions. Ensuring efficiency and safety is easy when patients come to the ED one at a time. However, patients arrive in the ED at different rates and with different acuities of illness. Facilitating efficiency and safety, triage is the process by which multiple patients are rapidly assessed for risk and queued for care by the ED providers. Patients assessed to be at the highest risk for deterioration or in need of immediate intervention are seen first, while patients with less urgent concerns may be asked to wait.

Thus, the role of triage is to take the patient who comes in crisis and make an initial attempt at determining whether the crisis represents an emergency. The crisis may be triggered by a catastrophic life event, like a relationship termination, an accident, or a natural disaster, or may be seemingly untriggered, like a panic attack in a case of panic disorder. The critical distinction is whether the crisis contains within it acute behavioral symptoms that impair the person's capacity for self-care and/or increase the risk of harm to self or others [1].

The physical organization of each individual emergency department influences this process. Some hospitals have dedicated psychiatric emergency services (PES) with an independent triage and evaluation process. Alternatively, the initial triage of patients with psychiatric complaints may be accomplished in a more general ED, where the medical ED physicians perform the initial evaluation, and the mental health service acts as consultants to assist in assessment and disposition. By its nature, the PES triage will be more attuned to making the distinction between crisis and emergency, whereas the general ED will have to make that distinction and also consider how to sequence and prioritize behavioral emergencies with other potential medical emergencies, like chest pain, shortness of breath, and so on. Similarly, PES triage will still need to perform an initial screening to see if there may be a medical emergency that would supersede the need for assessment and management of the presenting behavioral crisis.

Regardless of location, the staff responsible for triage should receive training in the assessment of mental health emergencies: what to determine before patient arrival, what to deter-

D. Ravindranath (✉)
Department of Psychiatry, Palo Alto Veterans Affairs Health Care System, Palo Alto, CA, USA
e-mail: divy.ravindranath@va.gov

M. Newman
Department of Psychiatry, University of Washington Medical Center, Seattle, WA, USA

L. S. Zun et al. (eds.), *Behavioral Emergencies for Healthcare Providers*,
https://doi.org/10.1007/978-3-030-52520-0_42

mine on arrival, how to manage the waiting room to keep patients safe, and what issues are specific to direct psychiatric admissions and interhospital ED-to-ED transfers. A cautionary section on patient handoffs is also provided.

What Can Be Determined Prior to Arrival

Before conducting an assessment and formulating a treatment plan with psychiatric patients in the ED, clinicians are encouraged to obtain information about the patient's thoughts and behavior before arrival at the ED whenever possible. Because some patients with emergent psychiatric complaints are unwilling or unable to report their medical or psychiatric histories, gathering collateral information can be extremely useful, especially if the patient's treatment record is not available to the ED.

A variety of sources can be used to obtain pre-arrival information, such as community providers, law enforcement personnel, and family members. Each source provides a slightly different perspective and can be contacted at any point during the ED encounter to solicit information. However, the triage professional is likely to have contact with at least one of these sources as the patient arrives. In this circumstance, information needed to prepare the ED for the patient should be obtained. Contact information for the referral source and other interested parties should also be recorded to facilitate gathering additional collateral information during the patient's stay.

Community Providers and Crisis Hotlines

Patients may already be involved with the community mental health system, substance-use disorder treatment clinics, or private therapists or psychiatrists. When these providers call the ED to advise that a patient is on the way, triage staff should document the reason for ED referral, the time course for the current crisis, the patient's baseline demeanor, and whether there is suspicion of substance misuse. Information about the patient's history of suicidal ideation and suicide attempts, history of homicidal ideation and other violent or dangerous behaviors, current mental health diagnoses, and medications should also be obtained.

Law Enforcement and Emergency Medical Services (EMS)

Law enforcement agents may become involved in a patient case secondary to a 911 or crisis-line call by the patient, a family member or friend, or the patient's outpatient treatment provider. These agents usually bring patients to the ED and can give a brief report upon arrival. This report should include details about the reason they became involved (i.e., the patient is intoxicated, behaviorally unstable, and/or suicidal or homicidal) and whether there are collateral sources that can be contacted for more information.

EMS personnel may similarly become involved and arrive at the ED with the patient. Beyond the reporting of vital signs and symptoms while en route, EMS personnel can also provide important information about a patient's initial presentation, cooperativeness, and medical status. This may include details about the condition of the patient's living environment and information transmitted from witnesses or family members. Again, a way to contact other collateral sources should be sought.

Friends and Family

Friends and family provide valuable information regarding the current mental status and past histories of patients. Spouses, children, and neighbors often have intimate knowledge of a patient's mental health history and baseline functioning. Determining any current psychosocial stressors such as pending legal issues, the recent death of a loved one, or the loss of a job will help the ED clinician assess the impact of situational factors on the patient's presentation.

What Can Be Determined at Arrival

Safety Assessment

Ambulatory patients with psychiatric complaints may present to triage alone or arrive with family or friends, and the degree of their cooperation can vary widely. It is advisable to have a protocol for determining the location of initial triage based on the circumstances of arrival. A patient who self-presents with a calm demeanor with no acute complaints can fill out paperwork and sit in the waiting room until triage staff is available. On the other hand, patients who arrive in an agitated state clearly require immediate de-escalation and medical assessment in a predesignated, secure triage area [2]. The challenging cases lay in between (i.e., a patient who is calm but brought in against their will for reporting suicidal ideation).

Initial Assessment

For cooperative patients, the triage process begins with ascertaining the chief complaint, gathering of basic demographic data, and patient registration. The patient should undergo a face-to-face interview with a triage clinician as soon as possible upon arrival to the ED. Rapid triage gathers at least a little bit of information with which to decide whether further evaluation of the patient should be expedited or whether the patient's concerns justify continued time in the waiting area.

This interview represents the formal triage process. It has been defined as "a brief intervention that occurs when a patient initially presents to the ED during which the patient is interviewed to help determine the nature and severity of his or her illness" [3]. This tightly focused assessment includes a brief history of chief complaint, brief mental status exam, vital signs, and targeted medical screening. The rest of this section provides further detail about this process and its implications for subsequent evaluation.

Indications for Restraint

One critical determination is the need for immediate behavioral management. This should be evaluated at presentation and periodically throughout a patient's ED visit. The fundamental consideration is the level of danger a patient poses to themselves or others. Agitated patients create such risk through actions like intimidating or threatening speech, striking walls, attempted elopement, and physical violence toward others. They also create a distraction for staff and a disturbing environment for other patients and families. Detailed management of agitated patients is covered elsewhere in this text; the focus here is on identification and immediate management of this behavior. Policies and procedures that outline the institution's approach to behavioral management are advisable.

The safety of patients and staff is the first priority. In cases where the risk is unclear or there is limited time for assessment, clinicians should always err on the side of safety, as patients can easily be removed from secure areas of the ED and/or restraints once they are calm. Patients brought in by police or EMS, particularly if agitated in the field, should be triaged in a contained environment if possible. Patients who arrive in restraints should remain in them during the initial assessment. Patients who arrive verbally or behaviorally agitated should be taken to a secure area of the ED immediately. Indications for restraint include repeated threatening comments or gestures, striking oneself, or lashing out at others.

Several methods exist to quantify agitation, such as the agitation subscale of the well-known Positive and Negative Syndrome Scale (PANSS). Brevity and ease of use are particularly important in fast-paced EDs, however. Schumacher et al. suggest using the Behavioral Activity Rating Scale (BARS). This is a single-item, seven-point scale initially developed to monitor behavioral activity in psychotic patients during pharmaceutical trials. It has demonstrated reliability and validity, and it takes minimal time to complete. In their investigation, a BARS score over 5 reliably

Table 42.1 Behavioral activity rating scale [5]

1	Difficult or unable to rouse
2	Asleep but responds normally to verbal or physical contact
3	Drowsy, appears sedated
4	Quiet and awake (normal level of activity)
5	Signs of overt (physical or verbal) activity, calms down with instructions
6	Extremely or continuously active, not requiring restraint
7	Violent, requires restraint

distinguished patients who required behavioral management but was not associated with subsequent psychiatric hospitalization [4] (Table 42.1).

Indications for Medical Evaluation

Another critical function of triage is to identify patients who, though their chief complaint may be psychiatric in nature, have medical issues that must be addressed. These patients fall into two broad categories: those with an acute medical condition manifesting with psychiatric symptoms and those with chronic but significant medical problems that are incidental to their current presentation. The high incidence of comorbid medical problems in patients with psychiatric complaints is well established, ranging from 25% to 40% in studies [6]. However, the practice of requiring a comprehensive "medical clearance" inclusive of screening labs and studies for all patients is inefficient and expensive, and exposes patients to unnecessary risk [7]. Instead, at a minimum, all patients should have a history of current crisis, a physical examination inclusive of assessment of mentation and cognition, and assessment of vitals, with labs and studies as needed to establish that the patient is stable and appropriate for treatment in a psychiatric setting. This approach to assessment for medical mimics and problems occurring in parallel to the psychiatric crisis should be tailored to fit the needs and capacities of the hospital ward to which the patient may eventually disposition [8].

Certain criteria should prompt immediate medical assessment and deferral of further psychiatric evaluation. Unstable vital signs are clearly a red flag, as are serious medical complaints such as chest pain, focal neurological deficits, or shortness of breath. Inebriated patients are not appropriate for psychiatric assessment, though there is no consensus on a specific blood alcohol content at which they can be interviewed [3]. In addition, new onset of altered mental status in a patient without psychiatric history should prompt an evaluation for organic causes before being attributed to a psychotic disorder. Similarly, visual hallucinations are more characteristic of organic disorders than primary psychosis [9, 10]. Finally, altered mental status in any elderly patient should be investigated medically due to the high incidence of delirium [10, 11].

Urgency of Psychiatric Evaluation

After addressing any acute medical issues or agitation, the urgency of patients' psychiatric complaints is assessed. Patients present to emergency services for many reasons, ranging from an interest in social services without specific psychiatric complaint to severe depression with acute suicidality. Consideration should be given to a formal triage process in which the urgency of need determines the timing of assessment, as is standard for patients with medical complaints. Five-level triage systems—such as the commonly used Emergency Severity Index (ESI) that is endorsed by the Emergency Nursing Association (ENA) and the American College of Emergency Physicians [12], or the Canadian ED Triage & Acuity Scale (CTAS)—define acceptable durations of waiting based on severity of presenting concern and, in the case of the ESI, availability of clinical resources. For example, a patient rated with a triage level of I in the CTAS protocol, such as an actively violent patient, should be seen immediately, whereas a patient with a level of V may be asked to wait for up to 120 minutes. Under the ESI system, a patient requiring immediate resuscitation should be in level I, a patient with a very urgent concern should be in level II, and other patients are assigned a level of III, IV, or V based on the number of clinical resources they may need [13].

Each emergency department has the latitude to choose which triage protocol to use, though calls for uniformity of approach in US EDs have resulted in widespread adoption of the ESI system. Unfortunately, the use of both patient characteristics and clinical resource usage is not validated for triage of mental health emergencies and results in a non-nuanced approach to mental health patients. Alternatively, the CTAS classifies an acutely psychotic and agitated patient as level II/emergent and a severely depressed patient without suicidal thoughts as level IV/semi-urgent [14]. A level II patient should be seen within 15 minutes, whereas a level IV patient can be seen within 60 minutes. Another system, the Australasian Triage Scale (ATS), has been adapted specifically for psychiatric emergencies into the Mental Health Triage Scale. It assigns patients with psychiatric complaints to five categories, as described in Table 42.2.

There are no quantitative criteria for assigning triage categories within the ATS. However, the developers recommend consideration of factors such as manifest behavioral disturbance; presence of or threatened deliberate self-harm; perceived or objective level of suicidal ideation; patient's current level of distress; perceived level of danger to self or others; need for physical restraint; accompaniment by police; disturbances of perception; manifest evidence of psychosis; level of situational crisis; descriptions of behavior disturbance in the community; current level of community support; and presence of caregiver/supportive adult. Even before the most recent revisions, this assessment tool was shown to decrease mean emergency waiting times and transit times in an Australian sample [16]. It is a valid assessment with no association found between triage rating and either perceived business of the ED or perceived patient cooperation [17].

Table 42.2 Australasian triage scale [15]

Category	Description	Patient characteristics
2	Emergency	Patient is an imminent risk to themselves or others. They have a police escort or require restraints
3	Urgent	Patient is intensely distressed, psychotic, likely to become aggressive, or acutely suicidal
4	Semi-urgent	Patient has a long-standing psychiatric disorder, with current exacerbation or other concern
5	Nonurgent	Patient has a long-standing psychiatric disorder without acute concerns

The ATS has been studied head-to-head against the CTAS protocol in an urban US patient sample. This study showed correlations between the ATS score, patient level of agitation, and some self-reported symptoms. Psychiatric patients were generally deemed less urgent using the ATS in comparison to the CTAS protocol. There was no difference in terms of patient waiting time or throughput time [18]. The same authors found that the ATS better predicted the wait times for a given patient over the CTAS. Of the 105 patients in their study, only 5 left without being seen or were determined to have a drug-use disorder or physical illness and were excluded from the study [19].

Other scales have been used for assessment, such as the Crisis Triage Rating Scale and the Brief Psychiatric Rating Scale. However, these studies focused on association with admission, rather than pure triage assessment [20, 21].

Regardless of the protocol used, patients should be assigned a level of acuity, queued for care in relation to other patients in the ED, and asked to wait as appropriate for their situation. The majority of patients will have to wait for at least a short amount of time before being seen for their concern.

How Can the Waiting Room and Waiting Intervals Be Managed?

As in any other area of medicine, continual reassessment of patient status is critical, especially as they wait for clinical care. After the initial triage and immediate management, a process must exist to monitor patients for new onset of medical issues, agitation, or self-injurious behavior. As always, safety is the primary concern in mental health emergencies. In addition, Clarke et al. noted that "an inherent mismatch exists between the needs of an individual or family experiencing a psychiatric emergency and the treatment norms in general hospital EDs" [22]. Patients without mental health concerns present to the emergency department with a reasonably clear goal in mind. However, psychiatric illness itself may cloud the patient's understanding of the need for treatment or their willingness to participate in treatment. Thus, a patient may appear safe for the waiting area after initial triage but become unsafe after having to wait, after encountering another person in the waiting area, after experiencing disturbing hallucinations, and so on. Moreover, a mental health patient may lack the wherewithal to report worsening of their state to staff and receive needed attention. This mismatch can be mitigated by appropriate training, proactive monitoring, and careful consideration of the process by which mental health patients are navigated through the ED.

Periodic Medical Re-evaluation

As with any other patient, individuals with psychiatric complaints should have a periodic brief review of systems to assess patient comfort. In addition, vital signs can be checked on a regular basis. Abnormal blood pressure and heart rate may simply result from anxiety, but they may also herald the onset of alcohol or benzodiazepine withdrawal. Finally, given the long lengths of stay often associated with behavioral emergencies, staff should inquire about scheduled, prescribed medications, both psychiatric and medical. It is all too easy for the patient and staff to forget their bedtime dose of a medication, but this mistake can be easily avoided with adequate communication.

Suicidality

Suicidality is a common reason for patients to present to emergency departments. Moreover, the Joint Commission on Accreditation of Health Care Organizations has recommended screening all patients for suicidal ideation using a standardized, evidence-based screening tool [23]. Of the tools they suggest, the ED-SAFE Patient Safety Screener was developed for use in the emergency department and has been used both at the triage phase of an ED encounter and at subsequent phases [24].

There are two major concerns associated with patients who screen positive for suicidal ideation at the triage phase: potential for elopement and potential for self-harm while in the ED. Careful observation can lessen, but not eliminate, both of these risks.

All patients presenting with suicidal ideation are at elevated risk of self-harm. While the full evaluation of risk is pending, the patient should not be allowed to leave the ED until they are cleared for discharge based on further clinical evaluation. There are various ways to achieve direct patient supervision and safety while the patients wait for the evaluation. Some psychiatric emergency rooms have locked areas where high-risk patients are boarded. Without such facilities, one approach is to mark high-risk patients with a wristband or other identifier to indicate that they are not to leave the ED [25]. If the patient does elope, security should be immediately notified and will be able to identify the patient by this marker.

Actual self-injurious behavior while in the ED is rare but difficult to predict. Patients with a history of such behavior, patients with psychosis, and those who are visibly anxious may be at higher risk. The use of a standardized screening instrument, like the Risk of Suicide Questionnaire [26], may help identify patients who are at particularly high risk for suicide and warrant additional monitoring while waiting for definitive assessment. Patients who are unable to keep themselves safe should be monitored directly. However, any patient identified as at risk for suicide should have their belongings held and their person searched for potential weapons. Increasing the level of observation throughout the ED, for instance by video monitoring, provides an additional layer of security. Finally, patients who harm themselves, or may attempt to do so, should be temporarily placed under direct observation or in restraints.

Agitation and Violence in the ED

Unfortunately, violence in emergency departments is not an uncommon phenomenon. While definitive statistics are hard to come by, several studies have revealed high lifetime prevalence of assaults toward staff. A 1999 survey of Canadian EDs found that 55% of employees, by self-report, had themselves been physically assaulted in some manner, and 86% had witnessed either a physical assault or threats of violence toward other staff [27]. Most violence occurred toward nursing and security personnel. Minimizing these incidents is imperative.

While high-quality evidence is lacking in this area, observational studies have suggested several steps to decrease the incidence of violence. The key themes are early identification and intervention. General steps include ensuring that the physical space is designed for safety, that staff have appropriate training in recognition of agitation and in de-escalation techniques, and that there are an adequate number of staff available to manage agitation should it occur [28]. The use of an objective measure of agitation, like the previously mentioned BARS scale, provides a uniform way of communicating the need for staff intervention. Completion of this scale does not require patient cooperation and can even be done via video monitoring. Periodically administering these measures to appropriate patients in the waiting area (and in the ED) can assist staff in managing potential agitation before it escalates, thus preventing assaults [29]. Should early identification of agitation and engagement in verbal de-escalation fail to prevent agitation and aggression, then the use of medications and, as a last resort, restraints can be considered [30].

How Can Handoffs Be Safer?

At various points in this chapter, we have discussed the movement of patients from one clinical environment to another. Each transition includes an attendant handoff between clinical providers. For example, a patient referred from the clinic to the ED will be seen by the ED clerk and the triaging provider, then by the ED physician, the bedside nurse, and perhaps a mental health professional associated with the ED. Thus, each patient may be transitioned through four or five professionals before the appropriate disposition.

Each transition point risks loss of critical information. Patient handoffs between providers are well documented to be high-risk times for medical errors [31]. An available technique to reduce the risk of error in handoff is the performance and documentation of a standardized protocol, or checklist [32].

It is also often the triaging provider's responsibility to collate information available about the patient's case, organizing it in an easily comprehensible package for use by the ED physician or mental health consultant. Opportunities abound for misplacement of information, unduly influencing the clinical decision-making of the rest of the team.

Standardizing the triage process can help mitigate these risks. For example, the ED could develop a flow sheet in the patient's medical record (electronic or paper record) used for jotting notes from telephone calls about patients referred to the ED. This can include prompts covering those topics listed in the first section of this chapter. This sheet could be available at the clerk's desk when the patient arrives, at which time it would be attached to another element of the medical record, prompting determination of chief complaint, vital signs, and necessary screening questions. These data can then determine whether the patient is safe to wait in the common waiting area, will need to be in a more secure space, or will need to be in restraints with immediate assessment by the physician. These documents would then be available for the physician to review before formally seeing the patient.

Direct Admissions and Transfers from Other EDs

At times, a patient will be sent to the emergency department en route to an inpatient psychiatric unit, for example, from a psychiatric clinic. These directly admitted patients have already been accepted to a psychiatric ward associated with the ED in question. However, there may be medical questions to be answered before admission. These patients may have disclosed dangerous behaviors to their outpatient clinician, and the clinic may lack the resources to ensure that the patient's medical conditions are stable enough for psychiatric admission. Thus, they are assessed in the ED prior to moving to the psychiatric ward. At arrival to the ED, these patients should be considered dangerous and should be afforded the same safety measures applied to any patient awaiting disposition to a mental health facility.

Since some hospitals lack the resources to formally assess the behavioral health of ED patients, an interhospital ED-to-ED or ED-to-emergency psychiatry services (EPS) transfer may be arranged. Deterioration may occur during transfer, which at times may be lengthy. When possible, these patients should receive necessary medical evaluation and clearance at the transferring hospital. Despite apparent stabilization, transferred patients should be afforded the same safety measures applied to any patient at high risk of dangerousness to self or others while awaiting full assessment at the receiving hospital.

In either circumstance, it is very helpful when the referring clinician contacts the ED/EPS with a report about the patient, including (at a minimum) the patient's identifying information, the clinical concern prompting referral, and details of the patient evaluation up to that point. Prior acceptance by the receiving ED physician or accepting psychiatrist is mandated by statute when patients are transferred from ED-to-ED, ED-to-EPS, or ED-to-inpatient. All emergency departments have structured procedures and documents to facilitate transfer of clinical information about patients between providers, and the mental health transfer is not exempt from these requirements.

Conclusion

This chapter has covered the details of mental health triage: the process by which the urgency of a patient's case is determined and cases are prioritized so as to maximize efficiency and safety. Based on this integration, the patient should be directed to the common waiting area, a more secure area of the ED with prioritized assessment by the physician, or into restraints with immediate assessment by the physician. Mental health patients may be uniquely unable to communicate deterioration to staff; therefore, each ED must have a system for periodic brief reassessment of mental health patients who are awaiting the next step in the assessment and disposition process. A standardized flow sheet, documenting the development of the patient's case, can minimize errors associated with patient handoffs. Direct admissions and ED-to-ED transfers constitute special cases.

Acknowledgments The authors thank Margaret Judd, LCSW, for her contributions and Kathy Adamson, RN, for her comments during the preparation of the first edition of this chapter.

References

1. Claassen CA, Hughes CW, Gilfillan S, McIntire D, Roose A, Lumpkin M, et al. Toward a redefinition of psychiatric emergency. Health Serv Res. 2000;35(3):735–54.
2. Nordstrom K, Zun LS, Wilson MP, Stiebel V, Ng AT, Bregman B, et al. Medical evaluation and triage of the agitated patient: consensus statement of the American Association of Emergency Psychiatry Project BETA Medical Evaluations Workgroup. West J Emerg Med. 2012;13(1):3–10.
3. Slade M, Taber D, Clarke MM, et al. Best practices for the treatment of patients with mental and substance use illnesses in the emergency department. Dis Mon. 2007;53:536–80.
4. Schumacher JA, Gleason SH, Holloman GH, McLeod WT. Using a single-item rating scale as a psychiatric behavioral management triage tool in the emergency department. J Emerg Nurs. 2010;36(5):434–8.
5. Swift RH, Harrigan EP, Cappelleri JC, Kramer D, Chandler LP. Validation of the behavioural activity rating scale (BARS): a novel measure of activity in agitated patients. J Psychiatr Res. 2002;36(2):87–95.
6. Carlson RJ, Nayar N, Sur M. Physical disorders among emergency psychiatric patients. Can J Psychiatry. 1981;42:99–102.
7. Anderson EL, Nordstrom K, Wilson MP, Peltzer-Jones JM, Zun L, Ng A, et al. American Association of Emergency Psychiatry Task Force on medical clearance of adults part I: introduction, review and evidence-based guidelines. West J Emerg Med. 2017;18(2):235–42.
8. Wilson MP, Nordstrom K, Anderson EL, Ng AT, Zun LS, Peltzer-Jones JM, et al. American Association for

Emergency Psychiatry Task Force on medical clearance of adult psychiatric patients. Part II: controversies over medical assessment, and consensus recommendations. West J Emerg Med. 2017;18(4):640–6.
9. Norton JW, Corbett JJ. Visual perceptual abnormalities: hallucinations and illusions. Semin Neurol. 2000;20(1):111–21.
10. Shah SJ, Fiorito M, McNamara RM. A screening tool to medically clear psychiatric patients in the emergency department. J Emerg Med. 2012;43(5):871–5.
11. Olshaker JS, Browne B, Jerrard DA, et al. Medical clearance and screening of psychiatric patients in the emergency department. Acad Emerg Med. 1997;4(2):124–8.
12. Fernandes CMB, Tanabe P, Gilboy N, et al. Five-level triage: a report from the ACEP/ENA five-level triage task force. J Emerg Nurs. 2005;31(1):39–50.
13. Gilboy N, Tanabe P, Travers DA, Rosenau AM, Eitel DR. Emergency severity index, version 4: implementation handbook. Rockville: AHRQ Publication 0046(2); 2005. Available at http://www.ahrq.gov/research/esi/
14. Bullard MJ, Unger B, Spence J, Grafstein E. Revisions to the Canadian emergency department triage and acuity scale (CTAS) adult guidelines. CJEM. 2008;10(2):136–42.
15. Australasian College for Emergency Medicine: G24—Guidelines for the implementation of the Australasian Triage Scale in Emergency Departments. 2005. Available at http://www.acem.org.au/media/policies_and_guidelines/G24_Implementation__ATS.pdf.
16. Smart D, Pollard C, Walpole B. Mental health triage in emergency medicine. Aust N Z J Psychiatry. 1999;33(1):57–66.
17. Happell B, Summers M, Pinikahana J. Measuring the effectiveness of the national Mental Health Triage Scale in an emergency department. Int J Ment Health Nurs. 2003;12(4):288–92.
18. Downey LA, Zun LS. Comparison of Canadian triage system to Australian triage system for psychiatric patients. San Francisco: American Psychiatric Association—Institute for Psychiatric Services; 2011.
19. Downey LA, Zun LS, Burke T. Comparison of Canadian triage acuity scale to Australian emergency mental health scale triage system for psychiatric patients. Int Emerg Nurs. 2015;23:138–43.
20. Brooker C, Ricketts T, Bennett S, Lemme F. Admission decisions following contact with an emergency mental health assessment and intervention service. J Clin Nurs. 2007;16(7):1313–22.
21. Hooten WM, Lyketsos CG, Mollenhauer M. Use of the brief psychiatric rating scale as a predictor of psychiatric admission for non-suicidal patients. Int J Psychiatry Med. 1998;28(2):215–20.
22. larke DE, Brown AM, Hughes L, Motluk L. Education to improve the triage of mental health patients in general hospital emergency departments. Accid Emerg Nurs. 2006;14(4):210–8.
23. The Joint Commission. Detecting and treating suicide ideation in all settings. Sentinel Event Alert. 2016;24:56.
24. Boudreaux ED, Camargo CA, Arias SA, Sullivan AF, Allen MH, et al. Improving suicide risk screening and detection in the emergency department. Am J Prev Med. 2016;50(4):445–53.
25. Macy D, Johnston M. Using electronic wristbands and a triage protocol to protect mental health patients in the emergency department. J Nurs Care Qual. 2007;22(2):180–4.
26. Folse VN, Hahn RL. Suicide risk screening in an emergency department. Clin Nurs Res. 2009;18(3):253–71.
27. Fernandes C, Bouthillette F, Raboud J, et al. Violence in the emergency department: a survey of health care workers. CMAJ. 1999;161:1245–8.
28. Richmond JS, Berlin JS, Fishkind AB, Holloman GH, Zeller SL, Wilson MP, et al. Verbal De-escalation of the agitated patient: consensus statement of the American Association for Emergency Psychiatry Project BETA De-escalation Workgroup. West J Emerg Med. 2012;13(1):17–25.
29. D'Orio BM, Purselle D, Stevens D, Garlow SJ. Reduction of episodes of seclusion and restraint in a psychiatric emergency service. Psychiatr Serv. 2004;55(5):581–3.
30. Knox DK, Holloman GH. Use and avoidance of seclusion and restraint: consensus statement of the American Association for Emergency Psychiatry Project BETA Seclusion and Restraint Workgroup. West J Emerg Med. 2012;13(1):35–40.
31. Philibert I. Use of strategies from high-reliability organizations to the patient hand-off by resident physicians: practical implications. Qual Saf Health Care. 2009;18(4):261–6.
32. Phillips A. The effect of a standardized form in guiding communication between peers during the hand-off of patients in a hospital setting. Stud Health Technol Inform. 2009;146:885.

Informed Decision-Making in the Emergency Department

43

Paul H. Desan

Introduction

Personnel in the emergency department are often called upon to make assessments of the patient's ability to make informed decisions to accept or refuse treatment. To understand medical decision-making, we must review two questions: what does it mean to make an informed decision about medical care, and then, what are the options when the patient cannot make an informed decision?

Case Example

A frail elderly man is admitted to the emergency department. He is mute, poorly responsive, disheveled, and homeless. His name is not known, and there are no known family members involved. The patient is febrile to 103 and appears to be gravely ill.

Terminology

Some clarification of terminology may be useful. Physicians tend to use the term "capacity" for informed decision-making. Capacity is dynamic and flexible. The patient may be able to make a certain simple decision but not a more complex decision. The patient may be able to make an informed decision now but not this evening when he is sun-downing. Lawyers tend to use the term "competence" for informed decision-making. Competence is all or none. When a patient has been found to be incompetent, the patient can legally not decide until a probate court judge determines that he or she is competent. When we ask whether a patient can make an informed decision in the medical context, we must distinguish between the concepts of capacity and competence. Here, capacity is what physicians assess, and competence is what probate court judges decide.

What Does It Mean to Make an Informed Decision?

Legal theorists agree that most state laws and scholarly analyses have referred to four elements that underlie informed decision-making. In a paper published three decades ago, two forensic psychiatrists explicated these four elements in the medical context, and their paper remains a classic [1]. A more theoretical legal discussion is available [2], as is a detailed, book-length account of related issues in medical consent [3] and a systematic, step-by-step protocol [4]. Understanding

P. H. Desan (✉)
Psychiatric Consultation Service, Yale New Haven Hospital, New Haven, CT, USA

Department of Psychiatry, Yale School of Medicine, New Haven, CT, USA
e-mail: paul.desan@yale.edu

L. S. Zun et al. (eds.), *Behavioral Emergencies for Healthcare Providers*,
https://doi.org/10.1007/978-3-030-52520-0_43

these four elements provides a widely accepted framework for understanding informed consent.

First, the patient must be able to make and express a choice. A patient who is comatose, a patient who cannot communicate, or a patient who will not communicate lacks the capacity for medical decision-making. A patient who cannot make up their mind or who changes their mind repeatedly also lacks the capacity for informed decision-making.

Second, the patient must know the facts. The patient must understand that they have a problem, and they must understand the range of options facing them. To be precise, the patient must understand what the medical system conveys as the likely outcome of choosing each of these options. An adult may make an informed decision to disregard the advice of the medical system. For example, a brilliant computer pioneer elected not to pursue resection of a nonmetastatic pancreatic tumor and instead to pursue holistic dietary treatment. If a probate judge had heard the case, the judge certainly would have found him competent to choose or reject mainstream medical thought. In an adult individual without cognitive impairment or mental illness, the legal system tends to respect any reasonable choice (an unreasonable choice that results in immediate serious or lethal harm is not likely to be respected by the legal system in any patient).

The patient needs to demonstrate an understanding of the essential facts regarding the situation he confronts. In practice, the accuracy of understanding is typically assessed by asking the patient to repeat back in their own words their conception of their medical situation. Alternatively, factual understanding may be assessed by asking questions to ascertain the patient's factual grasp. The patient does not need to understand the facts at the level of a physician. Legal standards exist, such as the prudent layperson standard or the local practice standard, but these standards are of limited use in actual day-to-day practice.

The third element of capacity is more subtle. The patient must not only know the facts but also appreciate the facts. The patient must know that the facts are real and apply to him. For example, an individual with psychosis may have normal cognition but be unable to make a sensible choice due to delusional beliefs. Similarly, a patient with a frontal cortex injury may be coherent and articulate but demonstrate a repeated pattern of being unable to conform their behavior to a prudent plan. The probate judges who decide competence are generally elected officials, well-educated lawyers, with standard cultural viewpoints. They are likely to share the typical American prejudices and attitudes about decision-making: psychosis, dementia, developmental disability, or brain injury are likely to be regarded as impairing informed decision-making, but addiction or personality may not be so regarded. It should be added that in some states, addiction is not a basis for incompetence. A probate judge is likely to allow a coherent and articulate patient to make their own medical decision, unless that decision can be definitively shown to be unreasonable. Thresholds for incompetence vary between jurisdictions, and experienced local practitioners may be informative about local thresholds.

The fourth element of capacity requires that the patient be able to manipulate facts in some logical or systematic way. There must be a process of decision-making that makes intelligible sense. It is not sufficient for the patient to repeat back that he knows a particular risk. The patient must demonstrate that there is some decision-making that yields a conclusion in some organized fashion. Perhaps, the most notable example of decision-making that is systematic is religious decision-making. For instance, millions of Jehovah's Witnesses believe that it is immoral to accept a blood transfusion, even if one were to die without the transfusion. This is a sincere and consistently held belief, and it is well respected by the medical system and by probate courts. (It should be noted that not all Jehovah's Witnesses agree with this opinion, and it should be noted that not all individuals who may be identified by family members as Jehovah's Witnesses are practicing members of the faith.)

We emphasize that just being able to state the risks of a decision does not constitute informed consent. There must be a decision process that is rational within some belief system—a process that demonstrates these four elements of capacity. Legal standards refer to overall function, more than simple knowledge. For example, in our state, the standards for conservatorship of the person and of the estate are a "mental, emotional or physical condition that results in such person being unable to receive and evaluate information or make or communicate decisions to such an extent" that the individual cannot "care for self" and cannot "manage his or her affairs" [5]. As a clinical example, a patient recovering from delirium may arrive at a state where the patient is coherent and oriented and able to repeat back simple facts, but is still not capable of using abstract thought to appreciate and manipulate those facts fully. Mental health professionals tend to apply higher standards for the appreciation and manipulation of facts [6].

We note that in practice, the approach to capacity is very different when the patient is making sensible decisions to accept needed care, as opposed to irrational decisions to reject what is appropriate and life-sustaining treatment. For example, a patient with mild dementia who requires surgery should face a low threshold for a determination of capacity. The patient must know what the surgery is for, must understand that the surgery may or may not work, and must understand that the surgery has certain risks. To consent to a procedure that virtually all unimpaired patients would readily accept should not require a detailed level of capacity. Conversely, a patient who is rejecting a standard and effective treatment, without which they are likely to face severe and immediate risks such as death, must meet a very high standard for decision-making capacity. In the same fashion, a patient accepting a risky and uncertain treatment must meet a much higher standard than a patient accepting an intervention of trivial risk. In the real world, both the medical and the legal system apply asymmetric thresholds for consent, rather than philosophical equipoise.

In rare cases, patients may be in an ambiguous zone at the edge of the capacity for informed consent. Our experience suggests that the strongest approach in these grey areas is for both the patient and the next of kin to agree to treatment. It is not clear whether the patient is consenting and the family assenting, or the family consenting and the patient assenting, but obtaining consent from both patient and family demonstrates a consensus to proceed.

What Are the Options When a Patient Cannot Make an Informed Decision?

When a patient is unable to make an informed decision, the laws of each state provide for alternatives. These laws differ somewhat from state to state, but in essence, at least four choices are recognized. When a patient is unable to make an informed decision, all states permit decisions by next of kin, by a healthcare representative appointed by the patient, or by a conservator appointed by a court. In a fourth situation, all states permit some form of decision-making in an emergency when none of these surrogates are available.

First, all states permit surrogate decisions by next of kin. In some states, these are recognized by elaborate statutes. For example, in certain states, there is a specific hierarchy of which next of kin is most appropriate as a surrogate decision-maker: the spouse, followed by adult children, followed by the parent, followed by the adult sibling, and so forth. The special role of a spouse is widely recognized in many states. In some states, there is no explicit statutory guidance, and medical teams must use their discretion. Obtaining a consensus of next of kin is always optimum. Any next of kin surrogate must demonstrate that they themselves are capable of making an informed decision. Medical teams are never forced to use an inappropriate individual. In some cases, there are too many informed decision-makers who do not agree with each other: inevitably, the most distant relative is the one who elects to continue inappropriate end-of-life care. The use of family or the significant other is surely the most common approach to decision-making for the hospitalized demented or confused patient. Hospital policies and state laws vary in detail. For example, in our hospital, a decision by a next of kin in a nonurgent situation is not accepted if the patient has mental status sufficient to object to the treatment, and we pursue the appointment of a legal decision-maker as described below.

Second, all state laws allow for an individual to appoint a surrogate decision-maker. In various states, this individual may be termed a healthcare representative, a healthcare proxy, a healthcare agent, or the like. Such appointments are a form of power of attorney, in which a competent individual gives the authority to some other individual to act on their behalf. In this case, the individual is appointing a durable power of attorney, who retains authority even after the appointing person has lost capacity. While an individual has the capacity, a power of attorney has no authority. A patient with capacity may change or end the power of attorney at any time. The appointment of a power of attorney is relevant only after the patient has lost capacity. The appointment is made by completing a form specified by state law, may require one or more witnesses, and may require notarization. In some states, these forms allow the individual to provide additional information about their wishes in various medical situations. The most authentic form of decision-making occurs when the patient has selected a trusted representative and discussed their preferences under different medical situations. We urge all individuals to appoint and brief a suitable healthcare representative before the need arises. Advance directives include a wide range of options by which a patient may record preferences. These range from code status decisions to informal notes by the patient to specific forms created by state law or healthcare providers. Research demonstrates that advance directives are often helpful but often not made [7].

In all states, a third option is a court-appointed conservator or guardian. Generally, such issues are handled by a probate court. The conservatorship may be divided into two roles: a conservator of the person makes medical decisions, and a conservator of the estate makes financial decisions. A probate court judge may choose to elect one or the other or both, and may appoint different individuals for these roles. Some state laws provide for a temporary conservator, who can be appointed relatively quickly, and for the appointment of a permanent conservator, which is likely to require more time. Once a probate court has determined that a patient is incompetent and appoints a conservator, the patient is not legally capable of making any decision, and all decisions must be deferred to the conservator. If the patient in the emergency department does have a conservator, that individual makes decisions for the patient. Unfortunately, in many jurisdictions, even obtaining a temporary conservator may entail substantial delay. If a patient does not already have a conservator, it is likely that such an appointment will not be obtained while the patient is in the emergency department.

Finally, there are emergency situations where no person is available with legal authority to consent for the patient. At that point, medical providers must act, and it must be stressed that most citizens in this country would elect standard medical care if admitted with an impaired mental state and an immediate need for life-sustaining care. Even in a medical emergency, modern views of substituted decision-making call for a reconstruction of the decision that the patient would have made if they were able. Respecting an individual's beliefs and values call for the physician to "don the mental mantle" of the patient. For example, a Jehovah's Witness who has clearly expressed a decision in the past to refuse a blood transfusion despite lethal consequences cannot be transfused against their will. Even in an emergency, we are obligated to investigate any available sources of information about the patient's previously expressed wishes.

Case Example, Continued

With this background, we can now return to our case. On presentation to the emergency department, the patient was mute, poorly responsive, and not able to make and express a choice. The patient could not make an informed decision, and there was no surrogate decision-maker available. Such instances of emergency medical decision-making are frequently encountered in the emergency department. The great majority of individuals with a life-threatening infection would want their condition evaluated and treated.

There was no reason to believe that the patient had made any previous informed decision to decline medical care. The patient was admitted to the intensive care unit, and IV antibiotics were started for a urinary tract infection and sepsis.

Two days later, the patient was verbal but confused, disoriented, and mostly incoherent. The patient was often agitated, poorly cooperative with treatment, and attempted to leave the unit.

At this stage, the patient was unable to meet the second element of capacity: to demonstrate knowledge of the facts. Intravenous antibiotics were continued.

After a further two days, the patient's mental state had improved markedly. The patient now was coherent and oriented, and provided his name. The patient stated that he understood that he had an infection, that he could die of an infection, and that antibiotics might be lifesaving. The patient also appeared suspicious of hospital staff. The patient asked to leave the hospital to feed his cat and stated that it was his right to decide whether to take antibiotics. He was unable to explain further how he might make such a choice. More detailed mental status examination disclosed deficits in concentration, memory, abstraction, and executive function.

Assessment at this point indicated that while the patient could express some knowledge of the facts, he displayed little appreciation of his situation, as well as a possible paranoid interpretation of reality. Nor did he display any sensible pattern of decision-making. This case reinforces that in recovery from delirium, some patients may become coherent and oriented but lack more sophisticated processing. Lower, but not higher, cortical functions have recovered. While in theory, a compliant patient with good supports could have been discharged on oral antibiotics with close medical follow-up, it was clear in this case that the patient would not be compliant with therapy and would be at lethal risk if discharged. A decision was made to retain the patient in the hospital and continue antibiotic treatment.

After seven days in the hospital, the patient appeared to have regained baseline mental status. The patient displayed a flat affect, an odd manner, and a preoccupation with the CIA. He thanked the hospital staff for their help. He admitted he did not own a cat. In the interim, it had been determined that the patient had a longstanding diagnosis of schizophrenia with limited compliance with treatment, and the local mental health authority had many years ago obtained a court-appointed conservator.

Had the existence of a conservator been known, that individual would have been consulted as the legal decision-maker for the patient. The conservator agreed with the plan to discharge the patient.

Conclusion

A useful framework for understanding the capacity for informed decision-making is based on four elements: The patient must be able to (1) make and express a choice, (2) know the facts, (3) appreciate the facts, and (4) manipulate the facts. When a patient is unable to make an informed decision, state laws permit next of kin, a healthcare representative previously appointed by the patient, or a conservator appointed by a court to serve as surrogate decision-makers. In some medical emergencies, these surrogates may be unavailable, and medical treaters must make their best efforts to reconstruct the decision the patient would have selected. Most cases in the emergency department will be clear instances of capacity or lack thereof. In those cases where capacity is partial and no legal decision-maker is available, the strongest approach is to obtain consent from both patient and next of kin.

Our discussion has focused on the legal options when the patient cannot be brought to make an informed decision. The first step is to seek a consensus among the patient, the medical treaters, and the family. In our experience, there is often a specific reason for an inappropriate decision, and sometimes addressing that factor can aid in improved decision-making. Most commonly, an adequate discussion of the alternatives has not been conducted, and a calm patient review secures an agreement. Patients may be overwhelmed by the sudden adverse medical news, and skillful reassurance may be critical to helping them navigate their medical decisions. Anxiety, pain, or insomnia may destabilize the patient's mental state and must be treated to return them to sensible decision-making capacity. Addicted individuals may be eager to leave the hospital because they are at risk of withdrawal from alcohol, heroin, or another drug. A clear commitment to the aggressive treatment of withdrawal is the correct approach to improve decision-making in these patients. Emotions such as anger with staff or a need for control may be driving an inappropriate decision and can also be explored. Medical teams may request a psychiatric consultation regarding capacity, but often the request is more about practical, ethical, and legal management [8, 9]. Our goal is always to avoid resorting to alternative decision-makers to force a decision on an unwilling patient.

References

1. Appelbaum PS, Grisso T. Assessing patients' capacities to consent to treatment. N Engl J Med. 1988;319:1635–8.
2. Berg JW, Appelbaum PS, Grisso T. Constructing competence: formulating standards of legal competence to make medical decisions. Rutgers Law Rev. 1996;48:345–96.
3. Kim SYH. Evaluation of capacity to consent to treatment and research (best practices for forensic mental health assessments). Oxford: Oxford University Press; 2009.
4. Grisso T, Appelbaum PS. Macarthur competence assessment tool for treatment (Maccat-T). Sarasota: Professional Resource Exchange; 1998.
5. Connecticut General Assembly. Connecticut General Statutes. Revision to 2017, Section 45a-644.
6. Ackerman S, Watkins MW, Kostial AF, Rabinowitz T. Urgent assessment of decision-making capacity in a patient with schizophrenia and an evolving myocardial infarction who is refusing care. Psychosomatics. 2015;56:89–93.
7. Silveira MJ, Kim SY, Langa KM. Advance directives and outcomes of surrogate decision making before death. N Engl J Med. 2010;362:1211–8.
8. Kornfeld DS, Muskin PR, Tahil FA. Psychiatric evaluation of mental capacity in the general hospital: a significant teaching opportunity. Psychosomatics. 2009;50:468–73.
9. Umapathy C, Ramchandani D, Lamdan RM, Kishel LA, Schindler BA. Competency evaluations on the consultation-liaison service: some overt and covert aspects. Psychosomatics. 1999;40:28–33.

Risk Management in the Emergency Department: Liabilities, Duties, and EMTALA

44

John S. Rozel and Mark Z. Zacharia

Introduction

Psychiatric emergencies create a number of clinical challenges, as well as direct and indirect legal risks. Issues relating to involuntary commitment, conditional confidentiality and duties to protect or warn third parties, and the frequency of autonomy subverting conditions make the Psychiatric Emergency Service (PES) a uniquely challenging setting from a medicolegal perspective. By consolidating resources and subject matter expertise into a designated PES, improved clinical outcomes and diminished liability may be attained by providers. A central concern should be mitigating the risk of malpractice claims: The PES creates a number of exposures relating to misdiagnosis, wrongful death after discharge, duties to third parties, and others. Additionally, the PES is exposed to all the "usual" medicolegal and business operation legal risks of health care, from the Emergency Medical Treatment and Active Labor Act (EMTALA) and Health Insurance Portability and Accountability Act (HIPAA) issues to billing and human resource risks. It is important to avoid litigation for medical malpractice and it is also important to avoid litigation because an employee sexually harassed another, improperly billed a payer, or stole a patient's identity.

Strategic Risk Management

Emergency and crisis settings create special challenges in risk management. Careful, thoughtful contemplation of facts, interpretations, and options can be confounded by complexity, the paucity of data, and time pressure. Adding to the challenge is the truism that containing short-term risk may escalate long-term risk, especially in patients with severe personality pathology, who can be frequent users of PES and emergency department (ED) services. A skilled clinician may need to accept some short-term risk to try to obtain meaningful long-term gains for the patient. Avoid risk when feasible, but not at the cost of valid clinical goals and needs. Some people will have moderate to high degrees of chronic risk, regardless of what we choose to do in the heat of the moment. A chronic risk may require different strategies, and the interventions that may work for acute risk can make chronic risk worse (Table 44.1).

Confounding our ability to understand and work with risk are cognitive biases and errors [1, 2]. Some of these are common to any profession, and some are specific to the psychological makeup

J. S. Rozel (✉)
Department of Psychiatry, University of Pittsburgh School of Medicine, Pittsburgh, PA, USA
e-mail: rozeljs@upmc.edu

M. Z. Zacharia
Corporate Legal Department, University of Pittsburgh Medical Center, Pittsburgh, PA, USA

L. S. Zun et al. (eds.), *Behavioral Emergencies for Healthcare Providers*,
https://doi.org/10.1007/978-3-030-52520-0_44

Table 44.1 Making decisions under pressure

Optimal decision-making	Emergency settings
Unrushed, opportunity for reflection	Ticking clock
Ample, reliable information	Limited information, unknown/unknowable reliability
Opportunity for consultation, research	Most cases are outside of typical business hours, limited resources
Easy-to-follow the rules	Rules may not exist for this situation, or there may be good reason to breach rules
Autonomous decision-making is ideal	Autonomous decision-making is challenged, imperfect, doubted, overridden
Can make use of elaborate, complex clinical, ethical, and operational concepts and rules	Decisions need to be made by frontline clinicians who may not be experts in relevant rules

of people who seek high-risk or high-stimulus work environments (i.e., emergency care) [3]. High-stress work itself adds to the risk of cognitive errors and distortions through fatigue and other factors. Personality factors of staff, including risk tolerance and competitiveness, can also play a role in decision-making styles. Awareness of the potential impact of these factors—and individual and organizational interventions to support staff wellness—can significantly improve the quality of high-pressure decisions.

Legal Foundations of Emergency Psychiatry

Legal aspects of emergency psychiatry generally focus on three issues: involuntary treatment and commitment, confidentiality and exceptions thereof, and duties to third parties. The legal structure of emergency psychiatry is broadly described by Supreme Court decisions, federal laws, or laws that are enumerated and administered on a state-by-state basis.

At default, a person is at liberty and is entitled to be free from undue restrictions on the movements, communications, and control of their body. In specific circumstances, where an accumulation of evidence is significant and appropriate procedures are followed, personal liberty interests can be limited by the state. *Parens patriae* powers allow the state to intervene when a person is a danger to themselves; police powers allow the state to intervene when a person is a danger to others. Generally, the initial criteria for commitment include behaviors that are potentially life-threatening, dangerousness, imminent, and associated with an identified mental illness. Commitment must be for a finite and reasonable period, with an opportunity for external review and legal representation for the patient. There are subtle variations between states, but these broad rules will be seen consistently across jurisdictions.

From the Constitution to the Clinic: The Hierarchy of Laws and Hospital Policies

Laws are created by the legislature, enforced by the executive branch, and when issues or ambiguities arise, may be reviewed by the judiciary. Laws and regulations issuing from a federal source generally override laws and regulations from states and municipalities. Statutes are laws enacted by the legislature. Regulations are rules proposed and enacted by government agencies, and are enforceable and binding for organizations subject to the oversight of such an agency. Case law consists of the opinions and rulings of judges, typically at an appellate or higher level, that establish rules and interpretations of existing laws. Practice guidelines, professional standards, and third-party standards (e.g., The Joint Commission) are less binding but may still be important to adhere to.

Hospital policies can often be used to clearly interpret laws and regulations that are conflicting, ambiguous, or simply too complex to be readily understood by frontline clinicians. No policy is perfect. Too broad, and they may not provide useful guidance; too specific, and the inevitable risk of deviation creating liability increases. Written hospital policies that are unclear, incongruent with the law, inconsistently followed, or not followed without clearly documented and plausible reasons become potential liabilities when litigation ensues.

Table 44.2 Common operational legal issues

Criteria and procedures for voluntary and involuntary commitment
Child abuse reporting
Elder abuse reporting
Institutional abuse reporting (misconduct by healthcare, law enforcement, education, or corrections professionals)
Duties to third parties (so-called "Tarasoff" duties)
Age of consent for children and adolescents to consent to mental, medical, substance use, and reproductive health care
Laws, standards, and procedures for carrying firearms in healthcare settings for patients, visitors/family, law enforcement, employees
Criteria and procedures for managing firearms possession during or after commitment/hospitalization
Guardianship laws
Impaired driver reporting to state DMV (e.g., due to severe symptoms, side effects, suicidality, dementia, etc.); also, consider the situation of an intoxicated patient, family member, etc., wishing to drive away from the facility
Medical and mental health advanced directives
Statute of limitations
Records retention

Routine Business Operational Issues Creating Legal Liability

PES programs face potential legal risk from issues unrelated to mental health emergencies. While the bulk of this chapter will focus on the issues most unique to the management of behavioral emergencies, there are a number of legal risks faced by other medical settings, as well as the PES that need to be considered. A PES located near multiple jurisdictions (e.g., near a state line) may need to be familiar with multiple sets of parallel legal rules that do not fully align (Table 44.2).

Law Enforcement Interactions

Emergency departments, and PESs in particular, have frequent and complex interactions with law enforcement around a number of issues. Proactive efforts to develop (or repair) a solid working relationship between the PES and the local police force is critical. Mishandling interactions with criminal justice systems—especially when hospital policies do not exist or are not followed—may open hospitals and providers to potential liability. Allowing law enforcement into the ED setting as they continue criminal investigations is common but must be handled with care, respecting prevailing criminal procedure and confidentiality standards [4]. Emergency departments have high rates of workplace violence and potential criminal activity; the presence of security or law enforcement, with or without firearms, requires a careful balancing of risks and benefits, and must be accompanied by careful delineations of roles, particularly in the context of managing agitation and behavioral emergencies [5]. Clinical staff are ultimately responsible for providing diagnosis and treatment, and not for serving as law enforcement themselves, although some cases may require collaboration. ED and PES leadership should consider policies developed proactively and revised periodically as applicable laws, regulations, clinical practices, or standards evolve. A list of suggested topics is in Table 44.3.

Table 44.3 Law enforcement interactions

Plan for law enforcement officer (LEO) drop-offs of people on commitment, people recently arrested with MH issues, or people simply brought in by officers, etc.
Plan for LEO pick-ups of people cleared by the PES, people who commit crimes in the ED, etc.
Plan for handling firearms worn by LEO when they respond to your site—accompanying patients, as patients, as visitors or family, etc. (Note that some LEOs carry an obvious sidearm and a back-up gun concealed under a shirt, ankle holster, etc.)
Consider also plans for firearms or other weapons brought by patients, visitors, staff, family, etc. who may or may not have concealed carry or other permits or licenses
Elopements, especially of patients felt to be at high risk for suicide or violence
Child and elder abuse reporting, including cases where the patient is not appropriate for admission and cannot safely be returned to their home, including scenarios where the caregiver abandons a dependent or insists on bringing a dependent home when it is not appropriate
Criminal investigations involving patients as victims or suspects
Criminal investigation involving staff as offenders, relating to patient complaints, or otherwise
Evacuations due to internal and external disasters, including actual or threatened severe violent acts
Evidence handling, especially for rape kits, victims of crime, and other scenarios

Table 44.4 Factors increasing the challenge and risk of ED and PES work compared to other clinical settings

Brief length of stay limits opportunity for patient and family engagement
Elevated clinical acuity and urgency
Less access to prior medical records or history
Frequent staff handoffs
Frequent multitasking/rapid task-switching
Increased frequency of inaccurate information or intentional deception by patients and others
Limited empirical evidence base for decision-making

Understanding Malpractice

Estimates are that even specialists in low-risk fields are more likely than not to be sued at least once before the end of their career. Emergency medicine is actually near the middle of the curve for malpractice probability, and psychiatry is near the low end in terms of risk [6]. That said, behavioral emergencies create special challenges and risks that need to be understood, and when possible, controlled (see Table 44.4).

Malpractice, or medical negligence, means that a provider failed to use reasonable care in the management of a patient, which directly led to a bad outcome that is compensable. Only an injured party or their representatives may make a claim; this plaintiff must prove their allegation in a civil court at a threshold of "more likely than not," or a preponderance of the evidence. Not all adverse outcomes are due to negligence, and not all successful litigation is based on actual malpractice. Most bona fide negligent adverse events do not lead to litigation [7].

Discussions of negligence risk usually focus on the proverbial four Ds: Duty, Dereliction, Direct causation, and Damages.

- *Duty*: Providers owe a duty of care to patients, that is, what a reasonable practitioner of our field would provide, including proper diagnosis, informed consent, appropriate treatment, and maintained boundaries [8].
- *Dereliction*: The provider must have either failed to do or recognize something a reasonable provider would have, or do something no reasonable provider would have.

Table 44.5 The dirty dozen of medical malpractice

What a jury needs believe, more likely than not, to make a finding of negligence	1. Duty 2. Dereliction 3. Direct causation 4. Damages
What drives a plaintiff to sue a healthcare provider	5. Disappointment 6. Disgust 7. Distrust
What an attorney also needs to see to incur the costs of pursuing a case	8. Deep pockets
What providers can do to reduce their risk of adverse events, litigation, or settlement	9. Documentation 10. Design for safety 11. De-escalation after adverse outcomes
What happens after adverse events, litigation, or settlement	12. Discovering that Adverse Medical events can Massively Impact the Team (DAMMIT)

- *Direct*: That dereliction must have directly (and, usually, foreseeably) caused the alleged harm; but for the error, the harm would not have occurred.
- *Damages*: The alleged harm must be financially compensable.

These four elements are what a jury or judge needs to believe to rule in favor of the injured party (plaintiff) in a medical malpractice case. To fully understand the cycle of malpractice risk, other factors also need to be understood (see Table 44.5).

Disappointment, Disgust, and Distrust

It is commonly said that bad feelings drive malpractice more than bad outcomes; there is substantial evidence to support this adage. A family or an individual facing the crisis of devastating harm or loss from an adverse medical event commonly feels sad or upset. It is often feelings of anger that motivate them to seek legal redress. Studies based on reviews of depositions have consistently found that negative feelings toward the treatment team are a major factor [9, 10]. Families and patients express that they feel the providers were not fully honest with them, were rude, or did not take them or their concerns seriously prior to the bad outcome. Improved communication with patients and families may help mitigate this risk. Time spent with patients and their families provides opportunities to assure their questions and concerns are addressed, and can be extremely helpful in creating positive relationships less likely to lead to litigation. Some studies suggest that a pattern of poor patient satisfaction scores—that is, a tendency not to get along with patients well—may be associated with increased risk of litigation [11]. Other studies suggest that the likelihood of malpractice lawsuits against ED providers is a product of the duration of practice and volume of patients seen, rather than provider-specific factors [12].

In general, psychiatrists are often quite good at developing and maintaining positive relationships with patients and their families. Often, however, the quick pace of the emergency setting and sometimes adversarial nature of involuntary evaluations make this substantially more challenging. Complex rules of confidentiality that limit a provider's ability to share information without a patient's permission can make it difficult to create a positive impression on the family.

Deep Pockets

Plaintiff malpractice attorneys work on a contingency basis: They offer services with the understanding that they will take a percentage (usually 33–40%) of any settlement or verdict award as payment for their services. Payments in psychiatric malpractice cases versus other specialties are infrequent and for relatively low settlement amounts [13]. Attorneys, in general, reject most potential malpractice cases they are presented with; in the absence of a likelihood of a high settlement price, they are likely to turn down even a case with clear liability [14, 15]. Put simply, the low potential payout in a psychiatric malpractice case makes such cases less desirable for attorneys. A malpractice case against a large medical center may be more appealing, however, and many PES programs are embedded in such programs.

Documentation

Providers can do several things to decrease liability exposure. First and foremost is solidifying documentation. Medical malpractice cases hinge on whether the provider's decision making was reasonable. Documentation provides a window into that process. Even if there is a bad outcome, if the decision-making process that led to it was reasonable, considerable allowance is given to the provider. Much like high school math, partial credit is given for showing your work. A medical record that reflects (1) that varying options were identified and considered, (2) that collateral or primary treatment providers' input was sought and supported the primary provider's decision, and (3) that clear instructions were given to the patient and family about future risk can be extremely helpful. For a useful discussion and examples of useful language, please see the chapter on suicide illness and risk assessment in this volume.

Design for Safety

Additionally, PES leadership should take efforts to design for safety. The physical layout should maximize staff and patient safety by minimizing blind spots, routes of elopement, and accessibility to potential weapons or ligatures while maintaining comfort, privacy, and dignity. Work processes and procedures should promote consultation and collaboration. Medical record systems that support an easy review of prior care and thorough but time-efficient documentation are vital.

De-escalation

Finally, de-escalation skills are critical for the PES [16]. The skills clinicians use to de-escalate an upset patient are the same that can be used to defuse hostility before complaints are filed and can engender effective apologies after bad outcomes [17]. Careful use of apologies and alternative dispute resolution can decrease the likelihood of litigation or at least decrease the sum and stress of the malpractice process for all involved [18, 19].

DAMMIT

Adverse outcomes are, of course, inevitable. And while it is difficult for providers to accept, some cases are settled or lead to a plaintiff verdict even in the absence of actual negligence. Every case has a settlement price; a number of factors including defense legal costs, optics, and experience may play a role [20]. The psychological impact on providers who are involved in adverse events or targets of malpractice suits is substantial; creating programs to help these "second victims" is critical [21, 22]. Preparing healthcare professionals to be ready for psychological stress and developing system-level plans for supporting staff after adverse events should be routine in an acute-care setting [23]. Even with the best resilience, adverse events and malpractice are still intensely stressful and may have an unavoidable impact on team dynamics and staff turnover.

Duties to Third Parties

Many jurisdictions recognize that a special duty or standard of care may arise when a clinician becomes aware of intentional harm against a known target that is reported by the patient. These duties to third parties vary significantly across jurisdictions. These duties generally spring from the Tarasoff II ruling, a California case decided in 1976 [24]. Sometimes, these duties derive from statute; other times, from case law. Some states have established a duty to warn or protect, and sometimes, permission to warn. Some states even have no duty at all. Every clinician should know their state standard and seek specific interpretive guidance from their legal counsel [25] (Table 44.6).

Table 44.6 Disambiguation of duties to third parties

Duty: An affirmative responsibility; one must act, and failure to act would be negligent
Permission: One may act, but is not obligated to do so; not acting does not necessarily create liability
Protect: Preventing harm from occurring; this may or may not include warning
Warn: Notifying a potential victim of potential harm or a threat; this may or may not protect

The Healthcare Insurance Portability and Accountability Act's (HIPAA) privacy regulations are not a barrier to fulfill duties to third parties; they allow for permission to warn insofar as such an action is consistent with professional ethical standards or the standards of the local jurisdiction. The HIPAA regulations are complex and, at times, difficult to interpret. The Office of Civil Rights—the enforcement arm of Health and Human Services for HIPAA violations—provides useful interpretive guidance on this and other mental health questions under HIPAA [26]. Note that, ultimately, you cannot be sued by a patient or family member for violating HIPAA, but you can be sued for a harmful breach of confidentiality that may be proven by evidence that you were not compliant with HIPAA standards. HIPAA enforcement is generally limited to larger breaches impacting the records of 500 or more patient records. HIPAA was never designed to support decision-making in complex, individual cases like these. Overall, litigation for good faith breach of confidentiality relating to warnings to third parties is rare, while a failure to warn or protect may be a more concerning liability.

Contract for Safety

It is important to note that the concept of a contract for safety is often used as a clinical intervention with people who may be at risk for suicide. With substantial variation in application, it is essentially an agreement by the patient to the provider that they will not kill themselves. Its use is strongly discouraged. No-suicide contracts are empirically less clinically effective than developing a person-centered safety plan [27]. Some providers falsely believe that a "contract for safety" inures them against potential liability; there is no evidence or legal reasoning to support this idea and more than a modicum of evidence to suggest it increases the risk of adverse outcomes [28, 29].

Skilled plaintiff attorneys and experts may make the use of "contract for safety" language in the medical record a specific issue during litigation.

The Emergency Medical Treatment and Active Labor Act (EMTALA)

Like all medical emergencies presenting to an emergency department, behavioral health emergencies require compliance with EMTALA. EMTALA is a set of federal regulations promulgated and enforced by CMS; in addition to the formal regulations, the interpretive guidelines can provide some added clarity [30, 31]. EMTALA is intrinsically complex, and hospital legal counsel should provide guidance and assistance.

EMTALA violations are usually investigated after a complaint is made to the Centers for Medicare and Medicaid Services Office of Inspector General, who may negotiate a settlement or levy a fine if violations are confirmed. Even confirmed violations infrequently lead to a formal financial penalty, although the repercussions and impact of the investigation and compliance agreements can be onerous [32]. Rarely, a civil action for an EMTALA violation may arise, but these are seldom successful for behavioral health emergencies [33].

EMTALA mandates that anyone seeking treatment or appearing to need treatment and on the hospital campus must be examined and treated or stabilized for transfer to a specialized facility to receive treatment. The hospital must conduct an emergency medical screening examination (MSE) done by a professional designated by the hospital to rule out an emergency medical condition (EMC) [31]. EMCs may include psychiatric disturbance, symptoms of substance abuse, suicidality, and aggression. The MSE must be appropriate and cannot be delayed or disparate due to the psychiatric nature of the illness or other factors such as insurance status or ability to pay. An MSE would be considered disparate if it was less complete or thorough not due to the clinical need for the assessment but due to potentially concerning or discriminatory criteria.

If an EMC is found, the hospital must treat the patient or the hospital must stabilize the patient to the best of its ability and transfer the patient to a specialized facility [34]. EMTALA is no longer applicable once the individual has been stabilized for transfer or has been admitted [31]. When a patient requires specialized care unavailable at the examining facility, the facility can initiate an appropriate transfer to an appropriate specialized receiving facility.

This appropriate transfer must be accepted by the receiving facility, and the specialized facility cannot reject the transfer so long as they have the capacity (i.e., space) and capability (i.e., skill) to treat the individual. A lack of beds is not per se a reason to reject a transfer if the facility has historically made other accommodations for patients when beds are full. Specific policies and guidelines relating to psychiatric boarding can assist the hospital in managing these challenges. The transferring facility must stabilize the patient within its ability, and the treating physician must certify that the benefit of treatment at the specialized facility outweighs the risk of transfer. The degree of clinical stability needed for transfer may be different from what is needed for discharge.

While EMTALA mandates a screening for and treatment of all emergency medical conditions, state involuntary commitment laws may have competing or conflicting requirements. State law will govern where an individual can be forced to undergo involuntary emergency examination and treatment of a psychiatric condition. State laws may not fully align with EMTALA requirements. An MSE done to comply with EMTALA may not satisfy the required examination under a state involuntary commitment law. Similarly, an involuntary psychiatric exam to comply with a state commitment statute should not be considered an MSE under EMTALA.

Another such conflict can be seen in the scope of the EMTALA and state commitment laws. All hospitals with an ED must comply with EMTALA, whereas not all hospitals with EDs may certify the need for involuntary psychiatric treatment under state law. State law may dictate that only facilities with inpatient psychiatric units can conduct a psychiatric exam to certify the need for inpatient psychiatric care for purposes of an involuntary commitment. Hospitals without inpatient psychiatric units may not be able to certify that the patient is in need of inpatient psychiatric treatment. Regardless, both EDs would still be mandated by EMTALA to conduct an emergency medical screen and stabilize a presenting psychiatric patient to the best of their ability.

Hospitals presented with a patient suffering from what seems to be a psychiatric emergency on their campus cannot immediately transfer the individual to a hospital having an inpatient psychiatric unit while forgoing the MSE and stabilization requirements. The hospital cannot cite state law as a defense for failing to conduct an MSE.

Additionally, issues of consent make compliance with both laws difficult. A patient arriving involuntarily at a hospital to be examined under the state involuntary commitment law has not consented to the MSE under EMTALA. What are medical professionals to do where a patient may refuse an MSE and subsequent treatment under EMTALA but is evaluated per state involuntary commitment law?

Treating psychiatric patients and complying with EMTALA and state commitment laws can be challenging, especially for receiving hospitals. An appropriate transfer under EMTALA will occur where the facility lacks the specialized capability to treat a psychiatric patient and the risk of transfer does not outweigh the benefit. Generally, a receiving facility must accept a transfer if they have the capacity and capability. The statute does not provide for a receiving facility to question the transferring facility's ability to treat the patient.

What if the facility has a psychiatric facility but lacks child beds? Questions arise as to what "stabilized" means—truly, a perennial debate in behavioral emergencies [35, 36]. Does an ED with a psychiatrist on call or access to a county mental health examiner lack the ability to diagnose and treat a patient having an emergency psychiatric medical condition? What about hospitals that have inpatient psychiatric units but no beds—is a transfer to another facility appropriate? Must that facility accept that patient if they have a bed? What if the transfer would require the patient to be sent across the state, hundreds of miles away from home and far from any family or community supports they may have?

Finally, a specialized facility must accept a transfer where the transferring facility lacks the capacity and capability. A facility that lacks capacity but not the specialized care providing capability cannot invoke an appropriate transfer in the name of EMTALA to a refusing specialized facility. Lateral transfers where the patient could be treated at either facility should not be considered appropriate transfer under EMTALA.

Conclusion

Let go of the illusion that there will always be a low-risk or no-risk option; often, it is risk versus risk. ED and PES programs should be designed, led, and operated fully accounting for the science and psychology of risk; intentional risk-taking can be essential in supporting some patients. Careful documentation and program design can be critical in supporting essential and effective clinical practices. Ultimately, optimal practices include a balance of thoughtful consideration of the complexities of behavioral emergencies in settings that support collaboration and good care, and proffer the needed clinical and legal expertise.

References

1. Kleespies PM. Decision making in behavioral emergencies: acquiring skill in evaluating and managing high-risk patients. Washington, D.C.: American Psychological Association; 2014.
2. Kahneman D. Thinking, fast and slow. New York: Farrar, Straus and Giroux; 2013.
3. Coates J. The hour between dog and wolf: risk-taking, gut feelings and the biology of boom and bust. New York: Penguin Press; 2012.
4. Jones PM, Appelbaum PS, Siegel DM, Massachusetts Work Group on Law Enforcement Access to Hospital Patients. Law enforcement interviews of hospital patients: a conundrum for clinicians. JAMA. 2006;295(7):822–5.
5. Rozel JS. Armed law enforcement in the emergency department: risk management considerations. ABA

Health ESource [Internet]. 2016 Nov 29;13(3) [cited 29 Nov 2016]. Available from: https://www.americanbar.org/publications/aba_health_esource/2016-2017/november2016/lawenforcement.html.
6. Jena AB, Seabury S, Lakdawalla D, Chandra A. Malpractice risk according to physician specialty. N Engl J Med. 2011;365(7):629–36.
7. Localio AR, Lawthers AG, Brennan TA, Laird NM, Hebert LE, Peterson LM, et al. Relation between malpractice claims and adverse events due to negligence. Results of the Harvard Medical Practice Study III. N Engl J Med. 1991;325(4):245–51.
8. Moffett P, Moore G. The standard of care: legal history and definitions: the bad and good news. West J Emerg Med. 2011;12(1):109–12.
9. Levinson W, Roter DL, Mullooly JP, Dull VT, Frankel RM. Physician-patient communication. The relationship with malpractice claims among primary care physicians and surgeons. JAMA. 1997;277(7):553–9.
10. Beckman HB, Markakis KM, Suchman AL, Frankel RM. The doctor-patient relationship and malpractice. Lessons from plaintiff depositions. Arch Intern Med. 1994;154(12):1365–70.
11. Fullam F, Garman AN, Johnson TT, Hedberg EC. The use of patient satisfaction surveys and alternative coding procedures to predict malpractice risk. Med Care. 2009;47(5):553–9.
12. Carlson JN, Foster KM, Pines JM, Corbit CK, Ward MJ, Hydari MZ, et al. Provider and practice factors associated with emergency physicians' being named in a malpractice claim. Ann Emerg Med. 2017;71:157.
13. Schaffer AC, Jena AB, Seabury SA, Singh H, Chalasani V, Kachalia A. Rates and characteristics of paid malpractice claims among US physicians by specialty, 1992-2014. JAMA Intern Med. 2017;177(5):710–8.
14. Trautner MN. Tort reform and access to justice: how legal environments shape lawyers' case selection. Qual Sociol. 2011;34(4):523–38.
15. Shepherd J. Uncovering the silent victims of the American medical liability system. Vanderbilt Law Rev. 2013;67(1):151.
16. Richmond JS, Berlin JS, Fishkind AB, Holloman GH, Zeller SL, Wilson MP, et al. Verbal De-escalation of the agitated patient: consensus statement of the American Association for Emergency Psychiatry Project BETA De-escalation Workgroup. West J Emerg Med. 2012;13(1):17–25.
17. Rozel JS, Sysak E. Difficult relationships: patients, providers and systems. Curr Emerg Hosp Med Rep. 2018;6:1.
18. Robbennolt JK. Apologies and legal settlement: an empirical examination. Mich Law Rev. 2003;102(3):460.
19. Soffer JI. Apologize first; mediate second; litigate never. Rev Litig. 2015;34:493.
20. Carroll AE, Parikh PD, Buddenbaum JL. The impact of defense expenses in medical malpractice claims. J Law Med Ethics. 2012;40(1):135–42.
21. Seys D, Wu AW, Gerven EV, Vleugels A, Euwema M, Panella M, et al. Health care professionals as second victims after adverse events a systematic review. Eval Health Prof. 2013;36(2):135–62.
22. Ullström S, Andreen Sachs M, Hansson J, Øvretveit J, Brommels M. Suffering in silence: a qualitative study of second victims of adverse events. BMJ Qual Saf. 2014;23(4):325–31.
23. Loeppke R, Boldrighini J, Bowe J, Braun B, Eggins E, Eisenberg BS, et al. Interaction of health care worker health and safety and patient health and safety in the US Health Care System: recommendations from the 2016 summit. J Occup Environ Med. 2017;59(8):803–13.
24. Tarasoff v. Regents of University of California. Vol. 551, P. 2d. 1976. p. 334.
25. National Conference of State Legislators. Mental health professionals' duty to warn [Internet]. 2015 [cited 1 Oct 2017]. Available from: http://www.ncsl.org/research/health/mental-health-professionals-duty-to-warn.aspx.
26. Office of Civil Rights. Sharing information related to mental health [Internet]. Health and Human Services. [cited 1 Oct 2017]. Available from: https://www.hhs.gov/hipaa/for-professionals/special-topics/mental-health/index.html.
27. Bryan CJ, Mintz J, Clemans TA, Leeson B, Burch TS, Williams SR, et al. Effect of crisis response planning vs. contracts for safety on suicide risk in U.S. Army Soldiers: a randomized clinical trial. J Affect Disord. 2017;212:64–72.
28. Simon RI. The suicide prevention contract: clinical, legal, and risk management issues. J Am Acad Psychiatry Law. 1999;27(3):445–50.
29. Edwards SJ, Sachmann MD. No-suicide contracts, no-suicide agreements, and no-suicide assurances: a study of their nature, utilization, perceived effectiveness, and potential to cause harm. Crisis. 2010;31(6):290–302.
30. Center for Medicare & Medicaid Services. State operations manual, appendix V – interpretive guidelines – responsibilities of Medicare participating hospitals in emergency cases [Internet]. Baltimore: Department of Health and Human Services; 2010. [cited 2017 Sep 17]. Available from: https://www.cms.gov/Regulations-and-Guidance/Guidance/Manuals/downloads/som107ap_V_emerg.pdf.
31. Center for Medicare & Medicaid Services. 42 CFR Parts 413, 482, and 489. Medicare Program; Clarifying policies related to the responsibilities of medicare-participating hospitals in treating individuals with emergency medical conditions [Internet]. Baltimore: Department of Health and Human Services; 2003. [cited 1 Oct 2017]. Report No.: CMS-1063-F RIN 0938-AM34. Available from: https://www.cms.gov/Regulations-and-Guidance/Legislation/EMTALA/Downloads/CMS-1063-F.pdf.
32. Zuabi N, Weiss LD, Langdorf MI. Emergency Medical Treatment and Labor Act (EMTALA) 2002-15: review of Office of Inspector General

Patient Dumping Settlements. West J Emerg Med. 2016;17(3):245–51.
33. Lindor RA, Campbell RL, Pines JM, Melin GJ, Schipper AM, Goyal DG, et al. EMTALA and patients with psychiatric emergencies: a review of relevant case law. Ann Emerg Med. 2014;64(5):439–44.
34. Emergency Medical Treatment and Active Labor Act [Internet]. The Public Health and Welfare. Sect. 1395dd. Available from: https://www.gpo.gov/fdsys/pkg/USCODE-2010-title42/pdf/USCODE-2010-title42-chap7-subchapXVIII-partE-sec1395dd.pdf.
35. Anderson E, Nordstrom K, Wilson M, Peltzer-Jones J, Zun L, Ng A, et al. American Association for Emergency Psychiatry Task Force on medical clearance of adults part I: introduction, review and evidence-based guidelines. West J Emerg Med. 2017;18(2):235–42.
36. Wilson MP, Nordstrom K, Anderson EL, Ng AT, Zun LS, Peltzer-Jones JM, et al. American Association for Emergency Psychiatry Task Force on medical clearance of adult psychiatric patients. Part II: controversies over medical assessment, and consensus recommendations. West J Emerg Med. 2017;18(4):640–6.

45 Delivery Models of Emergency Psychiatric Care

Scott L. Zeller and Jamie C. Christensen

Introduction

The volume of Emergency Department (ED) visits continues to rise in the United States, with 60% of ED physicians reporting that they believe the cause is an increase in psychiatric emergencies [1]. From 2006 to 2014, the rate of ED visits for mental health/substance abuse diagnoses increased by 44%, and out of all diagnosis types, ED visits with a diagnosis of suicidal ideation increased the most—by a staggering 414% [2].

According to the USA Federal Emergency Medical Treatment and Labor Act (EMTALA), patients with acute psychiatric conditions rendering them either a danger to themselves, or a danger to others, are considered to have Emergency Medical Conditions (EMCs), legally equivalent to serious physical ailments—and as such, they cannot be discharged until they are stable and safe, with no further emergent dangerousness [3]. Thus, all psychiatric emergencies at hospital EDs must be fully assessed, and treated as necessary, with appropriate and secure dispositions; the question is how to best meet these obligations within the limited resources and time constraints of the ED.

S. L. Zeller (✉)
Department of Psychiatry, University of California-Riverside, Emeryville, CA, USA

Department of Acute Psychiatry, Vituity, Reno, NV, USA

J. C. Christensen
Department of Acute Psychiatry, Vituity, Reno, NV, USA

Goals of Psychiatric Emergency Treatment

The main objectives of the evaluation and treatment of mental health crises can be summed up in what are known as the "Six Goals of Emergency Psychiatry" [4]:

1. Exclude medical etiologies of symptoms and ensure medical stability
2. Rapidly stabilize the acute crisis
3. Avoid coercion
4. Treat in the least restrictive setting
5. Form a therapeutic alliance
6. Formulate an appropriate disposition and aftercare plan

Exclude Medical Etiologies for Symptoms and Ensure Medical Stability

Since many medical conditions can present with symptoms that appear similar to psychoses, mania, or other acute psychiatric states, it is essential that medical etiologies be ruled out prior to commencing psychiatric treatment. A significant number of patients who present to emergency settings with apparent psychiatric disorders have acute medical illnesses either coexisting or at the root of their symptoms [5]; failure

L. S. Zun et al. (eds.), *Behavioral Emergencies for Healthcare Providers*,
https://doi.org/10.1007/978-3-030-52520-0_45

to recognize these conditions can lead to serious morbidity [6, 7]. For example, a mistaken diagnosis of psychosis in a patient suffering from an intracranial bleed, thyroid storm, or toxic delirium can place the patient at serious, perhaps life-threatening, risk. Even commonplace medical issues in psychiatric patients, such as diabetes, hypertension, and alcohol withdrawal, can have severe sequelae if not properly addressed.

At the very least, psychiatric emergency programs need to have access to patient evaluations by a qualified medical professional along with the measurement of vital signs prior to the commencement of psychiatric treatment.

Rapidly Stabilize the Acute Crisis

Once a patient's medical stability has been ensured, emergency psychiatry programs need to focus on prompt stabilization of the acute crisis. Every effort should be made to ensure safety and prevent danger to self and others, while simultaneously working to alleviate the patient's suffering. This includes timely triage and defined levels of staff observation based on the degree of acuity.

It is not uncommon in many acute care settings for emergency psychiatry patients to experience very long waits for evaluation and treatment, while other "more urgent" medical patients get more immediate assistance. And indeed, it can be difficult for many caregivers to recognize that the distress of a psychiatric crisis can be, in a way, just as crippling as more obvious conditions like asthma attacks or motor vehicle accidents. Some emergency department staff have even been heard to say that because there are no blood tests or X-rays which show psychiatric illness, it is hard to compare these symptoms to more straightforward cases.

Yet, there is another very common symptom that virtually everyone has experienced, which also cannot be detected on blood tests or X-rays, and that is "pain." Thus, we have often found that teaching healthcare personnel to think of psychiatric emergencies as analogous to their "worst headache ever"—something they can all relate to—helps them to empathize with the severity of the psychiatric emergency and understand that the patient is truly agonizing and needs relief as soon as possible.

Avoid Coercion, Treat in the Least Restrictive Setting, and Form a Therapeutic Alliance

Practitioners in the emergency setting are often the first contact a patient will have with mental health care. A bad experience during this initial mental health contact may lead to long-term problems in which consumers might fear, distrust, or dislike psychiatrists and other providers. Such issues might interfere with the consumer's desire to obtain help, continue in treatment, or willingness to take medications. During the early phases of psychiatric illnesses, even brief interactions can have enduring implications for a patient's long-term wellness.

In realizing this, it is extremely important that emergency professionals work with patients in a supportive and compassionate manner, creating with the patient what is known as a *therapeutic alliance*. A therapeutic alliance might be most simply described as a collaborative relationship between a patient and a clinician. Rather than the professional acting excessively authoritatively or giving the patient orders, a therapeutic alliance should instead involve clinicians' attempts to bond and empathize with patients, and treat them as partners in healing and recovery. This can lead to a working relationship with shared responsibility for achieving treatment goals in the acute setting, and often results in better outcomes. Results of studies have shown that the quality of the therapeutic alliance is a significant factor in predicting the likelihood of a patient becoming violent during psychiatric hospitalizations. In one predictive model, the quality of the therapeutic alliance was able to predict 78% of aggressive behavior in patients [8].

Working with a therapeutic alliance mindset also means avoiding *coercion*—the use of force or threats to make patients do things against their will. In Emergency Psychiatry, avoiding coercion includes the administration of oral medications willingly via informed consent, as opposed to forcible injections; verbal de-escalation of agitated individuals to calmness, instead of imposing physical restraints; and little or no infringement on a patient's rights when possible. Treating in the least restrictive level of care is another means of avoiding coercion.

The more restrictive the level of care, the more there is a propensity for a coercive experience, and thus less opportunity for a therapeutic alliance. Examples of levels of mental health care from most to least restrictive include physical restraints and/or seclusion rooms, locked clinical settings, and involuntary inpatient units and then, voluntary, unlocked facilities. The least restrictive settings are outpatient clinics where patients are free to come and go as they wish. Most individuals will do best in the appropriate level of care which is least restrictive; thus, avoiding hospital admissions, when possible, can be quite advantageous for patients.

Appropriate Disposition and Aftercare Plan

In Emergency Psychiatry, the duties of the treating professional are not complete merely with the cessation of the presenting crisis. It is strongly recommended that a patient be provided with an appropriate care plan for post-discharge. This includes appointments (when possible) with outpatient providers, referral to mental health clinics and/or substance abuse treatment programs, and instructions about what to do if crisis symptoms recur. Frequently, assistance with housing may be a part of the aftercare plan, as might be coordination of arrangements with loved ones or caregivers.

Appropriate aftercare planning can be of substantial benefit to the long-term stability of patients and help prevent recidivism. Individuals who do not have an outpatient appointment after discharge are two times more likely to be psychiatrically hospitalized in a year than patients who went to at least one outpatient appointment [9].

Simply put, the main goals in the evaluation and treatment of patients in mental health crises are to ensure medical stability, evaluate for safety, relieve the patient's distress as quickly as possible in a noncoercive, supportive, collaborative manner, and get the patient to the least-restrictive environment with a safe and well-communicated discharge plan, which will help individuals to avoid a return to crisis-level symptoms.

The models of care utilized by EDs and care systems in an attempt to meet the above goals are determined by a variety of factors, such as census, availability of psychiatric resources and professionals, local mental health laws, and, of course, financial considerations. Unsurprisingly, healthcare systems across the country have adopted idiosyncratic designs to fit their particular situations best; however, upon scrutiny, most are variations of several distinct models. This chapter will next review these most prominent paradigms of psychiatric emergency care, evaluating the pros and cons of each, and will include a discussion of several innovative and alternative models that have evolved more recently.

Mental Health Consultants in the Medical Emergency Department

It is recognized that some EDs have little or no opportunity for emergency psychiatric care beyond what can be provided by the general medical ED professional on duty. In those settings which do have access to separate psychiatric personnel, the use of a mental health professional to consult on patients within the general ED population is likely the most utilized emergency psychiatry care approach in the United States [10]. With this model, psychiatric patients are triaged alongside patients with general medical complaints; all receive a medical screening examination (MSE) by a licensed independent provider. If a psychiatric intervention is deemed necessary, a request will be made for a mental health consultant to assess the patient. Most commonly, the consultant is not on duty within the ED, but arrives from another location, typically another area of the hospital, on-call from the community, or, in some cases, via a municipal or regional mobile crisis team.

The preferred professional level for consultants is psychiatrists, but often these may be psychologists, social workers, or other mental health clinicians. Some facilities even employ psychiatric technicians or other practitioners with less than a Master's level training to perform consultations. However, the use of these less clinically qualified personnel has been described as an "insufficient" level of care for those in a psychiatric crisis [11].

The requested consultant will typically perform an assessment and may recommend a course of treatment, but most commonly his or her role is to make a determination as to the need for psychiatric hospitalization (as opposed to discharge). However, the attending ED physician remains the clinician ultimately responsible for the patient's care in this model, and, in most systems, is also the one who will make the final decision as to disposition—in some cases even over-ruling the mental health consultant's recommendations.

Pros and Cons

This design may be useful in EDs that encounter relatively few psychiatric patients in crisis, such as smaller community or rural hospitals, where the census is insufficient to justify round-the-clock onsite mental health personnel or a separate site for psychiatric patients. A benefit of the model is that comorbid medical issues will be addressed while the patient is in the ED, which allows for the treatment of medically compromised patients who might otherwise exceed the capability of a psychiatric-only program. This model is also typically the least expensive option for many hospitals, as no separate infrastructure for the psychiatric patient is needed.

Since the consultant is often not on-site when the consult is requested, though, patients may wait hours before the consultant arrives, occupying valuable space in the ED and impacting throughput. Also, during this time, there is frequently no treatment being provided [12]. Furthermore, patients who are in the midst of a severe psychiatric emergency may further decompensate or become agitated in the chaos of the ED, especially when untreated, and this may lead to an increase in the level of care required for them [13].

One of the most noteworthy shortcomings of this model is that disposition decisions are typically made as the result of a "snapshot" at the time of the initial consultation. This will not allow, for example, the opportunity to see if the patient might soon show a good response to medications, detoxify, have a change in perspective, or otherwise improve enough for clinicians to consider changing the disposition plans. The ability to "observe and re-evaluate later" is present in several of the other models, and those using this strategy appropriately will often have better diversion rates from hospitalization as a result [13].

If the consultant is not a psychiatrist or licensed prescriber, another major issue in this model may be that he or she cannot make medication or other physical care recommendations. In that case, the burden falls upon the ED physician to determine the course of treatment—often with little guidance or expertise to prescribe challenging psychopharmacologic regimens. As a result, too often, a patient might receive little more than sedation during their ED stay. Also, non-psychiatrist consultants may also lack the expertise to rule out organically caused symptoms that mimic psychiatric emergencies, such as delirium [14].

An additional concern about using non-physicians for psychiatric consultations is that such consultants might be viewed as "lesser authorities" by some emergency medicine physicians, who may thus feel justified in exerting undue influence on the consultant toward certain dispositions. This can happen even with the common practice of using psychiatry residents to do ED psychiatric consults, because the physicians-in-training may be understandably anxious about countermanding an ED attending-level physician's opinion.

There are EDs where the mental health consultation is provided by a visiting "intake" team from an area inpatient psychiatric facility. The impartiality of decisions by such teams may come into question, as there are perverse financial incentives for their employers regarding admissions, especially for those patients with attractive private insurance reimbursement potential.

Another compelling drawback of the consultant model is that medical ED staff may not be sufficiently trained to intervene with psychiatric emergencies, and may actually exacerbate patients' symptoms either with excessive coercion or by misunderstanding the needs of a person in crisis. Further, there have been instances where staff can be disdainful, condescending, or even derisive to these patients, seemingly from a mindset that the psychiatric afflictions are not "real" emergencies or perhaps should be the lowest priority for care. This phenomenon is considered part of the "stigma" of psychiatric illness that patients have referred to in their complaints about treatment in medical EDs [15].

Telepsychiatry

The newest version of the consultant model is the telepsychiatry model—accessing a psychiatrist via telemedicine. Most commonly, this service is provided in the ED via an "on-demand" format; the ED only requests a consultation when necessary, and then will access an off-site mental health professional consultant via video teleconferencing [16]. Online consultants are able to perform face-to-face assessments and make recommendations on treatment and disposition; efficacy, safety, and patient satisfaction have been shown to be roughly equivalent to interactions with a psychiatrist in the same room [17]. The use of telepsychiatry consultants is rapidly expanding, acting either as a complementary service when onsite clinicians are unavailable or as the sole source of ED psychiatric consultations. It has been successfully utilized in EDs across the state of South Carolina for several years [18], and is now available from multiple provider groups in most parts of the USA.

Pros and Cons

Studies to date demonstrate that telepsychiatry in the ED can substantially reduce ED crowding and delays in care, while improving access and timeliness of psychiatric interventions [19, 20]. Shortcomings of ED telepsychiatry consultation may be the significant dollar charge per consult, and the difficulties and costs in credentialing large groups of providers in each individual hospital when the service is provided by a large, external telepsychiatry team. An additional drawback is that the consulting psychiatrist may not be well informed about local resources, which can impact the recommendations for disposition.

Dedicated Mental Health Wing of the Medical Emergency Department

In this model, the ED has a separate area or room specifically for patients experiencing psychiatric emergencies. Typically, this area is a bit less chaotic than the main ED, and staff members are assigned who are knowledgeable in psychiatric care, especially psychiatric nurses, social workers, therapists, and even on-site psychiatrists. As the patient is still located within the ED proper, the patients will remain under the supervision of the emergency medicine attending physician, and involved professional staff in this wing may have simultaneous responsibilities in other areas of the ED or hospital.

Pros and Cons

These specialized sections for psychiatric emergencies tend to be more therapeutically appropriate for individuals in crisis, particularly when the staff is well trained to manage such patients; there may be dimmed lighting, soothing music, and artwork or color schemes conducive to calming. Patients will often have the opportunity for longer stays than in the consultant model, because they are not taking up beds allocated for traditional medical patients in the primary ED. The longer stays may allow time for healing, detoxification, and for medications to become effective, each of which might improve the chances for a patient to avoid inpatient hospitalization. In addition, since this area is part of the ED, medical emergency personnel are nearby, and any medical concerns can be dealt with quickly and efficiently. This arrangement thus permits psychiatric treatment to commence for patients with serious medical comorbidities, who might otherwise be considered medically unsuitable for standalone psychiatric programs.

However, while this separate area of the ED has its benefits, it certainly also has its potential drawbacks. For instance, despite the focus and adaptation for psychiatric care, the dedicated mental health wing is still in the midst of a bustling ED, with its cacophony of loud noises, hectic personnel activity, sirens, and enigmatic machinery. This can interfere with healing and increase anxiety. For the crisis patient, being separated from the main areas of the ED may lead to further marginalization or ostracization, along with lack of confidentiality, as other medical and nursing staff (and even other patients) might quickly identify the separated individuals as "the psych patients." Some EDs even dress their psychiatric patients in distinctive, different-colored gowns from the general population, with the idea being that this will assist the staff in recognizing "where patients belong" and help prevent elopements; however, this has often resulted in a serious stigma, as others in the ED quickly recognize "that color means a psych patient"—and it may be completely unnecessary with more modern options such as video monitoring or electronic wristbands [21]. Finally, on occasion, due to a high census in the general ED population, these psychiatric wings of the ED might be turned into "float" areas where non-psychiatric emergency patients will be housed, which may interfere or lead to less specialized care for the psychiatric patients.

Distinct Psychiatric Emergency Programs

Distinct Psychiatric Emergency Programs come in many shapes, sizes, and abbreviations. Names for these facilities include Emergency Psychiatric Assessment Treatment and Healing (emPATH) units, Psychiatric Emergency Services (PES), Psychiatric Urgent Care Centers (PsyUC), and Crisis Stabilization Units (CSU), among other monikers. These programs can be part of a hospital campus or completely free-standing and independent, and can vary in operations from simple screening processes and short-term interventions all the way up to comprehensive emergency psychiatric and medical diagnostic evaluation and treatment centers. Some sites even serve as the nexus of the region's acute mental health system, additionally housing such offerings as mobile crisis teams, outpatient clinics, and day treatment centers [22]. Some wide-ranging psychiatric emergency programs have even been described as comparable for psychiatric care to a Level 1 Trauma facility for emergency medical care [23].

Rather than attempt an all-encompassing overview of these varied distinct Psychiatric Emergency Programs, we will describe the basic models in order, from those with the lowest acuity capability and capacity to the most comprehensive and high-acuity sites. It should be understood that these descriptions are an attempt to categorize widely diverse operations, and there may be considerable overlap between the models suggested here at any particular site. For, as it is often said about emergency psychiatry programs, "When you've seen one, you've seen one."

Psychiatric Urgent Care/Voluntary Crisis Centers

Psychiatric urgent care centers may be found as part of a community mental health clinic or may be stand-alone programs funded by the local behavioral health agency. Some psychiatric hospitals have urgent-care drop-in units where patients might predominantly be screened for possible hospitalization onsite, but the service may also offer referrals to outpatient or medication refills for lower-acuity individuals.

These walk-in care centers may be beneficial for several reasons, especially from the patient's point of view. They are usually voluntary-only (meaning no patients held on involuntary psychiatric detention) and tend to focus on empathetic crisis counseling rather than acute medical interventions, so patients may feel they are in a more comfortable and supportive situation, without the stigma they may experience at a larger ED. The personnel are often therapists and social workers rather than nurses and doctors, although many of these programs also have access to prescribers to help clients obtain short-term medications or medication refills.

However, most urgent care centers will exclude individuals who are presently dangerous, have a history of dangerous behavior, or who are acutely hallucinating, medically compromised, intoxicated, or in substance withdrawal. Patients in those circumstances, which tend to be a substantial percentage of the overall urgent-needs patients in a region, will still need to go to an ED or a PES for a higher level of care, or the center may have to call 911 or summon police should more acute patients present at the site. This can limit the overall effectiveness of these programs in reducing ED utilization for acute psychiatric conditions.

Crisis Stabilization Units (CSU)

The concept of a "crisis stabilization unit" (CSU) has garnered varied meanings in different parts of the USA. Depending on the location, a CSU could be anything from a hospital-based outpatient department to a community counseling "drop-in" center, to a 30-day "halfway house"-style residential program [24, 25]. California's Medicaid Code defines a CSU as an outpatient "…service lasting less than 24 hours, to or on behalf of a beneficiary for a condition that requires more timely response than a regularly scheduled visit. Service activities include but are not limited to one or more of the following: assessment, collateral and therapy" [26]. Sometimes, a CSU aligned with this California description is referred to as a "23-hour program."

Most commonly across the USA, a CSU is a community-based, drop-in program with a focus on crisis intervention and primarily serving lower-acuity patients. This model often functions to provide more prompt access to counseling than a patient's regular provider can offer, or perhaps delivering brief respite from stressors or living situation issues, rather than as a site for active, high-acuity psychiatric intervention. Higher-acuity patients are more commonly referred to psychiatric hospitalization; in some cases, the design of these programs even calls for immediate referral for hospitalization as part of the CSU's paradigm for patients presenting with highly acute symptoms.

Many CSUs strive to create an environment that is more "home-like" than a typical hospital or ED, with comfortable furnishings and a setting that appears more like a clubhouse or hotel lobby than a clinic. It is believed that by making the treatment area a more welcoming, "less-restrictive" venue, patients will feel less stigma and anxiety, and be more relaxed, which will allow for calming and healing. A good example of this is with the "Living Room" concept, where in addition to the home-like setting, an emphasis is placed on using Peer Support Specialists (recovering mental health patients who have specialized training to work onsite in therapeutic and supportive roles) with individuals in crisis [27].

emPATH Units

*em*PATH units are a more recent development—a hospital-based program that combines the calming and comfortable 23-hour short-term setting of the community CSU with the capacity and capability to work with higher acuity patients, including those under both voluntary status and involuntary psychiatric detention, who otherwise would be relegated to hospital EDs or psychiatric inpatient units. *em*PATH units allow for hospital EDs to quickly medically screen individuals experiencing a psychiatric emergency, and then immediately move medically appropriate patients into the more therapeutic *em*PATH setting, where psychiatric assessment and treatment can take place, with the objective of prompt stabilization and avoiding inpatient hospitalization when possible.

The acronym "emPATH" stands for "*em*ergency Psychiatric Assessment, Treatment, and

Healing" unit. Accordingly, the objectives of this unit are closely tied to the "Six Goals" of Emergency Psychiatry previously outlined. Whereas the "dedicated mental health wing" is often more of an observation unit, or even limited to a "boarding" section where psychiatric patients await transfer to an inpatient hospital bed or other dispositions, in the *em*PATH unit, there is active engagement in treatment and constant reassessment of an individual's condition by the unit staff.

*em*PATH units differ from the "dedicated mental health wing of the ED" in that *em*PATH units are discrete programs, completely separate from the ED, operating in an alternate location of the hospital (or even on a different campus) with a goal of quickly evaluating and then treating a patient for up to 24 hours. Whereas the ED wing will usually be staffed by ED team members, and the patients remain under the jurisdiction of the ED emergency medicine attending, an *em*PATH unit is a thoroughly independent operation, with its own personnel, who are responsible for all of the assessment, treatment, and disposition of patients. However, an *em*PATH unit may not have a licensed independent medical provider on duty onsite at all times (though a psychiatrist will be available around the clock via telepsychiatry or on-call), and thus an *em*PATH unit, to be compliant with federal EMTALA laws, will be unable, in most designs, to accept presentations directly from the community or police. The most common *em*PATH unit model has all patients receiving a Medical Screening Examination at a general ED to rule out non-psychiatric emergency medical conditions, and, once cleared, promptly transferred to the *em*PATH unit for psychiatric evaluation.

In an *em*PATH unit, patients are not relegated to individual rooms or isolated "beds," but rather are treated concurrently in a large room known as the "milieu." Here, each patient will be allowed to choose a "sleeper chair" or recliner, which can be folded flat for a nap or set up as a chair to facilitate group or individual therapy. There is ample room to move about and no requirement to stay in a certain location, which can help to relax patients who lessen symptoms by walking or pacing around or who benefit from feeling less confined. Some *em*PATH units feature outdoor areas or gardens to further allow patients a spot for peacefulness and recovery.

To assist with the overall philosophy of a calming, restorative, environment which encourages meeting individual needs, patients are able to access food, beverages, and linens for themselves without asking permission from the staff. Rather than the staff being behind a walled-off nursing station, professionals are interspersed with the patients in the milieu, and thus will quickly recognize when a patient might need additional assistance. Unlocked "Calming Rooms" are available for individuals who might benefit from a period of privacy.

Because of the unit design and the overall focus on avoiding coercion, *em*PATH units have reported dramatically lower incidence of physical restraints, aggression, and assaults than more traditional units or EDs, even with a highly acute patient population under evaluation for dangerousness to self and/or others [28]. While some might question placing such individuals at risk into a common room rather than isolation, this group setting has been demonstrated to encourage interpersonal engagement and respect, and gives patients the feeling they have caring human contact rather than facing their troubles alone, with resulting positive outcomes [28]. As in some CSUs and Urgent Care programs, Peer Support Specialists are commonly also part of *em*PATH unit staffing, further enhancing the opportunity for therapeutic engagement.

A key part of the *em*PATH unit philosophy is that all newly arriving patients will receive an evaluation by a psychiatric provider as quickly as possible, with medications started immediately when indicated. Ensuring that upsetting symptoms are assessed and treated promptly will further reduce patient distress and improve the chances for stabilization within the 24-hour limit. *em*PATH units have successfully reported diversion from inpatient hospitalization in more than three-quarters of high-acuity patients treated [28].

*em*PATH units can be very effective in reducing their affiliated ED's overcrowding and shortening its throughput times, especially in those that follow the model of "accepting all the ED's medically-clear psychiatric patients promptly." However, their design still requires patients to be evaluated in a medical ED before transfer to the *em*PATH unit, and so this design still makes demands on the medical ED. Thus, there can be limits on overall utilization. For regions with a high volume of psychiatric emergency patients daily, it may be reasonable to consider a completely independent psychiatric emergency services program (PES).

Psychiatric Emergency Services (PES)

As opposed to an *em*PATH unit in which medical clearance is done prior to referral, a Psychiatric Emergency Services program (PES) is a separate ED-like operation that is solely dedicated to managing and treating psychiatric emergencies. A PES can accept patients directly from the field via police or ambulance or by self-presentation [29]. A PES is also "EMTALA-compliant," meaning it is a receiving facility with a physician or other licensed independent professional on duty at all times. In this regard, a PES can even be considered a mental health ED roughly analogous to a Level-One trauma center [30].

Similar to many CSUs and *em*PATH units, under the most common definitions, a PES is considered an emergency outpatient program, which is permitted to treat patients up to a maximum of 23 hours and 59 minutes. Any patients needing care beyond 24 hours should be admitted to an inpatient psychiatric hospital.

PES programs typically can provide psychiatric evaluations and treatment for both voluntary patients and those under involuntary psychiatric legal detentions. The designs can span from fully locked, partially locked, or completely unlocked facilities, depending on each unit's policies and requirements. Psychiatric emergency services may vary greatly depending on the scope of practice and exit resources, with some sites also offering such services as detox centers, crisis counseling, drop-in medication clinics, long-term or short-term housing referrals, site-based mobile crisis units, partial hospitalization, day treatment, and intensive outpatient case management [22].

Yet, despite the numerous differences between PES programs, there are many commonalities. PES programs usually consist of full-time staff dedicated to and trained for psychiatric emergencies, including psychiatrists, psychiatric nurses, therapists, social workers, and mental health technicians. Evaluation, medical screening, diagnosis, and treatment can all be initiated quickly onsite; the more prompt the interventions, the greater the possibility of stabilization within 24 hours and avoidance of hospitalization [13].

One of the chief advantages of a PES, since it can accept individuals directly from the community, is that patients can bypass the entire process of going to a separate general medical ED first. This subjects patients to less stress, delays, stigma, confusion, and redundancy, while allowing for prompt initiation of psychiatric care with knowledgeable personnel and in the appropriate setting. This paradigm also can mean substantial cost savings to the overall system, by reducing expensive visits to multiple locations and avoiding costly and time-consuming interfacility transfers; and it significantly reduces medical ED crowding and improves throughput, in that most psychiatric patients in such systems will be at the appropriate site from the beginning rather than adding to medical ED censuses.

PES programs can be located near hospital EDs, elsewhere on hospital campuses, or even as stand-alone operations outside hospital grounds. Many PES programs are directly affiliated with medical EDs or inpatient psychiatric hospitals, but neither of these is a requirement [11].

It is likely true that the great majority of emergency psychiatric patients can be stabilized, to the point of no longer requiring an acute or hospital level of care, in less than 1 day [31]. With a focus on prompt interventions, and with a philosophy of attempting stabilization for up to 24 hours prior to making a decision on hospitalization, it is not uncommon for PES programs to divert patients from hospital stays in 75% or more of their cases [32]. This not only can lead to better outcomes for patients but also can help preserve the limited numbers of available inpatient psychiatric beds for those individuals for whom there is truly no alternative.

The main drawback of PES programs is that given their 24/7 operational demands, they may be much more expensive to operate than other emergency psychiatry models. The expenditures required to operate a PES usually means that such a program should only be considered in systems with a volume of psychiatric emergencies in excess of 3000 patients per year [23]. Constructing a de novo PES facility can be a costly undertaking. Even if just remodeling an already-existing physical space, there must be adequate room for patient care as well as staff, administration, registration, and billing personnel. However, once constructed, a PES has ongoing budgetary issues associated with operations of a distinct program [33]. Another issue is the difficulty in recruiting and maintaining adequate and proper staffing around the clock. Twenty-four-hour staffing can be challenging for these facilities, as it is not uncommon for busy and demanding crisis programs to experience a high degree of employee turnover [33].

Furthermore, because PES programs are EMTALA-compliant, patients must receive a Medical Screening Examination and be stabilized to the point that they are no longer a danger to themselves or others before a discharge can occur. As noted before, psychiatric emergencies involving dangerousness qualify as Emergency Medical Conditions under EMTALA. However, it is important to note that although a PES must do a screening examination for medical concerns, it is not required to provide such services as advanced life support; EMTALA recognizes the existence of specialty emergency centers with limited capabilities, and permits transports from such sites to higher-level-of-care EDs [3]. Thus, despite having 24-hour physicians on duty, PES programs that are not co-located with a medical ED will typically not have the capability to stabilize serious medical conditions. A PES such as this will thus necessitate acute medical conditions be stabilized elsewhere prior to arrival and will need to rapidly transport out patients with medical emergencies arising or arriving onsite to a medical ED, even calling 911 in urgent situations.

Regional Dedicated PES Programs

Presently, most PES programs in the USA have a limited catchment area or are part of a specific medical center. However, there are a number of "Regional Dedicated Psychiatric Emergency Services" programs—which accept all emergency psychiatric patients from a defined widespread geographic area, directly from the field. Such programs also have a collaborative relationship with a number of otherwise-unaffiliated EDs, as the higher-level-of-care ED transfer destination for all their psychiatric emergency patients [34].

This regional design allows for a shorter duration of "boarding times" of psychiatric patients in medical EDs. One regional PES showed more than an 80% improvement over comparable boarding time state averages—remarkably, for an overall "cost per patient" less expensive than the average price tag of that same patient languishing those same hours in a medical ED, merely waiting for a disposition, when little or no psychiatric care is occurring [32]. Given the ability to bypass general EDs and present directly to the regional PES, the number of psychiatric emergencies evaluated in the area medical EDs is a much smaller percentage of the total that would be seen in systems without a regional PES [32]. As such, it not only allows for patients to receive treatment in an appropriate setting much more quickly, but also reduces ED crowding and overall expenditures that are incurred by areas with high censuses and lengthy boarding times.

Alternative Crisis Options

In addition to the emergency psychiatry models outlined above, there are several other alternative strategies for assisting those in psychiatric crisis, which are typically off hospital grounds: these include mobile crisis teams and acute diversion units such as crisis respite and crisis residential housing.

Mobile Crisis Teams

Mobile crisis teams are usually comprised of mental health professionals who travel via car or van to the site of a patient in crisis, instead of having police or emergency providers bring the patient to a fixed site. Mobile teams are found in many communities around the USA, and can provide a wide range of onsite crisis intervention, de-escalation, and conflict resolution services, as well as assistance with housing and access to more permanent care [35]. Some systems have police summon mobile teams as a consultation for possible involuntary psychiatric detentions, while others may ride along with specially trained police units known as Crisis Intervention Teams (CIT). Since mobile crisis teams are more focused on intervening in emerging situations in the field, they are not a replacement for ED or PES services, but they can often help resolve a patient's crisis without having to transport to a treatment center. Mobile crisis teams can be invaluable assistance for solving problems where they occur, and in the prevention of unnecessary ED presentations.

Acute Diversion Units (ADUs)/Crisis Respite/Crisis Residential Housing

Residential programs (sometimes called Acute Diversion Units or ADUs) are community-based facilities, which are often in actual private houses, allowing the care to take place in a setting that is comfortable and integrated into the outside world. These can be ideal for patients who would normally be thought to require several days of intensive mental health care, but are eager to engage in treatment, willing to participate in groups and activities, and have not reached a level of acuity or dangerousness that would necessitate hospitalization. Given the nonclinical setting, much of the stigma and difficulties some patients associate with hospitalization can be mitigated. Most commonly, these programs will take in 8–16 patients at a time for up to a maximum of 2 weeks [36]. Most ADUs require a prescreening from an ED or PES, but some may also accept patients from mobile crisis units or other community providers.

Summary

With the number of psychiatric emergencies on the rise, EDs often find themselves inundated with people in psychiatric crises. The needs of this population can often surpass most general medical ED personnel's expertise and capability, and will thus require more specialized interventions. While psychiatric consultation, including that done via telemedicine, can work well in EDs with a low volume of psychiatric crises, areas with a higher census of psychiatric emergencies will need to develop urgent care alternatives such as Crisis Centers, CSUs, *em*PATH units, and/or Psychiatric Emergency Services facilities. Surprisingly enough, although these emergency psychiatry programs can seem expensive when viewed in isolation, they can actually provide much-needed, targeted, immediate, and appropriate care for patients in crisis. This will actually save systems substantial dollars in other ways, by reducing ED utilization, eliminating boarding, and improving throughput times, all while successfully diverting patients away from unnecessary and costly hospital inpatient admissions.

References

1. Salinsky E, Loftis C. Shrinking inpatient psychiatric capacity: cause for celebration or concern? Issue Brief George Wash Univ Natl Health Policy Forum. 2007;(823):1–21.
2. Moore BJ, Owens PL. Trends in emergency department visits, 2006-2014. HCUP Statistical Brief #227 [Internet]. Rockville. 2017. Available from: http://www.hcup-us.ahrq.gov/reports/statbriefs/sb227-Emergency-Department-Visit-Trends.pdf.
3. Department of Health and Human Services. Centers for Medicare and Medicaid Services. State operations manual. Appendix V. Emergency Medical Treatment and Labor Act (EMTALA) Appendix V. Interpretive guidelines – responsibility of Medicare participating hospitals in emergency cases. 2010. https://www.cms.gov/Regulations-and-Guidance/Guidance/Manuals/Downloads/som107ap_v_emerg.pdf.
4. Holloman GH, Zeller SL. Overview of project BETA: best practices in evaluation and treatment of agitation. West J Emerg Med [Internet]. 2012;13(1):1–2; [cited 1 Sept 2017]. Available from: https://www.ncbi.nlm.nih.gov/pmc/articles/PMC3298232/.

5. Carlson RJ, Navar N, Sur M. Physical disorders among emergency psychiatry patients. Can J Psychiatry. 1981;26:65–7.
6. Citrome LL, Holt RI, Zachry WM. Risk of treatment-emergent diabetes mellitus in patients receiving antipsychotics. Ann Pharmacother. 2007;41:1593–603.
7. Kar SK, et al. Psychiatric manifestation of chronic subdural hematoma: the unfolding of mystery in a homeless patient. Indian J Psychol Med. 2015;37(2):239–42.
8. Beauford JE, McNiel DE, Binder RL. Utility of the initial therapeutic alliance in evaluating psychiatric patients' risk of violence. Am J Psychiatry. 1997;154:1272–6.
9. Nelson EA, Maruish ME, Axler JL. Effects of discharge planning and compliance with outpatient appointments on readmission rates. Psychiatr Serv. 2000;51:885–9.
10. Zeller SL. Treatment of psychiatric patients in emergency settings. Prim Psychiatry. 2010;17:35–41. http://primarypsychiatry.com/treatment-of-psychiatric-patients-in-emergency-settings.
11. Fishkind AB, Berlin JS. Structure and function of psychiatric emergency services. In: Glick RL, Berlin JS, Fishkind AB, Zeller SL, editors. Emergency psychiatry: principles and practice. Philadelphia: Wolters Kluwer Health/Lippincott Williams & Wilkins; 2008. p. 9–23.
12. Hoot NR, Aronsky D. Systematic review of emergency department crowding: causes, effects, and solutions. Ann Emerg Med. 2008;52:126–36.
13. Zeller SL. Psychiatric boarding: averting long waits in emergency rooms. Psychiatr Times. 2013;30:40. http://www.psychiatrictimes.com/psychiatric-emergencies/psychiatric-boarding-averting-long-waits-emergency-rooms.
14. Flaherty JA, Fichtner CG. Impact of emergency psychiatry training on residents' decisions to hospitalize patients. Acad Med. 1992;67:585–6.
15. Neauport A, Rodgers RF, Simon NM, Birmes PJ, Schmitt L, Bui E. Effects of a psychiatric label on medical residents' attitudes. Int J Soc Psychiatry. 2012;58:485–7.
16. Yellowlees P, Burke MM, Marks SL, Hilty DM, Shore JH. Emergency telepsychiatry. J Telemed Telecare. 2008;14:277–81.
17. Seidel RW, Kilgus MD. Agreement between telepsychiatry assessment and face-to-face assessment for Emergency Department psychiatry patients. J Telemed Telecare. 2014;20:59–62.
18. Narasimhan M, Druss BG, Hockenberry JM, Royer J, Weiss P, Glick G, et al. Impact of a telepsychiatry program at emergency departments statewide on the quality, utilization, and costs of mental health services. Psychiatr Serv. 2015;66:1167. http://ps.psychiatryonline.org/doi/pdf/10.1176/appi.ps.201400122.
19. Southard EP, Neufeld JD, Laws S. Telemental health evaluations enhance access and efficiency in a critical access hospital emergency department. Telemed J E Health. 2014;20:664–8.
20. Telepsychiatry program eases patient crowding in the ED, expedites mental health services to patients and providers. ED Manag. 2013;25:121–4.
21. Macy D, Johnston M. Using electronic wristbands and a triage protocol to protect mental health patients in the emergency department. J Nurs Care Qual. 2007;22:180–4.
22. Lee TS, Renaud EF, Hills OF. Emergency psychiatry: an emergency treatment hub-and-spoke model of psychiatric emergency services. Psychiatr Serv. 2003;54:1590–1,1594.
23. Allen MH. Level 1 psychiatric emergency services. The tools of the crisis sector. Psychiatr Clin North Am. 1999;22:13–34; vii.
24. Adams CL, El-Mallakh RS. Patient outcome after treatment in a community-based crisis stabilization unit. J Behav Health Serv Res. 2009;36:396–9.
25. Wolff A. Development of a psychiatric crisis stabilization unit. J Emerg Nurs. 2008;34:458–9.
26. Barclays Official California Code of Regulations. Title 9: Rehabilitative and developmental services. Division 1: Department of Mental Health. Chapter 11: Medi-Cal Specialty Mental Health Services. §1810.210: Crisis Stabilization. https://govt.westlaw.com/calregs/Document/IE4ACC7A0DF4A11E4A54FF22613B56E19?viewType=FullText&originationContext=documenttoc&transitionType=CategoryPageItem&contextData=(sc.Default).
27. Heyland M, Emery C, Shattell M. The living room, a community crisis respite program: offering people in crisis an alternative to emergency departments. Glob J Comm Psychol Pract. 2013;4(3):1–8.
28. Zeller SL. emPATH units as a solution for ED psychiatric patient boarding [Internet]. Psychiatry Advisor. 2017 [cited 1 Sept 2017]. Available from: http://www.psychiatryadvisor.com/practice-management/empath-mental-health-crisis-management-emergency-department-setting/article/687420/.
29. Allen MH, Forster P, Zealberg J, Currier G. Report and recommendations regarding psychiatric emergency and crisis services. A review and model program descriptions. Washington, DC: American Psychiatric Association Task Force on Psychiatric Emergency Services; 2002. http://www.emergencypsychiatry.org/data/tfr200201.pdf.
30. Allen MH, Currier GW. Medical assessment in the psychiatric emergency service. New Dir Ment Health Serv. 1999;(82):21–8.
31. Wilson MP, Zeller SL. Introduction: reconsidering psychiatry in the emergency department. J Emerg Med. 2012;43:771–2.
32. Zeller SL, Calma N, Stone A. Effects of a dedicated regional psychiatric emergency service on boarding of psychiatric patients in area emergency departments. West J Emerg Med. 2014;15:1–6.
33. Fishkind AB, Zeller SL, Snodgress M. Administration of psychiatric emergency services. In: Glick RL, Berlin

JS, Fishkind AB, Zeller SL, editors. Emergency psychiatry: principles and practice. Philadelphia: Wolters Kluwer Health/Lippincott Williams & Wilkins; 2008. p. 497–512.
34. Intriguing model significantly reduces boarding of psychiatric patients, need for inpatient hospitalization. ED Manag. 2015;27:1–5.
35. Geller JL, Fisher WH, McDermeit M. A national survey of mobile crisis services and their evaluation. Psychiatr Serv. 1995;46:893–7.
36. Patel RM. Crisis residential settings. In: Glick RL, Berlin JS, Fishkind AB, Zeller SL, editors. Emergency psychiatry: principles and practice. Philadelphia: Wolters Kluwer Health/Lippincott Williams & Wilkins; 2008. p. 393–412.

46 The Gun Talk: How to Have Effective Conversations with Patients and Families About Firearm Injury Prevention

John S. Rozel, Layla Soliman, and Abhishek Jain

Introduction

In fairness, few people present for clinical services identifying firearm ownership as their chief complaint. Nonetheless, firearms access is associated with a number of significant medical and social issues that may intersect with an emergency department (ED) or a psychiatric emergency service (PES), including suicide, homicide, assault, domestic violence, accidental injury, and shootings of law enforcement officers [1–5]. Some patients may present with emergencies that are obviously gun-related, such as injuries from firearms, threats of suicide, or aggression with a firearm. Others, however, may present with complaints that only indirectly raise questions regarding firearm safety, such as a history of an underlying psychiatric or substance use disorder, impulsivity in a juvenile, or cognitive impairment in an elderly person [6, 7]. In what may be a clinical presentation for a very different issue, clinicians may need to tactfully open a dialogue about firearm safety.

Recent legal minefields and controversies further complicate this delicate conversation. For example, in 2010, during routine health screening at a well-child visit, a pediatrician asked a parent about firearms at home. The family refused to answer, the conflict escalated, and the family was ultimately "fired" from the practice. The family went to a local chapter of a firearm advocacy group who, in turn, lobbied for legislation colloquially known as the "Docs vs. Glocks law" [8]. This law – formally, the Firearm Owner's Privacy Protection Act of 2011 – made inquiries about firearms a sanctionable disciplinary issue for licensed professionals. After numerous court cases and appeals, the most recent ruling struck down the law.

The United States has substantially more firearms than any other country with proportionately elevated risks for firearm suicides and homicides, including mass shootings [9–11]. Highly publicized incidents of firearm violence are often followed by periods of increased firearm sales, increased concealed carry permit applications, increased stock prices for firearm manufacturers, and decreased firearm regulation [12–14].

Thus, firearms are ubiquitous, potentially quite dangerous, and unlikely to be subject to significantly increased restrictions anytime in

J. S. Rozel (✉)
Department of Psychiatry, University of Pittsburgh School of Medicine, Pittsburgh, PA, USA
e-mail: rozeljs@upmc.edu

L. Soliman
Department of Psychiatry, Atrium Health Behavioral Health, Charlotte, NC, USA

A. Jain
Board Certified Forensic Psychiatrist, New York, NY, USA

L. S. Zun et al. (eds.), *Behavioral Emergencies for Healthcare Providers*,
https://doi.org/10.1007/978-3-030-52520-0_46

the foreseeable future. Nonetheless, when appropriate, health-care providers can play an important role in effectively and appropriately discussing firearm access with patients and their families [15–17]. Additionally, while evaluation of firearm access is only one aspect of violence and suicide risk assessment, it can be a vital component [18].

As clinical research continues and many legal considerations remain unresolved, in this chapter, we consider a practical approach to help providers engage patients regarding firearm safety, specifically by identifying and bridging cultural gaps through nonjudgmental interactions and the use of motivational interviewing. Embracing the concept of relative risks and harm reduction, an approach emphasizing safer storage, removal when possible (especially in the context of suicide and violence risk), and preservation of clinician-patient rapport is highlighted. We summarize the following: why clinicians should care about firearms, firearm access and ownership, recognizing and understanding gun culture, current clinical practices, initial screening for firearm access, using therapeutic approaches to encourage safer storage, and documentation.

Why Clinicians Should Care About Firearms

While gun ownership is a hot-button political issue and may not immediately be thought of as a health-care issue, firearm-related morbidity and mortality has a significant impact on the health-care system. Clinician knowledge of firearm prevalence and availability can play an important role in the overall care of a patient.

Over the previous few years, firearms have annually accounted for 10,000–12,000 homicides, 20,000–22,000 suicides, and 50,000–80,000 injuries [19, 20]. US firearm suicide rates are ten times as high, and homicide rates are 25 times as high as other developed countries [10]. Accidental and sublethal injuries with firearms occur with significant frequency; however, quantifying the full impact is challenging due to inconsistent reporting and coding standards [21, 22]. Nonetheless, studies show firearm injuries are extremely costly to the health-care system and disproportionately impact youth, minority, and uninsured populations [23]. Estimated annual costs for medical treatment of firearm injuries are as high as $2.8 billion with the majority of those costs absorbed by Medicare and Medicaid [23–25]. Furthermore, patients who survive often face frequent readmissions, lifelong disability, medical expenses, and elevated risks of subsequent violent injury or death [26, 27].

It should be noted that most firearm violence is personal (an altercation between a small number of people, usually two), whereas mass shootings, though devastating and frequently publicized, are actually quite rare in the United States (accounting for significantly less than 1% of firearm homicide incidents) and are even more rare in other developed nations [9, 28].

Firearm Access and Ownership

An estimated 270–350,000,000 firearms are in civilian hands in the United States [11, 29]. Of particular concern to clinicians may be that, according to recent evidence, households with more risk factors for violence and suicide are more likely to own firearms [30]. Furthermore, 18 states currently allow some firearm purchases or transfers without background checks. Recent research suggests that at least 22% are transferred privately in this manner [31], and another study approximates that 20% of firearms carried or owned by criminal offenders had been lawfully acquired [32]. Thus, the lack of universal background checks allows people – who may otherwise be stopped from purchasing possessing firearms from a licensed dealer (i.e., history of involuntary admission, severe substance use, certain felonies, permanent restraining orders) – to purchase firearms [33]. Additionally, most states do not have a process to confirm removal or actively remove firearms from a newly prohibited owner [34].

Accidental injuries and risk from firearm storage in homes with children can also be a significant concern. In one study of homes with children and firearms, more than two-thirds of the children knew where the firearm was stored, and one-third had handled the firearm without the parents' knowledge or permission [35]. In a laboratory study of children who had received firearm safety training, most located a hidden firearm in less than 15 minutes, and a third tried to fire the weapon; this was despite parents' near-unanimous belief that their children would not engage in such conduct [36]. One recent survey of licensed firearm dealer practices identified that education about suicide and domestic violence risk was provided in less than 10% of transactions and trainings offered to firearm purchasers [37].

Recognizing and Understanding Gun Culture

As with other culturally sensitive subjects (e.g., reproductive health, substance use, etc.), basic awareness of varying attitudes, behaviors, and beliefs surrounding gun ownership in the United States may help clinicians empathize and "meet the patient where they are." Firearm ownership in contemporary America is often a cultural issue with distinct political, social, and religious differences between owners and nonowners that impacts ownership, use, and storage [26, 38]. Additionally, there is significant heterogeneity of beliefs among firearm owners themselves, including about firearm policy [39]. The role of culture in driving these factors and legislative responses has been recognized for nearly 50 years and continues to play a major role in the public policy landscape [40]. It is important for clinicians to understand that there are distinct cultures and subcultures of firearm owners, and these can play a significant role in clinical interactions, such as how people perceive firearm risks and potential opportunities for counseling [41]. Similarly, reasons for owning firearms vary significantly – with two-thirds indicating ownership is for protection – while others indicate ownership is for hunting, sport shooting, collecting, or work [42]. A gun-naive clinician may not even realize cultural differences at play in their interactions with a patient or family until they have inadvertently damaged their rapport.

The authors are not aware of any controlled study of firearm ownership among doctors. There is some evidence that firearm-owning physicians are less likely to support safety counseling [43]. Clinical training about firearm issues is often limited to a "checklist" approach to asking about access [44]. This puts physicians, especially those without the personal experience of owning firearms, using firearms, or growing up in a "gun household," at a disadvantage in recognizing and working across the potential cultural divide. Specific continuing education and nonclinical exposure to firearms (e.g., going with a friend or colleague from hospital security to a firearm range) could be helpful means of addressing knowledge gaps.

Of concern, some groups recommend that firearm owners refuse to answer clinical questions about firearms, lie about ownership or storage, or challenge physicians with implied threats of litigation [45]. Training on firearm safety provided by dealers can also be quite limited, and seldom is delivered to other household members; few salespeople offer guidance on safer storage practices, and only 15% of purchasers or trainees receive any material about suicide risk [46, 47]. Reassuringly, most patients and most firearm owners, including those in ED settings, are open to inquiries or counseling if they are approached in a deliberate, respectful way [48].

Current Clinical Practices

Any time there is concern of suicide or violence risk, exploring access to lethal means, such as firearms, should be considered a prudent step [49, 50]. In fact, the Joint Commission recently advised screening for suicide risk in numerous settings (including emergency settings) with the included proviso that, for those at risk of suicide, access to firearms and other lethal means be assessed and removal or improved security be advised [51]. Additionally, the unfettered ability to screen and counsel about firearm access and storage has been identified as a major public health priority by a number of professional medical organizations [52]. That said, the nuances and

Table 46.1 Situations when firearm access may be explored in ED and PES settings

Suicidal or homicidal ideations, threats, or plans
Self-injury physical violence or related ideations, threats, or plans
Domestic or intimate partner violence
Substance use
Dementia and other progressive or acute cognitive issues
Anger issues
Any accidental injury in the home, especially involving children

optimal clinical approaches – beyond the broad advisory to explore access to firearms and counsel safe storage and removal – remains a matter of ongoing discussion, education, and research.

In the emergency setting, screening for firearm access and counseling about firearm safety may be considered when direct clinical concerns for suicide, homicide, or aggression emerge in a patient, particularly one who may be discharged to the community. Other clinical situations may also alert the clinician to explore firearm access (Table 46.1). It is important to highlight that although firearm access is appropriate to explore in the context of mental illness and that active symptoms of mental illness can increase the risk of both suicide and violent behavior, mental illness is more strongly linked with suicide and accounts for only a small portion of violence in the community [7]. It should also be noted that in and of itself, firearm access is not a robust risk factor and may not be an ideal target for intervention in the absence of pertinent risk factors.

Initial Screening for Firearm Access

Because inquiries about firearm access can lead to resistance, clinicians need to approach questioning sensitively. Similar to asking about other sensitive topics such as sexual behavior or substance use, phrasing matters [53]. First, timing is critical; broaching the topic before there is good clinical engagement can be off-putting. Embedding questions about firearm access into a list of other health survey type of questions may or may not be effective depending on the individual.

Optimally, look for an opportunity or an invitation to ask. Statements by a patient or family like "What can I do to keep myself/my child/my spouse safe?" or "How do I get through this illness?" may provide a good opportunity. Clinicians can respond with something like "Well, one thing to consider is doing everything we reasonably can to prevent something impulsive happening; may I ask you if there are any guns at home?"

Asking permission to ask is often a helpful strategy to diffuse resistance and encourage engagement. It may help to use prefatory statements as well. For example:

- "You initially came to our ED because you made some statements about wanting to kill yourself while you were drinking. Both of those issues raise some concerns about firearms. May I ask you some questions about your guns?"
- "You have an illness that can sometimes cause problems with emotions, decisions, and your sense of hope. Whenever this occurs, I am concerned about suicide and aggression as a risk, no matter how unlikely. You are too important to take chances with. May we talk about your access to guns?"

Note that the use of a gentle assumption – accepting the likely presence of firearms in the home – can be less stigmatizing than a question like "Are you a gun owner?" Additional suggested phrasing for questions about firearm access are listed in Table 46.2. Note that it is often preferable to ask about the firearms in the *home* rather than firearms that are *owned*; many households have only one or two "gun owners" but many people in the household.

A useful mnemonic to guide initial screening for risks related to weapon access for people with an elevated risk for violence is AEIOU (see Table 46.3). It is a helpful way to explore general firearm access and for other weapons as well.

For people with more extensive experience or access to firearms, some additional questions may be helpful. Firearms are complex tools, and while some basic functionality can be attained by

Table 46.2 General questions about firearms and weapons

How many guns are in your home? How do you store guns in your home? Why are guns important to you? What did you buy them for? Have those reasons changed over time? How hard is it for you to get your hands on a gun (in your neighborhood/family/community)? Do you have a gun or any other weapon with you now? When you get in fights, what kind of weapons have you used? Were they "opportunistic weapons" (e.g., picking up a 2 × 4 lying on the ground) or something you carried for that purpose (e.g., a gun or knife)? When there are fights at home, how often are guns brandished, used, or threatened with, implicitly or explicitly? What weapons do you have access to? Which would you use in [this situation]? I don't know much about guns. Would you please describe it to me so I can have a better idea of what we are talking about? How did you learn how to use that weapon? What do you do to practice with it? Has the frequency with which you carry a weapon increased recently? Are there weapons at home that you have moved recently (e.g., from the attic to the bedside table)? Where do your parents keep their guns? How are they secured?

Table 46.3 AEIOU: A weapons use mnemonic

Domain	What we are trying to learn
Access	How difficult is it for the patient to obtain a firearm for impulsive or deliberate violence?
Experience	How much experience do they have with handling firearms? Increased experience may increase risk of dangerous use or suicide. Tactical experience can certainly increase the magnitude and severity of any violent use.
Ideation and intent	How much thought, fantasy, or intent a person has about firearm use for violence can suggest fixation, a major risk factor for violence.
Operational plan	Impulsive use is concerning; detailed and specific plans are also concerning.
Unconcerned with consequences and suicidality	Suicidality and homicidality have similar risk factors, and the presence of one can significantly increase the risk of the other.

Table 46.4 PHASES mnemonic for advanced firearm users and violence risk

Domain	What we are trying to learn
Proximity change	Has the person made their firearms more readily accessible, i.e., moved them from a closet to their bedside table or their person? Are they carrying more frequently? Suggest increased perceived risk in the environment.
Hatefulness and hostility	Extremist/racist ideology or hate group affiliation may be associated with a lower threshold for violence. Hostile attributional style is a broad risk factor for ease of provocation into violence.
Acquisition despite exclusion	Obtaining a firearm despite being legally excluded and failing to relinquish firearms when required both demonstrate willingness to defy major laws about safe firearm use.
Substance use	Substance use in general, and especially while handling firearms, is a major risk factor for violence and suicide because of impaired judgement and affect regulation.
Escalating purchases	Purchasing more firearms at a time with decreased frequency or with increasing caliber may suggest preparation to attack others. (N.B., large purchases of ammunition may simply reflect a typical response to bona fide market scarcity.)
Suicidality and hopelessness	Presence of suicidality and hopelessness can increase violence risk

almost anybody, the impact of their use in skilled and experienced hands can be substantially greater. Consider the PHASES mnemonic for people with advanced access or knowledge about firearms (see Table 46.4).

Motivational Interviewing and Therapeutic Approaches to Encourage Safer Storage

Traditional approaches to counseling about firearm removal may be less effective than hoped. In a 2-year study of depressed adolescents at high risk for suicide, most firearm-owning families either did not remove the firearm after counseling or returned the firearm to the home while the adolescent was still at risk; one in six homes without a firearm acquired one during the period of the study [54]. In a study of adults involuntarily committed for suicidality or homicidality with access to a firearm who received extensive counseling and initially removed the firearms from the home, one-third of those reassessed within 2 years had reacquired access to firearms [55].

We highlight motivational interviewing (MI) as one helpful strategy in building alliance and moving people toward positive change [56]. MI has traditionally been used to engage patients regarding substance abuse but has also shown promise in early studies looking at means restriction in suicide prevention by counseling people at risk for suicide about the removal of dangerous implements including firearms [57]. Our ultimate goals are continued engagement and safer storage. Similar to the language used in reproductive health, consider framing storage options as safer storage, not safe storage, as any storage can potentially be breached [58, 59].

Motivational interviewing uses four basic stages – engaging, focusing, evoking, and planning – to help patients move through the Stages of Change toward a successful modification of behavior. Engaging means creating a meaningful clinical alliance with patients and families so that we understand their reasons for coming to the ED and PES and our role in helping them with that issue. Focusing allows us to make that subtle transition to exploring their firearm ownership, current practices for handling and storage, and our reasons for concern. The next step is helping the patient or family recognize the importance for change and what risks may be entailed with continued unsafe access to firearms. Finally, planning is the process of getting the patient and family to commit to safer storage, develop specific plans, and optimally create a plan to follow up and confirm removal. If, during a conversation, the clinician notices increased resistance, it is likely prudent to return to the engagement stage.

Long-term change is difficult to achieve and intimidating to contemplate. Clinicians should consider appealing to acuity concerns; no matter how chronic the illness or behavior, there is a reason that the patient is in the PES at this time. Note that many patients and families have had the firearm for many years (and, perhaps, never needed it for self-defense); that risk is stable. This is the acute phase of an illness that undermines rational decisions, hope, and impulse control. It is reasonable to make temporary changes in behavior to assure one's well-being. If the removal of the firearm becomes a "new normal" or newly tolerated habit, that may not be the worst outcome.

Once a patient or family member is engaged and willing to consider options for safer storage, first explore what ideas they may have. If they are open to your input, consider offering solutions as outlined in Table 46.5. Ultimately, removal is the safest intervention but may also be the option the person is most resistant to. To continue the safer sex metaphor, removal, like abstinence, may be highly effective but also less likely to be taken seriously or adhered to by the patient. Partial movement toward the goal of safety is preferable to frank refusal or false assurances of compliance. Of note, firearm theft from automobiles is quite common, and storage of firearms in vehicle should not be recommended [60]. It is important to note that there are a lot of ways to hurt and kill people without firearms. Clinicians must not assume that because there are no firearms, there is no risk. Do not forget to explore other types of weapon access, and do not lose sight of the fact that weapon access alone is not a meaningful risk factor or target for intervention in the absence of suicidality, aggression, or other risk factors.

Table 46.5 "May I offer some suggestions?"

Safer: Secure the firearm more safely in the home	Somewhere else: Store the firearm at another safe location	Sold: Sell, exchange, or transfer the firearm legally
Mechanical and "smart" trigger and chamber locks Gun safes Separated from ammunition	At work (if permitted by employer) Rental storage locker With a safe friend or relative	Licensed firearm dealers Community buyback programs Pawnshops

Documentation

In the event of adverse outcomes, a well-crafted medical record accurately reflecting clinical events and clinician decision-making is important. At the same time, the pace and volume of many ED and PES settings make extensively detailed documentation challenging. Ideally, documentation should clearly reflect patient or family responses to inquiries about firearm access, what role access plays in clinical decision-making (if any), what guidance (if any) was given to the patient or family, and how they appeared to receive such information.

Examples

We talked to Mr. and Mrs. Smith about Mr. Smith's depression and the fact that firearms access increases his risk of completed suicide. We recommended removal of firearms to a safe location. Mr. Smith reported that hunting with his brother is one of the few things that still gives him pleasure. He agreed to have his brother take possession of his rifle for now and continues to assess this issue with his therapist and intensive outpatient team. Though he does not currently meet criteria for involuntary commitment and is not actively suicidal, we remain concerned for his safety and encouraged him to find other outlets while he gets treatment for this acute depressive episode.

Miss Jones presented with symptoms of PTSD and passive death wish. She keeps a handgun for personal protection. Though she has a chronically elevated risk of suicide due to traumatic past, ongoing suicidal ideation, and past attempts, she does not currently meet criteria for involuntary commitment and declined voluntary admission. She declines our recommendation to remove the gun from her home. We have talked to her mother, who has no immediate safety concerns. We provided both the patient and her mother with our recommendation and the rationale, as well as alternatives for safer storage, such as mother keeping the gun locked in a combination safe in her room. These were also declined. We referred the patient for partial hospitalization programming and advised the treatment team in that clinic of the situation and recommendations.

In the event of involuntary commitment of a person who owns firearms, clinicians should consider how and when to inform patients and family members about potential restrictions on firearm access. And, of course, the clinicians should assure that they themselves have a reasonable understanding of such restrictions and rules. It may be appropriate for such a dialogue to be handled by an inpatient team or even by law enforcement involved in the commitment process depending on the context.

Use of prepared and vetted educational information for patients and families about firearm safety may be considered. The information may be better received if it targets specific high-risk situations or groups such as homes with children, acute psychiatric illness, or cognitive decline and dementia. Information that is provided to all ED patients – such as standard language in discharge instructions – may diminish any sense of stigmatization or being singled out. It also runs the risk of being information that is easily disregarded if it is embedded in long and detailed handouts.

Conclusion

Firearms are ubiquitous, are legally protected, and contribute to substantial morbidity, mortality, and health-care costs. Various ED and PES presentations – including aggression and suicidality – can raise concerns about a patient's gun access. Being able to navigate potential cultural barriers surrounding guns can help clinicians engage in constructive dialogues about strategies and safer storage with patients and their families. With appropriate therapeutic approaches, clinicians may be able to help mitigate risk of firearm-related injuries and death.

References

1. Anestis MD, Houtsma C. The association between gun ownership and statewide overall suicide rates. Suicide Life Threat Behav. 2018;48(2):204–17.
2. Anglemyer A, Horvath T, Rutherford G. The accessibility of firearms and risk for suicide and homicide victimization among household members: a sys-

tematic review and meta-analysis. Ann Intern Med. 2014;160(2):101–10.
3. Zeoli AM, Malinski R, Turchan B. Risks and targeted interventions: firearms in intimate partner violence. Epidemiol Rev. 2016;38(1):125–39.
4. Miller M, Azrael D, Hemenway D. Firearm availability and unintentional firearm deaths. Accid Anal Prev. 2001;33(4):477–84.
5. Swedler DI, Simmons MM, Dominici F, Hemenway D. Firearm prevalence and homicides of law enforcement officers in the United States. Am J Public Health. 2015;105(10):2042–8.
6. Branas CC, Han S, Wiebe DJ. Alcohol use and firearm violence. Epidemiol Rev. 2016;38(1):32–45.
7. Rozel JS, Mulvey EP. The link between mental illness and gun violence: implications for social policy. Annu Rev Clin Psychol. 2017;13(1):445–69.
8. Tomazic M. Docs v. Glocks: restricting doctor's professional speech in the name of firearm owner privacy – Wollschlaeger v. governor of Florida. Am J Law Med. 2015;41(4):680–3.
9. Lankford A. Public mass shooters and firearms: a cross-national study of 171 countries. Violence Vict. 2016;31(2):187–99.
10. Grinshteyn E, Hemenway D. Violent death rates in the US compared to those of the other high-income countries, 2015. Preventive Medicine. 2019;123:20–6.
11. Karp A. Estimating Global Civilian-Held Firearms Numbers. Small Arms Survey, Geneva. 2018. Available from: http://www.smallarmssurvey.org/fileadmin/docs/T-Briefing-Papers/SAS-BP-Civilian-Firearms-Numbers.pdf.
12. Gopal A, Greenwood BN. Traders, guns, and money: the effects of mass shootings on stock prices of firearm manufacturers in the U.S. Plos One. 2017;12(5):e0177720.
13. Studdert DM, Zhang Y, Rodden JA, Hyndman RJ, Wintemute GJ. Handgun acquisitions in California after two mass shootings. Ann Intern Med. 2017;166(10):698–706.
14. Luca M, Malhotra DK, Poliquin C. The impact of mass shootings on gun policy. Harv Bus Sch NOM Unit Work Pap [Internet]. 2016 [cited 2016 Jul 16];(16–126). Available from: http://papers.ssrn.com/sol3/Papers.cfm?abstract_id=2776657.
15. Betz ME, Wintemute GJ. Physician counseling on firearm safety: a new kind of cultural competence. JAMA. 2015;314(5):449–50.
16. Wintemute GJ, Betz ME, Ranney ML. Yes, you can: physicians, patients, and firearms. Ann Intern Med. 2016;165(3):205–13.
17. Betz ME, Wintersteen M, Boudreaux ED, Brown G, Capoccia L, Currier G, et al. Reducing suicide risk: challenges and opportunities in the emergency department. Ann Emerg Med. 2016;68(6):758–65.
18. Rozel JS, Jain A, Mulvey EP, Roth LH. Psychiatric assessment of violence. In: Sturmey P, editor. The Wiley handbook of violence and aggression. Chichester: Wiley; 2017. p. 697–709.
19. Wintemute GJ. The epidemiology of firearm violence in the twenty-first century United States. Annu Rev Public Health. 2015;36(1):5–19.
20. Fowler KA, Dahlberg LL, Haileyesus T, Annest JL. Firearm injuries in the United States. Prev Med. 2015;79:5–14.
21. Thiels CAD, Zielinski MD, Glasgow AEM, Habermann EB. The relative lack of data regarding firearms injuries in the United States. [Letter]. Ann Surg. 2018;268(6):e55–6.
22. Jacoby SF, Kollar LMM, Ridgeway G, Sumner SA. Health system and law enforcement synergies for injury surveillance, control and prevention: a scoping review. Inj Prev. 2018;24(4):305–11.
23. Peek-Asa C, Butcher B, Cavanaugh JE. Cost of hospitalization for firearm injuries by firearm type, intent, and payer in the United States. Inj Epidemiol. 2017;4(1):20.
24. Spitzer SA, Staudenmayer KL, Tennakoon L, Spain DA, Weiser TG. Costs and financial burden of initial hospitalizations for firearm injuries in the United States, 2006–2014. Am J Public Health. 2017;107(5):770–4.
25. Gani F, Sakran JV, Canner JK. Emergency department visits for firearm-related injuries in the United States, 2006–14. Health Aff (Millwood). 2017;36(10):1729–38.
26. Kalesan B. The cost of firearm violence survivorship. Am J Public Health. 2017;107(5):638–9.
27. Rowhani-Rahbar A, Zatzick D, Wang J, Mills BM, Simonetti JA, Fan MD, et al. Firearm-related hospitalization and risk for subsequent violent injury, death, or crime perpetration: a cohort study. Ann Intern Med. 2015;162(7):492.
28. Duwe G. The patterns and prevalence of mass murder in twentieth-century America. Justice Q. 2004;21(4):729–61.
29. Ingraham C. There are now more guns than people in the United States [Internet]. The Washington Post WonkBlog. 2015 [cited 2016 Jul 5]. Available from: https://www.washingtonpost.com/news/wonk/wp/2015/10/05/guns-in-the-united-states-one-for-every-man-woman-and-child-and-then-some/.
30. Ladapo JA, Elliott MN, Kanouse DE, Schwebel DC, Toomey SL, Mrug S, et al. Firearm ownership and acquisition among parents with risk factors for self-harm or other violence. Acad Pediatr. 2016;16(8):742–9.
31. Miller M, Hepburn L, Azrael D. Firearm acquisition without background checks: results of a national survey. Ann Intern Med. 2017;166(4):233–9.
32. Fabio A, Duell J, Creppage K, O'Donnell K, Laporte R. Gaps continue in firearm surveillance: evidence from a large U.S. city Bureau of Police. Soc Med. 2016;10(1):13–21.
33. Mueller DG, Frandsen R. Trends in firearm background check applications and denials. J Public Aff. 2017;17(3):n/a–n/a.
34. Roskam K, Chaplin V. The gun violence restraining order: an opportunity for common ground in the

gun violence debate section I. Dev Ment Health Law. 2017;36:1–22.
35. Baxley F, Miller M. Parental misperceptions about children and firearms. Arch Pediatr Adolesc Med. 2006;160(5):542–7.
36. Jackman GA, Farah MM, Kellermann AL, Simon HK. Seeing is believing: what do boys do when they find a real gun? Pediatrics. 2001;107(6):1247–50.
37. Hemenway D, Rausher S, Violano P, Raybould TA, Barber CW. Firearms training: what is actually taught? Inj Prev J Int Soc Child Adolesc Inj Prev. 2019;25(2):123–8.
38. Utter GH, True JL. The evolving gun culture in America. J Am Comp Cult. 2000;23(2):67–79.
39. comments KP. Among gun owners, NRA members have a unique set of views and experiences [Internet]. Pew Research Center. 2017 [cited 2017 Sep 15]. Available from: http://www.pewresearch.org/fact-tank/2017/07/05/among-gun-owners-nra-members-have-a-unique-set-of-views-and-experiences/.
40. Hofstadter R. America as a gun culture. Am Herit. 1970;21(6):4.
41. Braman D, Kahan DM, Grimmelmann J. Modeling facts, culture, and cognition in the gun debate. Soc Justice Res. 2005;18(3):283–304.
42. Parker K, Horowitz J, Igielnik R, Oliphant B, Brown A. America's complex relationship with guns: an in-depth look at the attitudes and experiences of U.S. adults [Internet]. Washington, D.C.: Pew Research Center; 2017 Jun [cited 2017 Jun 26]. Available from: http://assets.pewresearch.org/wp-content/uploads/sites/3/2017/06/22135403/Guns-Report-FOR-WEBSITE-PDF-6-21.pdf.
43. Becher EC, Cassel CK, Nelson EA. Physician firearm ownership as a predictor of firearm injury prevention practice. Am J Public Health. 2000;90(10):1626–8.
44. Puttagunta R, Coverdale TR, Coverdale J. What is taught on firearm safety in undergraduate, graduate, and continuing medical education? A review of educational programs. Acad Psychiatry J Am Assoc Dir Psychiatr Resid Train Assoc Acad Psychiatry. 2016;40(5):821–4.
45. Ammoland. What to do when your doctor asks about your guns [Internet]. AmmoLand.com. Shooting Sports News. 2015 [cited 2016 Mar 6]. Available from: http://www.ammoland.com/2015/06/what-to-do-when-your-doctor-asks-about-your-guns/.
46. Rowhani-Rahbar A, Lyons VH, Simonetti JA, Azrael D, Miller M. Formal firearm training among adults in the USA: results of a national survey. Inj Prev. 2018;24(2):161–5. https://doi.org/10.1136/injuryprev-2017-042352. Epub 2017 Jul 11.
47. Sanguino SM, Dowd MD, McEnaney SA, Knapp J, Tanz RR. Handgun safety: what do consumers learn from gun dealers? Arch Pediatr Adolesc Med. 2002;156(8):777–80.
48. Betz ME, Azrael D, Barber C, Miller M. Public opinion regarding whether speaking with patients about firearms is appropriate: results of a National Survey. Ann Intern Med. 2016;165(8):543–50.
49. Pinals DA, Appelbaum PS, Bonnie R, Fisher CE, Gold LH, Lee L-W. American Psychiatric Association: position statement on firearm access, acts of violence and the relationship to mental illness and mental health services: APA position statement on firearm access. Behav Sci Law. 2015;33(2–3):195–8.
50. Simon RI. Gun safety management with patients at risk for suicide. Suicide Life Threat Behav. 2007;37(5):518–26.
51. Patient Safety Advisory Group. Detecting and treating suicide ideation in all settings. Sentin Event Alert [Internet]. 2016 Feb 24 [cited 2017 Oct 15];(56). Available from: https://www.jointcommission.org/assets/1/18/SEA_56_Suicide.pdf.
52. Weinberger SE, Hoyt DB, Lawrence HC, Levin S, Henley DE, Alden ER, et al. Firearm-related injury and death in the United States: a call to action from 8 health professional organizations and the American Bar Association. Ann Intern Med. 2015;162(7):513–6.
53. Shea SC. My favorite tips for uncovering sensitive and taboo information from antisocial behavior to suicidal ideation. Psychiatr Clin North Am. 2007;30(2):253–9.
54. Brent DA, Baugher M, Birmaher B, Kolko DJ, Bridge J. Compliance with recommendations to remove firearms in families participating in a clinical trial for adolescent depression. J Am Acad Child Adolesc Psychiatry. 2000;39(10):1220–6.
55. Sherman ME, Burns K, Ignelzi J, Raia J, Lofton V, Toland D, et al. Firearms risk management in psychiatric care. Psychiatr Serv. 2001;52(8):1057–61.
56. Miller WR, Rollnick S. Motivational interviewing: helping people change. 3rd ed. New York: Guilford Press; 2013. 482 p. (Applications of motivational interviewing).
57. Britton PC, Bryan CJ, Valenstein M. Motivational interviewing for means restriction counseling with patients at risk for suicide. Cogn Behav Pract. 2016;23(1):51–61.
58. Shenassa ED, Rogers ML, Spalding KL, Roberts MB. Safer storage of firearms at home and risk of suicide: a study of protective factors in a nationally representative sample. J Epidemiol Community Health 1979-. 2004;58(10):841–8.
59. Ollam D. Safe to armed in seconds. In Las Vegas, Nevada; 2011 [cited 2017 Sep 30]. Available from: https://www.youtube.com/watch?v=3SVMT_zNlgA.
60. Hemenway D, Azrael D, Miller M. Whose guns are stolen? The epidemiology of Gun theft victims. Inj Epidemiol. 2017;4(1):11.

Disposition Decisions for Psychiatric Patients Presenting to the Emergency Setting

47

Steven W. Flynn and Leslie S. Zun

Introduction

Approximately one in four adults have a psychiatric disease, and annually, 5.3 million patients present to the emergency department (ED) with a psychiatric-related chief complaint [1]. It has been estimated that 50 inpatient psychiatric beds are needed per 100,000 people. Currently, some states have only 10 psychiatric beds per 100,000 people [2]. This demonstrates that less funding is being invested in inpatient psychiatric facilities and that there is a transition to more outpatient management [2]. Many of these patients present to EDs for evaluation and treatment and end up boarding in the ED waiting for an available psychiatric bed.

The emergency department is referred to as the gateway to the hospital. The public relies upon the ED to manage new acute medical problems or manage an exacerbation of their underlying chronic medical ailment. Many times, these patients, some with chronic mental illness, cannot be treated as an outpatient and, after evaluation in the ED, are deemed unsafe to be discharged home and must be admitted. Without objective admission measurements, such as a HEART (history, EKG, age, risk factors, troponin) score for major adverse cardiac events and CURB-65 (confusion, BUN, respiratory rate, blood pressure) for community-acquired pneumonia, determining which of these patients require admission can be a daunting task. The aim of this chapter is to review areas for improvement in patient evaluation and disposition of psychiatric complaints.

Psychosocial Factors Incorporated into Disposition Selection

Multiple factors need to be considered when making the decision to admit a psychiatric patient. In a general sense, the need for admission is based on danger to self, danger to others, or inability to care for one's self. However, the admission decision is not always an easy one because of illness severity, extenuating circumstances, and difficulty in assessment. These decisions may differ on the training and experience of the evaluator, time of evaluation in the disease process, and ability to obtain collateral information.

The symptoms and circumstances surrounding a psychiatric illness typically affect the admission decision [3]. Psychosocial factors should be collected to determine if the person has a safe place to go after discharge, if they are able to afford medication, if they can make it to

S. W. Flynn (✉)
Department of Emergency Medicine, Methodist Hospitals, Gary, IN, USA

L. S. Zun
Department of Emergency Medicine, Rosalind Franklin University of Medicine and Science/ The Chicago Medical School, North Chicago, IL, USA

L. S. Zun et al. (eds.), *Behavioral Emergencies for Healthcare Providers*,
https://doi.org/10.1007/978-3-030-52520-0_47

appointments, and if their living situation is contributing to their psychiatric condition. Finally, there should be a discussion with the patient and any significant others to determine disposition priorities. Although limited, studies have shown a correlation between patient preference for admission or discharge and actual disposition [4]. Collateral input can be very useful, especially if the patient is unable to answer appropriately. Through this collateral information, the emergency provider can gain a sense of what the patient is like outside of the hospital and collect details on events leading up to the patient's emergency presentation. Through discussion with the patient and family, a better relationship can be formed with the care provider. This may allow for open communication concerning care needs and what outcomes can be expected.

Admission Decisions

Admission decisions can be made by a number of mental health professionals including social workers, psychiatrists, psychologists, outsourced services, and others. These may be performed in person, telephonically, or using telemedicine. Despite whoever is doing this evaluation, the emergency provider is ultimately responsible for the patient's disposition.

Availability of a psychiatrist or other psychiatric professional can be a limiting factor affecting disposition time. On average, psychiatric patients wait 10 hours until being evaluated by a psychiatric professional [1]. Longer ED boarding time is associated with an escalation of symptoms and poorer outcome [2]. With such limited inpatient psychiatric facilities, if the emergency physician can make appropriate diagnosis and disposition, it would improve bed availability for other psychiatric patients presenting to the ED. This would also have a good financial impact on the patient and hospital by avoiding unnecessary admissions.

Disposition times could be improved if emergency physicians accurately recognized psychiatric issues warranting admission. Studies have looked into disposition selection between psychiatrists and emergency providers. When looking at psychiatric patients in the ED, the emergency provider's decision to admit psychiatric patients had a positive predictive value (PPV) of 87.3% and negative predictive value (NPV) of 66.7% compared to psychiatrists. Suicidal patients comprise a large proportion of these patients and the decision to admit had a PPV of 90% and NPV of 69.6% [1]. Emergency providers can identify patients requiring admission but do not do well with selecting which patients are safe to be discharged home.

Suicidal Patients

In 2007, 650,000 patients presented to the ED with suicidal thoughts as a chief complaint. It is listed as a top ten cause of death among all age groups [5]. Emergency providers are placed in a unique situation because the ED visit may be that the first-time patients with suicidal ideation are gaining access to psychiatric help. It is also important to note that not all depressed patients are suicidal and not all suicidal patients have depression. There are many tools to screen for suicidality, but these tools do not determine suicide risk. Although these tools evaluate degree of suicidal ideation, they do not accurately predict if a patient will attempt suicide and are not reliable in selecting disposition [5]. Although the Columbia Suicide Severity Rating Scale comes closest to a reliable risk assessment tool, it lacks reliability. Challenges in risk stratifying these patients clearly exist within emergency medicine as a specialty but also within psychiatry. A prospective study was performed to see which patients committed suicide following discharge from a psychiatric facility. The study showed that the psychiatrist did not foresee 44% of the completed suicides [6]. Since there are no reliable scoring systems, emergency providers must rely on patient history, static and dynamic risk factors, as well as protective factors in the determination. Patients are placed into low-, moderate-, and high-risk categories. The high-risk patients require obvious admission, and the low-risk category usually can be managed as an outpatient. Those in the moderate-risk category need further evaluation by a psychiatrist. High-risk factors include age, prior attempts, psychiatric illness, substance use disorder, sex, method that would be used, and sudden interest in death (books, movies, and websites). Protective factors include family and social support, ongoing relationship with mental health providers, and spirituality. If a patient is discharged home, then the emergency provider must document clearly in the medical record their assessment and thought process for patient discharge.

In the past, many EDs made "safety contracts" having the patient agree that they would call 911 or return to the ED immediately if the suicidal ideations persisted or if the patient was planning on committing suicide. These contracts have been shown to not work and have even been used against the physician in lawsuits [6].

Schizophrenic Patients

Schizophrenia is a spectrum disorder where symptoms may range from minor interference with functions to those that have difficulty taking care of their daily needs. In general, if the patient has no insight to their medical condition, is a danger to self or others, is grossly debilitated by their disease, and lacks essential social support or if this is their first psychotic episode, then admission is warranted to a psychiatric service [7, 8].

Patients presenting with worsening of underlying psychosis typically cannot be discharged especially if they lack insight and judgment. For insight, it is important to determine whether the patient (1) is aware of their psychiatric condition, (2) understands treatment options, and (3) is able to recognize manifestations of their disease (e.g., hallucinations). Judgment is best assessed with problem-solving scenarios such as asking what the person would do if they saw smoke coming from a building or what they would do if they found a stamped envelope [9]. Patients with poor insight and judgment will more likely need admission.

Bipolar Patients

Patients with bipolar illness need a complete mental status exam to determine their current functional abilities whether they are manic or depressed. The evaluation of insight and judgment as well as psychosis is especially important with these patients. Information from collateral resources is helpful in determining functional status and risky behaviors. Patients who have difficulty functioning and are suicidal or demonstrate dangerous behaviors usually need admission.

Decision-Making Tools

To date, there have been very limited studies to elucidate methods to risk stratify and select disposition. The severity of psychiatric illness (SPI) rating scale and the crisis triage rating scale (CTRS) provide some decision support.

The SPI score uses three features—suicide potential, harm to others, and severity of symptoms. Each feature is based on a 0–3 scale on symptom's severity and then plugged into two separate formulas to determine admission probability from 0 to 100. Any patient with an admission probability less than 80% could potentially be discharged [3, 10]. The SPI correctly determined disposition 73% of the time, which equates to a significant amount of inappropriate discharges and admissions. The moderate correlation with admission and cumbersome calculation makes this a challenging modality to use in the ED. A useful feature of the tool is a graded scale used to help determine high- and low-risk features of suicide potential.

Bengelsdorf and colleagues proposed the CTRS in 1984. It is a rating scale based off of three features: dangerousness to self/others, support system, and ability to cooperate. These three features are graded on a 1–5 score based on severity of symptoms and then added to determine a final score from 3 to 15. The initial prospective study showed scores 3–8 were found to have a high correlation with patients that required admission. Higher scores 10–15 were more likely to be discharged. Scores of 9 were intermediate, and the study showed about a 50/50 chance of being admitted [11]. Although a quick modality to determine inpatient vs. outpatient management, validation studies showed a moderately strong correlation rate with actual admission decision.

Table 47.1 Admission determination

Severity	Description	Suicidal	Disposition	Need for hospitalization
Stable	Functional, works	None	Outpatient	No
Low level	Medical or psych stressor	Low	Outpatient	OBS
Moderate	Decompensation, agitated	Moderate	Psych consultation	OBS or inpatient
Severe	Severe decompensation	High	Inpatient care	Yes

Based on these scales, a decision tool was developed to assist in the determination of whether patients need admission, discharge, or observation (Table 47.1). Further research and development of tools to determine the utility of an admission protocol is needed.

The CTRS using a cutoff score of 8 (<8 is admitted, 9 or greater in discharged) had a correlation of 62.2% with actual disposition decision [12]. With moderately strong correlation, this too leads to inappropriate admissions and discharges. Although not validated, Turner et al. found that a CTRS cutoff score of 9 had a correlation of 75.2%, and a cutoff score of 10 had correlation of 81.2% with actual disposition. This might be more easily utilized than the SPI in the ED based on quick addition of scores. If used, a higher cutoff score of 9 or 10 should be used.

Alternatives to Admission

Management and access to psychiatric care is not consistent across communities. It is important to know what is available in the community. Alternatives to ED admission include discussion with the patient's psychiatrist to be evaluated in clinic, crisis hotlines, observation units, day hospitals, and crisis housing. Studies have shown no difference in clinical outcome between inpatient hospital admissions vs. respite care and day hospitals [13–15]. There are advantages to outpatient care. These benefits may include the patient being managed in a more homelike setting where they are able to participate in ADLs to the extent of their functionality, a comfortable living situation, and less formality.

Patients across the whole spectrum of psychosis, mood disorders, and personality disorders can all be managed in these settings. Emergency providers are often not aware of these additional resources and should seek to find what alternatives our communities offer. Table 47.2 describes alternatives to inpatient management.

Table 47.2 Descriptions of outpatient facilities to manage psychiatric emergencies

Alternative to admission	
Day hospital	Facilities open during daytime hours, generally 9 AM–5 PM, that allow the patient to come for treatment and then go home or to a crisis center until they return to next day Offers psychotherapy, medication management, and counseling to improve interpersonal relationships and how best to manage emotional disturbances
Psychiatric urgent care	Similar to other medical urgent cares but specific for psychiatric emergencies. Allows for immediate counseling, medications, and other interventions for acute psychiatric emergencies. Referral for psychiatric follow-up is also given
Respite care	Housing unit that allows for small group of psychiatric patients to live in a home setting while receiving counseling and treatment. Case managers available to help with social issues outside of the facility to prevent decline of psychiatric condition. Length of stay can vary from days to weeks
Mobile crisis unit	Clinicians that respond to home, jail, hospital, etc. to perform evaluation of patient and offer counseling

Prior to Discharge

If the decision is made to discharge home, then medication adjustments and psychiatric follow-up should be determined. In general, it is best to communicate with their prescribing provider before any psychiatric medications are adjusted and to ensure that the patient has scheduled follow-up. Discharged patients should go home with a reliable family member or friend. It must also be clearly communicated to the patient and their family and friend, if appropriate, what medication changes have been made as well as when and where their follow-up appointments will be. They should also be given crisis resources such as the phone number for the National Suicide Prevention Hotline, local crisis support services and hotline, and possibly peer support groups.

Discharged suicidal patients require a safety plan. The Suicide Prevention Resource Center has developed a tool kit which includes a model safety plan. These safety plans/tool kits involve good follow-up, discussion with providers, phone calls to check in, and involvement of friends and family [16]. The phone number to the National Suicide Prevention Hotline should be part of the safety plan and discharge instructions.

Conclusion

Psychiatric disposition determination is a challenge to emergency and psychiatric physicians. To date, there are no reliable ways to score patient presentations to determine admission or discharge. Input from the patient and family is an invaluable resource to help guide disposition selection. SPI and CTRS need to be tested in the emergency department to determine its utility in the setting. More research is needed to create a quick scoring system that may be used to determine the need for hospitalization.

References

1. Chakravarthy B, Menchine M. Psychiatric patient disposition agreement between the emergency physician consultant. Crisis. 2013;34:354–62.
2. Wiler JL, Brown NA. Care of the psychiatric patient in the emergency department. Retrieved 19 Dec 2016, from ACEP: https://www.acep.org/uploaded-Files/ACEP/Clinical_and_Practice_Management/Resources/Mental_Health_and_Substance_Abuse/Psychiatric%20Patient%20Care%20in%20the%20ED% 202014.pdf.
3. Lyons JS, Colletta J. Validity of the severity of psychiatric illness rating scale in as sample of inpatients on a psychogeriatric unit. Int Psychogeriatr. 1995;7:407–16.
4. Way B. Relationship between patient, family and significant other disposition preferences in psychiatric emergency services and the clinical symptom rating and disposition decisions of psychiatrists. Psychiatr Rehabil J. 2005;29:132–7.
5. Kuo DC, Tran M. Depression and the suicidal patient. Emerg Med Clin North Am. 2015;33:765–78.
6. Colucciello SA. Mood disorders. In: Hockberger R-H, Marx JA, editors. Rosen's emergency medicine. Amsterdam: Elsevier; 2014. p. 1492–500.
7. Brown H. How to stabilize an acutely psychotic patient. Curr Psychiatr Ther. 2012;11:10–6.
8. Hockberger RS, R. J. Thought disorders. In: Hockberger R-H, Marx JA, editors. Rosens emergency medicine. Amsterdam: Elsevier; 2014. p. 1460–5.
9. Mental Status Exam. (n.d.). Retrieved Jan 2, 2017, from The Royal Children's Hospital Melbourne: http://www.rch.org.au/clinicalguide/guideline_index/Mental_State_Examination/
10. Lyons JS, Stutesman J. Predicting psychiatric emergency admissions and hospital outcome. Med Care. 1997;35:792–800.
11. Bengelsdorf H, Levy LE. A crisis triage rating scale: brief dispositional assessment of patients at risk for hospitalization. J Nerv Ment Dis. 1984;172:424–30.
12. Turner PM, Turner TJ. Validation of the crisis triage raring scale for psychiatric emergencies. Can J Psychiatr. 1991;36:651–4.
13. Sledge WH, Tebes J. Day hospital/crisis respite care versus inpatient care, part I: clinical outcomes. Am J Psychiatry. 1996;153:1065–73.
14. Goodwin R, Lyon JS. An emergency housing program as an alternative to inpatient admission. Psychiatr Serv. 2001;52:92–5.
15. Brooker CE. Admission decisions follow contact with an emergency mental health assessment and intervention service. J Clin Nurs. 2007;16:1313–22.
16. Support Safe Care and Transitions and Create Organizational Linkages. (2017). Retrieved January 14, 2017, from Suicide Prevention Resource Center: http://www.sprc.org/comprehensive-approach/transitions-lInkages.

Correction to: Depression in the Emergency Department

David Hoyer

Correction to:
Chapter 7 in: L. S. Zun et al. (eds.), *Behavioral Emergencies for Healthcare Providers*, https://doi.org/10.1007/978-3-030-52520-0_7

The chapter "Depression in the Emergency Department" by David Hoyer was originally published without open access. Following the author's decision to opt for open access, the copyright of the chapter was changed on 24 September 2024 to © The Author 2024, and the chapter is now distributed under the terms of the Creative Commons Attribution 4.0 International License (http://creativecommons.org/licenses/by/4.0/), which permits use, sharing, adaptation, distribution and reproduction in any medium or format, as long as you give appropriate credit to the original author(s) and the source, provide a link to the Creative Commons licence and indicate if changes were made.

The images or other third-party materials in this chapter are included in the chapter's Creative Commons licence, unless otherwise indicated in a credit line to the material. If material is not included in the chapter's Creative Commons licence and your intended use is not permitted by statutory regulation or exceeds the permitted use, you will need to obtain permission directly from the copyright holder. This Open Access publication was funded by "David Hoyer".

The updated version of this chapter can be found at https://doi.org/10.1007/978-3-030-52520-0_7

L. S. Zun et al. (eds.), *Behavioral Emergencies for Healthcare Providers*,
https://doi.org/10.1007/978-3-030-52520-0_48

Index

L. S. Zun et al. (eds.), *Behavioral Emergencies for Healthcare Providers*,
https://doi.org/10.1007/978-3-030-52520-0

E

GPSR Compliance

The European Union's (EU) General Product Safety Regulation (GPSR) is a set of rules that requires consumer products to be safe and our obligations to ensure this.

If you have any concerns about our products, you can contact us on ProductSafety@springernature.com

In case Publisher is established outside the EU, the EU authorized representative is:

Springer Nature Customer Service Center GmbH
Europaplatz 3
69115 Heidelberg, Germany

Batch number: 10731403

Printed by Printforce, the Netherlands